GET
THROUGH

Final FRCR 2A:
SBAs

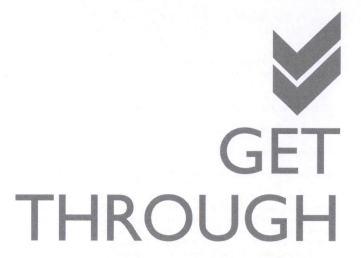

GET THROUGH

Final FRCR 2A:
SBAs

Teck Yew Chin, FRCR, MSc, MBChB

Susan Cheng Shelmerdine, MBBS, BSc, MRCS, PgCertHBE, FRCR

Akash Ganguly, MBBS, DMRD, FRCR

Chinedum Anosike, MBBS, MSc, FRCR

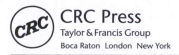

CRC Press
Taylor & Francis Group
Boca Raton London New York

CRC Press is an imprint of the
Taylor & Francis Group, an **informa** business

CRC Press
Taylor & Francis Group
6000 Broken Sound Parkway NW, Suite 300
Boca Raton, FL 33487-2742

© 2017 by Taylor & Francis Group, LLC
CRC Press is an imprint of Taylor & Francis Group, an Informa business

No claim to original U.S. Government works

Printed on acid-free paper

International Standard Book Number-13: 978-1-4987-3484-4 (Paperback); 978-1-1387-4399-1 (Hardback)

This book contains information obtained from authentic and highly regarded sources. While all reasonable efforts have been made to publish reliable data and information, neither the author[s] nor the publisher can accept any legal responsibility or liability for any errors or omissions that may be made. The publishers wish to make clear that any views or opinions expressed in this book by individual editors, authors or contributors are personal to them and do not necessarily reflect the views/opinions of the publishers. The information or guidance contained in this book is intended for use by medical, scientific or health-care professionals and is provided strictly as a supplement to the medical or other professional's own judgement, their knowledge of the patient's medical history, relevant manufacturer's instructions and the appropriate best practice guidelines. Because of the rapid advances in medical science, any information or advice on dosages, procedures or diagnoses should be independently verified. The reader is strongly urged to consult the relevant national drug formulary and the drug companies' and device or material manufacturers' printed instructions, and their websites, before administering or utilizing any of the drugs, devices or materials mentioned in this book. This book does not indicate whether a particular treatment is appropriate or suitable for a particular individual. Ultimately it is the sole responsibility of the medical professional to make his or her own professional judgements, so as to advise and treat patients appropriately. The authors and publishers have also attempted to trace the copyright holders of all material reproduced in this publication and apologize to copyright holders if permission to publish in this form has not been obtained. If any copyright material has not been acknowledged please write and let us know so we may rectify in any future reprint.

Library of Congress Cataloging-in-Publication Data

Names: Chin, Teck Yew, author. | Shelmerdine, Susan, author. | Ganguly, Akash, author. |
Anosike, Chinedum, author.
Title: Get through final FRCR 2A : SBAs / Teck Yew Chin, Susan Cheng Shelmerdine, Akash Ganguly,
Chinedum Anosike.
Other titles: Get through.
Description: Boca Raton, FL : CRC Press/Taylor & Francis Group, [2017] |
Series: Get through
Identifiers: LCCN 2016054175 (print) | LCCN 2016054780 (ebook) | ISBN 9781498734844 (pbk. : alk. paper) |
ISBN 9781138743991 (hardback : alk. paper) | ISBN 9781315382708 (Master eBook)
Subjects: | MESH: Radiology | Examination Questions
Classification: LCC RC78.15 (print) | LCC RC78.15 (ebook) | NLM WN 18.2 | DDC 616.07/57076--dc23
LC record available at https://lccn.loc.gov/2016054175

Visit the Taylor & Francis Web site at
http://www.taylorandfrancis.com

and the CRC Press Web site at
http://www.crcpress.com

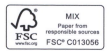

Printed and bound in Great Britain by
TJ International Ltd, Padstow, Cornwall

CONTENTS

PREFACE

The examination structure of the Fellowship of Royal College of Radiologists (FRCR) Final Part A examination (CR2A) in clinical radiology is reverting back from the current modular structure to a single examination. The RCR has approval from the General Medical Council (GMC) and the change will be effective from spring 2018.

From spring 2018, the examination will consist of two papers, to be taken on the same day, each consisting of 120 single best answer–type questions per paper. Each paper will be 3 hours long and will cover a broad range of topics from the radiology core curriculum covering all modalities.

This book is divided into seven test papers, consisting of 120 mixed SBA-type questions covering all modules (3 hours per paper for practice). The answers are in sequential order, followed by a short explanation and relevant discussion around the topic with appropriate references.

ACKNOWLEDGEMENTS

Vijay Kesavanarayanan
Grant Mair
Andrew Baird
Matthew Budak
Oliver Cram
Thomas Hartley
Laura Hinksman
Menelaos Philippou
Jo Powell
Calum Nicholson
Ewen G. Robertson
Nicola Schembri
Magdalena Szewczyk-Bieda
Richard D. White
Struan W.A. Wilkie
Nadeem A. Butt
Lauren L. Millar
Karim Samji
Euan G.C. Stubbs
André Stefan Gatt
Asha Neelakantan
Bappa Sarkar
Mubeen Chaudhry
Ramya G. Dhandapani

AUTHORS

Dr. Teck Yew Chin, MBChB, MSc, FRCR, is a consultant radiologist at Khoo Teck Puat Hospital, Singapore.

Dr. Susan Cheng Shelmerdine, MBBS, BSc, MRCS, PgCertHBE, FRCR, is a radiology research fellow at Great Ormond Street Hospital, London, UK.

Dr. Akash Ganguly, MBBS, DMRD, FRCR, is a consultant radiologist at Warrington Hospital, Warrington and Halton Hospitals NHS Foundation Trust, Warrington, UK.

Dr. Chinedum Anosike, MBBS, MSc, FRCR, is a consultant radiologist at Warrington Hospital, Warrington and Halton Hospitals NHS Foundation Trust, Warrington, UK.

ABBREVIATIONS

ABC – Aneurysmal Bone Cyst

ABPA – Allergic Bronchopulmonary Aspergillosis

AC – Acromio-clavicular

ACA – Anterior Cerebral Artery

ACE – Angiotensin Converting Enzyme

ACL – Anterior Cruciate Ligament

ACOM – Anterior Communicating Artery

ADC – Apparent Diffusion Coefficient

ADEM – Acute Disseminated Encephalomyelitis

AED/A&E – Accident and Emergency (department)

AFP – Alpha Fetoprotein

AICA – Anterior Inferior Cerebellar Artery

AIDS – Acquired Immunodeficiency Syndrome

ALP – Alkaline Phosphatase

ALPSA – Anterior Labroligamentous Periosteal Sleeve Avulsion

ALT – Alanine Aminotransferase

AML – Angiomyolipoma

AP – Anterior Posterior

ARDS – Acute Respiratory Distress Syndrome

ASD – Atrial Septal Defect

AST – Aspartate Aminotransferase

ATN – Acute Tubular Necrosis

AVM – Arteriovenous Malformation

AVN – Avascular Necrosis

BCG – Bacillus Calmette–Guerin

BPH – Benign Prostatic Hypertrophy

CA – Carbohydrate Antigen

CADASIL – Cerebral Autosomal-Dominant Arteriopathy with Subcortical Infarcts and Leukoencephalopathy

CBD – Common Bile Duct

CBF – Cerebral Blood Flow

CBV – Cerebral Blood Volume

CC – Coracoclavicular

CCAM – Congenital Cystic Adenomatoid Malformation

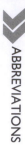

CDH – Congenital Diaphragmatic Hernia

CEA – Carcinoembryonic Antigen

CECT – Contrast-Enhanced CT

CF – Cystic Fibrosis

CFA – Common Femoral Artery

CHD – Common Hepatic Duct

Cho – Choline

CIN – Contrast-Induced Nephropathy

CJD – Creutzfeldt–Jakob Disease

CMV – Cytomegalo Virus

CNS – Central Nervous System

COAD – Chronic Obstructive Airway Disease

COP – Cryptogenic Organising Pneumonia

COPD – Chronic Obstructive Pulmonary Disease

CPAM – Congenital Pulmonary Airway Malformation

CPM – Central Pontine Myelinolysis

CPPD – Calcium Pyrophosphate Deposition Disease

Cr – Creatine

CRL – Crown Rump Length

CRM – Circumferential Resection Margin

CSF – Cerebrospinal Fluid

CT – Computerised Tomography

CTPA – Computed Tomography Pulmonary Angiogram

CXR – Chest X-Ray

DAD – Diffuse Alveolar Damage

DAI – Diffuse Axonal Injury

DCE – Dynamic Contrast Enhancement

DCIS – Ductal Carcinoma In-situ

DDH – Developmental Dysplasia of Hip

DIC – Disseminated Intravascular Coagulation

DIPJ – Distal Inter-Phalangeal Joint

DISH – Diffuse Idiopathic Skeletal Hyperostosis

DISI – Dorsal Intercalated Segment Instability

DJ – Duodenojejunal

DNET – Dysembryoplastic Neuroepithelial Tumour

DRUJ – Distal Radioulnar Joint

DWI – Diffusion-Weighted Imaging

ECG – Electrocardiogram

ENT – Ear Nose Throat

ERCP – Endoscopic Retrograde Chloangio-pancreatography

ESR – Erythrocyte Sedimentation Rate

ETT – Endotracheal Tube

EUS – Endoscopic Eltrasound

EVAR – Endovascular (Aortic) Aneurysm Repair

FAI – Femoroacetabular Impingement

FAPS – Familial Adenomatous Polyposis Syndrome

FB – Foreign Body

FCD – Fibrous Cortical Defect

FCL – Fibular Collateral Ligament

FD – Fibrous Dysplasia

FDG – F18 Fluorodeoxyglucose

FESS – Functional Endoscopic Sinus Surgery

FEV – Forced Expiratory Volume

FLAIR – Fluid Attenuation Inversion Recovery

FMD – Fibromuscular dysplasia

FNA – Fine Needle Aspiration

FNH – Focal Nodular Hyperplasia

GCA – Giant Cell Arteritis

GCS – Glasgow Coma Score

GCT – Giant Cell Tumour

GI – Gastrointestinal

GIST – Gastro Intestinal Stromal Tumour

GLAD – Glenolabral Articular Disruption

GRE – Gradient-Recalled Echo

GVHD – Graft Versus Host Disease

HCC – Hepatocellular Carcinoma

HCG – Hysterosalpingogram

HCM – Hypertrophic Cardiomyopathy

HELLP syndrome – Haemolysis, Elevated Liver enzyme Levels, and low Platelet syndrome

HHV – Human Herpes Virus

HIDA – Hepatobiliary Iminodiacetic Acid

HIV – Human Immunodeficiency Virus

HNPCC – Hereditary Non-Polyposis Colon Cancer Syndrome

HOCM – Hypertrophic Obstructive Cardiomyopathy

HRCT – High Resolution Computed Tomography

HSV – Herpes Simplex Virus

HU – Hounsfield Unit

IBD – Inflammatory Bowel Disease

ICA – Internal Carotid Artery

ICU – Intensive Care Unit

IJV – Internal Jugular Vein

INR – International Normalised Ratio

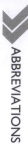

IPF – Idiopathic Pulmonary Fibrosis

IPMN – Intraductal Papillary Mucinous Neoplasm

IUCD – Intra-Uterine Contraceptive Device

IV – Intravenous

IVC – Inferior Vena cava

IVU – Intravenous Urogram

JVP – Juvenile Pilocytic Astrocytoma

KUB – Kidney, Ureters, Bladder

LA – Left Atrium

LAGBP – Laparoscopic Adjustable Gastric Banding Procedure

LAM – Lymphangioleiomyomatosis

LASA-P – Lipid-Associated Aialic Acid P

LCH – Langerhans Cell Histiocytosis

LCL – Lateral Collateral Ligament

LDH – Lactate Dehydrogenase

LFT – Liver Function Tests

LIP – Lymphocytic Interstitial Pneumonitis

LLL – Left Lower Lobe

LUL – Left Upper Lobe

LV – Left Ventricle

MAC – Mycobacterium Avian Complex

MCA – Middle Cerebral Artery

MCL – Medial Collateral Ligament

MCPJ – Metacarpophalangeal Joint

MCUG – Micturating Cysto-Urethrogram

MDA – Mullerian Duct Anomaly

MDT – Multi-disciplinary Team

MELAS – Mitochondrial Encephalomyopathy, Lactic Acidosis, and Stroke like episodes

MEN – Multiple Endocrine Neoplasia

MIBG – Metaiodobenzylguanidine

MPFL – Medial Patellofemoral Ligament

MR – Magnetic Resonance

MRA – Magnetic Resonance Angiography

MRCP – Magnetic Resonance Cholangio-Pancreatography

MRE – Magnetic Resonance Enterography

MRI – Magnetic Resonance Imaging

MRSA – Methicillin-Resistant *Staphylococcus aureus*

MRU – Magnetic Resonance Urography

MS – Multiple Sclerosis

MSSA – Methicillin-Sensitive *Staphylococcus aureus*

MTPJ – Metatarsophalangeal Joint

MTR – Magnetisation Transfer Ratio

MTT – Mean Transit Time

NAA – N-Acetylaspartate

NAFLD – Non-Alcoholic Fatty Liver Disease

NAHI – Non-Accidental Head Injury

NAI – Non-Accidental Injury

NASH – Non-Alcoholic Steatohepatitis

NF – Neurofibromatosis

NG(T) – Nasogastric (Tube)

NHL – Non-Hodgkins Lymphoma

NICE – National Institute for Health and Care Excellence

NOF – Non-Ossifying Fibroma

NPH – Normal Pressure Hydrocephalus

NSE – Neuron-Specific Enolase

NSIP – Nonspecific interstitial pneumonitis

OA – Osteoarthritis

OCD – Osteo-Chondral Defect

OCP – Oral Contraceptive Pill

OFD – Osteo Fibrous Dysplasia

OGD – Oesophago-Gastroduodenoscopy

OKC – Odontogenic Keratocyst

OM – Occipito-Mental/Osteomyelitis

PAN – Polyarteritis Nodosa

PCA – Posterior Cerebral Artery

PCKD – Polycystic Kidney Disease

PCL – Posterior Cruciate Ligament

PCOM – Posterior Communicating Artery

PCOS – Polycystic Ovarian Syndrome

PCP – Pneumocystis Pneumonia

PDA – Patent Ductus Arteriosus

PE – Pulmonary Embolism

PET – Positron Emission Tomography

PHACE syndrome – Posterior fossa malformations, Haemangioma Arterial anomalies, Cardiac defects, Eye abnormalities, sternal cleft and supra-umbilical raphe syndrome

PICA – Posterior Inferior Cerebellar Artery

PIN – Posterior Interosseous Nerve

PIPJ – Proximal Inter-Phalangeal Joint

PKU – Phenylketonuria

PMF – Progressive Massive Fibrosis

PML – Progressive Multifocal Leukoencephalopathy

PNET – Primitive Neuroectodermal Tumour

POEMS syndrome – Polyneuropathy, Organomegaly, Endocrinopathy, Monoclonal gammopathy, and Skin changes syndrome

PR – Per-Rectal

PSA – Prostate-Specific Antigen

PSC – Primary Sclerosing Cholangitis

PUJ – Pelvi-Ureteric Junction

PVA – Polyvinyl Alcohol

PVL – Periventricular Leukomalacia

PVNS – Pigmented Vilonodular Synovitis

PWI – Perfusion Weighted Imaging

RA – Right Atrium

RBILD – Respiratory Bronchiolitis Interstitial Lung Disease

RCC – Renal Cell Carcinoma

RFA – Radio Frequency Ablation

RLL – Right Lower Lobe

RML – Right Middle Lobe

RPF – Retroperitoneal Fibrosis

RRI – Renal Resistive Index

RRMS – Relapsing Remitting Multiple Sclerosis

RSV – Respiratory Syncytial Virus

RTA – Road Traffic Accident

RTC – Road Traffic Collision

RUL – Right Upper Lobe

RV – Right Ventricle

RVOT – Right Ventricular Outflow Tract

RYGBT – Roux-en-Y Gastric Bypass Surgery

SAH – Sub-Arachnoid Haemorrhage

SAPHO – Synovitis, Acne, Palmoplantar Pustulosis, Hyperostosis and Osteitis

SBC – Solitary Bone Cyst

SBO – Small Bowel Obstruction

SCC-A – Squamous Cell Carcinoma Antigen.

SCFE – Slipped Capital Femoral Epiphysis

SCM – Split Cord Malformation

SDH – Sub-dural Hemorrhage

SLAC – Scapholunate Advanced Collapse

SLAP – Superior Labrum Anterior Posterior

SLE – Systemic Lupus Erythematosus

SMA – Superior Mesenteric Artery

SMV – Superior Mesenteric Vein

SSPE – Subacute Sclerosing Panencephalitis

STIR – Short-Tau Inversion Recovery sequence

SUFE – Slipped Upper Femoral Epiphysis

SWI – Susceptibility Weighted Imaging

TA – Truncus Arteriosus

TACE – Transcatheter Arterial Chemoembolisation

TAG-72 – Tumour Associated Glycoprotein

TAPVR – Total Anomalous Pulmonary Venous Return

TB – Tuberculosis

TCC – Transitional Cell Carcinoma

TFC – Triangular Fibrocartilage

TGA – Transposition of Great Arteries

THR – Total Hip Replacement

TIPS – Transjugular Intrahepatic Portosystemic Shunt

TKR – Total Knee Replacement

TME – Total Mesorectal Excision

TOF – Tetralogy Of Falot/Time-Of-Flight

TRUP – Transurethral Resection of Prostate

TRUS – Trans Rectal Ultrasound

TS – Tuberous Sclerosis

TSH – Thyroid Stimulating Hormone

TT-TG – Tibial Tuberosity–Trochlear Groove

TURP – Transurethral Resection of the Prostate

TVS – Trans-Vaginal Scan

UAC – Umbilical Artery Catheter

UAE – Uterine Artery Embolisation

UBC – Unicameral Bone Cyst

UCL – Ulnar Collateral Ligament

UFE – Uterine Fibroid Embolisation

UIP – Usual Interstitial Pneumonia

UPJ – Uretero-Pelvic Junction

US – Ultrasound

UTI – Urinary Tract Infection

UVC – Umbilical Venous Catheter

VHL – Von Hippel–Lindau

VISI – Volar Intercalated Segment Instability

VNA – Vanillylmandelic Acid

VSD – Ventricular Septal Defect

VUJ – Vesico-Ureteric Junction

VUR – Vesico-Ureteric Reflux

XGP – Xanthogranulomatous Pyelonephritis

βhCG – beta Human Chorionic Gonadotropin

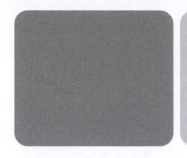

CHAPTER 1
TEST PAPER 1

Questions

Time: 3 hours

1. A 30-year-old man has been involved in an Road Traffic Accident (RTA). Aortic injury is suspected. CT angiogram shows a fusiform dilatation at the anteromedial aspect of the aortic isthmus with a steep contour superiorly, gently merging with the proximal descending thoracic aorta inferiorly. What is the likely diagnosis?
   A. Pseudoaneurysm
   B. Coarctation of the aorta
   C. Ductus diverticulum
   D. Aortic nipple
   E. Avulsed left subclavian artery

2. A 40-year-old man on the third cycle of chemotherapy for non-Hodgkin's lymphoma presents with dysphagia and odynophagia. A recent blood count revealed neutropenia. He is referred for a barium swallow, which shows several linear ulcers with 'shaggy borders' in the upper oesophagus. What is the most likely diagnosis?
   A. Candida oesophagitis
   B. CMV oesophagitis
   C. Post-radiotherapy stricture
   D. TB oesophagitis
   E. Pharyngeal pouch

3. A contrast CT scan shows an incidental renal cyst that is hyperdense with thick septations and a mural nodule. What is the Bosniak classification?
   A. Type 1
   B. Type 2
   C. Type 2F
   D. Type 3
   E. Type 4

4. A 33-year-old man with short stature and normal intelligence is being investigated for lower back pain. MRI of the thoracolumbar spine shows marked central stenosis with short pedicles. A comment of bullet-shaped vertebra with progressive narrowing of the lumbar interpedicular distance was noted on the report. Which of the following conditions is most likely?
   A. Hurler's syndrome
   B. Congenital pituitary dwarfism
   C. Achondroplasia
   D. Thanatophoric dysplasia
   E. Hunter's syndrome

5. A 75-year-old woman is admitted under the physicians with confusion and dementia. She has a history of spontaneous intracranial haemorrhage and has been diagnosed with amyloid angiopathy. The most specific MR sequence for diagnosis of multifocal intracranial cortical–subcortical microhaemorrhages in cerebral amyloid angiopathy is:
   A. T1W spin echo
   B. STIR
   C. T2W spin echo
   D. Gradient echo
   E. FLAIR

6. Regarding sporting injuries involving the upper limbs, all of the following statements are correct, except:
   A. Anomalous anconeus epitrochlearis muscle results in Posterior Interosseous Nerve (PIN) entrapment.
   B. Atrophy of extensor muscles can be seen in chronic PIN neuropathy.
   C. Partial thickness tears of the biceps can involve either the long or short heads.
   D. Cubital tunnel syndrome is the most common elbow neuropathy.
   E. Oedema of flexor carpi ulnaris and ulnar nerve thickening suggests cubital tunnel nerve entrapment.

7. An obese 25-year-old man presents with atypical chest pain. Cardiac MR demonstrates asymmetrical hypertrophy of the interventricular septum, primarily affecting the anteroinferior portion. What is the most likely diagnosis?
   A. Hypertrophic obstructive cardiomyopathy
   B. Restrictive cardiomyopathy
   C. Myocardial infarction
   D. Dilated cardiomyopathy
   E. Constrictive pericarditis

8. A 65-year-old diabetic with a history of alcohol excess is referred for a barium swallow following a history of dysphagia. The study shows several small, thin, flask-shaped structures along the cervical oesophagus oriented parallel to the long axis of the oesophagus. What is the most likely diagnosis?
   A. Feline oesophagus
   B. Pseudodiverticulosis
   C. Glycogenic acanthosis
   D. Traction diverticulum
   E. Idiopathic eosinophilic oesophagitis

9. A 21-year-old woman with infertility undergoes US that shows a 2-cm right adnexal mass with posterior acoustic enhancement. Another multilocular cyst is seen in the left ovary. Further evaluation with MR shows multiple small lesions in both the ovaries and pouch of Douglas, which were hyperintense on fat-suppressed T1W images with shading sign on T2W images. What is the likely diagnosis?
   A. Dermoid
   B. Endometrioid carcinoma of the ovary
   C. Endometriosis
   D. PCOS (polycystic ovarian syndrome)
   E. Pelvic inflammatory disease

10. A young man presents to the ENT clinic with deepening of the voice. Going through his history and clinical notes, the consultant reviews a recent plain radiograph report of his

hands, which describes cystic changes in the carpal bones along with enlarged phalangeal tufts and metacarpals. What is the next appropriate imaging investigation?
A. CT brain pre- and post-contrast
B. MRI brain
C. MRI pituitary pre- and post-contrast
D. Chest X-ray
E. Lateral view of the skull

11. A 77-year-old man with gradual onset dementia shows multifocal abnormalities on cranial CT and MRI. He has been recently diagnosed with amyloidosis. All of the following conditions may be present in central nervous system amyloidosis, except:
A. Occurrence in elderly patients
B. Multifocal subcortical intracranial haemorrhages
C. Cerebral and cerebellar atrophy
D. Non-communicating hydrocephalus
E. Typical occurrence in normotensive patients

12. An 11-year-old boy with left shoulder pain has a shoulder X-ray, which shows a lucent lesion in the metaphysis. This has distinct borders and lies in the intramedullary compartment. It is orientated along the long axis of the humerus. What is the most likely diagnosis?
A. Aneurysmal bone cyst
B. GCT
C. Simple bone cyst
D. Chondroblastoma
E. Non-ossifying fibroma

13. A 50-year-old secretary presents with epigastric pain, nausea and weight loss. She also complains of bilateral swollen ankles. She is referred for a barium meal as she is unable to tolerate an oesophago-gastroduodenoscopy (OGD). The examination shows thickened folds in the fundus and body of the stomach; the antrum was not involved. What is the most likely diagnosis?
A. Nephrotic syndrome
B. Lymphoma
C. Eosinophilic gastroenteritis
D. Leiomyoma
E. Ménétrier's disease

14. A 58-year-old woman undergoes an echocardiogram followed by cardiac MRI for investigation of exertional dyspnoea. The cardiac MRI was reviewed at the X-ray meeting, and the radiologist diagnosed concentric hypertrophic cardiomyopathy. Which of the following did the radiologist see?
A. Thickening of the interatrial septum at 7 mm
B. Thickening of the entire LV wall measuring 17 mm at end diastole
C. Nodular high signal in the interventricular septum on T2
D. Thickening of the LV wall measuring 14 mm with normal systolic function
E. Thickened LV with delayed hyperenhancement of midwall

15. A 50-year-old builder is involved in a high-speed RTA. CT is performed according to trauma protocol, demonstrating extra-peritoneal rupture of the bladder. Which of the following best describes this?
A. Contrast pooling in the paracolic gutters.
B. Contrast outlining small bowel loops.
C. Flame-shaped contrast seen in the perivesical fat.
D. CT cystogram is usually normal.
E. Intramural contrast on CT cystogram.

16. An elderly patient on long-term dialysis presents to the orthopaedic clinic with right shoulder pain. Plain films show juxta-articular swelling and erosions of the humerus, but the joint space is preserved. MRI shows a small joint effusion and the presence of low- to intermediate-signal soft tissue on all sequences covering the synovial membrane extending into the periarticular tissue. What is the likely diagnosis?
    A. Amyloid arthropathy
    B. Gout
    C. Calcium pyrophosphate deposition disease (CPPD)
    D. Pigmented villonodular synovitis (PVNS)
    E. Reticuloendotheliosis

17. A 33-year-old woman with recurrent episodes of optic neuritis with waxing and waning upper limb weakness is referred for an MRI brain with high suspicion of demyelination. All of the following are MR features of acute multiple sclerosis (MS) lesions of the brain, except:
    A. High signal intensity on FLAIR
    B. 'Black hole' appearance
    C. Incomplete ring-like contrast enhancement
    D. Increase in size of lesion
    E. Mass effect

18. A 14-year-old boy complains of left knee pain and limp. He also has medial thigh pain. On examination, he has full range of movement with some discomfort on internal rotation. AP and lateral X-rays of the knee and femur are normal. What is the next investigation?
    A. CT
    B. Bone scan
    C. MRI
    D. Frog leg lateral of the hips
    E. US

19. A 30-year-old woman presents with shortness of breath and fatigue. CT shows enlargement of the right atrium, right ventricle and pulmonary artery and normal appearance of the left atrium. What is the most likely diagnosis?
    A. VSD – Ventricular Septal Defect
    B. ASD – Atrial Septal Defect
    C. Bicuspid aortic valve
    D. Coarctation of the aorta
    E. Mitral valve disease

20. A 50-year-old man is referred to a gastroenterologist with a 6-month history of intermittent epigastric pain and nausea. He is referred for a barium meal test due to a failed OGD – oesophago-gastroduodenoscopy. The study shows an ulcer along the lesser curve of the stomach. Which of the following is a malignant feature of a gastric ulcer?
    A. The margin of the ulcer crater extends beyond the projected luminal surface.
    B. Carman meniscus sign.
    C. Hampton's line.
    D. Central ulcer within mound of oedema.
    E. The ulcer depth is greater than the width.

21. Which of the following characteristics is typical of prostate cancer?
    A. Low on T1   High on T2
    B. Low on T1   Low on T2
    C. Isointense on T1 High on T2

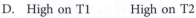

D. High on T1   High on T2
E. Isointense on T1   Isointense on T2

22. An eccentric expansile lesion in the metaphysis of the humerus is noted incidentally following a routine plain radiograph investigation in a young patient following a rugby tackle. MRI performed for further characterisation shows multiple cystic spaces, some with blood fluid level, with an intact low-signal periosteal rim. What is the diagnosis?
    A. Unicameral bone cyst
    B. Aneurysmal bone cyst
    C. Eosinophilic granuloma
    D. Enchondroma
    E. Fibrous dysplasia

23. A 34-year-old woman with previous history of upper limb weakness that resolved spontaneously and optic neuritis was referred for an MRI brain. MRI confirms the presence of bilateral periventricular hyperintensities on FLAIR with abnormal signal in the corpus callosum and middle cerebellar peduncles. MRI also shows signal abnormality in the right optic nerve. Which portion of the optic nerve does Multiple sclerosis (MS) most commonly affect?
    A. Intra-orbital.
    B. Intracanalicular.
    C. Intracranial.
    D. Chiasmatic.
    E. All portions are equally susceptible.

24. A newborn baby has US of the spine. At which level is the conus expected to be?
    A. Above L1
    B. Above T12
    C. L2 to L3
    D. L3 to L4
    E. S2

25. A middle-aged woman presents with cough and haemoptysis. Her chest X-ray reveals a large ovoid mass in the right lower lobe. She has a known history of Osler–Weber–Rendu syndrome. What is the most appropriate next imaging investigation that you will organise?
    A. MRA of the pulmonary artery
    B. CTPA
    C. CTPA with portal phase images covering the liver
    D. Chest HRCT
    E. Conventional pulmonary angiography

26. A nursing home resident is found to have a lung tumour and undergoes CT staging of the chest and abdomen. This reveals a discrete lesion medial to the second part of the duodenum with a fluid–fluid level. What is the most likely diagnosis?
    A. Duplication cyst
    B. Duodenal diverticulum
    C. Duodenal web
    D. Annular pancreas
    E. Adenocarcinoma of the duodenum

27. Which of the following is false?
    A. Skene cyst   Lateral to external urethral meatus
    B. Nabothian cyst   Lateral to the endocervical canal

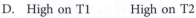

C.   Gartner's dust cyst   Posterolateral aspect of the upper vagina

D.   Bartholin's cyst   Posterolateral aspect of the vagina

E.   Urethral diverticulum   Posterolateral aspect of mid-urethra

28. A 31-year-old man who is known to the gastroenterologist and rheumatologist presents to the ophthalmology department with visual disturbances. A pelvic radiograph done a year ago in the emergency department showed whiskering of the ischial tuberosities and greater trochanters, with symmetrical sclerosis of both sacroiliac joints. What is the most likely diagnosis?
   A. Reiter syndrome
   B. Behcet's syndrome
   C. Ankylosing spondylitis (AS)
   D. Rheumatoid arthritis
   E. Systemic lupus erythematosus (SLE)

29. A 36-year-old woman with resolving limb weakness and previous history of optic neuritis is diagnosed as having relapsing remitting multiple sclerosis (RRMS). Which of the following statements concerning MS imaging is incorrect?
   A. Black holes correlate well with clinical outcome.
   B. Brain atrophy is higher in MS than normal ageing.
   C. The pattern of brain atrophy can mimic Alzheimer's disease.
   D. Diffusion tensor imaging demonstrates structural damage to the white matter.
   E. MS lesions have low MTR (Magnetisation Transfer Ratio) representing myelin loss.

30. A 3-year-old presents as acutely unwell with a maculopapular rash, lymphadenopathy and erythema of her palms. Her white cell count is normal, and a specific cause for her symptoms is not found. She improves on immunoglobulins and supportive treatment. A follow-up echocardiogram shows cardiomegaly and a coronary artery aneurysm. What is the likely diagnosis?
   A. Takayasu arteritis
   B. Kawasaki arteritis
   C. Moyamoya syndrome
   D. Henoch–Schonlein purpura
   E. Churg–Strauss syndrome

31. A 76-year-old male patient with chronic inflammatory disease and known history of secondary generalised multisystem amyloidosis showed an abnormal appearance of the heart on echocardiography. Dynamic enhanced cardiac MR imaging was advised for further characterisation. All of the following are imaging findings seen with cardiac amyloidosis, except
   A. Left ventricular wall hypertrophy
   B. Subendocardial delayed myocardial hyperenhancement
   C. Systolic dysfunction
   D. Granular echogenic myocardium
   E. Interatrial septal thickening

32. A taxi driver has had recurrent episodes of abdominal pain. On CT, a lesion is seen within the head of the pancreas. Pancreatic duct dilatation is noted with a normal CBD and atrophy of the body and tail of the pancreas. ERCP demonstrates thick mucous material discharging from the bulging papilla. What is the most likely diagnosis?
   A. Mucinous cystadenocarcinoma
   B. Serous cystadenocarcinoma

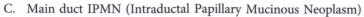

C. Main duct IPMN (Intraductal Papillary Mucinous Neoplasm)

D. Pancreatic pseudocyst

E. Pancreatic adenocarcinoma

33. A 55-year-old man with several episodes of epididymo-orchitis in the past has an ultrasound of the scrotum. The radiologist performing the scan notices several hypoechoic structures within the mediastinum testis and incidental epididymal cysts. There was no Doppler flow. What is the most likely diagnosis?

A. Lymphoma of the testes

B. Cystic dysplasia of the testis

C. Seminoma

D. Abscess

E. Cystic transformation of rete testis

34. An elderly woman presents with progressive atraumatic pain within her right knee over the course of the last month, particularly on the medial aspect, associated with functional impairment. Her clinical history includes a meniscal tear, which was treated arthroscopically 10 years ago with a good outcome. An MRI reveals florid marrow oedema within the medial femoral condyle associated with mild flattening of the weight-bearing surface. What is the diagnosis?

A. Perthe's disease

B. Sinding–Larsen's disease

C. Blount's disease

D. Spontaneous osteonecrosis of the knee

E. Osteochondral defect

35. A known MS patient has presented to the neurologist with clinical features of involvement of the spinal cord. An MRI of the whole spine has been requested with a view towards assessment of the cord for possible multiple sclerosis (MS) plaques. MS lesions in the spinal cord occur most commonly in the

A. Cervical segment.

B. Thoracic segment.

C. Lumbar segment.

D. Sacral segment.

E. All segments are equally affected.

36. A neonate presents with non-bilious vomiting with a palpable upper abdominal lump. Which of the following US findings would not be in keeping with pyloric stenosis?

A. Pyloric muscle thickness 3.5 mm

B. Target sign

C. Pyloric canal length 14 mm

D. Antral nipple sign

E. Cervix sign

37. A child with exertional dyspnoea and abnormal chest X-ray showing a boot-shaped heart and oligaemic lungs is diagnosed as suffering from tetralogy of Fallot. The pulmonary oligaemia is secondary to right ventricular outflow tract (RVOT) obstruction. Which of the following is the most common implicated cause for obstruction of RVOT?

A. Hypoplastic pulmonary annulus

B. Pulmonary valvular stenosis

C. Infundibular stenosis

D. Combined infundibular and pulmonary valvular stenosis

E. Overriding ventricular septum

38. A 50-year-old man presents with recurrent episodes of abdominal pain. Blood amylase is normal. Chronic pancreatitis is suspected. All of the following statements regarding MRI imaging in chronic pancreatitis are true, except
    A. MRI has a poor sensitivity for detecting parenchymal calcification in chronic pancreatitis.
    B. MRI allows evaluation of the ductal system for strictures and stones, debris within pseudocysts and fistula.
    C. MRI shows good sensitivity for the differential diagnosis of focal chronic pancreatitis from pancreatic carcinoma.
    D. Both focal chronic pancreatitis and pancreatic carcinoma demonstrate abnormal post-contrast enhancement on MRI.
    E. Both focal chronic pancreatitis and pancreatic carcinoma demonstrate low signal intensity of the pancreas on T1W fat-saturated images.

39. A 60-year-old heavy smoker presents with haematuria. US KUB shows a midline fluid-filled cavity with mixed echogenicity and calcification adjacent to the bladder wall. CT shows a focal low-attenuation enhancing mass along a cord-like structure extending from the bladder to the umbilicus. What is the most likely diagnosis?
    A. Complex urachal cyst
    B. Vescico urachal diverticulum
    C. Urachal adenocarcinoma
    D. Transitional cell carcinoma
    E. Urachal rhabdomyosarcoma

40. A 10 × 7 mm dense ossified focal lesion is noted in the neck of the right femur of a young man incidentally on a pelvic radiograph performed for an unrelated reason. The lesion has benign features and is consistent with a bone island (enostosis). No follow-up is suggested. All of the following are true of bone islands, except
    A. If more than 2 cm, they are classified as a 'giant' bone island.
    B. They have a sclerotic appearance on imaging.
    C. They show a characteristic brush border on plain films.
    D. They can be positive on a bone scan.
    E. Giant bone islands can be locally aggressive.

41. A patient recently diagnosed with MS has been sent for an MRI of the whole spine to detect possible spinal plaques. All of the following are MR features of spinal cord lesions in MS, except
    A. The sole site of involvement (in some cases).
    B. Imaging features similar to those of MS lesions in the brain.
    C. Most lesions are centrally located.
    D. The length rarely exceeds two vertebral segments.
    E. Dorsal column involvement.

42. Barium enema of a neonate shows an inverted cone shape at the rectosigmoid colon. There is marked retention of the barium on delayed post-evacuation films after 24 hours. The cause for this is
    A. Meconium ileus
    B. Meconium plug syndrome
    C. Hirschprung's disease
    D. Imperforate anus
    E. Hyperplastic polyp of colon

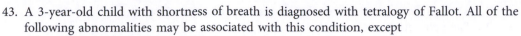

43. A 3-year-old child with shortness of breath is diagnosed with tetralogy of Fallot. All of the following abnormalities may be associated with this condition, except
    A. Transposition of great vessels (TGA)
    B. Patent ductus arteriosus (PDA)
    C. Anomalous origin of coronary arteries
    D. DiGeorge syndrome
    E. Right-sided aortic arch

44. A 40-year-old woman presents to her GP with right upper quadrant pain and is referred for an ultrasound of the abdomen. The scan demonstrates a thickened gall bladder wall with several intramural small echogenic foci showing 'comet tail artefacts'. A few gallstones are also noted. What is the most common diagnosis?
    A. Xanthogranulomatous cholecystitis
    B. Strawberry gallbladder
    C. Porcelain gallbladder
    D. Gallbladder adenomyomatosis
    E. Acute cholecystitis

45. A woman presents with infertility and undergoes a hysterosalpingogram. This demonstrates a uterus with two converging horns. A wide angle is seen at the roof of the uterus. Which uterine anomaly does the patient have?
    A. Uterine didelphys
    B. Septate uterus
    C. Arcuate uterus
    D. Bicornuate uterus
    E. Unicornuate uterus

46. A 53-year-old woman presents to the A&E department with acute knee pain. She has had two previous similar episodes in the past, which settled with analgesics and anti-inflammatory medications. Plain films show extensive degenerative change, which is worst at the patellofemoral joint with large subchondral cystic change and chondrocalcinosis of the knee menisci. She informs the attending doctor that she is under review with the endocrinologist. What is the likely diagnosis?
    A. Calcium pyrophosphate deposition disease (CPPD)
    B. Gout
    C. Rheumatoid arthritis
    D. Ochronosis
    E. Psoriasis

47. A 54-year-old man who developed brain metastases almost 9 years after resection of an acral lentiginous melanoma of the distal thumb shows two peripheral nodules in the right frontal lobe. All of the following are features of CNS metastatic melanoma, except
    A. Moderate to intense enhancement post-contrast administration
    B. Cystic components
    C. Subependymal nodules
    D. Multiple lesions at the gray–white matter junction
    E. Miliary pattern

48. A child presents with vomiting and sudden onset abdominal pain. Plain X-rays show a target sign in the right upper quadrant. US shows a pseudo kidney sign in keeping with intussusception. Which of the following is false regarding hydrostatic reduction?
    A. Free intraperitoneal air is a contraindication.
    B. A maximum of two attempts can be made.

C. Air is preferred to Gastrografin water solution in some institutions.

D. The perforation rate is 0.4%–3%.

E. Air enema is associated with a higher perforation rate.

49. Plain X-ray of a newborn shows a large tubular air shadow behind the trachea. The lungs are clear. The bowels are grossly distended with air. What is the likely type of tracheo-oesophageal fistula?

A. Type A

B. Type B

C. Type C

D. Type D

E. Type E

50. A 46-year-old American man who has come to the UK on a holiday trip arrives at the AED with worsening shortness of breath. Chest X-ray shows bilateral asymmetrical calcified mediastinal and hilar nodes, and chronic pulmonary histoplasmosis is provisionally diagnosed. The worsening symptoms are attributed to fibrosing mediastinitis. All the following conditions can occur as complications of fibrosing mediastinitis, except

A. SVC syndrome

B. Pulmonary arterial hypertension

C. Pulmonary venous stenosis

D. Tracheal stenosis

E. Aortic stenosis

51. A 70-year-old pensioner has been referred for an abdominal ultrasound as part of a routine medical examination. He is fit and well with no significant past medical history. The scan demonstrates a small focal well-defined hyperechoic area in the right lobe of the liver showing posterior acoustic enhancement. The most likely differential diagnosis is

A. Metastasis

B. Fatty infiltration

C. Liver cyst

D. FNH (Focal nodular hyperplasia)

E. Capillary haemangioma

52. The causes of medullary nephrocalcinosis include all, except

A. Hyperparathyroidism

B. Renal tubular acidosis

C. Medullary sponge kidney

D. Hypervitaminosis D

E. Alport's syndrome

53. A 56-year-old woman known to the endocrinologist has been going to her family doctor with a funny sensation in her right hand and fingers for the last few months. An MRI was organised along with nerve conduction studies by her family doctor. MRI revealed fusiform swelling of the median nerve in the distal forearm just before the entrance into the carpal tunnel with increased signal on T2. What is the likely diagnosis?

A. Cervical spondylosis

B. Ulnar tunnel syndrome

C. Carpal tunnel syndrome

D. Cervical rib with brachial plexus impingement

E. Neurofibroma of the median nerve

54. A 7-year-old boy with a history of a penetrating injury from a tree branch was sent for CT orbits for further assessment. Which of the following statements regarding the CT detection of intra-orbital foreign bodies is false?
   A. Size, type and location of glass foreign body (FB) affects detection.
   B. Wooden FB is hyperattenuating.
   C. Old wood can be mistaken for air.
   D. Attenuation of wood changes with water content.
   E. CT can demonstrate metal FB less than a millimetre.

55. A 56-year-old woman with an increase in shortness of breath comes to the A&E department and is assessed by the physicians. The ECG is low in voltage and a chest X-ray is organised. The chest X-ray shows a very large heart with sharply defined borders and a narrow pedicle, suggesting pericardial effusion. All of the following are associated, except
   A. Tuberculosis pericarditis
   B. Blunt trauma to the sternum
   C. Hyperthyroidism
   D. Radiation pericarditis
   E. Pericardial lymphoma

56. A 66-year-old joiner presents to his GP with jaundice and abdominal discomfort. He was subsequently referred to a gastroenterologist who requests a liver biopsy due to deranged liver function tests. Which of the following options is not a contraindication for percutaneous liver biopsy?
   A. INR above 1.6
   B. Platelets less than 60,000/mm^3
   C. Tense ascites
   D. Extra-hepatic biliary obstruction
   E. Suspected haemangioma

57. A 40-year-old man who is a known hypothyroid patient, presents with weight loss and dull pain in the flank and back. He undergoes an abdominal CT. Regarding retroperitoneal fibrosis, all of the following is seen on imaging, except
   A. Medial deviation of the ureters in the middle third, typically bilateral.
   B. CT shows soft-tissue mass displacing the aorta anteriorly.
   C. T2W MRI shows variable signal.
   D. PET CT has high sensitivity.
   E. Hydronephrosis is evident on CT urogram.

58. A 17-year-old teenager is under investigation for vague pain in the knee associated with a limp. A plain film radiograph shows an oval lucent lesion in the epiphysis of the distal femur. The pain was noticed following an injury sustained during a football match. What would be the next investigation of choice?
   A. CT
   B. MRI
   C. Bone biopsy
   D. Tc-99m bone scan
   E. No imaging necessary since it looks benign

59. Abnormal high density is noted in the vitreous on CT orbits, suggesting the presence of blood in the posterior chamber. All of the following conditions are potential causes of vitreous haemorrhage, except
   A. Intra-ocular tumour
   B. Abnormal vascularisation of the retina
   C. Terson syndrome

D. Corneal abrasion

E. Trauma

60. A 1-month-old baby presents with difficulty in feeding and shortness of breath. Chest X-ray shows cardiomegaly. She has an episode of seizure and undergoes cranial US, which shows a median tubular cystic space with high-velocity turbulent flow on Doppler. The ventricles are also mildly dilated. These findings are consistent with
    A. Pineal tumour
    B. Arachnoid cyst
    C. Colloid cyst
    D. Vein of Galen aneurysm
    E. Ventriculitis

61. A 66-year-old man with progressive shortness of breath and low-volume ECG shows an enlarged heart on chest X-ray. Echocardiogram confirms the presence of a moderately large pericardial effusion. The pericardial fluid is aspirated for symptomatic relief and sent off for cytology and culture. Cytology comes back as positive for malignant cells. Which of the following is the most common type of primary pericardial malignancy?
    A. Fibrosarcoma
    B. Pericardial angiosarcoma
    C. Fibromyxoid sarcoma
    D. Mesothelioma
    E. Epithelioid endothelioma

62. A 40-year-old man undergoes a CT KUB for renal colic, which shows an incidental finding of an 8-mm lesion in Segment VIII of the liver. Further characterisation of this lesion with MRI shows it to be low signal on T1W and high signal on T2W. On the dynamic phase, it shows peripheral nodular enhancement with centripetal filling. What is the most likely diagnosis?
    A. FNH
    B. Adenoma
    C. Haemangioma
    D. Early appearance of Hepatocellular Carcinoma (HCC)
    E. Cholangiocarcinoma

63. Of the normal uterus signal on MR, which is correct?

	Endometrium	Myometrium	Junctional zone
A.	High on T2	Intermediate on T2	High on T2
B.	High on T2	Intermediate on T2	Low on T2
C.	Isointense on T1	Isointense on T1	High on T1
D.	Isointense on T1	High on T1	Low on T1
E.	Low on T1	Low on T2	High on T2

64. A plain lumbar spine radiograph of a 45-year-old woman shows marked posterior scalloping of the vertebral bodies extending over several vertebral lengths. All of the following are diseases associated with this finding, except
    A. Marfan
    B. Neurofibromatosis
    C. Ependymoma
    D. Achondroplasia
    E. Hypothyroidism

65. A 58-year-old man with facial fractures shows deformity of the globe on unenhanced axial CT, but it is unclear if there is an open-globe injury. All of the following CT findings suggest an open-globe injury, except
   A. Intra-ocular air
   B. Lens dislocation
   C. Scleral discontinuity
   D. Flat tire sign
   E. Deep anterior chamber

66. An 18-month-old child is brought in by her mother with complaints of visual problems; on examination, the left eye is of normal size with a whitish mass behind the lens. US shows a heterogeneous hyperechoic solid intra-ocular mass with retinal detachment. There are fine focal calcifications with acoustic shadowing. The appearances suggest
   A. Persistent hyperplastic primary vitreous
   B. Coats disease
   C. Retinoblastoma
   D. Toxocara endophthalmitis
   E. Retrolental fibroplasia

67. A 35-year-old woman undergoes an X-ray in the A&E department with suspicion of chest infection. The X-ray reveals an abnormal mediastinal opacity but no evidence of chest infection. Review of two old films done 2 and 6 years ago shows the same abnormal mediastinal opacities with no significant interval change in size, shape, appearance or location. Judging by its location, the radiologist reports it as a simple pericardial cyst or spring water cyst. Which of the following statements concerning congenital simple pericardial cysts is false?
   A. They are homogenous and well defined on frontal chest X-ray.
   B. They are most commonly left-sided.
   C. On MRI, they are low on T1W and high on T2W images.
   D. Pericardial cysts can contain proteinaceous material.
   E. Pericardial cysts can occasionally calcify.

68. A 90-year-old man is admitted following intermittent episodes of bright red rectal bleeding. He is haemodynamically stable on initial assessment. OGD and flexible colonoscopy are normal. He subsequently has another bleed on the surgical ward and is then referred for a CT mesenteric angiogram. Which of the following statements is false regarding CT mesenteric angiography?
   A. Severe bleeding episodes, such as those manifesting with hemodynamic instability, decrease the pretest probability of a positive result for active bleeding at CT angiography.
   B. Active bleeding must be present during the time contrast is injected into the vascular system in order to demonstrate the site of bleeding.
   C. Portal venous phase imaging depicts extravascular blushes with higher sensitivity than arterial phase imaging does.
   D. Retention of previously administered barium in colonic diverticula may be mistaken for, or may obscure, acute extravasation of contrast material.
   E. Hyperattenuating material within the bowel lumen on the unenhanced scan without additional findings in the contrast-enhanced phases indicates recent haemorrhage.

69. A 25-year-old man undergoing abdominal CT shows the presence of bridging renal tissue across the midline at the level of the lower poles, consistent with a horseshoe kidney. All the following are recognised associations, except
   A. Bicornuate uterus
   B. Cardiac anomaly

C. Undescended testis

D. Tracheo-oesophageal fistula

E. Anorectal malformation

70. A young patient is followed up for a fractured tibia at the outpatient clinic. A repeat radiograph is acquired, which shows abnormal healing and callus formation at the fracture site. All the following are possible causes, except

A. Cushing's syndrome

B. Osteogenesis imperfecta

C. Osteopoikilosis

D. Paralytic state

E. Asthmatic on steroids

71. A 67-year-old man has been rushed to the stroke unit with features of acute stroke. All of the following are true about acute stroke imaging, except

A. CT source images correlate with infarct volume.

B. Matched CBV (Cerebral blood volume) and CBF (Cerebral blood flow) represent salvageable brain.

C. Diffusion-weighted MR imaging assesses the infarct core.

D. Mismatch between PWI (Perfusion weighted imaging) and DWI (Diffusion weighted imaging) volumes represents salvageable brain.

E. T2 shine through is seen as bright on DWI.

72. Neck US of a previously well 2-year-old girl shows a 3-cm thin-walled cystic structure with multiple septae of variable thickness in the left posterior triangle with extension into the mediastinum. The diagnosis is:

A. Third branchial cleft cyst

B. Cervical meningocoele

C. Cystic teratoma

D. Lymphangioma

E. Second branchial cleft cyst

73. A 34-year-old woman with chest pain, shortness of breath and collapse is brought to the A&E department. Initial chest X-ray is abnormal. Subject to the abnormal appearance of the cardiac contour, an MRI is obtained in the local cardiac centre on the following day, which confirms a large congenital pericardial defect. All of the following are imaging features, except:

A. Abnormal cardiac contour on plain chest X-ray.

B. Failure to identify pericardium on CT or MR is diagnostic.

C. Most commonly, a left-sided location.

D. Shift of cardiac axis to the left.

E. Association with ASD.

74. A 5-year-old boy involved in an RTA is referred for a trauma CT scan. The reporting radiologist does not find any acute abnormality. However, there are other incidental findings on the scan suggestive of malrotation. Which of the following options is the most specific feature of gut malrotation on CT?

A. SMV (superior mesenteric vein) anterior to the SMA (superior mesenteric artery)

B. SMV to the right of the SMA

C. Whirl sign around the SMA

D. DJ (duodenojejunal) flexure to the right of the midline

E. SMV to the left of the SMA

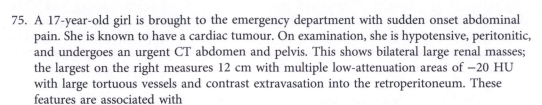

75. A 17-year-old girl is brought to the emergency department with sudden onset abdominal pain. She is known to have a cardiac tumour. On examination, she is hypotensive, peritonitic, and undergoes an urgent CT abdomen and pelvis. This shows bilateral large renal masses; the largest on the right measures 12 cm with multiple low-attenuation areas of −20 HU with large tortuous vessels and contrast extravasation into the retroperitoneum. These features are associated with
    A. Von Hippel–Lindau
    B. Neurofibromatosis type 1
    C. Sturge–Weber syndrome
    D. Tuberous sclerosis
    E. Amyloidosis

76. A young woman presents to the AED following a scuffle on a night out. On examination, there is a suspected fifth metacarpal fracture of her right hand. A plain radiograph is subsequently organised. This does not demonstrate a fracture, but it is noted that the patient has relatively short fourth metacarpal bones. Old chest films show bilateral inferior rib notching involving the third to sixth ribs bilaterally. What is the likely diagnosis?
    A. Noonan syndrome
    B. Turner syndrome
    C. Pseudohypoparathyroidism
    D. Marfan syndrome
    E. Achondroplasia

77. A 66-year-old man with acute onset of right upper limb weakness was brought to A&E within an hour of the onset of symptoms. All of the following are recognised features of early ischaemic change, except
    A. Insular ribbon sign
    B. Dense MCA sign
    C. Sulcal effacement
    D. Obscuration of the lentiform nucleus
    E. Dilatation of ventricle

78. In order of frequency, the most common location of congenital lobar emphysema is as follows:
    A. LUL, LLL, RUL
    B. LUL, RML, RUL
    C. RUL, RML, LLL
    D. LUL, RUL, RLL
    E. LUL, RML, RLL
    (LLL – left lower lobe, LUL – left upper lobe, RLL – right lower lobe, RML – right middle lobe, RUL – right upper lobe)

79. A 66-year-old woman with progressive shortness of breath, reduced exercise tolerance and occasional chest pain shows engorged neck veins and hepatomegaly on clinical examination. She is clinically thought to have constrictive pericarditis. All of the following are imaging features of constrictive pericarditis, except
    A. Pericardial thickness of more than 4 mm.
    B. Pericardial thickening may be limited to the right side of the heart.
    C. MR is better at demonstrating pericardial calcification.
    D. Sigmoid-shaped ventricular septum.
    E. Increased diameter of the IVC.

80. A 60-year-old woman presents with abdominal cramps and watery diarrhoea associated with flushing of the face. A CT colonography study is performed, as the patient is unable to tolerate optical colonoscopy. The colon and rectum are normal, but there is ileal thickening and a 2-cm partly calcified mass in the small bowel mesentery with surrounding desmoplasia. Carcinoid is suspected. Which of the following statements is true about small bowel carcinoid tumours?
    A. Carcinoid syndrome has higher morbidity and mortality than the tumour itself.
    B. Over 60% have carcinoid syndrome.
    C. Carcinoid tumours are associated with neurofibromatosis type II.
    D. They most commonly occur in the colon.
    E. They commonly cause osteolytic metastasis to bone.

81. The following are signs of a normal gestational sac, except
    A. Intradecidual sign.
    B. Cardiac activity seen with a CRL (crown-rump length) of 6 mm.
    C. Double decidual sign.
    D. Mean sac diameter increases by 1 mm/day.
    E. Embryo seen with a mean sac diameter of 10 mm.

82. A 17-year-old girl presents with a history of acute-on-chronic burning neck pain radiating into the right shoulder and arm. There is associated palmar paraesthesia, easy fatigability and loss of power, exacerbated by elevating the arm to the shoulder level. Sagittal T1W MRI obtained with the arm in the neutral position shows ample fat surrounding the subclavian vessels and brachial plexus. With the arm in abduction, there is compression of the subclavian vessels. What is the diagnosis?
    A. Subclavian artery stenosis
    B. Parsonage–Turner syndrome
    C. Median nerve entrapment
    D. Thoracic outlet syndrome
    E. Subclavian steal syndrome

83. A 67-year-old woman is imaged 3 hours after a witnessed sudden onset of a right hemiparesis. Transverse DWI ($b = 1,000$ sec/mm^2) demonstrates signal change in the subcortical region, including in the lenticular nucleus and corona radiate. Which of the following statements concerning diffusion-weighted MR imaging in cerebral infarction is false?
    A. It measures redistribution of water to intracellular space.
    B. DWI can remain positive for up to 3 weeks post-infarction.
    C. DWI is positive as early as 30 minutes post-infarction.
    D. Acute infarcts show hyperintense signal on ADC.
    E. Acute infarcts show hyperintense signal on DWI.

84. The most common structure to herniate in Bochdalek hernia is
    A. Stomach
    B. Spleen
    C. Omentum
    D. Left lobe of liver
    E. Pancreas

85. Which of the following statements regarding the normal pericardium is false?
    A. It consists of two inner serous layers of tissue and one outer fibrous layer.
    B. It is visualised on lateral chest X-ray as a fat pad sign.
    C. It is 1–2 mm thick on CT and may contain up to 30 ml of fluid.
    D. It is low in signal on T1W MRI.
    E. On frontal chest X-ray, it is visualised as a 2-mm stripe outlined by fat.

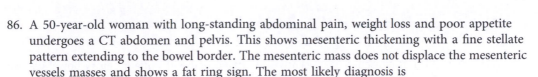

86. A 50-year-old woman with long-standing abdominal pain, weight loss and poor appetite undergoes a CT abdomen and pelvis. This shows mesenteric thickening with a fine stellate pattern extending to the bowel border. The mesenteric mass does not displace the mesenteric vessels masses and shows a fat ring sign. The most likely diagnosis is
    A. Retroperitoneal fibrosis
    B. Carcinoid
    C. Sclerosing mesenteritis
    D. Epiploic appendagitis
    E. Lymphoma

87. A 56-year-old man undergoing CT urogram displays an incidental lesion in his right adrenal gland. He is asymptomatic apart from pain in the left loin, which is currently being investigated. All these features suggest that adrenal carcinoma is more likely than a benign adenoma, except
    A. Size more than 5 cm
    B. Delayed washout
    C. HU value of <37 on delayed contrast enhanced CT
    D. Involvement of right kidney
    E. Peripheral nodular enhancement

88. What type of labral injury is not associated with an anterior shoulder dislocation?
    A. Bony Bankart lesion
    B. Perthes lesion
    C. Glenolabral articular disruption injury (GLAD)
    D. Superior labral anterior–posterior tear (SLAP)
    E. Anterior labroligamentous periosteal sleeve avulsion injury (ALPSA)

89. A 36-year-old woman with non-remitting headache is sent for an MRI brain by the neurologist to investigate the cause of her headache. The MRI brain is mostly unremarkable apart from showing areas of hyperintensity on FLAIR in subarachnoid spaces. All of the following conditions should be included in the differential diagnosis, except
    A. Pacchionian granulations
    B. Slow arterial flow due to vascular stenosis
    C. Subarachnoid haemorrhage
    D. Infectious meningitis
    E. Leptomeningeal melanosis

90. Which of the following is false regarding bronchopulmonary sequestration?

		Intralobar	Extralobar
A.	Pleural involvement	Visceral pleura	Own pleura
B.	Venous drainage	Pulmonary veins	Systemic veins
C.	Associated anomalies	Less common	More common
D.	Symptomatic	First 6 months	Adulthood
E.	Arterial supply	Aorta	Aorta

91. A 66-year-old man undergoing a routine staging contrast-enhanced CT chest shows a focal non-enhancing smoothly marginated homogeneous dumbbell-shaped mass of fat attenuation confined to the interatrial septum. All of the following features may be associated with lipomatous hypertrophy of the interatrial septum of the heart, except
    A. Fatty atrial septum exceeding 2 cm in transverse diameter.
    B. Related to chronic corticosteroid use.
    C. It is bright on T1 and dark on fat-suppressed images.

D. It is a recognised cause of SVC syndrome.

E. Enhances avidly post-contrast.

92. A 25-year-old music teacher has recently been diagnosed with inflammatory bowel disease. She has an MRI small bowel study for evaluation of her disease status. Regarding features of Crohn's versus ulcerative colitis on cross-sectional imaging, which of the following options is false?

		Crohn's	Ulcerative colitis
A.	Comb's sign	Yes	Yes
B.	Full thickness enhancement	Yes	No
C.	Fibro-fatty proliferation	Yes	No
D.	Enlarged lymph nodes	Yes	Yes
E.	Skip lesions	Yes	Yes

93. According to *Standards of Intravascular Contrast Agent Administration to Adult Patients*, second edition (RCR 2015), all are true regarding patients on metformin, except

A. Metformin need not be stopped prior to contrast enhanced CT if serum creatinine is normal.

B. Metformin need not be stopped prior to contrast examination if eGFR is >60.

C. If serum creatinine is above normal range, metformin should be withheld for 24 hours.

D. If eGFR is <60, the decision to withhold metformin should be made in consultation with the clinical team.

E. There is lack of evidence about whether lactic acidosis is really an issue post-iodinated contrast in metformin users.

94. A motorcyclist is brought into the A&E department with limb fractures and neck pain. Preliminary cervical spine radiographs review mild anterolisthesis (~10%) at C4/5 with slight overlap of the facet joints. CT shows a right 'naked facet' sign at this level.
What statement is false in regard to this injury?

A. It is an unstable injury.

B. Anterolisthesis is a common finding.

C. It is a stable injury.

D. There is widening of the interspinous space.

E. It is often associated with a neurological deficit.

95. A 76-year-old woman has been rushed to the stroke unit with features of acute stroke. A CT brain obtained in the A&E department on arrival is normal. A conventional MRI brain is performed. Which of the following statements regarding the imaging evaluation of an acute cerebral infarction by MR is false?

A. It may demonstrate parenchymal microhaemorrhages on SWI (susceptibility weighted imaging).

B. SWI shows intraparenchymal haemorrhage within hours.

C. SWI is based on homogeneity of magnetic field.

D. Deoxyhaemoglobin produces a non-uniform magnetic field.

E. Microbleeds on SWI are a risk factor for intracranial haemorrhage after stroke.

96. A 10-year-old boy presents with fever and eosinophilia. MRI of the head shows thickening of the infundibular stalk and a markedly enhancing mass in the superior aspect of the stalk. There is also enhancement in the sella extending along the left petrous temporal bone with poorly defined borders. The features are consistent with

A. Meningioma

B. Petrous apicitis

C. Histiocytosis X

    D. Craniopharyngioma

    E. Neuroblastoma metastasis

97. Follow-up CT chest done on a 71-year-old man with previous history of malignancy shows a mass lesion in the heart. It is new compared to previous CT scans and is determined to represent a metastatic deposit. Which of the following types of malignancy is most likely to be the primary in this case?

    A. Colonic

    B. Oesophageal

    C. Bronchogenic

    D. Renal cell

    E. Astrocytoma

98. A 30-year-old weightlifter presents with swelling in the right groin. Which of the following is false?

A.	Direct inguinal hernia	The hernial sac lies lateral to the inferior epigastric artery and above the pubic tubercle.
B.	Femoral hernia	The hernial sac lies medial and adjacent to the femoral vessels.
C.	Indirect inguinal hernia	The hernial sac lies lateral to the inferior epigastric artery and superior to the inguinal ligament.
D.	Obturator hernia	The hernial sac lies between the obturator externus and internus.
E.	Spigelian hernia	The hernial sac lies between the rectus abdominis medially and the semilunar line laterally.

99. A 43-year-old man has recently had a renal transplantation. All of the following are true regarding investigation of transplanted kidney, except

    A. ATN (acute tubular necrosis) is depicted by normal perfusion and reduced excretion.

    B. Normal perfusion and reduced excretion is non-specific.

    C. Reduced diastolic flow is specific for acute rejection.

    D. During acute rejection, T1W of renal cortex increases.

    E. Renal vein thrombosis causes characteristic waveform changes.

100. What is a role of ultrasound in the evaluation of a skier's thumb injury?

    A. To evaluate for the presence of a joint effusion

    B. To assess joint mobility on dynamic ultrasound

    C. To look for an Andersson lesion

    D. To look for a Stener lesion

    E. To look for associated extensor pollicis tenosynovitis

101. A 76-year-old woman with a recent episode of right-arm weakness is being followed up with an MRI a week after her presentation to the A&E department. The current MRI shows changes on T1W images, which were identified as cortical laminar necrosis at the stroke meeting. Which of the following statements regarding cortical laminar necrosis is false?

    A. Laminar necrosis is seen as serpiginous high signal on T1W MRI.

    B. It is thought to be due to lipid-laden macrophages.

    C. It can be seen 3–5 days after stroke.

    D. It is never seen beyond 2 weeks.

    E. SWI helps differentiate from haemorrhagic transformation.

102. Regarding Chiari II malformations, which of the following is true?

    A. Supratentorial abnormalities are uncommon.

    B. The tentorial attachment is usually normal.

    C. It is nearly always associated with failure of neural tube closure.

D. The severity of hydrocephalus nearly always improves after repair of the meningocoele.

E. Batwing appearance of the occipital horns.

103. A 42-year-old man presents with a high-grade fever, splenomegaly and abdominal pain. CT chest and abdomen done to look for a source of sepsis show multiple small cavitating lesions in both lungs with areas of hypo-attenuation in the spleen and kidneys. Which of the following is the most likely diagnosis?

A. Sarcoidosis

B. Carcinoid heart disease

C. Amyloidosis

D. Infective endocarditis

E. Rheumatic heart disease

104. A 50-year-old woman has a CT abdomen and pelvis for non-specific abdominal pain. The scan shows a 7-cm low-density lesion in segment VII of the liver with heterogeneous enhancement in arterial and portal venous phase. An MRI liver is performed for further characterisation and shows a large lobulated mass with low signal on T1W and intermediate to high signal on T2W. On the dynamic post-contrast T1 scans, it shows enhancement in the arterial phase with a non-enhancing central scar, which later enhances in the delayed phase. What is the most likely diagnosis?

A. Focal nodular hyperplasia

B. Fibrolamellar HCC

C. Adenoma

D. Haemangioma

E. Hepatocellular carcinoma

105. A 42-year-old woman is referred to the breast clinic and is due an ultrasound scan to evaluate a suspected lump in the breast. All of the following are ultrasonographic features of a benign breast mass, except

A. Feeding central vessel on Doppler imaging

B. Well-defined smooth margins

C. Three or fewer lobulations

D. Circumferential blood flow pattern on Doppler imaging

E. Uniform hyperechogenicity

106. A 6-year-old girl presents to her family doctor with fever and pain in the lower left leg. Blood tests reveal leucocytosis and anaemia. Plain X-ray of the leg shows a destructive lesion involving the fibular shaft with lamellated onion skin periosteal reaction, cortical destruction and large soft-tissue mass. What is the likely diagnosis?

A. Osteosarcoma

B. Ewing's sarcoma

C. Chondroblastoma

D. Chondromyxoid fibroma

E. Osteoid osteoma

107. A 67-year-old man with a history of head and neck cancer presents with acute stroke symptoms, and MRI is performed. SWI images show several tiny microbleeds in the basal ganglia at 48 hours. All of the following are true regarding haemorrhagic transformation in stroke, except

A. Microbleeds have worse prognosis than haematoma.

B. Fewer than five microbleeds does not contraindicate thrombolysis.

C. Parenchymal haemorrhage is common in the basal ganglia.

D. Haemorrhagic transformation is rare in the first 6 hours.

E. Parenchymal haemorrhages are rarer than microbleeds.

108. The following are diagnosed prenatally on ultrasound examination or MRI, except
    A. Pulmonary interstitial emphysema
    B. Bronchial atresia
    C. Pulmonary sequestration
    D. Congenital pulmonary airway obstruction
    E. Congenital diaphragmatic hernia

109. All of the following are causes of a right-sided cardiac thrombus, except
    A. DVT
    B. Behcet's syndrome
    C. Loffler syndrome
    D. Infective endocarditis
    E. Sarcoidosis

110. A 40-year-old woman with a known history of connective tissue disease presents to her gastroenterologist with non-specific upper abdominal pain and weight loss. She is referred for a barium follow-through, which shows that the small bowel folds are of normal morphology but distended and closely spaced together with delayed emptying of barium into the large bowel. There are also a number of jejunal diverticula. She had an X-ray of her left hand a few weeks earlier, which showed resorption of the distal tufts of her phalanges.
    What is the most likely unifying diagnosis?
    A. Hyperparathyroidism
    B. Whipple's disease
    C. Scleroderma
    D. Amyloidosis
    E. Coeliac disease

111. A 42-year-old woman is referred to the breast clinic and is due an ultrasound scan to evaluate a suspected lump in the breast. All of the following are ultrasonographic characteristics of breast malignancy, except
    A. Perpendicular radiating spiculations
    B. Anechoic mass
    C. Irregular margins of a mass
    D. Mass that is taller than it is wide
    E. Posterior acoustic shadow from a solid mass

112. A 70-year-old man with a history of a scaphoid fracture several years ago is referred to the orthopaedic clinic for increasing wrist pain. A plain X-ray is ordered to check for developing OA and assess the mid-carpal joints. Measurements based on the true lateral view reveal the capitolunate angle is >30° and the scapholunate angle is >80°. What is your diagnosis?
    A. Volar intercalated segment instability (VISI)
    B. Dorsal intercalated segment instability (DISI)
    C. Refracture of scaphoid
    D. Perilunate dislocation
    E. Scapholunate advanced collapse (SLAC) deformity

113. A 49-year-old woman with right lower extremity weakness and rigidity undergoes MRI with DWI, ADC map, FLAIR, T2W and T1W pre- and post-gadolinium images. Early hyperacute stroke is diagnosed. All of the following are true about the timing of stroke and MRI, except
    A. Low ADC signal suggests that the stroke is less than a week old.
    B. FLAIR hyperintensities are seen in 6–12 hours.

C. High signal on T2W MRI is seen >8 hours.

   D. Low signal on T1W MRI is seen >8 hours.

   E. Parenchymal enhancement generally doesn't persist beyond 8–12 weeks.

114. A neonate has an umbilical venous catheter inserted. On an abdominal X-ray, it has advanced up to the level of T10 at the midline. In which structure is the tip of the catheter?
   A. Left portal vein
   B. Right portal vein
   C. Ductus venosus
   D. Superior mesenteric vein
   E. Splenic vein

115. Which of the following statements concerning malignant cardiac masses is false?
   A. Cardiac metastasis outnumbers primary cardiac malignancy.
   B. Angiosarcomas have a high T1 signal due to methaemoglobin.
   C. Undifferentiated sarcomas mostly affect the left atrium.
   D. Primary cardiac lymphomas mostly affect the left side of the heart.
   E. Rhabdomyosarcoma commonly affects the valve.

116. A 30-year-old cab driver presents to his GP with malaise, jaundice and abdominal distension. Blood tests performed show deranged liver function tests. A provisional diagnosis of Budd–Chiari syndrome was made. All of the following are imaging features of Budd–Chiari syndrome, except
   A. Ultrasound demonstrates portal vein enlargement and change in flow dynamics.
   B. In acute Budd–Chiari, the liver is globally enlarged, with lower attenuation on CT.
   C. There is caudate lobe atrophy in chronic Budd–Chiari.
   D. CT shows non-homogenous liver enhancement with a predominantly central area of enhancement and delayed enhancement of the periphery.
   E. On MRI, the liver is low signal on unenhanced T1 and T2 and delayed enhancement post-contrast.

117. All of the following are major indications for ultrasound of the breast, except
   A. Delineation of cystic from solid breast masses
   B. Evaluation of a palpable breast mass in a mammographically dense breast
   C. Evaluation of nipple discharge in a mammographically dense breast
   D. Evaluation of breast lesions not well seen on mammography
   E. Routine breast screening

118. A 19-year-old man is reviewed at a clinic for a persistent ache in his lower back that has not improved for over 3 months. He is an avid mountain biker, but there is no history of significant trauma and there are no neurological deficits. The patient is found to have mild increase in thoracic kyphosis with mild wedging of the T4, T5 and T6 vertebrae. MRI reveals the presence of small scattered vertebral end plate lesions with signal characteristics identical to the adjacent intervertebral discs in several thoracic and lumbar vertebrae. What is the diagnosis?
   A. Spondylodiscitis with developing vertebral collapse
   B. Congenital kyphosis
   C. Metastatic deposits with early vertebral collapse
   D. Vertebral insufficiency fractures
   E. Scheuermann's disease

119. A 76-year-old man with known cerebral atrophy and dementia has been unsteady on his feet for the last 2–3 weeks following a fall down a flight of three steps. There is a small external cut

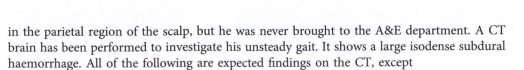

in the parietal region of the scalp, but he was never brought to the A&E department. A CT brain has been performed to investigate his unsteady gait. It shows a large isodense subdural haemorrhage. All of the following are expected findings on the CT, except

A. Fourth ventricle enlargement
B. Lateral ventricle compression
C. Effacement of the cortical sulci
D. Midline shift
E. White matter buckling

120. A 1-year-old boy is brought to the A&E department by his parents with head injury after falling off a sofa. The on-call paediatrician strongly suspects non-accidental injury. Which of the following features on unenhanced CT is most consistent with this?

A. Bilateral occipital extradural haemorrhage
B. Bilateral occipital subdural haemorrhage
C. Subarachnoid haemorrhage
D. Parietal skull fracture
E. Bilateral frontal subdural haemorrhage

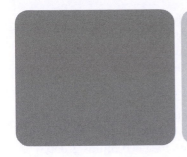

1. C. Ductus diverticulum

Ductus diverticulum is a focal bulge at the anteromedial aspect of the aortic isthmus, visualised in 9% of adults. It is critical to identify this normal variant and distinguish it from a post-traumatic false aneurysm, which also occurs most commonly at the aortic isthmus (88%). The classic ductus diverticulum has smooth, uninterrupted margins and gently sloping symmetric shoulders; in contrast, false aneurysms have a variety of shapes and sizes with sharp margins and often contain linear defects. Compared with the classic ductus diverticulum, the atypical ductus diverticulum has a shorter and steeper slope superiorly and a more classic gentle slope inferiorly. However, both shoulders have smooth, uninterrupted margins, an important feature that distinguishes this variant from true injury.

Other normal variants that can mimic injury include aortic spindle, which is a smooth circumferential bulge immediately distal to the aortic isthmus; infundibulum at the origin of aortic branches like the brachiocephalic and intercostal arteries, which are spherical or conical in shape but have a vessel at its apex, thereby differentiating them from false aneurysms.

Fisher RG, et al. 'Lumps' and 'bumps' that mimic acute aortic and brachiocephalic vessel injury. *Radiographics*. 1997;17(4):825–34.

2. A. Candida oesophagitis

Candida oesophagitis occurs in patients whose normal flora is altered by broad spectrum antibiotic therapy and in patients whose immune systems are suppressed by malignancy, immunosuppressive agents like chemotherapy and radiotherapy, and immunodeficiency states such as AIDS.

When the disease is superficial, the oesophageal mucosa may appear normal radiographically.

Early in the course of Candida oesophagitis, mucosal plaques are the most frequent finding. Later erosions and ulcerations may develop, which together with intramural haemorrhage and necrosis result in the 'shaggy' margin seen on esophagograms.

Roberts L Jr, et al. Adult oesophageal candidiasis: A radiographic spectrum. *Radiographics*. 1987;7(2):289–307.

3. D. Type 3

Type 3 cysts have thickened irregular/smooth walls or septa in which measurable enhancement is present. These need surgery in most cases, as neoplasm cannot be excluded. They include complicated haemorrhagic/infected cysts, multilocular cystic nephroma and cystic neoplasms.

Type 2F (F denotes follow-up) cysts may contain multiple hairline-thin septa. Perceived (not measurable) enhancement of a hairline smooth septum or wall can be identified, and there may be minimal thickening of the wall or septa, which may contain calcification that may be thick and nodular. There are no enhancing soft-tissue components; totally intrarenal non-enhancing high-attenuation renal lesions (>3 cm) are also included in this category. These lesions are generally well marginated and are thought to be benign but need follow-up.

Type 1 is a benign simple water attenuation cyst with a hairline-thin wall that does not contain septa, calcifications, or solid components and does not enhance.

Type 2 is a benign cystic lesion that may contain a few hairline septa in which perceived (not measurable) enhancement might be appreciated; fine calcification or a short segment of slightly thickened calcification may be present in the wall or septa. Uniformly high-attenuation lesions (<3 cm) that are sharply marginated and do not enhance are included in this group. No intervention is needed.

Type 4 are clearly malignant cystic masses that can have all of the criteria of Type 3 but also contain distinct enhancing soft-tissue components independent of the wall or septa; these masses need to be removed.

Israel GM, Bosniak MA. How I do it: Evaluating renal masses. *Radiology*. 2005;236:441–50.

4. C. Achondroplasia

Spinal stenosis from congenital short pedicles along with reducing interpedicular distance towards the lumbar spine is a classic finding of achondroplasia. Other associated findings include the 'champagne glass pelvis', bullet-shaped vertebra (cf. central vertebral beaking in Morquio syndrome and inferior vertebral beaking in Hurler's and Hunter's syndromes), trident hand and craniocervical stenosis from a small foramen magnum.

Platyspondyly, loss of vertebral height, specially affecting lumbar vertebra by 2–3 years of age, is a typical feature of Morquio syndrome (cf. vertebral height is normal in Hurler's syndrome).

Dähnert W. *Radiology Review Manual*, 6th edn. Philadelphia, PA: Lippincott Williams & Wilkins, 2007:122–4.
Weissleder R, et al. *Primer of Diagnostic Imaging*, 5th edn. St. Louis, MO: Elsevier Mosby, 2011:618.

5. D. Gradient echo

Cerebral microbleeds are increasingly recognised neuroimaging findings, occurring with cerebrovascular disease, dementia, hypertensive vasculopathy, cerebral amyloid angiopathy and normal ageing. Recent years have seen substantial progress in developing newer MRI methodologies for microbleed detection.

Hemosiderin deposits in microbleeds are super-paramagnetic and thus have considerable internal magnetisation when brought into the magnetic field of MRI, a property defined as *magnetic susceptibility*. Among available pulse sequences, T2*-weighted GRE MRI is most sensitive to the susceptibility effect.

Greenberg SM, et al. Cerebral microbleeds: A field guide to their detection and interpretation. *Lancet Neurol.* 2009;8(2):165–74.

6. A. Anomalous anconeus epitrochlearis muscle results in PIN entrapment

Cubital tunnel syndrome is the most common entrapment neuropathy of the elbow. It is seen in throwing sports, tennis and volleyball. Traction injuries to the ulnar nerve can occur secondary to the dynamic valgus forces. Compression of the ulnar nerve within the cubital tunnel occur secondary to direct trauma, repetitive stresses, or replacement of the overlying retinaculum with an anomalous anconeus epitrochlearis muscle. Recurrent subluxation of the nerve due to acquired laxity from repetitive stress or trauma can lead to friction neuritis. Finally, osseous spurring within the ulnar groove caused by overuse and posteromedial impingement in throwers can cause nerve irritation. Ulnar nerve thickening and increased T2-weighted signal are typical MRI features. Oedema-like signal changes or atrophy of the flexor carpi ulnaris and flexor digitorum profundus muscles may also be secondary to ulnar neuropathy.

Radial nerve entrapment at the elbow can be subdivided into two major categories: radial tunnel syndrome and posterior interosseous nerve syndrome. The posterior interosseous nerve is a deep branch of the radial nerve in the forearm that can be compressed from repetitive gripping combined with supination in weightlifters and swimmers. The superficial head of the supinator muscle along the arcade of Frohse is the most common site of nerve entrapment. It is important to note that a small percentage of radial neuropathy cases can be associated with tennis elbow. MRI manifestations of PIN includes thickening and increased T2-weighted signal of the nerve fibres, as well as oedema-like signal changes in the innervated extensor compartment musculature in the acute and subacute setting and atrophy in the chronic stages.

O'Dell MC, et al. Imaging sports-related elbow injuries. *Appl Radiol.* 2015;44(3):7–15.

7. A. Hypertrophic obstructive cardiomyopathy

Hypertrophic cardiomyopathy (HCM) is defined as a diffuse or segmental left-ventricular hypertrophy with a non-dilated and hyperdynamic chamber, in the absence of another cardiac or systemic disease explaining the degree of cardiac muscle hypertrophy. Dyspnoea on exertion is the most common symptom because the key functional hallmark of hypertrophic cardiomyopathy is an impaired diastolic function with impaired LV filling in the presence of preserved systolic function. Systolic dysfunction occurs at end-stage disease.

Asymmetric involvement of the interventricular septum is the most common form of the disease, accounting for an estimated 60%–70% of the cases of HCM. Other variants include apical, symmetric, midventricular, mass-like and non-contiguous

HCM is typically associated with hypertrophy of the muscle to 15 mm or thicker and a ratio of thickened myocardium to normal left-ventricular basal myocardium of 1.3–1.5. With MRI and multidetector computed tomography (CT), apical HCM has a characteristic spadelike configuration of the LV cavity at end diastole, appreciated on vertical long-axis views.

Chun EJ, et al. Hypertrophic cardiomyopathy: Assessment with MR imaging and multidetector CT. *Radiographics.* 2010;30(5):1309–28.
O'Donnell DH, et al. Cardiac MRI of non-ischemic cardiomyopathies: Imaging protocols and spectra of appearances. *Radiology.* 2012;262(2):403–22.

8. B. Pseudodiverticulosis

Oesophageal intramural pseudodiverticulosis is a condition of unknown cause characterised by flask-shaped outpouchings of the mucosa that extend into the muscular layer and show characteristic findings on oesophagograms. They are dilated excretory ducts of deep oesophageal mucous glands resulting from obstruction of excretory ducts by plugs of viscous mucus and desquamated cells or by extrinsic compression of the ducts by periductal inflammatory infiltrates and fibrotic tissue.

It occurs in all age groups predominantly in the sixth and seventh decades with slight male preponderance. It has been reported as a separate entity or in association with diseases such as diabetes, peptic strictures and oesophagitis.

Plavsic BM, et al. Intramural pseudodiverticulosis of the esophagus detected on barium esophagograms: Increased prevalence in patients with esophageal carcinoma. *AJR Am J Roentgenol.* 1995;165:1381–5.

9. C. Endometriosis

Endometriosis is a common multifocal gynaecologic disease that manifests during the reproductive years, often causing chronic pelvic pain and infertility. The ovaries are among the most common sites (20%–40% of cases). It manifests either as superficial fibrotic implants or as chronic retention cysts with cyclic bleeding (endometriomas). Endometriomas are thick-walled cysts with a dark, dense content that represents degenerated blood products. The cysts may be solitary or multiple, and they are bilateral in 50% of cases. Endometriomas may include peripheral nodules (blood clots) or fluid–fluid levels; in the latter, the non-dependent portion represents the freshest bleeding. A multilocular-appearing endometrioma may consist of multiple contiguous cysts. Endometriomas are a marker of severity of deeply infiltrating endometriosis. On MRIs, cystic cavities can appear as simple fluid, with high signal intensity on T2-weighted and low signal intensity on T1-weighted images. They also may show high signal intensity on T1-weighted and T1-weighted fat-saturated images because of their haemorrhagic content.

The shading sign, a common and unique feature of endometriomas, represents old blood products, which contain extremely high iron and protein concentrations. These haemorrhagic cysts typically show high signal intensity on T1-weighted images and low signal intensity on T2-weighted images. However, endometriomas also may show variable signal intensity on T2-weighted images.

Chamié LP, et al. Findings of pelvic endometriosis at transvaginal US, MR imaging, and laparoscopy. *Radiographics*. 2011;31(4):E77–100.

10. C. MRI pituitary pre- and post-contrast

The clinical history along with the radiographic findings points towards acromegaly, and in this case evaluating the pituitary gland for the presence of an adenoma along with correlating biochemistry blood profile would be appropriate investigations.

Osseous enlargement of the vertebrae with increased AP diameter can occur with premature loss of disc space. Expansion of the terminal phalangeal tufts and metacarpals contribute to the clinical finding of 'spadelike hands'. Other features include increased heel pad thickness >25 mm, premature OA, posterior vertebral scalloping, prognathism (elongated mandible), sellar enlargement and enlarged paranasal sinuses, mostly frontal sinus. In the case of pituitary macro adenomas, compression of the optic chiasm can often result in visual field defects.

Brower AC, Fleming DJ. *Arthritis in Black and White*, 3rd edn. Philadelphia PA: Elsiever Saunders, 1997:161.
Dähnert W. *Radiology Review Manual*, 6th edn. Philadelphia, PA: Lippincott Williams & Wilkins, 2007:43–4.

11. D. Non-communicating hydrocephalus

Cerebral amyloid angiopathy (CAA) is an important cause of spontaneous cortical–subcortical intracranial haemorrhage (ICH) in the normotensive elderly. On imaging, multiple cortical–subcortical haematomas are recognised. Prominence of the ventricular system and enlargement of the sulci representing generalised cerebral and cerebellar atrophy are non-specific imaging findings. CAA should be considered in the broad differential diagnosis of leukoencephalopathy (high signal intensity of white matter at T2-weighted MRI), especially if associated with cortical–subcortical haemorrhage or progressive dementia. Leukoencephalopathy may or may not spare U-fibres.

Chao CP, et al. Cerebral amyloid angiopathy: CT and MR imaging findings. *Radiographics*. 2006;26 (5):1517–31.

12. C. Simple bone cyst

SBC affects the young, aged 3–19 years, during the active phase of bone growth and has a slight male preponderance (M:F = 3:1). They are asymptomatic, unless fractured. They are commonly seen in the proximal femur or proximal humerus. They are solitary intramedullary lesions, centred at the metaphyses, adjacent to the epiphyseal cartilage (during the active phase) and migrating into diaphysis with growth (during the latent phase). They do not cross the epiphyseal plate. On a radiograph, they appear as an oval radiolucency with a long axis parallel to the long axis of the host bone, a fine sclerotic boundary and scalloping of the internal aspect of the underlying cortex. SBC appears as a photopenic area on a bone scan (if not fractured). Classic 'fallen fragment' sign if fractured (20%); centrally dislodged fragment falls into a dependent position.

Dähnert W. *Radiology Review Manual*, 7th edn. Philadelphia, PA: Lippincott Williams & Wilkins, 2011.

13. E. Ménétrier's disease

The hallmark of Ménétrier's disease is gastric mucosal hypertrophy, which may cause the rugae to resemble convolutions of the brain. The thickening of the rugae is predominantly caused by expansion of the epithelial cell compartment of the gastric mucosa. Patients with Ménétrier's disease most often present with epigastric pain and hypoalbuminemia secondary to a loss of albumin into the gastric lumen. Signs and symptoms of Ménétrier's disease include anorexia, asthenia, weight loss, nausea, gastrointestinal bleeding, diarrhoea, oedema and vomiting.

The disease has a bimodal age distribution. The childhood form is often linked to cytomegalovirus infection and usually resolves spontaneously. It usually occurs in children younger than 10 years (mean age 5.5 years), predominantly in boys (male-to-female ratio 3:1). The second peak occurs in adulthood, and the disease in adults tends to progress over time. The average age at diagnosis is 55, and men are affected more often than women.

A diagnosis of Ménétrier's disease is made by using a combination of upper gastrointestinal fluoroscopic imaging, endoscopic imaging and histologic analysis. On fluoroscopic images, Ménétrier's disease is characterised by the presence of giant rugal folds. Rugal folds should normally measure less than 1 cm in width across the fundus and 0.5 cm across the antrum, and they should be parallel to the long axis of the stomach.

Freidman J, et al. Best cases from the AFIP Ménétrier disease. *RadioGraphics*. 2009;29:297–301.

14. B. Thickening of the entire LV wall measuring 17 mm at end diastole

HCM should be differentiated from other causes of symmetric increased thickness of the LV wall, including athlete's heart, amyloidosis, sarcoidosis, Fabry disease and adaptive LV hypertrophy due to hypertension or aortic stenosis.

HCM is associated with hypertrophy of the muscle to 15 mm or thicker. In cardiac amyloidosis, the amyloid protein is deposited in the myocardium, which leads to diastolic dysfunction and restrictive cardiomyopathy. Because amyloidosis is a systemic process, involvement of all four chambers is common; thus, an increase in the thickness of the interatrial septum and right atrial free wall by more than 6 mm is seen. Dynamic enhanced MRI shows late enhancement over the entire subendocardial circumference.

Sarcoidosis is a non-caseating granulomatous disease that infiltrates any area of the body, but most of the morbidity/mortality is from involvement of the heart. MRI shows nodular or patchy increased signal intensity on both T2-weighted and enhanced images, which often involves the septum (more particularly, the basal portion) and the LV wall, whereas papillary and right-ventricular infiltration are rarely seen.

Fabry disease is a rare X-linked autosomal recessive metabolic storage disorder. At MRI, the LV wall is seen to be concentrically thickened, and delayed hyperenhancement is typically seen mid-wall and has been reported in the basal inferolateral segment.

Differentiation between compensatory hypertrophy and HCM is sometimes difficult. In comparison to HCM, patients with compensatory hypertrophy usually have normal systolic function, rather than hyperdynamic systolic function in HCM, and their LV wall rarely exceeds 15 mm in maximal thickness.

Athlete's heart can show increased LV wall thickness but end diastolic volume and ejection fraction are normal. Another feature of the cardiac remodelling in athletes is the lack of areas of delayed hyperenhancement within the LV myocardium at dynamic enhanced MRI.

Chun EJ, et al. Hypertrophic cardiomyopathy: Assessment with MR imaging and multidetector CT. *Radiographics*. 2010;30(5):1309–28.

15. C. Flame-shaped contrast seen in the perivesical fat

Sandler described five types of bladder injuries with conventional cystography.

Type 1: Contusion: Bladder contusion is defined as an incomplete or partial tear of the bladder mucosa. Findings at conventional and CT cystography are normal.

Type 2: Intraperitoneal rupture: CT cystography demonstrates intraperitoneal contrast material around bowel loops, between mesenteric folds and in the paracolic gutters.

Type 3: Interstitial injury: Interstitial bladder injury is rare. CT cystography may demonstrate intramural contrast material without extravasation.

Type 4: Extraperitoneal rupture: Extraperitoneal rupture is the most common type of bladder injury (80%–90% of cases) Extravasation is confined to the perivesical space in simple ruptures (Type 4a), whereas in complex ruptures, contrast extends beyond the perivesical space (Type 4b) and may dissect into thigh, perineum and properitoneal fat planes.

Type 5: Combined rupture: CT cystography usually demonstrates extravasation patterns that are typical for both types of injury.

Vaccaro JP, Brody JM. CT cystography in the evaluation of major bladder trauma. *Radiographics.* 2000;20(5):1373–81.

16. A. Amyloid arthropathy

Amyloid arthropathy most typically affects the shoulders, carpal bones and hips in a bilateral fashion. It is typically associated with long-term renal dialysis, which results in deposition of the beta-2 microglobulin. Affected joints demonstrate subchondral cystic lesions with juxta-articular swelling. The presence of low-to-intermediate signal soft tissue within and around the joint clinches the diagnosis, as this represents the signal characteristics of the deposited proteins (cf. other inflammatory/infectious arthropathies, which tend to produce higher water content than soft-tissue changes in the joint). Joint space is also typically preserved until the late stages of disease, similar to gout.

Dähnert W. *Radiology Review Manual*, 6th edn. Philadelphia, PA: Lippincott Williams & Wilkins, 2007:45.

Kiss E, et al. Dialysis-related amyloidosis revisited. *AJR Am J Roentgenol.* 2005;185:1460–7.

17. B. 'Black hole' appearance

MS lesions can occur anywhere in the central nervous system but are most common in the periventricular white matter. Typical lesions are ovoid, with the long axis perpendicular to the ventricles. They are better seen on PD and FLAIR than on T2-weighted images because of increased lesion–CSF contrast. Lesions of the corpus callosum, at callososeptal interface and subcallosal striations are characteristic. FLAIR is less sensitive than T2-weighted images to infratentorial lesions occurring in the brain stem and middle cerebellar peduncles. In the acute phase, lesions show increase in size and solid or ring enhancement with IV contrast, which can persist up to 3 months, but generally resolve in weeks. Large acute lesions, with associated oedema, mass effect and incomplete ring enhancement can mimic glioma (tumefactive MS).

MS lesions show reduced magnetisation transfer ratio (MTR), reflecting decreased myelin content. MTR is also reduced in normal-looking white matter, representing occult tissue damage. Such occult tissue damage is also detected by diffusion tensor imaging, showing reduced fractional anisotropy. Low-signal lesions on T1-weighted MRI (black holes), brain and spinal cord atrophy are seen in established MS.

Adam A, et al. *Grainger & Allison's Diagnostic Radiology: A Textbook of Medical Imaging*, 5th edn. New York: Churchill Livingstone, 2008:1337.

18. D. Frog-leg lateral of the hips

Diagnosis of SUFE (slipped upper femoral epiphysis) is made using anteroposterior (AP) pelvis and lateral frog-leg radiographs. CT is rarely needed, although it is very sensitive. MRI depicts the slippage earliest, and MRI can demonstrate early marrow oedema and slippage. It is also useful in identifying pre-slip changes in the opposite hip and shows differentials, for example, infection, tumour, synovitis and so on.

Although some institutions obtain a frog-leg lateral view, it is possible to further displace an acute or acute-on-chronic slip when the hips are placed in this position. Thus some institutions avoid them unless the request comes from an orthopaedic surgeon.

Phraseology is important in all investigation-related questions; while the next investigation is frog-leg lateral in several/most places, the best investigation or the most appropriate examination would be MRI because it will provide the most information and cover all differentials.

Boles CA, el-Khoury GY. Slipped capital femoral epiphysis. *Radiographics*. 1997;17(4):809–23.

Jarrett DY, et al. Imaging SCFE: Diagnosis, treatment and complications. *Pediatr Radiol*. 2013;43(Suppl 1): S71–82.

19. B. ASD – Atrial Septal Defect

	LA	LV	RA	RV
VSD	✓	✓		✓
Uncomplicated ASD			✓	✓
ASD with shunt reversal (Eisenmenger syndrome)	✓		✓	✓
Mitral valve disease	✓	✓		
Tricuspid valve disease			✓	✓
Pulmonary hypertension			✓	✓
PDA	✓	✓		✓

Adam A, et al. *Grainger & Allison's Diagnostic Radiology: A Textbook of Medical Imaging*, 5th edn. New York: Churchill Livingstone, 2008:427–9.

20. B. Carman meniscus sign

The Carman meniscus sign is a curvilinear lens-shaped intraluminal form of crater with convexity of crescent towards the gastric wall and concavity towards the gastric lumen.

Gastric ulcer		
Sign	Benign	Malignant
Crater	Round, ovoid	Irregular
Radiating folds	Symmetric	Nodular, clubbed, fused
Areae gastricae	Preserved	Destroyed
Projection	Outside lumen	Inside lumen
Ulcer mound	Smooth	Rolled edge

Dahnert W. *Radiology Review Manual*. 5th edn. Philadelphia, PA: Lippincott Williams & Wilkins, 2003: 826–7.

21. B. Low on T1   Low on T2

On T1-weighted MRI, the normal prostate gland demonstrates homogeneous intermediate to low signal intensity. T1-weighted MRI has insufficient soft-tissue contrast resolution for visualising the intraprostatic anatomy or abnormality. The zonal anatomy of the prostate gland is best depicted on high-resolution T2-weighted images. Prostate has a homogenous low-signal background on T1-weighted images. On T2-weighted images, prostate cancer usually demonstrates low signal intensity in contrast to the high signal intensity of the normal peripheral zone. Low signal intensity in the peripheral zone, however, can also be seen in several benign conditions, such as haemorrhage, prostatitis, hyperplastic nodules, or post-treatment sequelae (e.g., as a result of irradiation or hormonal treatment).

Claus FG, et al. Pretreatment evaluation of prostate cancer: Role of MRI and 1H MR spectroscopy. *Radiographics*. 2004;24(Suppl 1):S167–80.

22. B. Aneurysmal bone cyst

Aneurysmal bone cysts or ABCs are most commonly seen between the first and third decades of life. They are typically a metaphyseal lesion and are often located in the humerus, femur, or tibia. The presence of fluid–fluid levels along with bone expansion, a narrow zone of transition and metaphyseal location in a long bone is characteristic. Note that fluid–fluid levels can also be found in giant cell tumours, telangiectatic osteosarcomas and simple bone cysts, but the other associated locations and characteristics of the lesion would tend to be different from an ABC. Eosinophilic granulomas are associated with Langerhans cell histiocytosis. Enchondromas are typically located in the small long bones of the hands and in the proximal humerus and femur with non-expansile characteristics. Fluid–fluid levels are not typically associated with fibrous dysplasia, which takes on the commonly described 'ground glass' appearance.

Manaster BJ, et al. *Musculoskeletal Imaging: The Requisites*, 4th edn. Philadelphia, PA: Mosby Elsevier, 2013:449–50.

23. A. Intra-orbital

Typically, findings of optic neuritis in MS are seen in the retrobulbar intra-orbital segment of the optic nerve, which appears swollen, with high T2 signal. High T2 signal persists and may be permanent; chronically the nerve will appear atrophied rather than swollen. Contrast enhancement of the nerve is best seen with fat-suppressed T1-weighted coronal images, in >90% of patients if scanned within 20 days of visual loss.

Kupersmith MJ, et al. Contrast-enhanced MRI in acute optic neuritis: Relationship to visual performance. *Brain*. 2002;125(4):812–22.

24. C. L2 to L3

The conus normally lies at or above the L2 disc space. A normal conus located at the mid-L3 level may be identified, especially in preterm infants; this position is considered the lower limits of normal but is usually without clinical consequence. However, in a preterm infant with a conus that terminates at the L3 mid-vertebral body, a follow-up sonogram can be obtained once the infant attains a corrected age between 40 weeks' gestation and 6 months of age. In contrast, the thecal sac terminates at S2.

In the preterm group, more than 90% of conus medullaris cases lie above L2; in the term group, more than 92% lie above L2.

Kesler H, et al. Termination of the normal conus medullaris in children: A whole-spine magnetic resonance imaging study. *Neurosurg Focus*. 2007;23(2):E7.
Sahin F, et al. Level of conus medullaris in term and preterm neonates. *Arch Dis Child Fetal Neonatal Ed*. 1997;77(1):F67–9.

25. C. CTPA with portal phase images covering the liver

Hereditary haemorrhagic telangiectasia, also called Osler–Weber–Rendu syndrome, is an uncommon genetic disorder characterised by arteriovenous malformations in the skin, mucous membranes and visceral organs. The brain, gastrointestinal tract, skin, lung and nose are the primary sites affected. It is associated with the classic triad of epistaxis, telangiectasias and a family history.

Pulmonary AVMs are often discovered initially as a solitary pulmonary nodule or mass on plain chest films. If a pulmonary AVM is suspected, further imaging evaluation should be CT or conventional pulmonary angiography. Although conventional angiography is the gold standard, considering its invasive nature CT is considered a better method of diagnosis. This is more important when screening for AVM.

Portal venous-phase liver images are often obtained at the same time, in case the lesion does turn out to be a solid nodule.

Poole PS, Ferguson EC. Revisiting pulmonary arteriovenous malformations: Radiographic and CT imaging findings and corresponding treatment options. *Contemp Diagn Radiol*. 2010;33(8):1–5.

26. B. Duodenal diverticulum

Duodenal diverticulosis is a common entity first described by Chomel in 1710. Its prevalence varies depending on the mode of diagnosis. Diverticula are found in 6% of upper gastrointestinal series, 9%–23% of ERCP procedures and 22% of autopsies. Its occurrence has no sex predilection, and the age range for detection varies from 26 to 69 years. Duodenal diverticula may be congenital or acquired, with the latter being more common. Congenital or true diverticula are rare, contain all layers of the duodenal wall, and may be subdivided into intraluminal and extraluminal forms.

The CT appearance of a duodenal diverticulum includes a saccular outpouching, which may resemble a mass-like structure interposed between the duodenum and the pancreas that contains air, an air–fluid level, fluid, contrast material, or debris. A periampullary diverticulum may simulate a pseudocyst or tumour.

Pearl MS, et al. CT findings in duodenal diverticulitis. *AJR Am J Roentgenol*. 2006;187:W392–5.

27. C. Gartner's duct cyst   Posterolateral aspect of the upper vagina

Multiple paraurethral Skene's glands are related to the female urethra. There are paraurethral ducts that drain into the distal urethral lumen. Nabothian cysts are retention cysts in the cervix related to chronic cervicitis. Gartner's duct cysts are found at the anterolateral aspect of the proximal third of the vaginal wall. Bartholin's gland cysts affect the posterolateral aspect of the lower vaginal wall. Urethral diverticulum occurs at the posterolateral aspect of the mid-urethra.

Dähnert W. *Radiology Review Manual*, 7th edn. Philadelphia, PA: Lippincott Williams & Wilkins, 2011:934, 1032, 1062.

28. C. Ankylosing spondylitis (AS)

AS is characterised by the hallmark of bilateral and symmetrical sacroiliac joint involvement, though there may be unilateral involvement in the early stages of disease. Other common findings include periostitis with whiskering of the pelvic bones and the typical 'bamboo' spine appearance from syndesmophyte formation. Up to 10% of AS cases are associated with inflammatory bowel disease, and iritis is common in up to 40% of patients. Ninety-six percent of patients are HLA-B 27 positive, the antigen associated with the other seronegative spondyloarthropathies of psoriasis, Reiter's syndrome and inflammatory bowel disease–associated spondyloarthritis.

Behcet's syndrome affects the chest and gastrointestinal tracts and doesn't involve the skeleton primarily.

Dähnert W. *Radiology Review Manual*, 6th edn. Philadelphia, PA: Lippincott Williams & Wilkins, 2007:46–7.
Rudwaleit M, Baeten D. Ankylosing spondylitis and bowel disease. *Best Pract Res Clin Rheumatol*. 2006;20(3):451–71.

29. C. The pattern of brain atrophy can mimic Alzheimer's disease

The T1 lesion load including enhancing lesions or black holes is correlated more closely than T2 lesion load with clinical outcome. Another imaging hallmark of MS is brain atrophy. Brain atrophy in MS usually appears as enlarged ventricles and reduced size of the corpus callosum. The rate of brain atrophy is higher in MS than in the normal ageing process. Significant loss of white matter rather than grey matter is seen in the early stage of MS, suggesting a different mechanism of atrophy compared to neurodegenerative diseases such as Alzheimer's disease. MS lesions show reduced Magnetisation transfer ratio (MTR), reflecting decreased myelin content. MTR is also reduced in normal-looking white matter, representing occult tissue damage. MS lesions usually have a more reduced MTR as compared with ischaemic lesions in small vessel diseases. Such occult tissue damage is also detected by diffusion tensor imaging, showing reduced fractional anisotropy (representing microstructural damage).

Ge Y. Multiple sclerosis: The role of MR imaging. *AJNR Am J Neuroradiol*. 2006;27(6):1165–76.

30. B. Kawasaki arteritis

Kawasaki disease is a systemic vasculitis that is more severe in small and medium arteries, and veins to a lesser extent, with inflammatory lesions in virtually all organs. It is a leading cause of acquired heart disease in childhood. The aetiology of KD remains unknown, although the clinical presentation – self-limiting illness manifested by an abrupt onset of fever, rash, exanthema, conjunctival injection and cervical adenopathy – and the epidemiological features – a seasonal peak in winter and spring, age distribution and a geographic wave-like spread of illness during epidemics – strongly suggest an infectious cause.

Fever is usually the first sign of KD. Rash is non-specific and mostly maculopapular. Cervical lymphadenopathy is the last common of the main manifestations. Cardiovascular complications include coronary artery aneurysms, myocarditis, pericarditis with pericardial effusion, systemic arterial aneurysms, valvular disease, mild aortic root dilatation and myocardial infarct.

Takayasu arteritis (TA), also known as *pulseless disease*, is a granulomatous large vessel vasculitis that predominantly affects the aorta and its major branches, with increased prevalence in Asian women <50 years of age.

Churg–Strauss syndrome is a small-to-medium vessel necrotising pulmonary vasculitis, affecting patients in the third and fourth decades with asthma, eosinophilia and systemic symptoms like purpura and arthralgia.

Moyamoya disease is an idiopathic, non-inflammatory, non-atherosclerotic, progressive vasculo-occlusive disease involving the circle of Willis, typically the supraclinoid internal carotid arteries. It has a bimodal age distribution, affecting children and adults. In children, ischaemic strokes are most pronounced, whereas in adults haemorrhage from the abnormal vessels is more common.

Dähnert W. *Radiology Review Manual*, 7th edn. Philadelphia, PA: Lippincott Williams & Wilkins, 2011.
Duarte R, et al. Kawasaki disease: A review with emphasis on cardiovascular complications. *Insights Imaging*. 2010;1(4):223–31.

31. C. Systolic dysfunction

In cardiac amyloidosis, the amyloid protein is deposited in the myocardium, which leads to diastolic dysfunction that progresses to restrictive cardiomyopathy. Because amyloidosis is a systemic process, involvement of all four chambers is common; thus, an increase in the thickness of the interatrial septum and right atrial free wall by more than 6 mm has been shown to be a specific finding for cardiac amyloidosis. Through the use of dynamic enhanced cardiac MRI, a distinct pattern of late enhancement, which was distributed over the entire subendocardial circumference, has been shown to have high specificity and sensitivity for cardiac amyloidosis

Echocardiogram shows concentric LV hypertrophy, with hyperechoic granular sparkling of the ventricular wall.

Chun EJ, et al. Hypertrophic cardiomyopathy: Assessment with MR imaging and multidetector CT. *Radiographics*. 2010;30(5):1309–28.

32. C. Main duct IPMN (Intraductal Papillary Mucinous Neoplasm)

IPMNs are a group of neoplasms in the biliary duct or pancreatic duct that causes cystic dilatation from excessive mucin production and accumulation. The true incidence of IPMNs is unknown because many are small and asymptomatic. However, in a series of 2,832 consecutive CT scans of adults with no history of pancreatic lesions, 73 cases of pancreatic cysts (2.6%) were identified. Many of these cases likely were IPMNs, given that IPMNs account for 20%–50% of cystic pancreatic neoplasms. There are three main types of pancreatic IPMNs: main duct, branch duct and combined. A main duct IPMN commonly causes dilatation of the papilla, with bulging of the papilla into the duodenal lumen. Filling defects caused by mural nodules or mucin may be seen at MRCP or ERCP. At CT and MRI, filling defects caused by mural nodules enhance, while filling defects caused by mucin do not enhance.

Nikolaidis P, et al. Imaging features of benign and malignant ampullary and periampullary lesions. *RadioGraphics*. 2014;34:624–41.

33. E. Cystic transformation of rete testis

Cystic transformation of rete testis is a benign condition, also known as *tubular ectasia*, resulting from partial or complete obliteration of the efferent ductules that causes ectasia and, eventually, cystic transformation. The location of the lesion in or adjacent to the mediastinum testis and the presence of epididymal cysts are characteristic. Cystic dysplasia of the rete testis is a rare benign testicular tumour that is found mainly in the paediatric population. Abscesses are usually secondary to epididymo-orchitis; however, they appear cystic with shaggy, irregular walls; intratesticular location; low-level internal echoes; and occasionally hypervascular margins. Teratomas are the most frequent to manifest as cystic masses; however, cystic tumours are rare and, when present, usually have an abnormal rind of parenchyma with increased echogenicity surrounding the cystic lesion.

Dogra VS, et al. Benign intratesticular cystic lesions: US features. *Radiographics*. 2001;21:S273–81.

34. D. Spontaneous osteonecrosis of the knee

Spontaneous osteonecrosis of the knee (SONK) is a rapid and painful condition in elderly patients that ultimately results in subchondral collapse of the weight-bearing portion of the medial femoral condyle. It is often idiopathic but can be associated with minor trauma. It is now also increasingly recognised as a subchondral insufficiency fracture resulting in rapid secondary subchondral collapse. Perthes disease is a childhood disease with avascular necrosis of the femoral head. Sinding–Larsen disease is essentially tendinosis of the proximal origin of the patella tendon. Blount's disease is a growth disorder of the tibia resulting in a 'bow leg' deformity from disturbance to the medial proximal tibial epiphysis. An osteochondral defect is a traumatic injury involving the articular cartilage and adjacent subchondral bone.

Manaster BJ, et al. *Musculoskeletal Imaging: The Requisites*, 4th edn. Philadelphia, PA: Mosby Elsevier, 2013:212–13.

35. A. Cervical segment

MS can show multiple lesions in the spinal cord. Typical spinal cord lesions in MS are relatively small and peripherally located.

They are most often found in the cervical cord and are usually less than two vertebral segments in length.

Bot JC, et al. Spinal cord abnormalities in recently diagnosed MS patients: Added value of spinal MRI examination. *Neurology*. 2004;62:226–33.

36. C. Pyloric canal length of 14 mm

Ultrasound is the modality of choice because of its advantages of directly visualising the pyloric muscle and no ionising radiation. The hypertrophied muscle is hypoechoic, and the central mucosa is hyperechoic. Normal measurements of the pylorus are as follows:

Pyloric muscle thickness (i.e., the diameter of a single muscular wall on a transverse image):
   <3 mm (most accurate)
Length (i.e., longitudinal measurement): <15–17 mm

Pyloric volume: <1.5 cc

Pyloric transverse diameter: <13 mm

Abnormal features on US includes target sign (hypoechoic ring of hypertrophied pyloric muscle around echogenic mucosa centrally on cross section), cervix sign (indentation of muscle mass on fluid-filled antrum on longitudinal section) and antral nipple sign (redundant pyloric channel mucosa protruding into gastric antrum). Other features include increased antral peristalsis and delayed gastric emptying.

Infantile pyloric spasm also shows increased peristalsis and delayed gastric emptying with pyloric muscle thickness between 1.5 and 3 mm.

Dähnert W. *Radiology Review Manual*, 7th edn. Philadelphia, PA: Lippincott Williams & Wilkins, 2011.

37. C. Infundibular stenosis

Tetralogy of Fallot (TOF) is the most common form of cyanotic congenital heart disease. This disease accounts for approximately 10% of all congenital heart defects, affecting men and women equally. In addition, TOF is the most common cyanotic heart disease that survives to adulthood.

The four components of TOF, first described in 1888 by French physician Etienne-Louis Arthur Fallot, are interventricular communication (ventricular septal defect), right-ventricular outflow tract (RVOT) obstruction, concentric right-ventricular hypertrophy (RVH) and deviation of the origin of the aorta to the right.

Combined infundibular and pulmonary valvular stenosis is the second most common cause.

Chang EY, Stark P. Imaging of tetralogy of fallot: A continuum from infancy to adulthood. *Contemp Diagn Radiol.* 2009;32(12):1–6.

38. C. MRI shows good sensitivity for the differential diagnosis of focal chronic pancreatitis from pancreatic carcinoma.

The diagnosis of chronic pancreatitis on MRI is based on signal intensity and enhancement changes as well as on morphologic abnormalities in the pancreatic parenchyma, pancreatic duct and biliary tract. The imaging features of chronic pancreatitis can be divided into early and late findings. Early findings include low-signal-intensity pancreas on T1-weighted fat-suppressed images, decreased and delayed enhancement after IV contrast administration, and dilated side branches. Late findings include parenchymal atrophy or enlargement, pseudocysts, and dilatation and beading of the pancreatic duct often with intraductal calcifications.

Differentiating between an inflammatory mass due to chronic pancreatitis and pancreatic carcinoma on the basis of imaging criteria remains difficult. Decreased T1 signal intensity with delayed enhancement after gadolinium administration as well as dilatation and obstruction of the pancreaticobiliary ducts can be seen in both diseases. Irregularity of the pancreatic duct, intraductal or parenchymal calcifications, diffuse pancreatic involvement, and normal or smoothly stenotic pancreatic duct penetrating through the mass ('duct penetrating sign') favour the diagnosis of chronic pancreatitis over cancer. In distinction, a smoothly dilated pancreatic duct with an abrupt interruption, dilatation of both biliary and pancreatic ducts ('double-duct sign') and obliteration of the perivascular fat planes favour the diagnosis of cancer.

Miller FH, et al. MRI of pancreatitis and its complications: Part 2, Chronic Pancreatitis. *AJR Am J Roentgenol.* 2004;183:1645–1652.

39. C. Urachal adenocarcinoma

Urachal adenocarcinoma is characteristically located at the dome of the bladder in the midline or slightly off midline. Ninety percent of masses occur close to the bladder, with the remainder along the course of the urachus or at the umbilical end. A midline, infra-umbilical, soft-tissue mass with calcification is characteristic and is considered to be urachal adenocarcinoma until proved otherwise. Eighty percent of urachal cancers are adenocarcinoma. At CT, the tumour is mixed solid and cystic in 84% of cases and solid in the remainder. CT is the most sensitive modality for calcification, which is present in 72% of cases and is more commonly peripheral than stippled. On T2-weighted MRI, focal areas of high signal intensity from mucin are highly suggestive of urachal adenocarcinoma. The solid portions of the tumour are isointense to soft tissue on T1-weighted images and enhance with intravenous contrast material.

Wong-you-cheong JJ, et al. From the archives of the AFIP: Neoplasms of the urinary bladder: Radiologic-pathologic correlation. *Radiographics*. 2006;26(2):553–80.

40. E.   Giant bone islands can be locally aggressive

Bone islands are benign entities and represent compact bone within the medullary space. They do not exhibit aggressive features regardless of size. Classically they are sharply defined with thorny radiations (brush border). Then can occasionally show increase or decrease in size (about a third of them) (cf. osteoblastic metastasis, which shows aggressive features, cortical break/destruction, periosteal reaction or soft-tissue component; osteoid osteoma is associated with typical pain and a nidus).

Dähnert W. *Radiology Review Manual*, 6th edn. Philadelphia, PA: Lippincott Williams & Wilkins, 2007:54.

41. C.   Most lesions are centrally located.

Occurrence of spinal cord abnormalities is largely independent of brain lesions in MS. Both focal and disuse lesions affecting the cord are described, though multiple focal lesion (median 3) is the most common finding. Patients with focally involved spinal cords mostly show multiple small lesions. Focal lesions have an elongated configuration along the axis of the spinal cord and affect the peripheral part of the cord. Cervical cord is the most commonly affected segment and the lesions usually extend over fewer than two vertebral segments in length.

Bot JC, et al. Spinal cord abnormalities in recently diagnosed MS patients: Added value of spinal MRI examination. *Neurology*. 2004;62(2):226–33.

42. C.   Hirschprung's disease

Hirschprung's disease, also called *aganglionosis of the colon* (absence of parasympathetic ganglia in muscle and submucosal layers secondary to an arrest of craniocaudal migration of neuroblasts), results in relaxation failure of the aganglionic segment. It affects full-term infants during the first weeks of life, mainly boys. It is extremely rare in premature infants. It usually affects the rectosigmoid junction and results in short-segment disease (80%). Long-segment disease (20%) and total colonic aganglionosis (5%) are less common.

Barium enema shows a 'transition zone' (aganglionic segment), which appears normal in size with dilatation of large and small bowel proximally with marked retention of barium on delayed films after 24 hours. Normal children show a rectosigmoid ratio of >1, as the rectum is larger in diameter than the sigmoid; in the case of Hirschprung's disease, the ratio is reversed (rectosigmoid ratio <1).

Dähnert W. *Radiology Review Manual*, 7th edn. Philadelphia, PA: Lippincott Williams & Wilkins, 2011.

43. A.   Transposition of great vessels (TGA)

A number of associated features can occur in patients with Tetralogy of Falot (TOF). Right sided aortic arch is the most common variant, known as *Corvisart syndrome*. Coronary artery anomalies, such as the left anterior descending artery arising from the right coronary artery (whose course may run directly across the right ventricular outflow tract) can occur. Other associations include patent ductus arteriosus, multiple ventricular septal defects and complete atrioventricular septal defect. Approximately 15% of patients have extracardiac anomalies, including chromosomal abnormalities such as Down's syndrome, DiGeorge syndrome and Alagille syndrome.

Chang EY, Stark P. Imaging of tetralogy of fallot: A continuum from infancy to adulthood. *Contemp Diagn Radiol*. 2009;32(12):1–6.

44. D. Gallbladder adenomyomatosis

Adenomyomatosis is a benign hyperplastic cholecystosis. It is a relatively common condition, identified in at least 5% of cholecystectomy specimens. There is no definite racial or sex predilection. Most diagnoses are made in patients in their fifties, but the age range is wide and case reports exist of paediatric adenomyomatosis. Adenomyomatosis is most often an incidental finding, has no intrinsic malignant potential, and usually requires no specific treatment. It frequently coexists with cholelithiasis, but no causative relationship has been proved. Adenomyomatosis occasionally produces abdominal pain, and in some cases cholecystectomy may be indicated for relief of symptoms. Cholesterol accumulation in adenomyomatosis is intraluminal, as cholesterol crystals precipitate in the bile trapped in Rokitansky–Aschoff sinuses, intramural diverticula lined by mucosal epithelium. Gallbladder wall thickening and intramural diverticula containing bile with cholesterol crystals, sludge, or calculi are the pathologic correlates of the distinctive multimodality imaging features of adenomyomatosis.

US is a primary modality for biliary imaging, and adenomyomatosis of the gallbladder is frequently identified at sonography. The non-specific finding of gallbladder wall thickening is well demonstrated with US, as are sludge and calculi, when present. Echogenic intramural foci from which emanate V-shaped comet tail reverberation artefacts are highly specific for adenomyomatosis, representing the unique acoustic signature of cholesterol crystals within the lumina of Rokitansky–Aschoff sinuses.

Boscak AR, et al. Best cases from AFIP. Adenomyomatosis of the Gallbladder. *RadioGraphics*. 2006;26:941–6. Published online.

45. D. Bicornuate uterus

While the presence of a divided rather than triangular uterine cavity at Hysterosalpingogram (HSG) may suggest the presence of an Mullerian duct anomaly (MDA), it is not possible to differentiate between subtypes. MRI and US provide greater anatomic detail; both of these imaging methods provide information on the external uterine contour, which is an important diagnostic feature of MDAs. Furthermore, both MRI and US may be used to assess for concomitant renal anomalies; renal anomalies occur at a higher rate among MDA patients. Unicornuate uterus appears as a small, oblong, off-midline structure on US and MRI. Uterus didelphys results from complete failure of Müllerian duct fusion. Each duct develops fully with duplication of the uterine horns, cervix and proximal vagina. A fundal cleft greater than 1 cm has been reported to be 100% sensitive and specific in differentiation of fusion anomalies (didelphys and bicornuate) from reabsorption anomalies (septate and arcuate). Bicornuate uterus involves duplication of the uterus with possible duplication of the cervix (bicornuate unicollis or bicornuate bicollis). HSG demonstrates opacification of two symmetric fusiform uterine cavities (horns) and fallopian tubes. Historically, an intercornual angle of greater than 105° was used for diagnosis of bicornuate uterus. Septate uterus is the most common form of MDA, accounting for approximately 55% of cases. Historically, an angle of less than 75° between the uterine horns has been reported to be suggestive of a septate rather than bicornuate uterus. However, considerable overlap occurs between septate and bicornuate uteri; as such, the angle measurement is not a reliable diagnostic feature. Arcuate uterus at HSG shows a single uterine cavity with a broad saddle-shaped indentation at the uterine fundus.

Behr SC, et al. Imaging of müllerian duct anomalies. *Radiographics*. 2012;32(6):E233–50.

46. A. Calcium pyrophosphate deposition disease (CPPD)

This is a typical description of CPPD, which can be idiopathic or associated with endocrinological problems such as hyperparathyroidism and hypothyroidism. The joints of the knee, wrist and second/third MCP joints of the hand are most frequently involved. Differentials would also include gout, but the distribution of erosions are different, with gouty erosions tending to be juxta-articular and punched out ('rat-bitten') rather than subchondral. Joint space is also typically preserved in gout until the late stages. Psoriasis produces enthesitis and periostitis with new bone formation. Ochronosis, or alkaptonuria, is a metabolic disorder whereby there is abnormal build-up of homogentisic acid in connective tissue with pigmentation of the sclera and urine appearing dark in colour. Diffuse multilevel vertebral disc calcification and early OA changes in multiple joints are associated with this condition.

Manaster BJ, et al. *Musculoskeletal Imaging: The Requisites*, 4th edn. Philadelphia, PA: Mosby Elsevier, 2013:298–9.

47. B.   Cystic components

Metastatic malignant melanoma is a commonly encountered neoplasm in the head. Typical appearance of a lesion is high signal intensity on T1-weighted images and low signal on T2-weighted images (melanotic pattern). The other described pattern is the amelanotic pattern. In this pattern, the lesion is hypointense or isointense to the cortex on T1-weighted images and hyperintense or isointense to the cortex on T2-weighted images. Metastatic melanoma presents as multiple brain metastasis, which are located predominantly in the cortex and at the grey matter–white matter junction. They can also present in miliary form or as subependymal nodules. The lesions often appear hyperdense on unenhanced CT. The lesions show moderate to intense contrast enhancement, although larger lesions can show non-enhancing or hypoenhancing necrotic areas. Prominent perilesional oedema is seen.

Escott EJ. A variety of appearances of malignant melanoma in the head: A review. *Radiographics*. 2001;21(3):625–39.

48. B.   Maximum of two attempts can be made.

Intussusception is one of the most common causes of acute abdomen in infancy.

Perforation may already have occurred before enema therapy or may occur during the reduction process.

There is no agreement on the number and duration of reduction attempts, the efficacy of premedication or sedation, the use of rectal tubes with inflatable retention balloons, or the use of transabdominal manipulation. The classic 'rule of threes' is that the number of reduction attempts is capped at three, lasting 3 min each. This rule has been discarded at some institutions, and some authors use a nearly unlimited number of attempts. Use of sedation, rectal tube with balloons and the Valsalva manoeuvre are said to improve the reduction rate achieved.

Absolute contraindications to enema therapy are shock not readily corrected with IV hydration and perforation with peritonitis. Criteria that are linked to a lower reduction rate and a higher perforation rate are age less than 3 months or greater than 5 years, long duration of symptoms, especially if greater than 48 hours, passage of blood via the rectum, significant dehydration, small bowel obstruction and visualisation of the dissection sign during enema therapy. Air enema produces excellent results but is also associated with maximum perforation rates.

del-Pozo G, et al. Intussusception in children: Current concepts in diagnosis and enema reduction. *Radiographics*. 1999;19(2):299–319.

49. C.   Type C

Different types of oesophageal atresia are identified on the basis of the presence (and location) or absence of a tracheo-oesophageal fistula.

Type A is pure oesophageal atresia without fistula, and Type B is oesophageal atresia with a fistula between the proximal pouch and the trachea. Type C is oesophageal atresia with a fistula from the trachea or the main bronchus to the distal oesophageal segment. Type D is oesophageal atresia with both proximal and distal fistulas, and Type E is an H-shaped tracheo-oesophageal fistula without atresia. Of these five types, Type C is by far the most common. Oesophageal atresia is generally suspected on the basis of polyhydramnios, inability to swallow saliva or milk, aspiration during early feedings, or failure to successfully pass a catheter into the stomach. Feeding difficulties with choking occur in infants with Type E (fistula without atresia), but the diagnosis may not be made until several years later when the patient presents with a cough while swallowing, recurrent pneumonia and a distended abdomen.

In Types A and B, there is a complete absence of gas in the stomach and intestinal tract, whereas in Types C and D the gastrointestinal tract commonly appears distended with air.

Berrocal T, et al. Congenital anomalies of the upper gastrointestinal tract. *Radiographics.* 1999;19(4):855–72.

50. E. Aortic stenosis

Chronic histoplasmosis may lead to two well-described complications: fibrosing mediastinitis and broncholithiasis. Fibrosing mediastinitis is a fibrotic immune response to histoplasma antigens. The abnormal fibrosing process encases and narrows vital mediastinal structures, which can lead to superior vena cava syndrome, precapillary pulmonary arterial hypertension from pulmonary arterial stenosis, post-capillary pulmonary arterial hypertension owing to pulmonary vein stenosis, atelectasis from bronchial obstruction, tracheal stenosis, or dysphagia from oesophageal obstruction. The imaging appearance can mimic infiltrating metastatic disease or lymphoma; however, the presence of mediastinal calcifications often provides a clue to the diagnosis. Broncholithiasis results from erosion of a calcified hilar lymph node into an adjacent bronchus. Affected patients present with chronic cough and haemoptysis and even occasionally with lithoptysis. Typical imaging features include endobronchial calcification with atelectasis of the associated pulmonary segment or lobe.

McAdams HP, et al. Thoracic mycoses from endemic fungi: Radiologic-pathologic correlation. *Radiographics.* 1995;15:255–70.
Saket RR, et al. Intrathoracic fungal diseases: A guide to classification and pictorial review part I: Endemic fungi. *Contemp Diagn Radiol.* 2009;32(1):1–7.

51. E. Capillary haemangioma

The classic haemangioma is an asymptomatic lesion that is discovered at routine examination or autopsy. At US, the typical appearance is a homogeneous, hyperechoic mass with well-defined margins and posterior acoustic enhancement.

The CT findings consist of a hypoattenuating lesion on non-enhanced images. After intravenous administration of contrast material, arterial-phase CT shows early, peripheral, globular enhancement of the lesion. The attenuation of the peripheral nodules is equal to that of the adjacent aorta. Venous-phase CT shows centripetal enhancement that progresses to uniform filling. This enhancement persists on delayed-phase images.

At MRI, haemangiomas are characterised by well-defined margins and high signal intensity on T2-weighted images, which is identical to that of cerebrospinal fluid. Specificity is improved by using serial gadolinium-enhanced gradient-echo imaging. The gadolinium intake is similar to the intake of iodinated contrast material during enhanced CT. With T2-weighted spin-echo and dynamic gadolinium-enhanced T1-weighted gradient-echo sequences, the sensitivity and specificity of MRI are 98% and the accuracy is 99%. The imaging features of a haemangioma depend on its size; typical haemangiomas are mostly less than 3 cm in diameter.

Vilgrain V, et al. Imaging of atypical haemangiomas of the liver with pathologic correlation. *RadioGraphics.* 2000;20:379–97.

52. E. Alport's syndrome

Causes of medullary nephrocalcinosis include hyperparathyroidism, sarcoidosis, myelomatosis, primary or secondary hyperoxaluria (Crohn's disease), hyperthyroidism, osteoporosis, idiopathic hypercalciuria, renal tubular acidosis, medullary sponge kidney and drug-induced (hypervitaminosis D, milk-alkali syndrome).

Alport's syndrome is an autosomal dominant condition also called *chronic hereditary nephritis*, associated with ocular abnormalities, deafness, small kidneys, cortical calcification and progressive renal failure without hypertension.

Adam A, et al. *Grainger & Allison's Diagnostic Radiology: A Textbook of Medical Imaging*, 5th edn. New York: Churchill Livingstone, 2008:882.

53. C. Carpal tunnel syndrome

Imaging of carpal tunnel syndrome is controversial and diagnosis is primarily made on clinical grounds and nerve conduction studies. However, there are some imaging findings that can be associated with the syndrome. These include the 'pseudo-neuroma' appearance of the median nerve (swelling of the median nerve just before the carpal tunnel entrance), increased T2 signal changes and increased post-contrast enhancement. It is associated with acromegaly. Neurofibroma of the median nerve can account for the symptoms but would tend to be more distinct as a lesion and sometimes associated with a low-signal central region.

Dähnert W. *Radiology Review Manual*, 6th edn. Philadelphia, PA: Lippincott Williams & Wilkins, 2007:56.
Luchetti R, Amadio P. *Carpal Tunnel Syndrome*. New York: Springer, 2007:76.

54. B. Wooden FB is hyperattenuating.

CT is a very sensitive imaging modality that can demonstrate metal fragments less than 1 mm in size. Non-metallic foreign bodies are more problematic; not only the size of the glass fragment but also the type of glass and its location affect detection rates. Wooden foreign bodies usually appear hypoattenuating on CT images. Because of their low attenuation, they can be mistaken for air. If the low-attenuation collection on CT displays a geometric margin, wood or organic FB should be suspected. The attenuation of wood changes over time as the water content changes, older wood being drier than fresh green wood.

Kubal WS. Imaging of orbital trauma. *Radiographics*. 2008;28(6):1729–39.

55. C. Hyperthyroidism

Inflammation of the pericardium (pericarditis) occurs in response to a variety of stimuli. It results in cellular proliferation or the production of fluid (pericardial effusion), either alone or in combination. Causes include myocardial infarction (acute or post-myocardial infarction Dressler syndrome), pericardiotomy, mediastinal irradiation, infection (viral or bacterial), connective-tissue disease (rheumatoid arthritis, SLE), metabolic disorders (uraemia, hypothyroidism rather than hyperthyroidism), pericardial neoplasia, trauma and AIDS.

Chest X-ray shows increased cardiac size, 'flask' or 'water bottle' configuration, filling of retrosternal space, effacement of cardiac borders and thickening of anterior pericardial stripe. Echocardiography is the investigation of choice for diagnosis.

Adam A, et al. *Grainger & Allison's Diagnostic Radiology: A Textbook of Medical Imaging*, 5th edn. New York: Churchill Livingstone, 2008:263.

56. E. Suspected haemangioma

Contraindications for liver biopsy include the following:

1. Uncooperative patient
2. Extrahepatic biliary duct dilatation (except if benefit outweighs the risk)
3. Bacterial cholangitis (relative contraindication due to risk of septic shock)
4. Abnormal coagulation indices (having a normal INR or PT is not a reassurance that the patient will not bleed; however, there is increased incidence of bleeding with INR above 1.5)
5. Thrombocytopenia (platelet count below 60,000/mm^3)

6. Presence of ascites

7. Cystic lesion

Guidelines on the use of liver biopsy in clinical practice. *BSG Guidelines in Gastroenterology*. 2004.
   Available at: www.bsg.org.uk/pdf_word_docs/liver_biopsy.pdf.

57. B. CT shows soft-tissue mass displacing the aorta anteriorly

Intravenous urography usually demonstrates the classic triad of medial deviation of the middle third of the ureters, tapering of the lumen of one or both ureters in the lower lumbar spine or upper sacral region, and proximal unilateral or bilateral hydroureteronephrosis with delayed excretion of contrast material. CT and MRI is the mainstay of non-invasive diagnosis of Retroperitoneal fibrosis (RPF). CT allows comprehensive evaluation of the morphology, location and extent of RPF and involvement of adjacent organs and vascular structures. Moreover, abdominal CT allows detection of diseases often associated with idiopathic RPF (e.g., autoimmune pancreatitis) or demonstrating an underlying cause in cases of secondary RPF (e.g., malignancy). CT shows a well-defined mass, usually anterior and lateral to the aorta, sparing the posterior aspect and not causing aortic displacement. Idiopathic RPF typically has low signal intensity on T1-weighted images. The signal intensity on T2-weighted images is variable and reflects the degree of associated active inflammation (hypercellularity and oedema). After administration of contrast material, early soft-tissue enhancement mirrors the degree of inflammatory activity observed at T2-weighted imaging. The sensitivity of ^{18}F-FDG PET is very high, which allows detection and quantification of the metabolic activity of retroperitoneal lesions. Although sensitivity is high, specificity is low and aortic wall in the elderly can show FDG uptake.

Caiafa RO, et al. Retroperitoneal fibrosis: Role of imaging in diagnosis and follow-up. *Radiographics*. 2013;
   33(2):535–52.

58. B. MRI

A main differential for a symptomatic lesion in the epiphysis of a long bone in an unfused skeleton is a chondroblastoma. MRI will reveal the presence of marked reactive surrounding marrow oedema. In a fused skeleton, the differentials would include clear cell chondrosarcoma, giant cell tumours and other benign causes like subarticular cyst and intraosseous ganglion.

Chondroblastomas are very well defined with sclerotic margin on plain X-ray and low-signal rim on MRI (cf. Langerhans cell histiocytosis, which appears less well defined with variable margins). Often definitive diagnosis requires surgical biopsy.

Dähnert W. *Radiology Review Manual*, 6th edn. Philadelphia, PA: Lippincott Williams & Wilkins, 2007:56.

59. D. Corneal abrasion

Vitreous haemorrhage is common, with varied clinical manifestations and causes. The most common causes include proliferative diabetic retinopathy, vitreous detachment with or without retinal breaks, and trauma. Less common causes include vascular occlusive disease, retinal arterial macroaneurysm, haemoglobinopathies, age-related macular degeneration, intra-ocular tumours and others. Terson syndrome is the occurrence of a vitreous haemorrhage of the human eye in association with subarachnoid haemorrhage.

Goff MJ, et al. Causes and treatment of vitreous hemorrhage. *Compr Ophthalmol Update*. 2006;7(3):97–111.

60. D. Vein of Galen aneurysm

Vein of Galen aneurysmal malformations (VGAMs) are rare congenital vascular malformations characterised by shunting of arterial flow into an enlarged cerebral vein dorsal to the tectum. Most of these malformations present in early childhood, often causing congestive heart failure in the neonate.

Antenatal ultrasound scans demonstrate the venous sac as a sonolucent mass located posterior to the third ventricle. Ultrasonic demonstration of pulsatile flow within it helps in differentiating

VOGMs from other midline cystic lesions. Associated venous anomalies can often be visualised. Evidence of hydrocephalus and cardiac dysfunction can also be obtained on antenatal ultrasonography. Contrast-enhanced axial CT scan of the brain usually demonstrates a well-defined, multilobulated, intensely enhancing lesion located within the cistern of velum interpositum. Dilatation of the ventricular system and periventricular white matter hypodensities, as well as diffuse cerebral atrophy, are the commonly associated findings.

Davel L, et al. MRI imaging of vein of Galen malformations at Steve Biko Academic Hospital: A mini case series. *SA J Radiol.* 2011;15:53–5.
Jones BV, et al. Vein of Galen aneurysmal malformation: Diagnosis and treatment of 13 children with extended clinical follow-up. *AJNR Am J Neuroradiol.* 2002;23(10):1717–24.

61. D. Mesothelioma

Malignant mesothelioma is the most common primary pericardial malignancy. A causal relationship with asbestosis is uncertain because of low prevalence of this neoplasm. Mesothelioma may present as a well-defined single mass, multiple nodules, or diffuse plaques involving the visceral and parietal pericardium and wrapping around the cardiac chambers and great vessels.

Other malignant primary tumours include lymphoma, sarcoma, pheochromocytoma and liposarcoma. Teratomas of the pericardium may also be malignant and are most commonly seen in children.

Pericardial metastases are much more common than primary pericardial tumours. Breast and lung cancers are the most common sources of metastases in the pericardium, followed by lymphomas and melanomas.

Adam A, et al. *Grainger & Allison's Diagnostic Radiology: A Textbook of Medical Imaging*, 5th edn. New York: Churchill Livingstone, 2008:265.
Wang ZJ, et al. CT and MR imaging of pericardial disease. *Radiographics.* 2003;23:S167–80.

62. C. Haemangioma

The classic haemangioma is an asymptomatic lesion that is discovered at routine examination or autopsy. At US, the typical appearance is a homogeneous, hyperechoic mass with well-defined margins and posterior acoustic enhancement.

The CT findings consist of a hypoattenuating lesion on non-enhanced images. After intravenous administration of contrast material, arterial-phase CT shows early, peripheral, globular enhancement of the lesion. The attenuation of the peripheral nodules is equal to that of the adjacent aorta. Venous-phase CT shows centripetal enhancement that progresses to uniform filling. This enhancement persists on delayed-phase images.

At MRI, haemangioma are characterised by well-defined margins and high signal intensity on T2-weighted images, which is identical to that of cerebrospinal fluid. Specificity is improved by using serial gadolinium-enhanced gradient-echo imaging (6). The gadolinium intake is similar to the intake of iodinated contrast material during enhanced CT. With T2-weighted spin-echo and dynamic gadolinium-enhanced T1-weighted gradient-echo sequences, the sensitivity and specificity of MRI are 98% and the accuracy is 99%. The imaging features of a haemangioma depend on its size; typical haemangiomas are mostly less than 3 cm in diameter.

Vilgrain V, et al. Imaging of atypical haemangiomas of the liver with pathologic correlation. *RadioGraphics.* 2000;20:379–97.

63. B. High on T2   Intermediate on T2   Low on T2

On T1-weighted images, normal pelvic musculature and viscera demonstrate homogenous low-to-intermediate signal intensity. Zonal architecture is best demonstrated on T2-weighted MRI.

T2 signal reflects the water content, which is highest in the endometrium, intermediate in the myometrium and least in the junctional zone.

Adam A, et al. *Grainger & Allison's Diagnostic Radiology: A Textbook of Medical Imaging*, 5th edn. New York: Churchill Livingstone, 2008:1219.

Dähnert W. *Radiology Review Manual*, 7th edn. Philadelphia, PA: Lippincott Williams & Wilkins, 2011:1042.

64. E. Hypothyroidism

A common cause of localised posterior vertebral scalloping is increased intraspinal pressure secondary to an expanding mass. Widening of the interpediculate distance and alteration of the configuration of the pedicles are associated signs. Relatively large, slow-growing lesions that originate during a period of active skeletal growth (such as ependymomas) are most likely to give rise to posterior vertebral scalloping. Dural ectasia is thought to cause posterior vertebral scalloping due to loss of the normal protection provided to the vertebral body by a strong, intact dura. Dural ectasia classically occurs in association with inherited connective-tissue disorders such as Marfan syndrome (classical) and Ehlers–Danlos syndrome. Posterior vertebral scalloping is also commonly seen in patients with neurofibromatosis, most likely due to dural ectasia but also secondary to neurofibromas or a thoracic meningocoele. It has also been reported in patients with AS; in these cases, the development of associated arachnoid cysts may give rise to cauda equina syndrome. Acromegaly has been described as a further cause of diffuse posterior vertebral scalloping, probably because of a combination of soft-tissue hypertrophy in the spinal canal and increased bone resorption.

Wakely SL. The posterior vertebral scalloping sign. *Radiology*. 2006;239(2):607–9.

65. B. Lens dislocation

In blunt traumas, ruptures are most common at the insertions of the intra-ocular muscles where the sclera is thinnest. CT findings suggestive of an open-globe injury include a change in globe contour, an obvious loss of volume, the 'flat tire' sign, scleral discontinuity, intra-ocular air and intra-ocular foreign bodies. A deep anterior chamber has been described as a clinical finding in patients with a ruptured globe and can also be a clue on CT.

Kubal WS. Imaging of orbital trauma. *Radiographics*. 2008;28(6):1729–39.

66. C. Retinoblastoma

Retinoblastoma, a small round-cell tumour arising from neuroepithelial cells, is the most common childhood intra-ocular malignancy. Diagnosis is typically by ophthalmologic examination, prompted by leukocoria or 'white reflex'.

Retinoblastoma appears as an echogenic soft-tissue mass with various degrees of calcification. The vascularity indicates tumour activity; that is, lesions are hypervascular at diagnosis and when active. Vascularity regresses with treatment. CT detects intra-ocular, extra-ocular and intracranial disease extension; excels at delineation of bony abnormalities; and readily depicts tumoural calcifications. On CT, retinoblastoma is characterised by an intermediate-density enhancing soft-tissue mass or masses, with varying degrees of calcification; calcification increases with therapeutic response. The vitreous may be abnormally dense from debris, haemorrhage, or increased globulin content. Retinoblastoma is a heterogeneously enhancing soft-tissue mass with various degrees of calcification on MRI. Lesions are typically hyperintense to vitreous on T1-weighted sequences and hypointense to vitreous on T2-weighted sequences. The vitreous may be abnormally bright on T1-weighted sequences because of increased globulin content and a decreased ratio of albumin to globulin that occurs with malignancy.

The other choices are all differentials for white reflex, but do not show a solid mass with calcification.

Kaste SC, et al. Retinoblastoma. *AJR Am J Roentgenol*. 2000;175(2):495–501.

67. B.   They are most commonly left-sided.

The most common congenital pericardial anomaly is a pericardial cyst. Chest pain is the most common presenting symptom, but most patients with pericardial cysts are asymptomatic. On plain chest radiographs, pericardial cysts present as well-defined, round, homogeneous soft-tissue densities and are most commonly found at the right pericardiophrenic angle. Pericardial cysts are visualised most easily using CT or MRI. With MRI, simple pericardial cysts are characterised by low signal intensity on T1-weighted images or high signal intensity on T2-weighted images. With CT, pericardial cysts are usually of water density, but when they contain sufficient proteinaceous material the attenuation may be greater than that of water. Occasionally, pericardial cysts may calcify and simulate thymic cysts.

Kisler T, et al. Multimodality imaging of the pericardium: 2007 update. *Contemp Diagn Radiol.* 2007;30(19):1–6.

68. A.   Severe bleeding episodes, such as those manifesting with haemodynamic instability, decrease the pretest probability of a positive result for active bleeding at CT angiography.

Severe bleeding episodes, such as those manifesting with haemodynamic instability, increase the pretest probability of a positive result for active bleeding at CT angiography.

Artigas JM, et al. Multidetector CT angiography for acute gastrointestinal bleeding: Technique and findings. *Radiographics.* 2013;33:1453–70.

69. D.   Tracheo-oesophageal fistula

Horseshoe kidney is the most common fusion anomaly of the kidneys. There is recognised association with cardiovascular, skeletal, CNS, genitourinary anomalies (undescended testes, bicornuate uterus, duplication of ureter, hypospadias, etc.), anorectal malformations, trisomy 18 and Turner syndrome. Vesico-ureteric reflux, hydronephrosis secondary to PUJ obstruction and increased frequency of complications like renal stones and infection are recognised.

Dähnert W. *Radiology Review Manual*, 7th edn. Philadelphia, PA: Lippincott Williams & Wilkins, 2011:948.

70. C.   Osteopoikilosis

Patients with co-morbidities like diabetes, anaemia and malnutrition can suffer from impaired bone fracture healing. Drug therapy like corticosteroids and NSAIDs can also produce similar problems. Osteogenesis imperfecta is a connective-tissue disorder with resultant abnormal bone density and structure, resulting in poor mineralisation and fragile, brittle bones. Osteopoikilosis is a benign condition and usually found incidentally. It is a form of sclerosing bone dysplasia with multiple enostoses. It is not associated with impaired fracture healing.

Sim E. Osteopoikilosis and fracture healing. *Unfallchirurgie.* 1989;15(6):303–5.

71. B.   Matched CBV (Cerebral blood volume) and CBF (Cerebral blood flow) represent salvageable brain.

An important advance in stroke imaging is the development of CT perfusion imaging. CT angiography source images (CTA-SI) represent cerebral blood volume that is reduced in the core infarct and correlates with infarct volume as seen on DWI (Diffusion Weighted Imaging).

CBF (cerebral blood flow), CBV (cerebral blood volume), and MTT (mean transit time) are three parameters that can distinguish infarcted tissue from potentially salvageable penumbra. Ischemic but non-infarcted tissue will have decreased CBF, elevated MTT, and normal or high CBV (mismatch). Once infarcted, there will also be a persistent decrease in CBV (matched defect). Sensitivity and specificity of DWI for stroke detection is very high. DWI bright signals do not necessarily represent irreversibly infarcted tissue but reflect redistribution of water from the extracellular to the intracellular space in ischaemic tissue. It is necessary to analyse maps of ADC (apparent diffusion coefficient) to distinguish the effects of reduced water diffusibility (dark on ADC) from T2 'shine-through' (bright on ADC). Both features lead to the DWI bright signals seen in ischaemia. The volumetric mismatch between the PWI and DWI volumes is a marker of potentially salvageable tissue at risk. Overall DWI provides the best estimate of infarcted core.

Sá de Camargo EC, Koroshetz WJ. Neuroimaging of ischemia and infarction. *NeuroRx.* 2005;2(2):265–76.

72. D. Lymphangioma

A cystic hygroma is the most common form of lymphangioma and constitutes about 5% of all benign tumours of infancy and childhood. On US scans, most cystic hygromas manifest as a multilocular predominantly cystic mass with septa of variable thickness. The echogenic portions of the lesion correlate with clusters of small, abnormal lymphatic channels. Fluid–fluid levels can be observed with a characteristic echogenic, haemorrhagic component layering in the dependent portion of the lesion. Prenatal US may demonstrate a cystic hygroma in the posterior neck soft tissues. On CT images, cystic hygromas tend to appear as poorly circumscribed, multiloculated, hypoattenuated masses. They typically have characteristic homogeneous fluid attenuation. Usually, the mass is centred in the posterior triangle or in the submandibular space.

A third branchial cleft cyst most commonly appears as a unilocular cystic mass centred in the posterior cervical space on CT and MRI. At US, a second branchial cleft cyst is seen as a sharply marginated, round to ovoid, centrally anechoic mass with a thin peripheral wall that displaces the surrounding soft tissues. The 'classic' location of these cysts is at the anteromedial border of the sternocleidomastoid muscle. The first branchial cleft cyst appears as a cystic mass either within, superficial to, or deep to the parotid gland.

Koeller KK, et al. Congenital cystic masses of the neck: Radiologic-pathologic correlation. *Radiographics.* 1999;19(1):121–46.

73. B. Failure to identify pericardium on CT or MR is diagnostic.

Congenital pericardial defects are uncommon. They range from small defects to complete absence of the pericardium. Both small pericardial defects and complete absence of the pericardium most often are left-sided. They can be recognised on plain chest radiographs because there is abnormal cardiac contour due to protrusion of all or part of the cardiac chamber, for example, the left atrial appendage, through the defect. Shift of the cardiac axis to the left and posteriorly is seen with complete absence or large pericardial defects. With CT or MRI, failure to visualise a portion of the pericardium does not necessarily indicate a pericardial defect, however, because the pericardium over the left atrium and ventricle may not always be visualised in normal subjects.

Patients with pericardial defects also may have one or more associated congenital abnormalities, including atrial septal defect, patent ductus arteriosus, mitral valve stenosis, or TOF, which also are detectable on CT or MRI.

Kisler T, et al. Multimodality imaging of the pericardium: 2007 update. *Contemp Diagn Radiol.* 2007;30(19): 1–6.
Wang ZJ, et al. CT and MR imaging of pericardial disease. *Radiographics.* 2003;23:S167–80.

74. E. SMV to the left of the SMA

SMV positioned to the left of SMA is the most specific sign of malrotation on CT (80%). Other signs on CT include the 'whirl sign' around the SMA and large intestine on the left with small intestine on the right.

Abnormal position of the caecum and duodenum with duodeno-jejunal junction over the right pedicle is the most specific sign of malrotation on barium meal studies.

Dähnert W. *Radiology Review Manual*, 7th edn. Philadelphia, PA: Lippincott Williams & Wilkins, 2011:869–70.

75. D. Tuberous sclerosis

Tuberous sclerosis (TS) is an autosomal, dominant, inherited neurocutaneous syndrome characterised by a variety of hamartomatous lesions in various organs. Classically, TS demonstrates a triad of clinical features (Vogt triad): mental retardation, epilepsy and adenoma sebaceum. Recently advocated criteria for diagnosis of TS consist of both major and minor diagnostic features.

Major features include facial angiofibromas, hypomelanotic macules, cortical tubers and subependymal nodules (frequent); retinal hamartoma, LAM (lymphangioleiomyomatosis), renal AML (angiomyolipoma), and cardiac rhabdomyomas (common); and shagreen patches, ungual fibroma and subependymal giant cell tumours (uncommon). Minor features include dental enamel pits and hamartomatous rectal polyps (frequent); bone cysts, renal cysts, gingival fibromas and cerebral white matter radial migration lines (common); and confetti skin lesions and retinal achromatic patches (uncommon). Definite diagnosis requires two major or one major and two minor criteria.

Umeoka S, et al. Pictorial review of tuberous sclerosis in various organs. *Radiographics*. 2008;28(7):e32.

76. B. Turner syndrome

Turner syndrome is a female, sex chromosome abnormality from the deletion of one X chromosome (45 XO). It is characterised by a webbed neck and short stature. Skeletal manifestations include short fourth metacarpals and Madelung's deformity. 5–20% of patients with Turner syndrome have coarctation of the aorta, which would account for the additional finding of rib notching. Pseudohypoparathyroidism and pseudopseudohypoparathyroidism can exhibit a short fourth metacarpal, but they are not associated with coarctation of the aorta. Noonan's syndrome is associated with short stature and characteristic facies, along with other congenital cardiopulmonary anomalies, but shortening of the fourth metacarpal is not a feature of this entity. Marfan syndrome is associated with pectus excavatum and aortic root dilatation with the increased risk of aortic dissection.

Dähnert W. *Radiology Review Manual*, 6th edn. Philadelphia, PA: Lippincott Williams & Wilkins, 2007:174.
Mazzanti L, Cacciari E. Congenital heart disease in patients with Turner's syndrome. *J Pediatr*. 1998;133(5):688–92.

77. E. Dilatation of ventricle

Non-contrast CT is usually the first neuroimaging examination performed in acute stroke assessment. In addition to detecting haemorrhage, modern non-contrast CT can reveal early ischaemic change, such as hypo-attenuation of the parenchyma and grey matter with loss of grey–white differentiation (insular ribbon sign, obscuration of the lentiform nucleus, brain swelling with sulcal effacement) and compression of the ventricular system and basal cisterns, the dense artery (MCA) sign and the MCA dot sign.

Sá de Camargo EC, Koroshetz WJ. Neuroimaging of ischemia and infarction. *NeuroRx*. 2005;2(2):265–76.

78. B. LUL, RML, RUL

Congenital lobar emphysema represents a condition of progressive over-distension of one or multiple pulmonary lobes secondary to deficiency/immaturity of bronchial cartilage, endobronchial obstruction, or extrinsic compression. It is more common in boys.

Preferential involvement is LUL (left upper lobe) > RML (right middle lobe) > RUL (right upper lobe) > two lobes.

Initial chest X-ray shows opacification of lobe secondary to delayed clearing of pulmonary fluid; this is followed by progressive features of air trapping, hypertranslucent lung and mediastinal shift.

Dähnert W. *Radiology Review Manual*, 7th edn. Philadelphia, PA: Lippincott Williams & Wilkins, 2011.

79. C. MR is better at demonstrating pericardial calcification.

Patients with constrictive pericarditis present with symptoms of heart failure. The most frequent causes are cardiac surgery and radiation therapy. Other causes include infection (viral or tuberculous), connective-tissue disease, uraemia, neoplasm, or idiopathic condition.

Transthoracic echocardiography is not very accurate in the depiction of pericardial thickening. Transoesophageal imaging allows better visualisation of the pericardium, and Doppler techniques are particularly useful in the diagnosis; however, the transoesophageal approach has a narrow field of view and is invasive.

Both CT and MRI demonstrate the pericardium very well. Normal pericardial thickness is less than 2 mm. Pericardial thickness of 4 mm or more indicates thickening and, when accompanied by features of heart failure, is suggestive of constrictive pericarditis. Constrictive pericarditis and restrictive cardiomyopathy are differentiated on the basis of thickened pericardium.

Pericardial thickening may be limited to the right side of the heart or an even smaller area, such as the right atrioventricular groove. An additional advantage of CT is its high sensitivity in depicting pericardial calcification. It is important to remember, however, that neither pericardial thickening nor calcification is diagnostic of constrictive pericarditis unless the patient also has symptoms of physiologic constriction or restriction.

At both CT and MRI, the right ventricle tends to have a reduced volume and a narrow tubular configuration. In some patients, a sigmoid-shaped ventricular septum or prominent leftward convexity in the septum can be observed. Systemic venous dilatation particularly inferior vena cava (IVC), hepatomegaly and ascites also are frequently seen.

Wang ZJ, et al. CT and MR imaging of pericardial disease. *Radiographics*. 2003;23:S167–80.

80. A. Carcinoid syndrome has higher morbidity and mortality than the tumour itself.

Carcinoid is the most common tumour of the small bowel and appendix. Seven percent of small bowel carcinoids are associated with carcinoid syndrome. There is no association with NF2. Carcinoid tumours most commonly occur in the appendix (30%–45%) and small bowel (25%–35%). Carcinoid syndrome has higher morbidity and mortality than the tumour itself. Common sites of metastasis are liver, lungs, lymph nodes and bone (osteoblastic).

Dähnert W. *Radiology Review Manual*, 7th edn. Philadelphia, PA: Lippincott Williams & Wilkins, 2011:826–8.

81. E. Embryo seen with a mean sac diameter of 10 mm.

The gestational sac is first identifiable on transvaginal ultrasound at 4.5 weeks. It appears as a round 2–3 mm fluid collection. It is located in the central echogenic part of the endometrium (decidua). In some cases, it is surrounded by two echogenic rings corresponding to the two layers of decidua, described as the double decidual sac sign of intrauterine pregnancy. Sometimes the gestational sac is eccentrically located on one side of a thin white line corresponding to the collapsed uterine cavity, called the *intradecidual sign*.

The yolk sac is the first structure visualised on TVS (trans vaginal scan) within the sac at 5.5 weeks. Yolk sac is evident when sac diameter is 10 mm. Heartbeat is evident when crown–rump length (CRL) is 5 mm. On TVS, an embryo is seen when the mean sac diameter is 18 mm. Mean sac diameter increases by approximately 1 mm per day. Lack of foetal pole in a gestational sac with diameter more than 20 mm is suggestive of an anembryonic or nonviable pregnancy.

Adam A, et al. *Grainger & Allison's Diagnostic Radiology: A Textbook of Medical Imaging*, 5th edn. New York: Churchill Livingstone, 2008:1205.
Doubilet PM. Ultrasound evaluation of the first trimester. *Radiol Clin North Am.* 2014;52(6):1191–9.

82. D. Thoracic outlet syndrome

Thoracic outlet syndrome involves the brachial plexus and the subclavian artery or vein at three anatomic levels where they are vulnerable to entrapment; the interscalene space, the costoclavicular space and the retropectoralis minor space. Thoracic outlet syndrome may result from post-traumatic fibrosis of the scalene muscles, compression secondary to activities like backpacking, and clavicular fractures with callus formation and exercise-related muscle hypertrophy affecting weightlifters, swimmers, tennis players and so on. Other causes include mass lesions such as lipomas, neurogenic tumours, accessory muscles and fibrous bands.

MRI can help identify specific muscle denervation patterns. Muscle oedema may occur within 24–48 hours. In contrast, fatty atrophy reflects chronic denervation and manifests several months later. In this setting, MRI has an advantage over electromyography, which does not demonstrate signs of muscle denervation until 2–3 weeks after nerve impairment.

Radiographs may reveal a cervical rib or a prominent C7 transverse process. Narrowing has been reported in the costoclavicular and retropectoralis minor spaces during imaging with postural manoeuvres during dynamic MRI. Sagittal T1-weighted MRI sequences are particularly useful in demonstrating the presence of denervation-related fatty atrophy of muscles, effacement of fat planes around the compressed plexus and an abnormal intramuscular course of the components of the brachial plexus. The retropectoralis minor space is not frequently affected by entrapment and is more often involved by mass lesions.

Linda DD, et al. Multimodality imaging of peripheral neuropathies of the upper limb and brachial plexus. *Radiographics*. 2010;30(5):1373–400.

83. D. Acute infarcts show hyperintense signal on ADC.

Sensitivity and specificity of DWI for stroke detection is very high. DWI bright signals do not necessarily represent irreversibly infarcted tissue but reflect redistribution of water from the extracellular to the intracellular space in ischaemic tissue. It is necessary to analyse maps of ADC to distinguish the effects of reduced water diffusibility (dark on ADC) from T2 'shine-through' (bright on ADC). Both features lead to the DWI bright signals seen in ischaemia.

DWI is already positive in the acute phase (as early as 30 minutes) and then becomes brighter with a maximum at 7 days. DWI in brain infarction will be positive for approximately for 3 weeks after onset. ADC is of low signal intensity with a maximum at 24 hours and then increases in signal intensity and finally becomes bright in the chronic stage.

Sá de Camargo EC, Koroshetz WJ. Neuroimaging of ischemia and infarction. *NeuroRx*. 2005;2(2):265–76.

84. C. Omentum

Bochdalek hernia represents the commonest type of congenital diaphragmatic hernia. It is more common on the left. The most common structure to herniate on the left is omental fat; on the right is the liver.

Dähnert W. *Radiology Review Manual*, 7th edn. Philadelphia, PA: Lippincott Williams & Wilkins, 2011.

85. E. On frontal chest X-ray, it is visualised as a 2-mm stripe outlined by fat.

The pericardium is composed of an outer layer of fibrous tissue and two inner layers of serous tissue. The normal pericardium is not usually seen on plain film chest radiography on the frontal projection, but it may be identified on a lateral projection as an opaque line bordered by mediastinal and subepicardial fat termed the *fat pad sign*. With high-resolution CT, the pericardium may be visualised as a 1- to 2-mm band of soft-tissue attenuation. With T1-weighted MRI, the pericardium is a dark band bordered by high-intensity fat. The pericardial sac normally contains 15–30 mL of fluid lying between the parietal and visceral layers of the serous pericardium.

The fibrous pericardium is anchored to the diaphragm by the pericardiophrenic ligament and the central tendons; the sternopericardial ligaments provide anterior attachment. The outer layer of the pericardium extends to and fuses with the root of the aorta, the right and left pulmonary arteries, the superior vena cava and the pulmonary veins. The visceral pericardium reflects from the heart along the great vessels onto the parietal pericardium. Pericardial extensions, recesses, or sinuses are formed at these reflections.

Kisler T, et al. Multimodality imaging of the pericardium: 2007 update. *Contemp Diagn Radiol*. 2007;30 (19):1–6.

86. C. Sclerosing mesenteritis

Sclerosing mesenteritis is a rare condition of unknown cause that is characterised by chronic mesenteric inflammation. The process usually involves the mesentery of the small bowel, especially at its root, but can occasionally involve the mesocolon. On rare occasions, it may involve the peripancreatic region, omentum, retroperitoneum, or pelvis. Although the cause of sclerosing mesenteritis is unknown, the disorder is often associated with other idiopathic inflammatory disorders such as retroperitoneal fibrosis, sclerosing cholangitis, Riedel thyroiditis and orbital pseudotumour. The CT appearance of sclerosing mesenteritis can vary from subtle increased attenuation in the mesentery to a solid soft-tissue mass. Sclerosing mesenteritis most commonly appears as a soft-tissue mass in the small bowel mesentery, although infiltration of the region of the pancreas or porta hepatis is also possible. The mass may envelop the mesenteric vessels, and over time collateral vessels may develop. There may be preservation of fat around the mesenteric vessels, a phenomenon that is referred to as the *fat ring sign*. This finding may help distinguish sclerosing mesenteritis from other mesenteric processes such as lymphoma, carcinoid tumour, or carcinomatosis.

Karen M, Horton MD. CT findings in sclerosing mesenteritis (panniculitis): Spectrum of disease. *RadioGraphics*. 2003;23(6):1561–7.

87. C. HU value of <37 on delayed contrast enhanced CT

Features suggestive of adrenal carcinoma on imaging include large size (>5 cm); invasion of other organs like liver, kidney, IVC, or diaphragm; calcification; central heterogeneous area of low density (tumour necrosis); peripheral nodular enhancement on contrast-enhanced images; and delayed washout. A HU of <37 on contrast-enhanced CT at 5–15 minutes after contrast injection is diagnostic of a benign adrenal lesion.

Dähnert W. *Radiology Review Manual*, 7th edn. Philadelphia, PA: Lippincott Williams & Wilkins, 2011:937–8.

88. D. Superior labral anterior–posterior tear (SLAP)

The anteroinferior glenoid labrum is typically injured in an anterior shoulder dislocation. All of the aforementioned injuries except for the superior labral anterior–posterior (SLAP) tear involve the anteroinferior labrum. The glenolabral articular disruption (GLAD) lesion is a partial tear of the anteroinferior labrum with an associated glenoid cartilage injury. Perthes lesion is a complete tear of the labrum, which is still attached to the glenoid periosteum. An anterior labroligamentous periosteal sleeve avulsion (ALPSA) injury is similar to the Perthes lesion but with medial displacement of the torn labrum, which is still attached to the glenoid scapula periosteal sleeve.

Manaster BJ, et al. *Musculoskeletal Imaging: The Requisites*, 4th edn. Philadelphia, PA: Mosby Elsevier, 2013:82–92.

89. A. Pacchionian granulations

Hyperintensity on FLAIR in subarachnoid spaces has been well described in a wide range of pathologic conditions, such as subarachnoid haemorrhage (SAH), infectious or malignant meningitis, leptomeningeal spread of malignant disease, Leptomeningeal melanosis (part of the neurocutaneous melanosis congenital phakomatosis), vascular hyperintensity in the subarachnoid space produced by severe (>90%) vascular stenosis or occlusion of major cerebral vessels with resulting slow flow and fat-containing tumours like lipoma of subarachnoid space. Retrograde slow flow of engorged pial arteries through leptomeningeal anastomoses is also seen as high signal intensity in the subarachnoid space on FLAIR in patients with Moyamoya disease, called *ivy sign*. Other, less common, causes of subarachnoid FLAIR hyperintensity are artefacts.

Stuckey SL, et al. Hyperintensity in the subarachnoid space on FLAIR MRI. *AJR Am J Roentgenol*. 2007;189(4):913–21.

90. D. Symptomatic First 6 months Adulthood
Bronchopulmonary sequestration

	Intralobar	Extralobar
Prevalence	75%	25%
Pleural involvement	Visceral pleura	Own pleura
Venous drainage	Pulmonary veins	Systemic veins
Associated anomalies	Less common (15%)	More common (50%)
Symptomatic	Adulthood	First 6 months
Arterial supply	Thoracic aorta	Thoracic aorta
Aetiology	Acquired	Developmental

Dähnert W. *Radiology Review Manual*, 7th edn. Philadelphia, PA: Lippincott Williams & Wilkins, 2011.

91. E. Enhances avidly post-contrast

Lipomatous hypertrophy of the interatrial septum is defined as wedge-shaped expansion of the interatrial septum by adipose tissue exceeding 2 cm in transverse diameter.

The incidence increases with age and body mass and is also associated with chronic corticosteroid therapy. Patients are usually asymptomatic, but they may have arrhythmias or superior vena cava syndrome when the superior vena cava is encased. Lipomatous hypertrophy of the interatrial septum, in contrast to cardiac lipoma, does not have a capsule. Because lipomatous hypertrophy of the interatrial septum spares the fossa ovalis, it often has a dumbbell-shaped appearance. Lipomatous hypertrophy of the interatrial septum has the same density and signal intensity as fat on CT and MR, respectively. Lipomatous hypertrophy of the interatrial septum is hypointense on fat saturation sequences and does not enhance post-contrast.

François CJ, et al. CT and MR imaging of primary, metastatic, and nonneoplastic cardiac masses. *Contemp Diagn Radiol.* 2006:29(24):1–6.

92. E. Skip lesions Yes Yes

In patients with proved or suspected Crohn's disease, cross-sectional images should be analysed specifically for the presence and character of a pathologically altered bowel segment (wall thickness, pattern of attenuation, degree of enhancement, length of involvement), stenosis and prestenotic dilatation, skip lesions, fistulas, abscess, fibrofatty proliferation, increased vascularity of the vasa recta (comb sign), mesenteric adenopathy and other extra-intestinal disease involvement.

Furukawa A. Cross sectional imaging in Crohn's disease. *RadioGraphics.* 2004;24:689–702.

93. C. If serum creatinine is above normal range, metformin should be withheld for 24 hours.

Metformin is not recommended for use in diabetics with renal impairment because it is excreted exclusively via the kidneys. Accumulation of metformin may result in the development of lactic acidosis – a serious complication. There is lack of any valid evidence that lactic acidosis is really an issue after administration of iodinated contrast media in patients taking metformin. The problems caused to patients and clinicians by stopping the drug and its increasing use in poorly controlled diabetic patients regardless of renal function have been considered when formulating this advice. It does, however, remain the case that renal function should be known in patients taking metformin who require intravenous or intra-arterial iodinated contrast medium administration. There is no need to stop metformin after contrast in patients with serum creatinine within the normal reference range and/or eGFR >60 ml/min/1.73 m^2. If serum creatinine is above the normal reference range or eGFR is below 60, any decision to stop metformin for

48 hours following contrast medium administration should be made in consultation with the referring clinic.

Standards for Intravascular Contrast Administration to Adult Patients, 3rd edn. Royal College of Radiologists, 2015. BFCR(15)1.

94. A. It is an unstable injury.

Unilateral facet joint dislocation occurs from a flexion/distraction injury with a rotatory component. It is a stable form of facet joint dislocation (cf. with highly unstable bilateral facet joint dislocation). The naked facet sign is seen involving one facet joint on CT, and on plain radiograph there is often an overlapping appearance to the facet joints. Mild anterolisthesis and widening of the interspinous space at the level of injury is a common finding. Up to 30% of patients have a neurological deficit.

Shapiro SA. Management of unilateral locked facet of the cervical spine. *Neurosurgery.* 1994;33(5):832–7.

95. C. SWI is based on homogeneity of magnetic field.

Gradient-echo and susceptibility-weighted sequences are the most sensitive sequences for depicting haemorrhagic transformation in patients with ischaemic stroke, particularly susceptibility-weighted imaging.

Susceptibility-weighted MRI utilises magnetic artefacts generated by in-homogeneities of the magnetic field. Deoxyhaemoglobin produces a non-uniform magnetic field, which accounts for signal changes seen in acute haemorrhages and for the blood oxygen level–dependent effect. With SWI, intraparenchymal haemorrhages can be seen within the first hour of bleeding, with high sensitivity and accuracy. SWI enables the visualisation of multiple cerebral microbleeds, which have been shown to be a risk factor for intracranial haemorrhage after stroke, both with and without thrombolytic therapy.

Sá de Camargo EC, Koroshetz WJ. Neuroimaging of ischemia and infarction. *NeuroRx.* 2005;2(2):265–76.

96. C. Histiocytosis X

Space-occupying lesions affect the hypothalamic-neurohypophyseal axis, which is the central nervous system site most commonly and often earliest involved in Langerhans cell histiocytosis. MRI findings have been correlated with symptoms of diabetes insipidus, which is a clinical hallmark of the condition. Typically, the formation of Langerhans cell histiocytosis granulomas leads to a loss in the normally high signal intensity of the posterior neurohypophysis on T1-weighted images. Furthermore, the hypothalamus, the pituitary stalk or both are frequently enlarged and demonstrate gradually increasing homogeneous enhancement after an intravenous injection of gadolinium, without subsequent washout. The differential diagnosis includes other infundibular diseases, such as adenohypophysitis, which can be differentiated from Langerhans cell histiocytosis by a sharp increase in contrast enhancement and rapid washout after the administration of the intravenous contrast medium. Granulomatous diseases such as sarcoidosis, Wegener disease and leukaemia must also be considered in the differential. Rarer differentials are germ cell tumours (germinoma, teratoma) and haemangioblastoma. These produce the same MRI features, with the same pattern of enhancement at dynamic imaging.

The second most frequent pattern of central nervous system involvement in Langerhans cell histiocytosis is characterised by intra-axial neuro-degenerative changes. Bilateral symmetric lesions in the cerebellum, especially the dentate nucleus, basal ganglia, or brainstem, are most often observed. The differential diagnosis includes ADEM, acute multiphasic disseminated encephalitis, disseminated encephalitis, various metabolic and degenerative disorders, leukoencephalopathy secondary to chemotherapy or radiation therapy, and paraneoplastic encephalitis.

Less frequently, Langerhans cell histiocytosis granulomas, which resemble tumours, are observed in the extra-axial space (in the meninges, pineal gland, choroid plexus and spinal cord).

Schmidt S, et al. Extraosseous langerhans cell histiocytosis in children. *Radiographics*. 2008;28(3):707–26.

97. C. Bronchogenic

Pericardial metastases are much more common than primary pericardial tumours. Breast and lung cancers are the most common sources of metastases in the pericardium, followed by lymphomas and melanomas.

Wang ZJ, et al. CT and MR imaging of pericardial disease. *Radiographics*. 2003;23:S167–80.

98. A. Direct inguinal hernia   The hernial sac lies lateral to the inferior epigastric artery and above the pubic tubercle.

There are several sites on the abdominal wall prone to herniation.

The first site is the deep inguinal ring, where an indirect inguinal hernia occurs. Here, herniated structures enter the inguinal canal lateral to the inferior epigastric artery and superior to the inguinal ligament, extending for a variable distance through the inguinal canal.

A second site of herniation is at the inferior aspect of the Hesselbach's triangle, where a direct inguinal hernia usually occurs. This weakened area is just lateral to the conjoint tendon and medial to the inferior epigastric artery, in contrast to the indirect inguinal hernia, which originates lateral to the inferior epigastric artery.

A third weakened area is inferior in relation to the inguinal ligament and lateral to the lacunar ligament, where a femoral hernia occurs, typically medial and adjacent to the femoral vessels. The fourth area is at the lateral margin of the rectus abdominis muscle, superior to the inferior epigastric artery as it crosses the linea semilunaris, where a spigelian hernia occurs. Indirect inguinal hernias are most common regardless of sex; femoral hernias are more common in women.

Jamadar DA. Jamadar sonography of inguinal region hernias. *AJR Am J Roentgenol*. 2006;187:185–90.

99. C. Reduced diastolic flow is specific for acute rejection.

Acute rejection is a cell-mediated reaction seen within 1–4 weeks. Doppler shows decreased diastolic flow, causing a high resistance index (>0.8) and low pulsatility index. However, it is a non-specific finding also seen with acute tubular necrosis, cyclosporine toxicity, acute pyelonephritis, obstruction, renal vein thrombosis and compression by perirenal collections. A high resistive index, more than 0.9, is relatively specific for acute rejection. Some centres use pulsatility index. A PI of more than 1.5 is used for diagnosing rejection. MRI shows increased cortical signal intensity and loss of corticomedullary differentiation on T1-weighted scans.

Acute tubular necrosis is common in the early post-operative period and results in reduced function, which gradually recovers over the next few weeks to months. There is no graft tenderness or fever, unlike acute rejection. The scintigraphic findings are abnormal immediately after surgery. The perfusion phase is relatively maintained well; later phases show slow washout and persistent isotope accumulation. In contrast, if the isotope study is normal in the early post-operative phase and becomes abnormal subsequently, acute rejection can be diagnosed confidently.

Thrombosis of the renal vein is rare and typically occurs in the early post-operative phase. The transplant appears swollen and hypoechoic on US. Doppler US shows the absence of flow in the veins and sharp systolic waves, with reversed diastolic flow. Resistivity index is markedly elevated.

Cyclosporine is nephrotoxic and causes a dose-dependent reduction of renal function. The imaging findings are non-specific. The perfusion phase of the 99m Tc-DTPA study is normal, but there is prolonged clearance of 99 m Tc MAG3. Normal perfusion and delayed excretion are also seen in obstruction.

Rajiah P, et al. Renal transplant imaging and complications. *Abdom Imaging.* 2006;31:735–46.

100. D. To look for a Stener lesion

Skier's thumb, otherwise known as *gamekeeper's thumb*, is an injury to the ulnar collateral ligament (UCL) of the first MCP joint. Most of the injuries to the UCL are managed conservatively. However, in complete tears, the UCL may retract and slip to lie superficial to the adductor pollicis aponeurosis or muscle. This prevents healing of the UCL as the adductor pollicis aponeurosis/muscle is now interposed between the torn ends of the UCL, which is known as a *Stener lesion*. Ultrasound is primarily performed to identify this abnormality, as this requires surgical correction. *Andersson lesion* refers to the vertebral end plate changes seen in rheumatic spondylodiscitis.

Manaster BJ, et al. *Musculoskeletal Imaging: The Requisites*, 4th edn. Philadelphia, PA: Mosby Elsevier, 2013:139.

101. D. It is never seen beyond 2 weeks.

Cortical laminar and pseudolaminar necrosis cause serpiginous cortical T1 shortening, which is not caused by calcium or haemoglobin products; rather, it presumably results from some other unknown substance or paramagnetic material, possibly lipid-laden macrophages. High cortical signal intensity may be seen on T1-weighted images 3–5 days after stroke, and in many cases it is seen about 2 weeks after stroke. Thereafter, it increases in intensity and fades after about 3 months, but in some cases it may persist for more than a year. In patients with suspected cortical laminar necrosis, susceptibility-weighted imaging may help differentiate it from haemorrhagic transformation.

Allen LM, et al. Sequence-specific MR imaging findings that are useful in dating ischemic stroke. *Radiographics.* 2012;32(5):1285–97.

102. C. It is nearly always associated with failure of neural tube closure.

Chiari II malformation is characterised by a caudally displaced fourth ventricle and brain stem, as well as tonsilar/vermian herniation through the foramen magnum.

Spinal anomalies are extremely common: lumbar meningomyelocele (>95%) and syringohydromyelia. Supratentorial abnormalities are common: dysgenesis of corpus callosum (>80%), obstructive hydrocephalus following closure of meningocoele, absent septum pellucidum, to name a few.

CT and MRI show colpocephaly (enlarged occipital horn and atria), 'batwing' configuration of frontal horns on coronal view (pointing inferiorly secondary to enlarged caudate nucleus), 'hourglass ventricle', excessive cortical gyration (stenogyria), interdigitation of medial cortical gyri, 'cerebellar peg sign', thin elongated fourth ventricle exiting below the foramen magnum, dysplastic tentorium, towering cerebellum, tethered cord and cervico-medullary kink among multiple other cranial and spinal anomalies.

It is not associated with basilar impression/C1 assimilation/Klippel-Feil deformity.

Dähnert W. *Radiology Review Manual*, 7th edn. Philadelphia, PA: Lippincott Williams & Wilkins, 2011.

103. D. Infective endocarditis

Extracardiac Complications of Infective Endocarditis

Central nervous system	Embolic stroke, intracranial haemorrhage, intracranial mycotic aneurysm, brain abscess, meningitis
Thoracic	Septic pulmonary emboli, pulmonary oedema, pulmonary abscess, pleural effusion/empyema, pneumothorax

Abdominal	Renal infarction, renal failure, splenomegaly, splenic infarction, hepatic infarction, mesenteric ischaemia
Musculoskeletal	Spondylodiscitis, osteomyelitis, septic arthritis, peripheral soft-tissue abscess
Vascular	Major arterial emboli, mycotic aneurysm (including aortic aneurysm), vasculitis (including aortitis)

Colen TW, et al. Radiologic manifestations of extra-cardiac complications of infective endocarditis. *Eur Radiol.* 2008;18:2433–45.

104. A. Focal nodular hyperplasia

Focal nodular hyperplasia (FNH) is the second most common benign liver tumour after haemangioma. FNH is classified into two types: classic (80% of cases) and non-classic (20%). Distinction between FNH and other hypervascular liver lesions such as hepatocellular adenoma, hepatocellular carcinoma and hypervascular metastases is critical to ensure proper treatment. An asymptomatic patient with FNH does not require biopsy or surgery. MRI has higher sensitivity and specificity for FNH than does US or CT. Typically, FNH is iso- or hypointense on T1-weighted images, is slightly hyper- or isointense on T2-weighted images, and has a hyperintense central scar on T2-weighted images. FNH demonstrates intense homogeneous enhancement during the arterial phase of gadolinium-enhanced imaging and enhancement of the central scar during later phases.

Hussain SM, et al. Focal nodular hyperplasia: Findings at state-of-the-art MR imaging, US, CT, and pathologic analysis. *RadioGraphics.* 2004;24:3–19.

105. A. Feeding central vessel on Doppler imaging.

US features characteristic of benign lesions have been described. These include hyperechogenicity compared to fat, an oval or well-defined, lobulated, gently curving shape and the presence of a thin echogenic pseudocapsule. Doppler examination of benign lesions shows displacement of normal vessels around the edge of the lesion. In contrast, malignant lesions show abnormal vessels that are irregular and centrally penetrating.

Adam A, et al. *Grainger & Allison's Diagnostic Radiology: A Textbook of Medical Imaging*, 5th edn. New York: Churchill Livingstone, 2008:1180.

106. B. Ewing's sarcoma

The main differential in such findings would be between infection and a primary bone tumour. Because infection has not been given as an option, the choices would be between osteosarcoma and Ewing's sarcoma. Ewing's sarcoma tends to occur in both the appendicular and axial skeleton equally, whereas osteosarcoma mostly occurs in the appendicular skeleton. Ewing's sarcoma usually begins in the diaphysis of the long bones, whereas osteosarcoma tends to occur in the metaphysis. Ewing's sarcoma may also have a large extra osseous component. The two are often differentials of each other, as each can have a large overlap of imaging findings, but the above traits can help one sway towards the other.

Dähnert W. *Radiology Review Manual*, 6th edn. Philadelphia, PA: Lippincott Williams & Wilkins, 2007:75.
Kan JH, Klienman PK. *Pediatric and Adolescent Musculoskeletal MRI – A Case Based Approach*. Secaucus, NJ: Springer-Verlag, 2007: 23–4.

107. A. Microbleeds have a worse prognosis than haematoma.

Haemorrhagic transformation demonstrates a spectrum of findings ranging from small microbleeds to large parenchymal haematoma. Several studies have reported that microbleeds are present in one-half to the majority of patients with ischaemic stroke and are seen around 48 hours after onset of symptoms. Studies have shown that these areas of microbleeding are not associated with a worse outcome, and guidelines state that the presence of fewer than five areas of microbleeding on initial MRIs does not contraindicate thrombolysis.

Parenchymal haematoma is a rarer type of haemorrhagic transformation that results from vessel wall rupture caused by high reperfusion pressure. It is more common with cardio-embolic events, is associated with hyperglycaemia, most commonly occurs in the basal ganglia, and confers a much worse prognosis.

Haemorrhagic transformation is rare in the first 12 hours after stroke onset (the hyperacute stage), particularly within the first 6 hours. When it occurs, it is usually within the first 24–48 hours and, in almost all cases, is present 4–5 days after stroke. Studies have reported that the presence of early parenchymal enhancement within 6 hours of stroke is associated with a higher risk for clinically significant haemorrhagic transformation.

Allen LM, et al. Sequence-specific MR imaging findings that are useful in dating ischemic stroke. *Radiographics*. 2012;32(5):1285–97.

108. A.   Pulmonary interstitial emphysema

MRI's excellent tissue contrast resolution allows easy differentiation between organs, allowing prenatal diagnosis of congenital diaphragmatic hernia. MRI is also useful in the evaluation of foetal lung maturation through volume and signal intensity.

Congenital cystic adenomatoid malformation (CCAM) is the most commonly diagnosed lung malformation. In CCAM, abnormal branching of the immature bronchioles and lack of normal alveolar development results in a solid/cystic intrapulmonary mass.

Most pulmonary sequestrations detected prenatally are extralobar, with an anomalous vein that drains into the systemic circulation. On T2-weighted images, they are seen as well-defined hyperintense masses with or without hypointense septa. Intralobar sequestration may be difficult to differentiate from CCAM.

MRI is also useful for evaluating other pulmonary and thoracic anomalies. Bronchogenic cysts are identified as hyperintense lesions on T2-weighted sequences; they are usually single lesions, located in the lung or mediastinum. Oesophageal duplication cysts are also identified as hyperintense mediastinal lesions. Congenital lobar emphysema can be difficult to distinguish from intralobar sequestration and from CCAM.

Pulmonary interstitial emphysema refers to the abnormal location of air within the pulmonary interstitium, resulting from rupture of over-distended alveoli following barotrauma in infants who have surfactant deficiency lung disease.

Martin C, et al. Fetal MR in the evaluation of pulmonary and digestive system pathology. *Insights Imaging*. 2012;3(3):277–93.

109. E.   Sarcoidosis

Cardiac thrombus tends to occur in older adults with a history of atrial fibrillation or ventricular aneurysm due to prior myocardial infarction. Right ventricular thrombus has been reported in patients with deep venous thrombosis, Behcet's syndrome, Loffler syndrome, endocarditis, Churg–Strauss syndrome and right atrial aneurysms. Cardiac thrombus appears as a lobular, intracavitary mass. The density and signal intensity depend on the age of the thrombus. Cardiac thrombus does not enhance. Patients with cardiac thrombus are treated with anticoagulation.

François CJ, et al. CT and MR imaging of primary, metastatic, and nonneoplastic cardiac masses. *Contemp Diagn Radiol*. 2006;29(24):1–6.

110. C.   Scleroderma

Systemic sclerosis, or scleroderma, is characterised by excessive collagen production, autoimmune disease–induced inflammation, and microvascular injury. It is divided into two subtypes: limited cutaneous systemic sclerosis and diffuse cutaneous systemic sclerosis. Limited cutaneous systemic sclerosis typically manifests as CREST syndrome, which stands for calcinosis cutis, Raynaud phenomenon, oesophageal dysmotility, sclerodactyly and telangiectasia and is generally anticentromere–antibody positive.

The systemic manifestations of systemic sclerosis are diverse. Abnormalities of the circulatory system (most notably Raynaud phenomenon) and involvement of multiple organ systems – such as the musculoskeletal, renal, pulmonary, cardiac and gastrointestinal systems – with fibrotic or vascular complications are most common. Nearly 90% of patients with systemic sclerosis have evidence of gastrointestinal involvement, which is, ultimately, a substantial cause of morbidity. The underlying pathologic change consists of smooth muscle atrophy and fibrosis caused by collagen deposition primarily in the tunica muscularis. Oesophageal involvement typically affects the distal two-thirds of the oesophagus because of the lack of striated muscle in the upper one-third. Findings of oesophageal involvement include decreased or absent oesophageal peristalsis combined with prominent gastroesophageal reflux from an incompetent lower oesophageal sphincter. Oesophagitis is frequently present, and associated complications such as oesophageal stricture or Barrett metaplasia are fairly common. Small bowel findings include hypomotility from smooth muscle atrophy and fibrosis, which leads to stasis, dilatation and pseudo-obstruction. The 'hide-bound' sign of valvular packing is a fairly specific finding and may be seen in as many as 60% of patients with scleroderma.

Bhavsar AS. Abdominal manifestations of neurologic disorders. *RadioGraphics*. 2013;33:135–53.

111. B. Anechoic mass

Carcinomas are irregular in outline, ill-defined and hypoechoic compared to the surrounding fat. They are taller than wide (AP dimension more than transverse dimension). There may be an ill-defined echogenic halo around the lesion, particularly the lateral margins, and distortion of the adjacent breast tissue, akin to spiculations, may be evident. Posterior acoustic shadowing is frequently observed, due to attenuation of the US beam by dense tissue. Doppler examinations of malignant lesions show abnormal vessels that are irregular and centrally penetrating.

Adam A, et al. *Grainger & Allison's Diagnostic Radiology: A Textbook of Medical Imaging*, 5th edn. New York: Churchill Livingstone, 2008:1184.

112. B. Dorsal intercalated segment instability (DISI)

DISI and VISI injuries refer to malalignment of the carpal rows with emphasis of the relation of the lunate to the capitate. In DISI (associated with tear of scapholunate ligament), the lunate is tilted dorsally with an increased scapholunate angle (>60 degrees) and capitolunate angle (>30 degrees). In VISI (associated with tear of the luno-triquetral ligament), there is a volar tilt of the lunate with decreased scapholunate angle (<30 degrees) and increased capitolunate angle (>30 degrees).

Manaster BJ, et al. *Musculoskeletal Imaging: The Requisites*, 4th edition. Philadelphia, PA: Mosby Elsevier, 2013:130.

113. D. Low signal on T1W MRI is seen >8 hours.

A good rule of thumb is that if the signal intensity on ADC maps is low, the stroke is less than 1 week old. Most literature indicate that in patients with ischaemic stroke, findings on FLAIR images are positive 6–12 hours after onset of symptoms. Sometimes the presence of restricted diffusion with negative findings at FLAIR imaging alone has been enough to initiate treatment.

High signal intensity is not usually seen at T2-weighted imaging until at least 8 hours after the initial ischaemic insult and continues into the chronic phase. Low signal intensity is not usually seen at T1-weighted imaging until 16 hours after the onset of stroke and persists into the chronic phase.

The pattern of contrast enhancement may help determine the age of the stroke. In ischaemic stroke, enhancement may be arterial, meningeal, or parenchymal. Arterial enhancement, dubbed the 'intravascular enhancement' sign, usually occurs first and may be seen as early as 0–2 hours after the onset of stroke. Meningeal enhancement is the rarest type of enhancement.

It occurs within the first week after onset of stroke. If parenchymal enhancement persists longer than 8–12 weeks, a diagnosis other than ischaemic stroke should be sought.

Allen LM, et al. Sequence-specific MR imaging findings that are useful in dating ischemic stroke. *Radiographics.* 2012;32(5):1285–97.

114. C. Ductus venosus

The single umbilical vein extends from the umbilicus to the left portal vein. When blood from the umbilical vein reaches the left portal vein, it is directed to the ductus venosus, which originates from the left portal vein immediately opposite the insertion site of the umbilical vein and courses cephalad to the inferior vena cava. The preferred location of the tip of the umbilical venous catheter is typically in the cephalad portion of the inferior vena cava or at the inferior vena caval–right atrial junction.

An umbilical venous catheter can be distinguished from an umbilical arterial catheter as the UVC travels cranially in the umbilical vein while the UAC travels caudally in an umbilical artery to reach a common iliac artery.

Schlesinger AE, et al. Neonates and umbilical venous catheters: Normal appearance, anomalous positions, complications, and potential aid to diagnosis. *AJR Am J Roentgenol.* 2003;180(4):1147–53.

115. D. Primary cardiac lymphomas mostly affect the left side of the heart.

Secondary malignancies involving the heart are 20–40 times more frequent than primary cardiac neoplasms.

Angiosarcoma is the most common primary cardiac malignancy of adulthood. The tumour typically involves the right atrium, and so presenting symptoms are related to obstruction to right cardiac filling and pericardial tamponade. They are heterogeneously high signal on T1 and T2-weighted images with heterogeneous enhancement.

Undifferentiated sarcoma mostly arises in the left atrium, although they can also involve the cardiac valve. It appears as an isointense irregular mass infiltrating the myocardium.

Primary cardiac lymphomas are exceedingly rare, are typically of the non-Hodgkin B-cell type and are confined to the heart or pericardium. They most commonly involve the right side of the heart, in particular the right atrium, with frequent involvement of more than one chamber and invasion of the pericardium. At MRI, they are isointense on T1-weighted images and heterogeneously hyperintense on T2-weighted images; they demonstrate heterogeneous enhancement after administration of gadolinium contrast material.

Rhabdomyosarcomas do not arise from any specific chamber, but they are more likely than any other primary cardiac sarcomas to involve the valves.

Sparrow PJ, et al. MR imaging of cardiac tumors. *Radiographics.* 2005;25(5):1255–76.

116. C. There is caudate lobe atrophy in chronic Budd–Chiari.

Budd–Chiari syndrome is a heterogeneous group of disorders characterised by hepatic venous outflow obstruction at the level of the hepatic veins, the IVC, or the right atrium. Budd–Chiari syndrome has variable imaging features. Hepatic vein or IVC thrombosis, with resultant changes in liver morphology and enhancement patterns, venous collaterals, varices, and ascites may be directly observed.

Duplex Doppler US is a useful method for detecting Budd–Chiari syndrome because it allows easy assessment of hepatic venous flow and detection of hepatic parenchymal heterogeneity. CT and MR imaging also can depict hepatic venous flow or thrombosis and IVC compression or occlusion.

In the presence of acute disease, the imaging features correspond with histologic findings of liver congestion and oedema. The liver is globally enlarged, with lower attenuation on CT images, decreased signal intensity on T1-weighted MRIs, and heterogeneously increased signal intensity on

T2-weighted MRIs, predominantly in the periphery. Differential contrast enhancement between the central and peripheral areas of liver parenchyma is a feature of acute Budd–Chiari syndrome. The more oedematous and congested peripheral regions demonstrate decreased contrast enhancement, whereas stronger enhancement is seen in the central parenchyma. After the administration of contrast material, increased enhancement is seen in areas of venous drainage that are less affected, such as the caudate lobe. The development of intra- and extrahepatic collateral veins in subacute Budd–Chiari syndrome permits the egress of venous flow, producing a more homogeneous enhancement pattern with persistent signs of oedema. In chronic Budd–Chiari syndrome, there is atrophy of the affected portions of the liver, and the parenchymal oedema is replaced by fibrosis, which results in decreased T1- and T2-weighted signal intensity at unenhanced MRI and in delayed enhancement in contrast-enhanced studies. Hypertrophy of the caudate lobe, irregularities of the liver contour, and regenerative nodules are prominent features of chronic Budd–Chiari syndrome.

Cura M. Diagnostic and interventional radiology for Budd-Chiai syndrome. *RadioGraphics*. 2009;29:669–81.

117. E. Routine breast screening

Ultrasound is not a screening tool. It is used for assessment of a palpable lump, particularly in young patients (below 30 years) and mammographically dense breasts, and in characterisation of a mammographic or palpable mass as solid or cystic. It is used for evaluation of mammographically uncertain lesion or for confirmation of lesion seen on a single projection. It is used for assessing breast discharge, suspected silicone leaks, follow-up of lesions seen on US and for guiding cyst aspiration, biopsy or wire localisation.

Dähnert W. *Radiology Review Manual*, 7th edn. Philadelphia, PA: Lippincott Williams & Wilkins, 2011:573–5.

118. E. Scheuermann disease

Scheuermann disease is a spinal disorder named after Dr Holger Scheuermann, who, in 1921, first described a structural thoracic kyphosis mainly affecting adolescents. Its best-known manifestations are multiple wedged vertebrae and thoracic kyphosis known as Scheuermann kyphosis. Its classic diagnostic criterion was '3 or more consecutive wedged thoracic vertebrae'. However, the pathological changes also include disc and end plate lesions, primarily Schmorl node and irregular vertebral end plate. Therefore, the diagnosis of 'atypical Scheuermann disease' was proposed for patients with only one or two wedged vertebrae and no notable kyphosis but characteristic disc/end plate lesions. Because atypical Scheuermann disease tends to affect the lumbar or thoracolumbar junction region instead of the thoracic spine, it is also called *lumbar Scheuermann disease*.

Liu N, et al. Radiological signs of Scheuermann disease and low back pain. Retrospective categorization of 188 hospital staff members with 6-year follow-up. *Spine*. 2014;39(20):1666–75.

119. A. Fourth ventricle enlargement

Isodense subdural haematoma are a recognised pitfall on CT, which is often difficult to recognise. Indirect signs are hence critical, midline shift; compression of the ipsilateral lateral ventricle; effacement of cerebral sulci; medial displacement of junction of grey and white matter (white matter buckling); and dilatation of contralateral lateral ventricle, which is a bad prognostic sign. In case of bilateral collections, the frontal horns lie closer than normal, giving 'rabbit ear' appearance.

Adam A, et al. *Grainger & Allison's Diagnostic Radiology: A Textbook of Medical Imaging*, 5th edn. New York: Churchill Livingstone, 2008:1343–4.

120. B. Bilateral occipital subdural haemorrhage

Subdural haemorrhage (SDH) and subarachnoid haemorrhage (SAH) are common abusive injuries. Epidural haematoma is much more often accidental. Probably the most common location of inflicted SAH, and SDH diagnosed radiologically is a layer of hyperattenuating material adjacent to the falx; bleeding at this site represents an interhemispheric extra-axial haemorrhage. In this location, it is often difficult, radiologically, to distinguish SAH from SDH, and SDH and SAH may coexist.

Lonergan GJ, et al. From the archives of the AFIP. Child abuse: Radiologic-pathologic correlation. *Radiographics.* 2003;23(4):811–45.

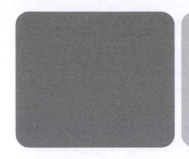

CHAPTER 3
TEST PAPER 2

Questions

Time: 3 hours

1. An intracardiac mass was incidentally detected during echocardiography in a patient undergoing preoperative assessment. Chest X-ray was non-specific, showing an enlarged heart. Which one of the following statements regarding primary benign cardiac tumours is false?
   A. Cardiac fibromas are homogenously low on T2W MRI.
   B. Cardiac lipomas are high on T1W MRI.
   C. Cardiac rhabdomyomas are associated with tuberous sclerosis.
   D. Cardiac fibroelastomas usually arise from the pericardium.
   E. Cardiac myxomas show heterogeneous signal on MRI.

2. A 40-year-old man undergoes a CT scan of the abdomen for recurrent abdominal pain. The precontrast scan showed bilateral renal calculi. A post-contrast scan showed several pancreatic lesions, measuring between 1 and 2 cm. What is the likely unifying diagnosis?
   A. MEN I
   B. MEN II A
   C. Insulinoma
   D. Glucagonoma
   E. NF1

3. A 45-year-old woman presents with a rapidly enlarging mildly painful breast mass over a period of few months. An urgent ultrasound is performed. The ultrasound shows that the mass measures 7 cm, filling up almost the entire breast with fluid-filled clefts in the tumour. What is the diagnosis?
   A. Inflammatory carcinoma
   B. Cystosarcoma phylloides
   C. Complex breast cyst
   D. Invasive lobular carcinoma
   E. Breast lymphoma

4. Osteoid osteomas:
   A. Are aggressive bone lesions with malignant potential
   B. Are referred to as *osteoblastomas* when larger than 3 cm
   C. Are typically cortical rather than subcortical-based lesions
   D. Typically require surgical curettage and resection
   E. Are more common in women

5. A 67-year-old known alcoholic man with acute onset neurological symptoms has been referred for an urgent CT brain to exclude haemorrhage. CT shows an isodense subdural on the right, but the history of trauma was 24 hours earlier with no previous history of head

injury or fall. All of the following are causes of isodense subdural haematoma on CT following head trauma, except

A. A 2-week-old head injury with subdural haemorrhage
B. Acute subdural haematoma in a patient with Hb 7.5 g/dL
C. Chronic haematoma in a patient with coagulopathy
D. Patient with an associated arachnoid tear
E. Patient with leptomeningeal metastasis

6. A child presents with intermittent abdominal pain, vomiting, and a right upper-quadrant mass. On clinical examination, blood is noted on rectal examination. A clinical diagnosis of intussusception is made. Where is the most common site of intussusception in this population group?

A. Ileoileal
B. Ileocolic
C. Ileoileocolic
D. Colocolic
E. Jejunoileal

7. A 29-year-old woman with fever, malaise, fatigue, intermittent pain and numbness in both hands and feet, and normal chest radiograph is referred for MRI thorax. MRI shows wall thickening of the origin of the right subclavian artery and both carotid arteries. What is the diagnosis?

A. Moyamoya disease
B. Takayasu arteritis
C. Churg–Strauss disease
D. PAN
E. Wegener's granulomatosis

8. A slimly built 60-year-old woman presents with anorexia, diarrhoea, and weight loss. Barium meal shows multiple filling defects in the stomach with thickened gastric rugae. Colonoscopy shows multiple colonic polyps. The top differential is

A. Peutz–Jeghers syndrome
B. Familial adenomatous polyposis
C. Cronkhite–Canada syndrome
D. Cowden syndrome
E. Turcot's syndrome

9. A middle-aged woman presents to the breast clinic with a few weeks' history of vague breast pain and lumpiness. On further direct questioning, she reveals a history of trauma to the breast a few months ago. Mammogram shows a well-defined circular mass with central translucency and eggshell calcification. What is the most likely diagnosis?

A. Cystosarcoma phylloides
B. Complex breast cyst
C. Invasive lobular carcinoma
D. Fat necrosis
E. Fibroadenoma

10. A 60-year-old patient is admitted for progressive thoracic back pain with a low-grade fever, which has been going on for several weeks. Routine chest radiograph reveals no abnormality. An MRI of the spine reveals minimal intervertebral disc space reduction at T4/5 with hyperintensity of the disc. There is adjacent vertebral end plate oedema and irregularity. A well-defined and

predominantly high T2W signal collection is noted, extending beneath the anterior longitudinal ligament and cranially to reach the level of T2. What is the most likely diagnosis?

A. Pyogenic discitis

B. Insufficiency fracture with ongoing collapse, complicated by chronic vertebral osteomyelitis

C. Degenerative disc disease with Modic Type II end plate changes

D. Pott disease

E. Vertebral lymphoma

11. A 16-year-old boy with progressive extra-pyramidal symptoms, dementia and positive family history was sent for an MRI brain by his neurologist. MRI showed bilaterally symmetric hyperintense signal changes in the anterior medial globus pallidus with surrounding hypointensity in the globus pallidus on T2W images, commonly described as 'eye of the tiger' sign. Caudate was normal and no other areas of signal change was demonstrated. What is the diagnosis?

A. Wilson disease

B. Huntington disease

C. MELAS

D. Hallervorden–Spatz disease

E. CADASIL

12. A 2-year-old boy presents with a large abdominal mass and there is suspicion of an underlying neuroblastoma. Which feature would be supportive of this diagnosis with the highest confidence?

A. Calcification is uncommon.

B. Well circumscribed.

C. Displaces major vessels rather than encasing them.

D. Encases major vessels but does not invade them.

E. Claw of renal tissue extends partially around the mass.

13. A 73-year-old woman with previous history of myocardial infarction was referred for a chest radiograph by her GP to exclude chest infection. No infective focus was identified but a focal bulge was noticed in the left heart border, with curvilinear calcification along the edge. What is the diagnosis?

A. Myocardial calcification

B. Right atrial calcification

C. Mitral annulus calcification

D. Calcified vegetations

E. Left ventricular aneurysm calcification

14. A 70-year-old man presents with rectal bleeding. Flexible sigmoidoscopy shows a circumferential tumour in the upper third of the anal canal. An MRI performed for staging shows locoregional lymphadenopathy. The lymph node group most likely to be involved is

A. Superficial inguinal

B. Common iliac

C. Pudendal

D. External iliac

E. Paraortic

15. A fit and healthy 25-year-old woman presents to the breast clinic with a small mobile non-tender breast lump that she noticed incidentally. An ultrasound is deemed as the first-line

investigation; it reveals an extremely well-defined homogenous, hypoechoic oval mass with posterior acoustic shadowing. What is the most likely diagnosis?
A. Cystosarcoma phylloides
B. Fibroadenoma
C. Complex breast cyst
D. Invasive lobular carcinoma
E. Fat necrosis

16. A 35-year-old weightlifter presents to the orthopaedic clinic with pain in the right shoulder. An initial radiograph is normal and no abnormality is identified on US. An MRI is suggested for further evaluation; it reveals increased T2W signal changes with fatty atrophy of the teres minor muscle. What is the likely diagnosis?
A. Parsonage–Turner syndrome
B. Spinoglenoid notch paralabral cyst
C. Duchenne's muscular dystrophy
D. Quadrilateral space syndrome
E. Acute rotator cuff tear

17. A 45-year-old male patient with low back pain, rectal bleeding and faecal incontinence is investigated with CT and MRI. CT shows an enhancing soft-tissue mass replacing the sacrum with areas of amorphous calcifications. On MRI, the lesion shows low to intermediate signal on T1W and high signal on T2W images. What is your diagnosis?
A. Sacral meningocoele
B. Sacral chordoma
C. Central dural ectasia
D. Rhabdomyosarcoma
E. Sacrococcygeal teratoma

18. A 3-year-old girl presents with a cough, temperature and hyperinflated left lower zone, elevating the left hilum. What is the likeliest diagnosis?
A. Congenital lobar emphysema
B. Viral pneumonia
C. Cystic fibrosis
D. Pulmonary sequestration
E. Inhaled foreign body

19. A 72-year-old man presents to the vascular surgeon with abdominal pain 4 months after endovascular repair of an abdominal aortic aneurysm. An emergency dual phase contrast-enhanced CT is performed. The unenhanced images reveal high-density material interposed between the stent and the wall of the aorta. There is further enhancement of this high-density area on arterial phase images. The graft and the attachments look intact. What is the most likely diagnosis?
A. Type I endoleak
B. Type II endoleak
C. Type III endoleak
D. Type IV endoleak
E. Type V endoleak

20. A 76-year-old woman with 6 months' history of progressive weight loss and altered bowel habits is referred for a CT scan of the abdomen and pelvis. The examination shows several hypoattenuating lesions on Segments II and III of the liver that are highly suspicious for malignancy. Blood biochemistry with tumour markers shows a normal AFP and CA 19–9 but raised CEA. LFTs are minimally deranged. The case is discussed at MDT.

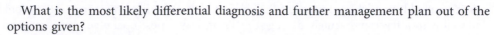

What is the most likely differential diagnosis and further management plan out of the options given?
A. Primary hepatocellular carcinoma – liver biopsy
B. Hepatic adenoma – liver resection
C. Probable lung cancer – CT chest
D. Metastatic renal carcinoma – renal biopsy
E. Metastasis from colonic adenocarcinoma – colonoscopy

21. A late-middle-aged woman undergoes an MRI breast with contrast to investigate a clinically palpable nodularity. Fat-suppressed 3D images show a 3-cm well-defined abnormality with peripheral enhancement. Which of the following statements regarding enhancement pattern is incorrect?
A. Rim enhancement is a non-specific finding.
B. Fat content is a sign of benignity.
C. Homogenous enhancement is a sign of benignity.
D. Centripetal spread of contrast is more common in carcinomas.
E. Homogenous high T2 signal suggests malignancy.

22. Which statement is not associated with transient patellar dislocation?
A. The medial patellar retinaculum frequently demonstrates high T2W signal changes.
B. A tibial tuberosity to trochlear groove distance of <1.5 cm.
C. Trochlear dysplasia is a predisposing condition.
D. There is an increase in the ratio of the patellar tendon to the patellar length.
E. Bone contusions of the anterolateral aspect of the lateral femoral condyle.

23. A 45-year-old patient with chronically progressive low back pain is referred for an MRI scan. Sagittal T1W and T2W MRI lumbar spine show dehydration of the L4/5 disc, with low signal to the disc on T2. High signal is noted in the adjacent end plates of the L4 and L5 vertebra on both the T1W and T2W sequences. There is no cortical destruction. How would you report the finding?
A. Modic Type I end plate change
B. Modic Type II end plate change
C. Andersson lesion
D. Modic Type III end plate change
E. Discitis

24. A 4-year-old boy falls off his bike and complains of neck pain. Which of the following features is worrying for a serious injury on plain cervical X-rays?
A. Atlanto-axial distance <5 mm
B. Displacement of 6 mm of the lateral masses relative to the dens
C. Absence of lordosis
D. Disruption of the spinolamellar line
E. Anterior subluxation of C2 on C3

25. A 77-year-old man is brought into A&E with progressive increase in back pain. There is a history of known moderately large aortic aneurysm in the notes. A contrast CT is organised because the patient is haemodynamically stable. CT does not show any evidence of a ruptured aneurysm. All of the following are findings of pending rupture, except
A. Drape sign
B. Tangential calcium sign
C. Focal discontinuous intimal calcification
D. Retroperitoneal haematoma
E. High attenuation crescent

26. A 56-year-old man with a history of PSC has an orthotopic liver transplant. He becomes unwell with a fever and acutely deranged LFTs on Day 4 post-operative. An ultrasound is subsequently performed. What is the likely cause of his symptoms?
    A. Hepatic vein thrombosis
    B. Portal vein thrombosis
    C. Hepatic artery thrombosis
    D. CBD ligation and cholangitis
    E. Gangrenous cholecystitis with perforation

27. A young woman with a palpable nodule in the breast undergoes a contrast-enhanced MRI breast for further evaluation. MRI demonstrates typical multiple non-enhancing internal septations. What is the diagnosis?
    A. Fibrocystic change
    B. Abscess
    C. Atypia
    D. Fibroadenoma
    E. Hydatid cyst

28. A 21-year-old man presents with an acute knee injury following a violent tackle in a game of ice hockey. He is unable to weight-bear. Plain film reveals a small elliptical bone fragment just adjacent to the lateral tibial plateau on the AP view. There is also an accompanying suprapatellar joint effusion. Based on the plain film findings and the mechanism of injury, what is the most commonly injured structure in this injury pattern?
    A. Medial meniscus
    B. Lateral meniscus
    C. Anterior cruciate ligament
    D. Posterior cruciate ligament
    E. Lateral collateral ligament

29. A 36-year-old male patient with acute exacerbation of low back pain shows an 8×5 mm intermediate signal fragment lying in the epidural space with signal characteristics closely matching the lower lumbar discs. However, no definite continuity can be established with any of the local discs. Inflammatory markers and white cell count are normal. The most likely cause for this appearance would be
    A. Disc extrusion
    B. Disc protrusion
    C. Meningioma
    D. Schmorl node
    E. Sequestrated disc

30. A young boy undergoes an MCUG, which shows reflux of contrast into the right ureter and pelvicalyceal system. The ureter and pelvicalyceal system are not dilated. What grade is the reflux?
    A. 1
    B. 2
    C. 3
    D. 4
    E. 5

31. A 66-year-old man with central chest pain radiating to the back is brought into the A&E department. A chest X-ray is read as unremarkable and a contrast CT is organised. The contrast CT shows an acute dissection flap in the aortic arch at the origin of the left common carotid trunk extending through the descending thoracic aorta, into the proximal

abdominal aorta at the level of the renal arteries. Which of the following best classifies this dissection type?
- A. DeBakey 1 – Stanford A
- B. DeBakey 2 – Stanford A
- C. DeBakey 3 – Stanford A
- D. DeBakey 1 – Stanford B
- E. DeBakey 2 – Stanford B

32. A 22-year-old man with mucocutaneous skin pigmentation around the lips and hand presents to the A&E department with acute colicky abdominal pain. Plain radiograph and subsequent CT of the abdomen show multiple dilated loops of small bowel with a transition point in the distal ileum associated with an ileo-ileal intussusception. What is the most likely diagnosis?
- A. Gardner's syndrome
- B. Peutz–Jeghers syndrome
- C. Cowdens syndrome
- D. Turcot syndrome
- E. TAR syndrome

33. All of the following are accepted indications for MRI breast in breast cancer imaging, except
- A. Response to chemotherapy
- B. Patients with breast augmentation
- C. High-risk screening
- D. Differentiate residual disease from post-surgical scar
- E. Breast cancer recurrence

34. A 66-year-old woman presents with back pain that radiates down the left anterior thigh towards the medial aspect of the knee. What are the MRI lumbar spine findings that you may expect based on the clinical history?
- A. L1/2 generalised disc bulge with left lateral recess stenosis
- B. L1/2 disc bulge with left foraminal stenosis
- C. L2/3 generalised disc bulge with left lateral recess stenosis
- D. L2/3 generalised disc bulge with left neural foraminal stenosis
- E. L3/4 generalised disc bulge with left lateral recess stenosis

35. A CT abdomen done on a 38-year-old woman with pancreatitis incidentally shows the presence of split cord syndrome with a central bony bridge in the vertebra. A horseshoe kidney is evident. All of the following are other well-described associations seen in patients with diastematomyelia, except
- A. Thickened filum
- B. Club foot
- C. Cord tethering
- D. Chiari malformation
- E. Congenital dislocation of hips

36. Which of the following is false?
- A. Posterior oesophageal impression and normal trachea — Right aortic arch with aberrant left subclavian artery
- B. Normal trachea and anterior oesophageal indentation — Aberrant right subclavian artery
- C. Posterior tracheal and anterior oesophageal indentation — Pulmonary artery sling

D.	Anterior tracheal and posterior oesophageal indentation	Double aortic arch
E.	Reverse '3' indentation of the oesophagus and normal trachea	Coarctation of the aorta

37. An 8-week old boy presents with profound cyanosis with associated congestive cardiac failure. Imaging demonstrates a localised concurrent aortic coarctation. The likeliest underlying diagnosis would be
   A. Tetralogy of Fallot
   B. Truncus arteriosus
   C. Transposition of the great arteries
   D. Hypoplastic left heart syndrome
   E. Tricuspid atresia

38. All the following are useful features for differentiating true lumen from false lumen, except
   A. In case of lumen wrapping, the inner lumen is true.
   B. Beak sign indicates a false lumen.
   C. A false lumen is often larger than a true lumen.
   D. A cobweb sign demarcates the true lumen.
   E. Intimal calcification surrounds the true lumen.

39. Contrast-enhanced CT performed on a 52-year-old man showed a hypodense liver with low attenuation rim around the portal tracts. The following differential diagnoses are recognised causes of periportal halo sigh, except
   A. Blunt trauma to the liver
   B. Hepatitis
   C. Congestive heart disease
   D. Obesity
   E. Cardiac tamponade

40. All of the following are technical requirements for performing an MRI breast, except
   A. Supine position
   B. Breast coil
   C. Intravenous contrast
   D. Thin slices
   E. T1W images

41. A 74-year-old man presents with neck pain, with right upper-arm pain and radicular symptoms at the lateral aspect of the forearm and tingling in the thumb. What is the most likely finding on the MRI?
   A. Central disc bulge at C3/4 with severe cord compression
   B. Right foraminal disc osteophyte at C2/3
   C. Right foraminal disc osteophyte at C4/5
   D. Right foraminal disc osteophyte at C5/6
   E. Right foraminal disc osteophyte at C3/4

42. A 35-year-old man involved in a major RTA undergoes a lateral view of the cervical spine in the resus on arrival. All of the following are features associated with atlanto-occipital dislocation, except
   A. Soft-tissue swelling anterior to C2 by >10 mm.
   B. Basion dens interval >12 mm.
   C. Odd's ratio >1.
   D. X-ray can often be normal.
   E. Incongruity of articular surface of atlas and occipital condyles.

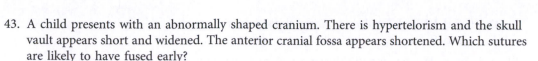

43. A child presents with an abnormally shaped cranium. There is hypertelorism and the skull vault appears short and widened. The anterior cranial fossa appears shortened. Which sutures are likely to have fused early?
    A. Sagittal
    B. Coronal
    C. Metopic
    D. Lambdoid
    E. Unilateral coronal and lambdoid

44. A 37-year-old woman with newly diagnosed hypertension undergoes an MRA, which shows alternate areas of stricture and dilatation to the right renal artery, sparing the origin. Which of the following is the least likely association?
    A. String-of-beads appearance of the contralateral renal artery
    B. String-of-beads appearance of the extracranial internal carotid artery
    C. String-of-beads appearance of the retinal artery
    D. String-of-beads appearance of the vertebral artery
    E. String-of-beads appearance of the SMA

45. A 40-year-old man with a known history of primary haemochromatosis was referred for assessment of the liver with an MRI scan. Which option shows the expected signal characteristics of the liver with iron deposition?
    A. Hyperintense liver relative to spleen on T1 and T2
    B. Hypointense liver relative to spleen on T1 and T2
    C. Isointense liver relative to spleen on T1 and T2
    D. Signal drop-out in the liver on out-of-phase T1 imaging
    E. High-signal liver on the high B-value diffusion-weighted sequences

46. A 47-year-old woman presents to the breast clinic with a palpable lump. Mammography shows a well-circumscribed round mass with mixed dense and radiolucent areas surrounded by a thin radiopaque capsule. Targeted ultrasound performed in the clinic shows a sharply defined, encapsulated, round, heterogeneous mass with echo texture similar to surrounding breast. MRI breast reveals a lesion heterogeneous on T1W and T2W images. What findings on MRI confirm the diagnosis?
    A. Non-enhancing internal septations
    B. Slowly enhancing peripheral rim
    C. Solid homogenous enhancing lesion with well-defined margins
    D. Peripheral hyperintense cystic spaces on T2W images
    E. Thin hypointense pseudocapsule and fat content on T1W images

47. What is the primary role of a T2W fluid-sensitive sequence in an MRI shoulder arthrographic study with intra-articular administration of gadolinium?
    A. To check for glenoid labral tears
    B. To check for articular cartilage integrity
    C. To check for extra-articular fluid
    D. To determine whether there is a full-thickness rotator cuff tear with communication to the bursae
    E. To increase the visual contrast of the soft-tissue structures

48. A 35-year-old man involved in a major RTA undergoes a facial series due to marked swelling and bruising of the face. All of the following are true of Lefort fractures, except
    A. By definition, the pterygoid plates have to be fractured.
    B. Lefort I involves the maxilla and medial wall of the orbit.
    C. Lefort III involves the maxilla and the medial and lateral wall of the orbit.

D. Lefort III is also called *craniofacial disjunction.*

E. Lefort II fracture is also called *pyramidal fracture.*

49. A 46-year-old woman with Marfan's syndrome presents to the A&E department with progressive worsening of central chest pain radiating to the back. Clinically, there is a differential blood pressure between the two arms, and aortic dissection is strongly suspected. CECT chest confirms the dissection and shows its distribution involving the arch of the aorta and ascending aorta. Which one of the following complications is least likely to occur with this type of dissection?

A. Aortic valve insufficiency

B. Haemopericardium

C. Mitral valve insufficiency

D. Cardiac tampondae

E. Myocardial infarction

50. A 38-year-old man with a 6-month history of dark coloured urine presents to his GP. He has a history of inflammatory bowel disease. LFTs are found to be deranged on blood work-up and he is then referred for an US liver. US shows non-specific coarsening of liver echotexture suspicious for cirrhosis. A subsequent MRCP shows multiple focal strictures in the intrahepatic bile ducts alternating with normal calibre. What is the likely diagnosis?

A. Primary biliary cirrhosis

B. Primary sclerosing cholangitis

C. Haemochromatosis

D. Glycogen storage disease

E. Cholangiocarcinoma

51. A 30-year-old woman who is 36 weeks pregnant is being evaluated with targeted ultrasound to investigate a recently noticed breast lump. Ultrasound images are reported to show a well-circumscribed, wider than tall, hypoechoic, solid mass corresponding to the abnormality. Follow-up imaging to assess stability shows progressive regression in size of the mass post-partum. What is the likely diagnosis?

A. Fibrocystic change

B. Fat necrosis

C. Inflamed intramammary node

D. Lactating adenoma

E. Breast hamartoma

52. A 17-year-old Afro-Caribbean boy presents with multiple painful soft-tissue masses around the right hip, some of which are ulcerating whitish fluid. Plain radiograph reveals a dense lobulated calcified mass with normal underlying bones at the right hip. His blood biochemistry is normal and there is no known history of renal or metabolic disease. What is the likely diagnosis?

A. Renal osteodystrophy

B. Lympocele with infection

C. Scleroderma

D. Burkitt's lymphoma

E. Tumoural calcinosis

53. A 38-year-old man with back pain and sensory deficit in both lower limbs shows widening interpedicular distance on plain radiograph of the lumbar spine extending over four vertebral lengths. MRI reveals a hypointense rim around a well-defined lesion on T2W images, with intense enhancement on post-gadolinium images. What is the diagnosis?

A. Astrocytoma

B. Ganglioglioma

C. Neurofibroma

D. Ependymoma

E. Subependymoma

54. Chest X-ray of a boy shows shift of the heart and mediastinum to the right. There is also a tubular structure parallel to the right heart border with its maximum width close to the diaphragm. The finding suggests

A. ASD

B. Scimitar syndrome

C. Total anomalous pulmonary venous return

D. Intralobar sequestration

E. Inhaled foreign body

55. A 67-year-old woman with 5.5 cm atherosclerotic abdominal aortic aneurysm is being worked up for a potential aortic endograft repair. All of the following are important imaging observations to be determined prior to treatment, except

A. Tortuosity of the aorta

B. Diameter of aortic aneurysms

C. Non-thrombosed residual lumen of the aneurysm

D. Flow characteristic at the aneurysm neck

E. Length of proximal and distal landing zones

56. A 16-year-old girl presents to a gastroenterologist with intermittent episodes of diarrhoea, weight loss and abdominal discomfort over the past 2 years. A full blood count done shows macrocytic anaemia. She is referred for a barium small bowel follow-through examination to assess the small bowel. The barium study reveals several discontinuous ileal strictures with alternate areas of dilatation. The terminal ileum is distinctly abnormal, with ulceration with 'cobblestoning'. What is the most likely diagnosis?

A. Ulcerative colitis

B. Coeliac disease

C. Whipple's disease

D. Crohn's disease

E. Tuberculosis

57. With regard to mammography and MRI breast, which is incorrect?

	Mammography	Breast MRI
A.	Less expensive	More expensive
B.	Poor tissue resolution	Better tissue resolution
C.	No information on vascularity	Information regarding vascularity
D.	Poorer visualisation of posterior breast tissue	Better visualisation of posterior breast tissue
E.	Needs IV contrast	Does not need IV contrast

58. A 52-year-old man with painful hands and feet is referred for plain film imaging by his family doctor. Radiographs of both hands demonstrate bilateral resorption of the distal phalangeal tufts of the hands and feet. All the conditions below are differentials, except for

A. Psoriasis

B. Diffuse idiopathic skeletal hyperostosis

C. Scleroderma

D. Thermal injury

E. Raynaud disease

59. A 53-year-old woman with known retinal lesion undergoes an MRI of the spine in a regional neuroimaging centre. The MRI reveals a well-defined hyperintense lesion on T2W sequences with internal flow voids and intense enhancement in association with syringohydromyelia. What is the diagnosis?
    A. Ependymoma
    B. Astrocytoma
    C. Haemangioblastoma
    D. Lymphoma
    E. Metastasis

60. A 6-year-old boy presents with increasing pain within his upper back, which came on insidiously over a few weeks. The child is otherwise well. A radiograph of his thoracic spine reveals collapse of the T9 vertebral body. The disc spaces are preserved; there is no kyphosis and no involvement of the posterior elements. Which of the following is the most likely diagnosis?
    A. Ewing's sarcoma
    B. Metastasis
    C. Tuberculosis
    D. Fracture
    E. Langerhans cell histiocytosis

61. A 72-year-old man with a 5.8 cm aortic aneurysm increasing at a rate of 1.2 cm every year is being worked up for an EVAR. Planning CT with multiformatted images and 3D volume–rendered reconstructed images have been obtained. All of the following measurements need to be provided at the MDT by the vascular radiologist, except
    A. Size of aorta at the level of the renal artery
    B. Size of aorta at the bifurcation
    C. Largest diameter of the aneurysm
    D. Size of the common iliac artery
    E. Distance from aortic bifurcation to common iliac bifurcation

62. A 47-year-old admitted with acute diverticulitis becomes more unwell with swinging pyrexia, right upper-quadrant pain, and acutely deranged LFTs. US liver shows several ill-defined hypoechoic areas with very little posterior acoustic enhancement and some floating internal echoes. What is the diagnosis?
    A. Hydatid disease
    B. Liver metastasis
    C. Multifocal HCC
    D. Pyogenic liver abscess
    E. Infected simple cysts

63. Which of the following is malignant calcification in the breast?
    A. Stellate
    B. Pleomorphic
    C. Punctate
    D. Curvilinear
    E. Popcorn

64. Scaphoid waist fracture healing is often complicated by avascular necrosis, non-union, or delayed union. Which of the following is the primary reason for this?
    A. The blood supply to the distal pole enters at the proximal pole.
    B. The blood supply of the proximal pole enters at the waist.
    C. It is a difficult fracture to immobilise.

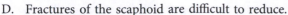

D. Fractures of the scaphoid are difficult to reduce.

E. Fractures are often comminuted.

65. A 72-year-old man with a known malignancy undergoes a spinal MRI for characterisation of multilevel vertebral collapse identified on plain radiograph. All of the following are true about malignant vs osteoporotic causes of vertebral fractures, except

A. The involved vertebra are low on T1W images.

B. Paraspinal mass is useful in differentiating metastatic from benign fracture.

C. DWI can differentiate between malignant and benign compression fracture.

D. Posterior bulging of collapsed vertebral body suggests metastasis.

E. Acute osteoporotic fractures show intense enhancement post-contrast.

66. A 4-year-old child presents with short stature and failure to grow. Plain radiographs reveal multiple abnormalities, including generalised increased density of long bones with thickened cortices, widened cranial sutures, Wormian bones, hypoplastic mandible and shortened pointed distal phalanges. Which of the following is the most likely diagnosis?

A. Pyknodysostosis

B. Osteopetrosis

C. Cleidocranial dysostosis

D. Osteosclerosis

E. Kinky hair syndrome

67. An 83-year-old man with a history of bladder cancer and myocardial infarction was referred for radiofrequency ablation (RFA) because of his co-morbidities. All of the following are true regarding RFA, except

A. RFA uses high frequency alternating current to generate heat and high temperature to cause cell death.

B. Cell death occurs by denaturation of proteins (coagulative necrosis).

C. The tip of the electrode is placed in the centre of the lesion.

D. The heat sink effect results in a poor outcome in larger lesions.

E. Cell death starts at 49 degrees.

68. A 76-year-old woman with anorexia, weight loss, and obstructive LFTs worsening over a period of 6 months presents to a gastroenterologist. She has been referred for an MRCP, which shows extensive dilatation of the intrahepatic bile ducts secondary to a long segment stricture at the proximal CBD. Distal CBD and pancreatic duct are normal. The most likely diagnosis is

A. Post-infective stricture

B. Cholangiocarcinoma

C. Intraductal stones

D. Mirizzi syndrome

E. Ampullary carcinoma

69. A 53-year-old woman presents to the breast clinic with a palpable left axillary node. Biopsy reveals adenocarcinoma, likely secondary to breast primary. Clinical examination is unremarkable. This is followed by a normal ultrasound and a mammogram, which was interpreted to be normal. MRI demonstrated a 1.5 cm slightly irregular heterogeneously enhancing lesion in the left breast and a second smaller enhancing nodule. What management should the reporting radiologist suggest?

A. Likely benign disease. Follow-up imaging in 6 months.

B. Ignore. Routine follow-up.

C. Masses only visible on MRI and not on mammogram; does not require biopsy.

D. Suspicious masses need biopsy.

E. Advanced disease. Straight to mastectomy.

70. A 24-year-old man presents to his family doctor with chronic hindfoot pain. Plain radiographs reveal elongation of the anterior dorsal calcaneus on lateral projection of the foot, often described as *anteater's nose*. What is the diagnosis?

A. Talocalcaneal coalition

B. Calcaneonavicular coalition

C. Talonavicular coalition

D. Calcaneocuboid coalition

E. Cubonavicular coalition

71. All of the following tumours are associated with drop metastasis, except

A. Medulloblastoma

B. PNET

C. Ependymoma

D. Melanoma

E. Pineocytoma

72. A female child with short stature presents with gradual onset hearing loss. Diagnostic work-up reveals micromelic dwarfism, diffuse demineralisation and thinning of cortical bone, mild scoliosis, and old fractures of the vertebral bodies and long bones. There is evidence of poor dentition. Which of the following is the most likely diagnosis?

A. Hypophosphatasia

B. Osteogenesis imperfecta

C. Paget's disease

D. Osteoporosis

E. Achondroplasia

73. A 66-year-old man with hepatocellular carcinoma is being worked up for transcatheter arterial chemoembolisation (TACE) of the liver. All of the following are correct regarding TACE of the liver, except

A. TACE is useful in patients with Child–Pugh Class C Cirrhosis.

B. It is essential to assess patency of the portal vein.

C. Biliary surgery increases complications.

D. Normal liver receives only a third of its blood from the hepatic artery.

E. Diffuse involvement of the liver results in a poor outcome.

74. A 67-year-old man with a family history of colorectal cancer and a background history of COPD has been referred for a screening barium enema, which shows multiple small filling defects throughout the descending and sigmoid colon but no colonic mass. The most likely diagnosis is

A. Hereditary non-polyposis syndrome

B. Ulcerative colitis

C. Crohn's disease

D. Colonic serosal metastasis

E. Pneumatosis coli

75. A 42-year-old man with known ankylosing spondylitis presents to the A&E department with blood in the urine and right loin pain. CT urogram performed out-of-hours showed calyceal horns and signet ring appearance on excretory phase study. The most likely cause would be

A. Renal TB

B. Acute pyelonephritis

C. Acute tubular necrosis

D. Right renal stone

E. Renal papillary necrosis

76. A 44-year-old man presents to the A&E department with acute exacerbation of knee pain and recurrent episodes of locking. Plain radiograph performed in the A&E department showed multiple calcified/ossified loose bodies in the suprapatellar pouch and behind the knee with underlying tricompartmental OA (osteoarthritis) like changes. What is the diagnosis?

A. CPPD

B. Primary synovial osteochondromatosis

C. Secondary synovial osteochondromatosis

D. Gout

E. Haemophilia

77. A 63-year-old man with worsening bilateral leg pain has been sent for an MRI. The MRI report stated secondary spinal canal stenosis at multiple levels involving the lumbar spine. All the following are causes of acquired canal stenosis, except

A. Ligamentum flavum hypertrophy

B. Facet joint hypertrophy

C. Epidural lipomatosis

D. Congenital short pedicles

E. Disc herniation

78. A 10-year-old girl of Jewish descent presents with pain in her left thigh. A radiograph reveals diffuse medullary osteoporosis, a 'flask shaped' distal femur, a serpentine area of sclerosis within the femoral metaphysis, and a sharply circumscribed endosteal lytic lesion in the distal femur with a pathological fracture. Clinical examination reveals splenomegaly. Which of the following is the most likely diagnosis?

A. Thalassaemia

B. Osteopetrosis

C. Diaphyseal aclasis

D. Gaucher disease

E. Rickets

79. All of the following statements regarding post-embolisation syndrome following a TACE procedure are true, except

A. It depends on the histology of the tumour being treated.

B. It is caused by tumour necrosis or damage to liver tissue.

C. There is elevation of hepatic transaminase levels.

D. Abdominal pain, fever, malaise and vomiting are reported.

E. It does not prolong hospital stay.

80. A 45-year-old man with a known history of a polyposis syndrome presents to the emergency department with abdominal distention and bloating. A CT scan of the abdomen and pelvis reveals a large soft-tissue density mass within the small bowel mesentery displacing the bowel loops and compressing the right ureter with resultant hydronephrosis. Which of the following options describes the likely tumour and underlying polyposis syndrome?

A. Desmoid tumour – Gardner's syndrome

B. Desmoid tumour – Turcot syndrome

C. Desmoid tumour – Cronkhite–Canada syndrome

D. Carcinoid syndrome

E. Desmoid tumour – MEN syndrome

81. All the following are correct regarding the use of MR urography (MRU) except
   A. Cine MRU is useful for assessing stenosis.
   B. Diuretic administration improves the quality of MR excretory urogram.
   C. Diuretic administration reduces the time during which images can be obtained.
   D. Motion suppression is critical for MR urography.
   E. Oral hydration can reduce quality due to fluid-filled bowel loops on T2 FSE.

82. When performing an MR arthrogram, what is the correct concentration of gadolinium (Gd-DTPA, Magnovist) that should be injected into the joint prior to imaging?
   A. 0.01 mmol/L
   B. 0.1 mmol/L
   C. 2.0 mmol/L
   D. 20 mmol/L
   E. 200 mmol/L

83. Plain radiograph of a 9-month-old baby girl shows a large soft-tissue mass in the pelvis with punctate calcification. MRI reveals a large, lobulated, sharply demarcated tumour with extremely heterogeneous signal on T1W images. What is the diagnosis?
   A. Anterior sacral meningocoele
   B. Sacrococcygeal teratoma
   C. Caudal regression syndrome
   D. Rhabdomyosarcoma
   E. Rectal duplication

84. A skeletal survey was performed on a 2-year-old boy with short stature. The lateral film of the spine revealed abnormal vertebral bodies with a central anterior 'beak' and generalised flattening. Radiographs of the hands showed a pointed proximal fifth metacarpal base with a notch at the ulnar aspect. Which of the following is the most likely diagnosis?
   A. Hunter syndrome
   B. Hurler syndrome
   C. Morquio syndrome
   D. Achondroplasia
   E. Nail–patella syndrome

85. A middle-aged woman underwent uterine fibroid embolisation (UFE) recently. All of the following statements regarding prognosis are correct, except
   A. The enhancement pattern correlates well with treatment response.
   B. Pedunculated fibroids with narrow pedicle are unfavourable.
   C. Fibroids more than 15 cm in size may continue to give bulk symptoms.
   D. Progressive liquefaction of fibroid post-treatment results in a high signal on T2W images.
   E. Fibroids with high T1 signal pretreatment respond better to UFE.

86. A 66-year-old woman with chronic right upper-quadrant pain, anorexia and weight loss is referred by her GP for a CT scan of her abdomen and pelvis. The scan shows an irregular hypodense mass replacing the gallbladder, with infiltration into the surrounding liver and enlarged periportal nodes. The following are risk factors for gallbladder carcinoma, except
   A. Chronic gallbladder inflammation
   B. Porcelain gallbladder
   C. Choledochal cyst
   D. Cirrhosis
   E. Ulcerative colitis

87. A 23-year-old woman with large bilateral low-density renal lesions on CT is also known to have a large posterior fossa brain tumour. Review of the old notes reveals that she has

had several visits to the ophthalmology department. The condition that she is most likely to be suffering from is

A. Tuberous sclerosis
B. Von Hippel–Lindau syndrome
C. Wunderlich syndrome
D. NF1
E. No syndrome – the findings are unrelated

88. A 32-year-old runner presents to the sports clinic with acute exacerbation of right heel pain. He is referred for an MRI study to investigate a potential underlying cause. The MRI reveals a poorly defined hypointense lesion inferior to the calcaneum on both T1W and T2W sequence. A further smaller lesion is noted beneath the first metatarsal head. There is marked contrast enhancement on the post-gadolinium sequences. What is the likely diagnosis?

A. Haemangioma
B. Mortons neuroma
C. Plantar fibromatosis
D. Abscess
E. Neurofibroma

89. An unenhanced CT brain performed on a young man with sudden severe occipital headache shows acute subarachnoid haemorrhage with most of the blood at the foramen magnum. Considering that the source is a ruptured aneurysm, what is the most likely location for the aneurysm in this patient?

A. ACOM
B. PCOM
C. ACA
D. AICA
E. PICA

90. A 4-year-old girl presents with progressive enlargement of her right thigh, with episodes of unprovoked bleeding from pigmented lesions over her right thigh, which have been present since birth. A lower limb venogram of the right leg demonstrates absence of the deep venous system, with varicose veins on the lateral aspect of the right leg. Which of the following is the most likely diagnosis?

A. Klippel–Trénaunay syndrome
B. Neurofibromatosis
C. Beckwith–Wiedemann syndrome
D. Macrodystrophia lipomatosis
E. Maffuci syndrome

91. Regarding uterine artery embolisation (UAE) for treatment of uterine fibroids, all of the following are correct, except

A. MRI is used to delineate arterial anatomy prior to treatment.
B. PVA or embospheres are used to embolise a fibroid.
C. Gel foam or coils are preferred in post-partum haemorrhage.
D. Endometritis shows signal void in the uterine cavity on all sequences.
E. Ovarian dysfunction after UAE is more common in women under 45 years.

92. A 62-year-old man with known hepatocellular carcinoma on a background of long-standing liver cirrhosis is scheduled to have a TACE procedure. Which one of the following is an absolute contraindication to TACE therapy for hepatocellular carcinoma in a cirrhotic patient?

A. Contrast medium allergy
B. Replacement of 25% of the liver by the tumour

C. Total bilirubin greater than 2 mg/dL

D. Biliary tree obstruction

E. Child–Pugh Class C cirrhosis

93. A 33-year-old woman on immunosuppressant medication presents to the urology clinic with haematuria. Review of old notes reveals a history of treated pulmonary tuberculosis. All the findings suggest renal/ureteric TB, except
A. Hydrocalyx with infundibular stenosis
B. Amorphous parenchymal calcification
C. Sawtooth ureter
D. Bilateral involvement in 75%
E. Distal ureteric calcification

94. A 60-year-old man complaining of pain at multiple sites for several months is referred for skeletal evaluation. A whole-body bone scan demonstrates diffusely increased uptake in the axial skeleton, with minimal uptake in the appendicular skeleton, soft tissues and kidneys. Which of the following is the most likely diagnosis?
A. Diffuse bone metastasis
B. Hypoparathyroidism
C. Hypothyroidism
D. Osteoporosis
E. Normal physiological uptake

95. A 65-year-old man undergoing a CT brain for right-sided weakness shows a unilocular thin-walled extra-axial CSF density lesion replacing the anterior portion of the right temporal lobe. No calcification or contrast enhancement is seen, although there is a mass effect in the form of erosion of the inner table of the skull vault. What is your diagnosis?
A. Meningioma
B. Arachnoid cyst
C. Epidermoid cyst
D. Dermoid cyst
E. Porencephalic cyst

96. A 5-year-old male child is found to have ataxic gait and multiple cranial nerve palsies. A CT scan of the brain shows an infratentorial hypodense mass with ring enhancement indenting the fourth ventricle posteriorly. Which of the following is the most likely diagnosis?
A. Lymphoma
B. Vascular malformation
C. Metastasis
D. Brainstem glioma
E. Haemangioma

97. All of the following are recognised indications for transjugular intrahepatic portosystemic shunt (TIPS), except
A. Right heart failure
B. Budd–Chiari
C. Refractory ascites
D. Acute variceal bleeding
E. Portal hypertensive gastropathy

98. A 55-year-old woman with rectal cancer diagnosed on colonoscopy undergoes a staging MRI. The scan reveals direct extension of the tumour into the vagina and spreading to five

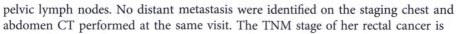

pelvic lymph nodes. No distant metastasis were identified on the staging chest and abdomen CT performed at the same visit. The TNM stage of her rectal cancer is

A. T1 N2 M0
B. T2 N0 M0
C. T3 N2 M0
D. T3 N1 M0
E. T4 N2 M0

99. A 57-year-old man with known staghorn calculus was brought to the A&E department acutely unwell. Urgent CT abdomen out-of-hours showed enlarged heterogeneous right kidney with fatty masses replacing the parenchyma. Extensive fat stranding was also seen in the peri- and pararenal spaces. The most likely diagnosis is

A. Xanthogranulomatous pyelonephritis
B. Emphysematous pyelonephritis
C. Ruptured kidney
D. Acute non-specific pyelonephritis
E. Acute papillary necrosis

100. A 9-year-old girl was taken to her family doctor with fever and painful knee and wrists. The GP noticed a skin rash, hepatosplenomegaly and lymphadenopathy. Plain X-ray of the knee and wrist shows expansion of bones around the knee and advanced carpometacarpal arthritis. What is the likely diagnosis?

A. Still disease
B. Haemophilia
C. Sickle-cell disease
D. Psoriasis
E. Lyme disease

101. A 7-year-old boy undergoes a plain CT brain for recent trauma, which reveals a cystic lesion in the cerebellum with a mural nodule laterally. No calcification is evident, but enhancement of the mural nodule is seen in post-contrast images. What is the most likely diagnosis in this patient?

A. Haemangioblastoma
B. Pilocytic astrocytoma
C. Giant cell astrocytoma
D. Pleomorphic xanthoastrocytoma
E. Lymphoma

102. A 10-year-old child is admitted with headache, visual disturbance and short stature. A suprasellar mass that is hyperintense on T1 and heterogeneous on T2 is identified. Which of the following is the most likely diagnosis?

A. Rathke cleft cyst
B. Pituitary macroadenoma
C. Pituitary microadenoma
D. Craniopharyngioma
E. Medulloblastoma

103. A 67-year-old man with several episodes of acute variceal bleeding is being investigated prior to TIPS procedure. Which one of the following is not a contraindication to TIPS?

A. Tricuspid regurgitation
B. Severe congestive cardiac failure
C. Multiple hepatic cysts
D. Severe portal hypertension
E. Unrelieved biliary obstruction

104. Which of the following is not a limitation of CT imaging in staging of rectal cancer?
    A. Poor tissue characterisation.
    B. Inability to identify T4 tumour.
    C. Non-visualisation of the mesorectal fascia.
    D. Low sensitivity, specificity and accuracy in the detection of local nodal metastasis.
    E. Sensitivity, specificity and accuracy are much lower in post-radiation evaluation.

105. A 73-year-old woman undergoing a CT urogram shows multiple filling defects in the lower third of the ureter. All of the following are possibilities, except
    A. Malakoplakia
    B. Pyeloureteritis cystica
    C. Non-radio-opaque calculi
    D. Endometriosis
    E. Retrocaval ureter

106. A 56-year-old woman with previous history of a distal radius fracture presents to her GP with progressive swelling and pain of the right hand and digits. Plain radiograph shows a healed fracture but also reveals diffuse osteopaenia involving all the small bones of the right hand with subperiosteal resorption at places. A three-phase bone scan demonstrates diffuse increased and uniform uptake involving the whole wrist. What is the likely diagnosis?
    A. Soft-tissue infection
    B. Osteomyelitis
    C. Reflex sympathetic dystrophy
    D. Vitamin D deficiency
    E. Scurvy

107. A 56-year-old man undergoes a CT brain for recent trauma, revealing a 2 × 2 cm well-defined hyperintense focus in the right frontal lobe without any mass effect or surrounding oedema. MR shows a well-defined, mulberry-shaped area of mixed signal intensity with a hypointense rim on T2W images. What is the diagnosis?
    A. Capillary telangiectasia
    B. Cavernous angioma
    C. AVM
    D. Diffuse axonal injury
    E. Evolving haematoma

108. Which one of the following is the most common intracranial tumour in children?
    A. Metastasis
    B. Astrocytoma
    C. Haemangioblastoma
    D. Craniopharyngioma
    E. None of the above

109. A 56-year-old woman post-renal transplant is being evaluated by renal ultrasound. A small amount of fluid is noted around the graft. All of the following facts are true regarding renal and vascular complications post-transplant, except
    A. Loss of corticomedullary differentiation is a feature of reduced renal function.
    B. Reversal of diastolic flow is specific for renal vein thrombosis.
    C. Extrarenal arteriovenous fistulas are related to surgical technique.
    D. Intrarenal arteriovenous fistulas are the result of percutaneous biopsy.
    E. Crescentic peritransplant fluid collections immediately post-transplantation are not usually significant.

110. A 76-year-old man with mid-rectal tumour rectal cancer who has had neoadjuvant chemoradiotherapy has been referred for a pelvic MRI to assess local treatment response. Which of the following findings on rectal MRI are predictors of disease recurrence post-treatment for rectal cancer?
    A. Mesorectal facial involvement
    B. Peritoneal reflection involvement
    C. Spiculated tumour nodules in the perirectal fat
    D. Tumour involvement of pelvic wall lymph nodes
    E. All of the above

111. An 82-year-old man complaining of increased urgency of micturition shows a markedly reduced bladder volume on ultrasound. All the following are possible explanations, except
    A. TB cystitis
    B. Schistosomiasis
    C. Previous surgery
    D. Enlarged prostate
    E. History of pelvic radiation

112. A wrist arthrogram is performed for instability and 5 mL of contrast is injected into the radiocarpal joint. The contrast is seen to extend lateral to the lunate into the mid-carpal joint. Which of the following is this diagnostic of?
    A. Contrast extravasation secondary to the large volume of contrast injected
    B. Scapholunate ligament tear
    C. Lunatotriquetral ligament tear
    D. Distal radioulnar joint (DRUJ) disruption
    E. Triangular fibrocartilage (TFC) tear

113. A 52-year-old obtunded patient is admitted to ICU with severely deranged blood electrolytes, in particular very low sodium, and has been on intravenous fluids for 24 hours. MR brain performed to find a cause for developing spastic quadriparesis shows a central area of low T1, high T2 signal in the pons. What is your diagnosis?
    A. Pontine infarct
    B. Osmotic myelinolysis
    C. MS
    D. Pontine haemorrhage
    E. Pontine glioma

114. A child is admitted to the A&E department following head injury. A CT scan of the head is performed and, incidentally, a well-defined lobulated heterogeneous mass containing calcification is seen to arise from the floor of the fourth ventricle. Which of the following is the most likely diagnosis?
    A. Glioma
    B. Pilocytic astrocytoma
    C. Medulloblastoma
    D. Ependymoma
    E. Brainstem glioma

115. On post-transplant renal graft, the ultrasound resistive index can be increased by all, except
    A. Infection
    B. Acute rejection
    C. Acute tubular necrosis
    D. Renal artery stenosis
    E. Extrinsic compression

116. A 31-year-old man with known history of Crohn's disease needs imaging for assessment of his disease status. The gastroenterologist had requested MR enterography, but the patient is reluctant to have this due to claustrophobia. A CT enterography has been booked instead. All of the following statements regarding CT enterography for Crohn's disease are true, except

    A. The CT features of active Crohn's disease include mucosal hyperenhancement, wall thickening (thickness >3 mm), mural stratification with a prominent vasa recta (comb sign) and mesenteric fat stranding.
    B. Mural enhancement is the most sensitive indicator of active Crohn's disease.
    C. Prominence of the vasa recta adjacent to the inflamed loop of bowel (comb sign), along with increased mesenteric fat attenuation, is the most specific CT feature of active Crohn's disease.
    D. Findings that might be seen in active long-standing Crohn's disease include submucosal fat deposition, pseudosacculation, surrounding fibro-fatty proliferation and fibrotic strictures.
    E. CT enterography has high sensitivity for the detection of bowel strictures occurring as a complication of Crohn's disease.

117. MR angiogram performed on a patient with fibromuscular dysplasia shows a small renal artery aneurysm. Which of the following statements regarding rupture of renal artery aneurysm is incorrect?

    A. Size greater than 2 cm increases the risk of rupture.
    B. There is debate over whether calcification reduces risk of rupture.
    C. Risk of death is high in renal artery aneurysm rupture in non-pregnant patients.
    D. Pregnancy is associated with increased risk of rupture.
    E. Kidney salvage may be possible in some patients.

118. An MRI knee of a 65-year-old woman with known osteoarthritis shows a 6 × 5 cm well-defined cystic area, posteromedial to the tibiofemoral joint on axial images. A narrow neck is identified extending between the medial head of the gastrocnemius and semimembranosus tendon to communicate with the knee joint. No significant joint effusion is evident. What is the likely diagnosis?

    A. Pes anserinus bursitis
    B. Baker's cyst
    C. Large parameniscal cyst
    D. Tibiofibular cyst
    E. Cruciate cyst

119. All of the following are associations of Chiari I malformation, except

    A. Basilar impression
    B. Klippel Feil anomaly
    C. Hydrocephalous
    D. Myelomeningocele
    E. Syringomyelia

120. A 7-year-old child is noticed to have difficulty walking. A central mass is suspected, and MRI demonstrates a large cystic mass in the right cerebellar hemisphere, with an intensely enhancing nodule on post-gadolinium images. Which of the following is the most likely diagnosis?

    A. Haemangioblastoma
    B. Cerebellar pilocytic astrocytoma
    C. Medulloblastoma
    D. Ependymoma
    E. Arachnoid cyst

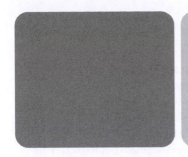

CHAPTER 4
TEST PAPER 2

Answers

1. D. Cardiac fibroelastomas usually arise from the pericardium.

Most lipomas appear to be subepicardial, expanding into the pericardial space. They typically have high signal on T1-weighted images and low signal on fat-suppressed images.

Fibroelastomas occur on cardiac valves, making them the most common neoplasm of the valves. They are hypointense mobile masses situated away from the free edge of the valves.

Fibroma is a neoplasm primarily of infants and children. Fibromas are homogeneously hypointense on T2-weighted images and show variable enhancement.

Rhabdomyomas are the most common benign cardiac tumour of childhood associated with tuberous sclerosis. They originate within the myocardium, typically in the ventricles, may be multiple, and are high on T2-weighted images.

The majority of myxomas manifest in adulthood between the fourth and seventh decades. A minority will constitute part of an autosomal dominant syndrome known as *Carney complex*, characterised by myxomas, hyperpigmented skin lesions and extracardiac tumours such as pituitary adenomas, breast fibroadenomas and melanotic schwannomas. The classic triad of symptoms attributed to myxomas include cardiac obstructive symptoms related to obstruction to blood flow, embolic events and constitutional symptoms such as fever, malaise and weight loss. At MR imaging, the vast majority of myxomas demonstrate heterogeneous signal intensity.

The main differential diagnoses for myxoma include atrial thrombus or papillary fibroelastoma. Myxomas are more likely to arise anteriorly from the interatrial septum, whereas thrombus is more likely located posteriorly in the left atrium. In addition, myxomas enhance with gadolinium contrast material, whereas thrombi, in most cases, do not.

Sparrow PJ, et al. MR imaging of cardiac tumours. *Radiographics*. 2005;25(5):1255–76.

2. A. MEN I

Multiple endocrine neoplasia Type 1 is also known as *Wermer syndrome*. Inheritance is autosomal dominant with high penetrance. The male-to-female ratio is 1:1. Organ involvement includes parathyroid hyperplasia (97%), pancreatic islet cell tumour (30%–80%), anterior pituitary gland tumour (15%–50%) and adrenocortical hyperplasia (33%–40%).

MEN	Type 1	Type 2	Type 3
Pituitary adenoma	+		
Parathyroid adenoma	+	+	
Medullary thyroid carcinoma		+	+
Pancreatic islet cell tumour	+		
Phaeochromocytoma		+	+
Ganglioneuromatosis			+

Dähnert W. *Radiology Review Manual*, 7th edn. Philadelphia, PA: Lippincott Williams & Wilkins, 2011:728–9.

3. B. Cystosarcoma phyllodes

Phylloides tumour (PT) is a rare breast fibroepithelial neoplasm. It is now generally accepted that PTs can be classified as benign, borderline or malignant. Mammography and ultrasound are notorious for their inability to distinguish the benign or malignant histologic nature of PTs. On US, they can be indistinguishable from fibroadenoma. They appear as an inhomogeneous, solid-appearing mass. A solid mass containing single or multiple, round or cleft-like cystic spaces and demonstrating posterior acoustic enhancement strongly suggests a diagnosis of PTs. Solid components of the tumour show vascularity on Doppler. On MRI, well-defined margins with a round or lobulated shape and a septate inner structure have been described as characteristic morphologic signs. They are usually low on T1-weighted images and vary from low to very high signal on T2-weighted images. Some have described a silt-like pattern on MRIs of benign PTs; these appear as hyperintense slit-like fluid-filled spaces on T2-weighted images, with a low signal after enhancement. Solid areas of the tumour show enhancement with contrast.

Tan H, et al. Imaging findings in phyllodes tumours of the breast. *Eur J Radiol.* 2012;81(1):e62–9.

4. C. Are typically cortical rather than subcortical-based lesions

Osteoid osteomas are benign and aggressive bone tumours that are more common in men and usually present clinically in patients less than 30 years of age. They are most commonly based within the cortex, although they can also occur in any other area of the bone. When larger than 2 cm, they are regarded as osteoblastomas. Radiofrequency ablation is now a common and viable treatment for these lesions throughout the UK.

Dähnert W. *Radiology Review Manual*, 6th edn. Philadelphia, PA: Lippincott Williams & Wilkins, 2007:136.

5. E. Patient with leptomeningeal metastasis

CT attenuation of blood in the subdural space remains denser than brain for 1 week and is less dense after 3 weeks. There is an interim period of 2 weeks when it is isodense to brain tissue.

In addition to variation in appearance over time, subdural haemorrhage may have a variable appearance in a setting of systemic disease like anaemia and coagulopathy. An acute SDH can appear isodense in the following settings: anaemia with a haemoglobin concentration of <10 g/dL, admixture of CSF in the subdural space caused by an associated tear to the arachnoid layer and disseminated intravascular coagulation. If there is chronic CSF leakage of venous blood, for example, if the patient has coagulopathy or is on anticoagulants/antiplatelet agents, chronic haematoma may look isodense rather than hypodense.

Meningeal metastasis may appear as hyperdensity on gyri and mimic subarachnoid haemorrhage.

Adam A, et al. *Grainger & Allison's Diagnostic Radiology: A Textbook of Medical Imaging*, 5th edn. New York: Churchill Livingstone, 2008:1344.

Zasler ND, et al. *Brain Injury Medicine, 2nd Edition: Principles and Practice*. III Neuroimaging and Neurodiagnostic Testing. New York: Demos Medical publishing, 2013:200.

6. B. Ileocolic

Intussusception is one of the most common causes of acute abdomen in infancy. Intussusception occurs when a portion of the digestive tract becomes telescoped into the adjacent bowel segment. This condition usually occurs in children between 6 months and 2 years of age. In this age group, intussusception is idiopathic in almost all cases. The vast majority of childhood cases of intussusception are ileocolic.

US is highly accurate in the diagnosis of intussusception with a sensitivity of 98%–100% and a specificity of 88%–100%. US is also good at demonstrating alternative pathology. Hence, enema could be reserved for therapeutic purposes when US is available.

del-Pozo G, et al. Intussusception in children: Current concepts in diagnosis and enema reduction. *Radiographics*. 1999;19(2):299–319.

7. B.   Takayasu arteritis

Takayasu arteritis is a form of granulomatous vasculitis affecting large and medium-sized arteries, characterised by ocular disturbances and weak pulses in the upper extremities (pulseless disease). It is associated with fibrous thickening of the aortic arch with narrowing of the origins of the great vessels at the arch. Takayasu arteritis can be limited to the descending thoracic and abdominal aorta. It is seen in young and middle-aged patients, especially Asian and women. The diagnosis is confirmed by a characteristic arteriographic pattern of irregular vessel walls, stenosis, post-stenotic dilatation, aneurysm formation, occlusion and evidence of increased collateral circulation.

Polyarteritis nodosa is a fibrinoid necrotising vasculitis that mainly involves small and medium-sized arteries of the muscles. Multiple aneurysm formation is a characteristic finding. The kidney is most commonly involved, followed by the GI tract, liver, spleen and pancreas. Positive ANCA titres (usually pANCA type) are found in variable percentages of patients.

Wegener's granulomatosis is a distinct clinicopathologic entity characterised by granulomatous vasculitis of the upper and lower respiratory tract together with glomerulonephritis.

Churg–Strauss syndrome is characterised by granulomatous vasculitis of multiple organ systems, particularly the lung, and involves both arteries and veins as well as pulmonary and systemic vessels.

Moyamoya disease is a progressive vasculopathy leading to stenosis of the main intracranial arteries. Characteristic angiographic features of the disease include stenosis or occlusion of the arteries of the circle of Willis, as well as the development of collateral vasculature that produces a typical angiographic image called 'clouds of smoke' or 'puff of cigarette smoke'.

Ha HK, et al. Radiologic features of vasculitis involving the gastrointestinal tract. *Radiographics*. 2000; 20(3):779–94.

Tarasów E, et al. Moyamoya disease: Diagnostic imaging. *Pol J Radiol*. 2011;76(1):73–9.

8. C.   Cronkhite–Canada syndrome

Cronkhite–Canada syndrome occurs in older patients with an average age of 60 with no familial predisposition. The histologic appearance of the GI polyps resembles that of juvenile polyps, and they are characteristically distributed throughout the stomach. They are commonly small, sessile and characterised by cystic dilatation of the glands and inflammation of the lamina propria. Patients commonly present with abdominal pain, protein-losing diarrhoea, anorexia and weight loss. Dystrophic nail changes and alopecia usually appear after the onset of GI symptoms.

Cho G, et al. Peutz-Jeghers syndrome and the harmatomatous polyposis syndromes: Radiologic-pathologic correlation. *Radiographics*. 1997;17:785–91.

9. D.   Fat necrosis

Fat necrosis is a frequently encountered cause of benign calcification, particularly when there is a history of trauma. It appears well circumscribed with translucent areas in the centre (homogenous fat density of the oil cyst). Occasionally, it shows curvilinear or eggshell calcification in the wall. On US, it appears as a hypoechoic or anechoic mass with ill- or well-defined margins, with or without acoustic shadowing or as a complex cyst.

Dähnert W. *Radiology Review Manual*, 7th edn. Philadelphia, PA: Lippincott Williams & Wilkins, 2011:577–8.

10. D.   Pott disease

Infection usually begins in the anterior part of the vertebral body adjacent to the end plate. Subsequent demineralisation of the end plate results in loss of definition of its dense margins on conventional radiographs. These end plate changes allow the spread of infection to the adjacent intervertebral disk, resulting in a classic pattern of involvement of more than one vertebral body together with the intervening disks. It also allows spread into the paraspinal tissues, resulting in the formation of a paravertebral abscess. However, if there is anterior subligamentous involvement of the spine, infection can extend both superiorly and inferiorly, with sparing of the intervertebral disks. A normal chest radiograph is present in up to 50% of cases. In the later stages of disease, there is often vertebral collapse with a gibbus deformity.

Tuberculosis rarely affects the posterior vertebral elements (including the pedicles), in contrast to metastatic disease. Anterior scalloping seen with subligamentous spread of infection can also be seen with paravertebral lymphadenopathy, secondary to metastases or lymphoma. In differentiating tuberculosis from pyogenic infection, the clinical picture is as important as the radiologic features, with insidious onset of symptoms, a normal erythrocyte sedimentation rate, relevant respiratory symptoms and slow disease progression favouring a diagnosis of tuberculosis. Radiologic features that favour this diagnosis include involvement of one or more segments; a delay in destruction of the intervertebral disks; a large, calcified paravertebral mass; and the absence of sclerosis. Sarcoidosis can produce multifocal lesions of vertebrae and disks, along with paraspinal masses that appear identical to tuberculosis.

Burrill J, et al. Tuberculosis: A radiologic review. *Radiographics*. 2007;27(5):1255–73.

11. D. Hallervorden–Spatz disease

The 'eye of the tiger' sign represents marked low signal intensity of the globus palladi on T2-weighted MRI, surrounding a central, small hyperintense area. The sign is seen in what was once known as Hallervorden–Spatz (HS) syndrome but is now called *neurodegeneration with brain iron accumulation* (NBIA) or *pantothenate kinase II (PANC2)-associated neurodegeneration*. The low signal is a result of excessive iron accumulation and the central high signal is attributed to gliosis, increased water content and neuronal loss with disintegration. Iron levels in blood and CSF are normal. HS is a neurodegenerative disorder associated with extrapyramidal dysfunction and dementia. The sign can also be seen in other extrapyramidal Parkinsonian disorders such as cortical-basal ganglionic degeneration, Steele–Richardson–Olszewski syndrome, and early onset levodopa-responsive Parkinsonism.

High signal in the basal ganglia, thalamus and midbrain is seen in Wilson disease. Caudate is atrophic in Huntington disease. CADASIL shows extensive white matter signal change and MELAS shows multiple focal white matter signal changes.

Chavhan GB, Shroff MM. Twenty classic signs in neuroradiology: A pictorial essay. *Indian J Radiol Imaging*. 2009;19(2):135–45.

12. D. Encases major vessels but does not invade them.

Neuroblastoma (NBL) is the most common extracranial tumour in childhood and commonly presents as an abdominal mass. Abdominal and pelvic tumours are usually large and heterogeneous, and approximately 80%–90% demonstrate calcification on CT scans. Low attenuation areas of necrosis or haemorrhage are frequently noted at CT. Vascular encasement and compression of the renal vessels, splenic vein, inferior vena cava, aorta, celiac artery and superior mesenteric artery may occur, and vascular invasion is rare. Regional invasion of the psoas and paraspinal musculature may occur, and invasion of the neural foramen into the epidural space is also frequent; these are better evaluated at MR imaging, as is regional organ invasion. Metastatic disease of the liver and lung are readily evaluated with CT. They are typically heterogeneous, variably enhancing and of relatively low signal intensity on T1-weighted images and high signal intensity on T2-weighted images.

Wilms tumour demonstrates a 'claw' of normal renal tissue around the tumour. In contrast to neuroblastoma, vessels are displaced rather than encased and vascular invasion occurs in approximately 5%–10% of cases.

Dumba M, et al. Neuroblastoma and nephroblastoma: An overview and comparison. *Cancer Imaging*. 2014; 14(Suppl 1):O15.
Lonergan GJ, et al. Neuroblastoma, ganglioneuroblastoma, and ganglioneuroma: Radiologic-pathologic correlation. *Radiographics*. 2002;22(4):911–34.

13. E. Left ventricular aneurysm calcification

A cardiac false aneurysm is defined as a rupture of the myocardium that is contained by pericardial adhesion. It usually represents a rare complication of myocardial infarction, but it may also occur after cardiac surgery, chest trauma and endocarditis. True left ventricular aneurysms are discrete, dyskinetic areas of the left ventricular wall with a broad neck. Unlike a true aneurysm, which contains some myocardial elements in its wall, the walls of a false aneurysm are composed of organised haematoma and pericardium only. Both demonstrate focal bulge to the cardiac contour and can calcify.

Marked delayed enhancement of the pericardium on dynamic enhanced MRI may help in differentiating a false aneurysm from a true one.

Konen E, et al. True versus false left ventricular aneurysm: Differentiation with MR imaging-initial experience. *Radiology*. 2005;236(1):65–70.

14. A. Superficial inguinal

Metastatic spread to regional lymph nodes represents the most common mode of tumour spread from cancer of the anal canal and margin. Nodal metastasis is more likely in cases of larger tumour size or a poorly differentiated anal tumour. Metastasis most commonly occurs to the perirectal nodes, with inguinal nodal spread being the second most common location of nodal metastasis.

McMahon CJ, et al. Lymphatic metastases from pelvic tumours: Anatomic classification, characterization, and staging. *Radiology*. 2010;254(1):31–46.

15. B. Fibroadenoma

Fibroadenomas are the most common cause of benign solid mass in the breast. On US, they appear round or oval, wider than tall, hypoechoic, well-defined and mostly homogenous and show a 'hump and dip' sign (small focal bulge to the contour with a contagious small sulcus), a thin echogenic pseudocapsule and rarely either posterior acoustic enhancement (17%–25%) or posterior acoustic shadow (9%–11%).

Dähnert W. *Radiology Review Manual*, 7th edn. Philadelphia, PA: Lippincott Williams & Wilkins, 2011:578–9.

16. D. Quadrilateral space syndrome

The anatomy of the suprascapular nerve renders it particularly susceptible to compression at the suprascapular notch and spinoglenoid notch. The pattern of muscle denervation provides information about the duration of entrapment and can identify the site of neurologic compromise. Acute denervation presents as hyperintensity of the supraspinatus and infraspinatus or of the infraspinatus muscle alone on fluid-sensitive sequences. Chronic compression is shown as a reduction in muscle bulk and fatty infiltration of the involved muscles. Involvement of both the supra- and infraspinatus muscles reflects proximal compression at the suprascapular notch, whereas isolated infraspinatus denervation suggests compression at the spinoglenoid notch. Quadrilateral space syndrome is a rare condition referring to an isolated compressive neuropathy of the axillary nerve. It generally results in isolated atrophy of the teres minor and, less commonly, of the deltoid, which appears as a reduction in muscle bulk and fatty infiltration with chronic compression. Parsonage–Turner syndrome is an uncommon, self-limiting disorder characterised by sudden onset of non-traumatic shoulder pain associated with progressive weakness of the shoulder girdle musculature. MRI is the technique of choice in patients with shoulder pain and weakness. It is sensitive for the detection of signal abnormalities in the shoulder girdle musculature related to denervation injury. MRI is also useful in excluding intrinsic shoulder abnormalities that can produce symptoms similar to Parsonage–Turner syndrome such as rotator cuff tears, impingement syndrome and labral tears.

None of the findings or history would be compatible with an acute rotator cuff tear or Duchenne's muscular dystrophy.

Yanny S, Toms AP. MR patterns of denervation around the shoulder. *AJR Am J Roentgenol.* 2010;195:2.

17. B. Sacral chordoma

A chordoma is a tumour that derives from notochordal remnants. At imaging, it typically manifests as a large, destructive sacral mass with secondary soft-tissue extension. Radiographs may show sacral osteolysis with an associated soft-tissue mass and calcifications. CT shows bone destruction with an associated lobulated midline soft-tissue mass. Areas of low attenuation within the mass reflect the myxoid properties (high water content) of the tissue. Areas of punctate calcification often are noted.

At MR imaging, the most striking feature is the high signal intensity seen on T2-weighted images. High T2 signal intensity is a non-specific feature; however, the combination of high T2 signal intensity and a lobulated sacral mass that contains areas of haemorrhage and calcification is strongly suggestive of a chordoma. Chordomas tend to show hypointense or isointense signal relative to that in muscle on T1-weighted images, and contrast-enhanced images show a modest degree of heterogeneous enhancement in the soft-tissue components of the tumour. Areas of intrinsic T1 signal hyperintensity typically represent areas of haemorrhage or mucinous material. The tumour may cross the sacroiliac joint.

Farsad K, et al. Sacral chordoma. *Radiographics.* 2009;29(5):1525–30.

18. E. Inhaled foreign body

Most inhaled foreign bodies are organic and may not be visible on chest X-ray. It is recognised that chest X-ray can be normal with inhaled foreign bodies and clinical suspicion needs to be high. The most common findings are unilateral, distal obstructive emphysema, followed by normal X-ray. Lower lobes are most commonly involved. Long-standing unrecognised foreign body may present with recurrent or non-resolving consolidation or unexplained segmental collapse.

Passàli D, et al. Foreign body inhalation in children: An update. *Acta Otorhinolaryngol Ital.* 2010;30(1):27–32.

19. B. Type II endoleak

In a Type I endoleak, there is poor apposition between one of the attachment sites of a stent graft and the native aortic or iliac artery wall, and blood leaks through this defect into the aneurysm sac. A Type I endoleak can be seen immediately after stent-graft deployment. On CT, dense contrast collection is usually seen centrally within the sac and is often continuous with one of the attachment sites.

Type II endoleaks are the most common. They occur when there is retrograde flow of blood into the aneurysm sac via an excluded aortic branch, most commonly IMA or a lumbar artery. Many Type II endoleaks close spontaneously over time. CT shows peripheral or central location of acute haemorrhage.

Leakage of blood through the body of a stent graft results in a Type III endoleak. Type III endoleaks manifest as collections of haemorrhage or contrast material centrally within the aneurysm sac, usually distant from the attachment sites or native vessels.

Opacification of the aneurysm sac immediately after placement of a stent graft without a discernible source of leakage is designated a Type IV endoleak.

A Type V endoleak, or endotension, is characterised by continued growth of an excluded aneurysm sac without direct radiologic evidence of a leak.

Bashir MR, et al. Endoleaks after endovascular abdominal aortic aneurysm repair: Management strategies according to CT findings. *AJR Am J Roentgenol.* 2009;192(4):178–86.

20. E. Metastasis from colonic adenocarcinoma – colonoscopy

	Associated malignancy	
Tumour marker	Primary	Other malignancies
Oncofoetal antigens		
AFP	Primary HCC	Teratoblastomas of the ovaries and testes
CEA	Colorectal carcinoma	Various carcinomas
Hormones		
β-hCG	Choriocarcinoma	Testicular cancers (non-seminomatous), trophoblastic tumours
Calcitonin	Medullary carcinoma	Cancer of the thyroid, liver cancer, renal cancer
Metanephrines	Pheochromocytoma	Neuroblastoma, ganglioneuromas
Chromogranin A	Pheochromocytoma, neuroblastoma	MEN, small-cell lung cancer, carcinoid tumours
IGF-1	Pituitary cancer	Insulinoma
Glycoproteins		
CA 15-3	Breast cancer	Various carcinomas
CA 19-9	Pancreatic and gastric carcinomas	Various carcinomas
CA 72-4	Gastric carcinoma	Various carcinomas
CA 125	Ovarian carcinoma	Various carcinomas
Isoenzymes		
PSA	Prostate cancer	
NSE	Small-cell lung carcinoma	Neuroblastoma, kidney tumours
Cellular components/products		
LASA-P		Various carcinomas, leukaemia, lymphoma, Hodgkin's disease
SCC-A		Squamous cell carcinoma of the uterus, cervix, lung, and head and neck
TAG 72	Gastric carcinoma	Colorectal, lung, pancreatic and ovarian cancers
Immunoglobulins	Multiple myeloma	Gammopathies

AFP: alpha foetoprotein; β-hCG: beta human chorionic gonadotropin; CA: carbohydrate antigen; CEA: carcinoembryonic antigen; HCC: hepatocellular carcinoma; LASA-P: lipid-associated sialic acid P; MEN: multiple endocrine neoplasia; NSE: neuron-specific enolase; PSA: prostate-specific antigen; SCC-A: squamous cell carcinoma antigen.

Sharma S. Tumor markers in clinical practice: General principles and guidelines. *Indian J Med Paediatr Oncol.* 2009;30(1):1–8.

21. E. Homogenous high T2 signal suggests malignancy.

Smooth margins, characterised by well-defined and sharply demarcated borders, are the feature with the highest benign lesion predictive value. Round and oval shapes have also been found to be predictive of benignity. Homogeneous enhancement is highly suggestive of benign nature. Fat content is specific to benign lesions, such as hamartoma, fibroadenoma, intramammary lymph nodes or fat necrosis. In the case of fat necrosis, even if the lesion appears irregular in both shape and margin, with rim enhancement, the key to diagnosis is a fat internal signal on unenhanced sequences without fat suppression. Strong hypersignal on non-fat-suppressed T2-weighted sequences is classically considered to be a clear sign of fibroadenoma, but it is non-specific and is seen in mucinous carcinomas, invasive ductal carcinomas, metaplastic carcinomas and intracystic papillary carcinomas (although it does not have a homogenously high T2 signal as fibroadenoma). Although rim enhancement is regarded as suggestive of malignancy, a regular enhanced rim, which may be thick, may be seen around cysts, seroma (both of which are high T2 fluid signal) and fat necrosis (high T1 signal). In relation to enhancement kinematics, a centrifugal contrast uptake pattern may help in diagnosing a fibroadenoma, whereas a centripetal spread of contrast is more common in carcinomas.

Millet I, et al. Pearls and pitfalls in breast MRI. *Br J Radiol.* 2012;85(1011):197–207.

22. B. A tibial tuberosity to trochlear groove distance of <1.5 cm.

Transient patellar dislocation is the dislocation of the patella laterally and subsequent relocation. Trochlear dysplasia, patella alta (increase in the ratio of the patella tendon to the patella length) and an increase in the tibial tuberosity–trochlear groove (TT-TG) distance are associated factors. TT-TG >20 mm is abnormal and 15–20 mm is considered borderline change. TT-TG less than 15 mm is within normal limits.

Contusional marrow oedema is often seen in the medial patellar facet and the lateral femoral condyle. The medial patellar retinaculum and/or medial patellofemoral ligament (MPFL) may be torn or show a pattern of strain injury.

Dähnert W. *Radiology Review Manual*, 6th edn. Philadelphia, PA: Lippincott Williams & Wilkins, 2007:69.

23. B. Modic Type II end plate change

Modic described three types of reactive changes in the cancellous bone adjacent to the vertebral end plates. Type I change is low on T1 and high on T2, representing oedema secondary to acute fibrovascular tissue invasion. Type 2 change represents fatty replacement of red marrow, bright on T1 and T2. This leads to bony sclerosis, low on T1 and T2. Occasionally the end plates become irregular and the degenerative process progresses to a destructive discovertebral lesion, simulating infective discitis. The key differentiation is signal of the disc, which is high in discitis and low in degeneration.

Andersson lesions refer to inflammatory involvement of the intervertebral discs by spondyloarthritis.

Adam A, et al. *Grainger & Allison's Diagnostic Radiology: A Textbook of Medical Imaging*, 5th edn. New York: Churchill Livingstone, 2008:1375.

24. D. Disruption of the spinolamellar line

The atlantoaxial interval is defined as the distance between the anterior aspect of the dens and the posterior aspect of the anterior ring of the atlas. This distance should be 5 mm or less. Pseudospread of the atlas on the axis ('pseudo–Jefferson fracture') can be seen on anterior open-mouth radiographs. Up to 6 mm of displacement of the lateral masses relative to the dens is common in patients up to 4 years old and may be seen in patients up to 7 years old. On extension radiographs, overriding of the anterior arch of the atlas onto the odontoid process can be seen in 20% of healthy children.

In children, the C2–3 space and, to a lesser extent, the C3–4 space have a normal physiologic displacement. The absence of lordosis, although potentially pathologic in an adult, can be seen in children up to 16 years of age when the neck is in a neutral position.

In children, the flexion manoeuvre can increase the distance between the tips of the C1 and C2 spinous processes. Normal posterior intraspinous distance is a good indicator of ligamentous integrity and should not be more than 1.5 times greater than the intraspinous distance one level either above or below the level in question. Anterior wedging of up to 3 mm of the vertebral bodies should not be confused with compression fracture. Such wedging can be profound at the C3 level.

A prevertebral space of less than 6 mm at the level of C3 is considered normal in children. In paediatric patients, widening of the prevertebral soft tissues can be a normal finding that is related to expiration.

Disruption of the spinolamellar line is a sign of injury.

Lustrin ES, et al. Pediatric cervical spine: Normal anatomy, variants, and trauma. *Radiographics*. 2003; 23(3):539–60.

25. D. Retroperitoneal haematoma

A retroperitoneal haematoma adjacent to an abdominal aortic aneurysm is the most common imaging finding of abdominal aortic aneurysm rupture.

The most common finding predictive of rupture is increase in aneurysm size, and thus it is the most common indicator for elective surgical management. Decreasing thrombus–lumen ratio is also predictive of increasing aneurysm size. The rest include drape sign, tangential calcium sign, focal discontinuous intimal calcification and high attenuation crescent.

High attenuation crescent represents an internal dissection of blood into either the peripheral thrombus or the aneurysm wall. It is one of the earliest and most specific imaging manifestations of the rupture process.

Rakita D. Spectrum of CT findings in rupture and impending rupture of abdominal aortic aneurysms. *Radiographics*. 2007;27(2):497–507.

Singh A. *Emergency Radiology: Imaging of Acute Pathologies. Imaging of Acute Aortic Conditions*. New York: Springer Science & Business Media; 2013.

26. C. Hepatic artery thrombosis

In the early post-operative period (<72 hours after transplantation), increased hepatic artery resistance (resistive index of >0.8) is a frequent finding, but resistance ordinarily returns to a normal level within a few days. Increased hepatic artery resistance is associated with older donor age and a prolonged period of ischaemia. The estimated incidence of hepatic artery thrombosis among liver transplant recipients is 4%–12% in adults and 42% in children. This is one of the most feared complications, as it may lead to fulminant hepatic necrosis. In addition, in liver grafts, biliary ducts are supplied exclusively by small branches of the hepatic artery; therefore, arterial thrombosis may lead to biliary ischaemia and necrosis. Prompt diagnosis of hepatic artery thrombosis is extremely important because early intervention (with thrombectomy, hepatic artery reconstruction or both) may allow graft salvage. However, most patients ultimately require retransplantation. Even after retransplantation, the mortality rate approaches 30%. Risk factors for hepatic artery thrombosis include a significant difference in hepatic artery calibre between the donor and the recipient, an interpositional conduit for the anastomosis, a previous stenotic lesion of the celiac axis, excessive duration of cold ischaemia time, ABO blood type incompatibility, cytomegalovirus infection and acute rejection.

Caiado AHM, et al. Complications of liver transplantation: Multimodality imaging approach. *RadioGraphics*. 2007;27:1401–17.

27. D. Fibroadenoma

Non-enhancing internal septations were initially described to have a high specificity in fibroadenoma diagnosis; however, this feature has recently been described in PTs and cancers and thus has little value when considered alone. Although morphological findings are important in lesion characterisation, breast cancers may have a benign appearance. In particular, 30% of familial breast cancers revealed a mass showing benign morphological features with a round or oval shape, smooth margins and homogeneous internal enhancement. It should be considered that all enhancing masses in women with genetic risks are suitable for biopsy when there is a lack of typical cyst or fat necrosis findings.

Millet I, et al. Pearls and pitfalls in breast MRI. *Br J Radiol*. 2012;85(1011):197–207.

28. C. Anterior cruciate ligament

This is a classic plain film appearance of a Segond fracture. Segond fracture is an avulsion fracture at the proximal, non-articular aspect of the lateral tibia. The presence of this fracture is strongly associated with injury to other knee structures like the medial meniscus. However, it is the anterior cruciate ligament that is most commonly injured (75%–100%).

Dähnert W. *Radiology Review Manual*, 6th edn. Philadelphia, PA: Lippincott Williams & Wilkins, 2007:90.

29. E. Sequestrated disc

Protrusion is present if the greatest distance between the edges of the disc material presenting outside the disc space is less than the distance between the edges of the base of that disc (wider than tall). Extrusion is present when, in at least one plane, any one distance between the edges of the disc material beyond the disc space is greater than the distance between the edges of the base of the disc material or when no continuity exists between the disc material beyond the disc space and that within the disc space (taller than wide). The latter form of extrusion is best specified as sequestration if the displaced disc material has lost continuity completely with the parent disc. The term *migration* may be used to signify displacement of disc material away from the site of extrusion. Herniated discs in the craniocaudal (vertical) direction through a gap in the vertebral end plate are referred to as intravertebral herniations (Schmorl nodes).

Fardon DF, et al. Lumbar disc nomenclature: Version 2.0: Recommendations of the combined task forces of the North American Spine Society, the American Society of Spine Radiology and the American Society of Neuroradiology. *Spine J*. 2014;14(11):2525–45.

30. B. 2

Grading of reflux:

Grade I: Reflux into distal ureters
Grade II: Reflux into collecting system (without calyceal dilatation/blunting)
Grade III: All of the above, plus mild dilatation of the pelvis and calices
Grade IV: All of the above, plus moderate dilatation (clubbing of calices)
Grade V: All of the above, plus severe tortuosity of the ureter
Prognosis: Grades I–III VUR resolve with maturation of the ureterovesical junction; Grades IV and V require surgery to avoid renal scarring, renal impairment and/or hypertension.

Dähnert W. *Radiology Review Manual*, 7th edn. Philadelphia, PA: Lippincott Williams & Wilkins, 2011.

31. A. DeBakey 1 – Stanford A

Site of dissection	DeBakey	Stanford
Both ascending and descending aorta	Type I	Type A
Ascending aorta and arch only	Type II	Type A
Descending aorta only, distal to left subclavian artery	Type IIIa	Type B
Descending aorta only, distal to left subclavian artery	Type IIIb	Type B

Adam A, et al. *Grainger & Allison's Diagnostic Radiology: A Textbook of Medical Imaging*, 5th edn. New York: Churchill Livingstone, 2008:557.

32. B. Peutz–Jeghers syndrome

Peutz–Jeghers syndrome is a disorder characterised by mucocutaneous pigmentation and gastrointestinal harmatomas. The syndrome is an autosomal, dominant, inherited trait and occurs with equal frequency in male and female subjects. Mucocutaneous pigmentation, a characteristic feature of this syndrome, is manifested by melanotic deposits around the nose, lips and buccal

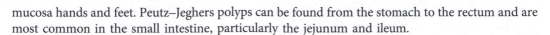

mucosa hands and feet. Peutz–Jeghers polyps can be found from the stomach to the rectum and are most common in the small intestine, particularly the jejunum and ileum.

Cho G, et al. Peutz-Jeghers syndrome and the harmatomatous polyposis syndromes: Radiologic-pathologic correlation. *Radiographics*. 1997;17:785–91.

33. D.   Differentiate residual disease from post-surgical scar

MRI of the breast has evolved into an important adjunctive tool with multiple indications in breast imaging, as recommended by US and European guidelines. Breast MRI is currently the most sensitive detection technique for breast cancer diagnosis. The indications are staging before treatment planning, screening of high-risk women, evaluation of response to neoadjuvant chemotherapy, patients with breast augmentation or reconstruction, occult primary breast cancer, breast cancer recurrence, identifying residual tumour in positive surgical margins and characterisation of equivocal findings. Differentiating early post-operative scarring from residual breast tumour is not possible because of similar enhancement characteristics of post-surgical scarring.

Millet I, et al. Pearls and pitfalls in breast MRI. *Br J Radiol*. 2012;85(1011):197–207.

34. C.   L2/3 generalised disc bulge with left lateral recess stenosis

Medial aspect of the knee corresponds to the L3 dermatome. Lateral recess stenosis at L2/3 will affect the transiting L3 nerve root, whereas foraminal stenosis will affect the exiting L2 nerve root.

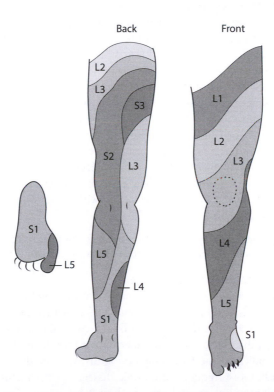

Netter FH. Dermatomes of lower limb. Lower limb. In: *Atlas of Human Anatomy*, 5th edn. E O'Grady and M Thiel (eds.). Philadelphia, PA: Saunders Elsevier, 2011:470.

35. E.   Congenital dislocation of hips

Split cord malformations (SCMs) are relatively rare forms of occult spinal dysraphism and tethered spinal cord syndrome. SCMs are of two types. Type I consists of two hemicords, each contained within its own dural sheath and separated by a median bony spur, and Type II consists of two hemicords housed in a single dural tube separated by a fibrous median septum.

There are recognised associations with myelomeningocele, Chiari malformation, tethering of cord, hypertrichosis, nevus, lipoma, dimple or haemangioma overlying the spine, clubfoot (50%), muscle wasting and progressive scoliosis.

Borkar SA, Mahapatra AK. Split cord malformations: A two years experience at AIIMS. *Asian J Neurosurg.* 2012;7(2):56–60.

36. B.   Normal trachea and anterior oesophageal indentation   Aberrant right subclavian artery

Aberrant right subclavian artery with a left-sided aortic arch or aberrant left-sided subclavian artery with a right-sided aortic arch both result in posterior impression on the oesophagus on a barium swallow, with normal appearance of the trachea. An aberrant left pulmonary artery or pulmonary vascular sling runs in between the trachea and oesophagus, resulting in an anterior indentation on the oesophagus and a posterior indentation on the trachea. Other entities that can result in anterior indentation on the oesophagus are a bronchogenic cyst, trachea-oesophageal node or a tracheal neoplasm extending posteriorly.

Anterior tracheal, posterior tracheal and lateral oesophageal impression occurs with double aortic arch. The right arch is higher than the left, resulting in an S-shaped oesophagogram on AP view. Reverse '3' indentation of the oesophagus and normal trachea occurs with coarctation of the aorta.

Dähnert W. *Radiology Review Manual*, 7th edn. Philadelphia, PA: Lippincott Williams & Wilkins, 2011.

37. D.   Hypoplastic left heart syndrome

Hypoplastic left heart syndrome presents with early onset (days) of cyanosis and heart failure, leading to collapse and death in a few weeks of life. Associated cardiac malformations include pre- and post-ductal coarctation of the aorta, PDA, VSD, patent foramen ovale and so on.

Truncus arteriosus presents with minimal cyanosis in newborn infants; signs of heart failure are usually absent. Heart failure is evident in older infants.

Tetralogy of Fallot presents in early infancy with cyanosis, usually not present in early infancy, leading to clubbing; dyspnoea, heart failure, failure to thrive and paroxysmal hypercyanotic spells. X-ray shows a boot-shaped heart with oligaemic lungs.

Transposition of the great arteries is a medical emergency. Infants usually present in the first few hours or days with worsening duct-dependent cyanosis. Hypoxia is severe, but heart failure is not a feature. X-ray shows an 'egg on end' or 'egg on string' appearance.

Tricuspid atresia presents in the first few days of life with increasing cyanosis; other clinical features are dependent on associated PDA or VSD.

Bardo DM, et al. Hypoplastic left heart syndrome. *Radiographics.* 2001;21(3):705–17.
Tasker RC, et al. *Oxford Handbook of Paediatrics.* Oxford: Oxford University Press, 2008.

38. D.   A cobweb sign demarcates the true lumen.

The beak sign and a larger cross-sectional area were the most useful indicators of the false lumen for both acute and chronic dissections. Features generally indicative of the true lumen included outer wall calcification and eccentric flap calcification. In cases showing one lumen wrapping around the other lumen in the aortic arch, the inner lumen was invariably the true lumen. Outer wall calcification always indicated the true lumen on scans of acute dissections. False lumen thrombus was significantly more frequent in chronic dissections than acute dissections. Cobwebs are specific for the false lumen but are only rarely observed.

LePage MA. Aortic dissection: CT features that distinguish true lumen from false lumen. *AJR Am J Roentgenol.* 2001;177(1):207–11.

39. D.   Obesity

Periportal halos are defined as circumferential zones of decreased attenuation identified around the peripheral or subsegmental portal venous branches on contrast-enhanced CT. These halos probably represent fluid or dilated lymphatics in the loose areolar zone around the portal triad structures. While this CT finding is non-specific, it is abnormal and should prompt close scrutiny of the liver in search of an underlying aetiology.

Periportal halos, which may be due to blood, are commonly seen in patients with liver trauma. Periportal oedema may cause this sign in patients with congestive heart failure and secondary liver congestion, hepatitis, or enlarged lymph nodes and tumours in the porta hepatis, which obstruct lymphatic drainage. This CT sign has also been observed in liver transplants (probably secondary to disruption and engorgement of lymphatic channels) and in recipients of bone marrow transplants, who might develop liver oedema from microvenous occlusive disease. Although the precise pathophysiologic basis of periportal tracking has not been proven, it represents a potentially important CT sign of occult liver disease.

Lawson TL, et al. Periportal halo: A CT sign of liver disease. *Abdominal Imaging.* 1993;18(1):42–6.

40. A.   Supine position

There are several prerequisites for maximising the sensitivity and specificity of breast MRI, including the following:

- High magnetic field strength with a highly homogeneous magnetic field.
- Bilateral image acquisition with a prone-positioning bilateral breast coil.
- Unenhanced imaging with a T2-weighted and 3D T1-weighted pre- and post-IV gadolinium.
- Selection of a phase-encoding direction minimises artefacts.
- Homogeneous fat suppression.
- Thin-section acquisitions (section thickness of 3 mm or less).
- Pixel size of less than 1 mm in each in-plane direction.
- Temporal resolution of less than 2 minutes for imaging of both breasts.

Rausch DR, Hendrick RE. How to optimize clinical breast MR imaging practices and techniques on your 1.5-T system. *Radiographics.* 2006;26(5):1469–84.

41. D.   Right foraminal disc osteophyte at C5/6

Lateral aspect of the forearm and the thumb corresponds to the C6 dermatome. Foraminal osteophyte at C5/6 will impinge upon the exiting C6 nerve root. (cf. foraminal osteophyte at a thoracic or lumbar level, e.g., T4/5 or L4/5, which will impinge upon the exiting T4 or L4 nerve roots, subject to the discrepancy between number of cervical vertebra and cervical roots. Note that the exiting root at C7/T1 is C8.)

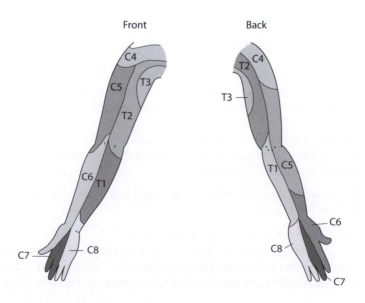

Netter FH. Dermatomes of upper limb. Upper limb. In: *Atlas of Human Anatomy*. 5th edn. E O'Grady and M Thiel (eds.). Philadelphia, PA: Saunders Elsevier, 2011:401.

42. D.   X-ray can often be normal.

Atlanto-occipital dislocation shows the following on lateral radiograph of the cervical spine: >10 mm soft-tissue swelling anterior to C2, with pathological convexity (80%), basion-dens interval of >12 mm, odd's ratio (distance between the basion and the posterior arch of the atlas divided by opisthion and anterior arch of atlas) >1, and basion–posterior axial line interval >12 mm anterior/>4 mm posterior to axial line.

Direct signs include loss of congruity of articular surfaces of atlas and occipital condyle. Normal X-ray in the presence of atlanto-occipital dislocation is rare.

Dähnert W. *Radiology Review Manual*, 6th edn. Philadelphia, PA: Lippincott Williams & Wilkins, 2007:203.

43. B.   Coronal

The appearance here describes brachycephaly. Craniosynostosis is the premature fusion of cranial sutures and may be isolated or may present as part of a craniofacial syndrome. It typically alters the shape of the cranial vault. Broad categories include simple craniosynostosis, involving only one suture, or compound craniosynostosis, where two or more sutures are involved.

Deformity	Suture involved
Dolichocephaly	Sagittal
Scaphocephaly	Sagittal
Brachycephaly	Bicoronal
Anterior plagiocephaly	Unicoronal
Turricephaly	Bilateral lambdoid
Posterior plagiocephaly	Unilateral lambdoid
Trigonocephaly	Metopic
Oxycephaly	Sagittal and coronal
Kleeblattschädel	Sagittal, coronal and lambdoid

Khanna PC, et al. Pictorial essay: The many faces of craniosynostosis. *Indian J Radiol Imaging*. 2011; 21(1):49–56.

44. C.   String-of-beads appearance of the retinal artery

Fibromuscular dysplasia (FMD) is an idiopathic, segmentary, non-inflammatory and non-atherosclerotic disease that can affect all layers of both small- and medium-calibre arteries. Vascular loops, fusiform vascular ectasia and a string-of-beads aspect are typical presentations. Arterial dissection, aneurysm and subarachnoid haemorrhage are less typical radiologic presentations.

The affected arteries are mainly the renal arteries, extracranial carotid and vertebral arteries, mesenteric arteries and intracranial carotid arteries. Central retinal artery occlusion is a rarely recognised feature of fibromuscular dysplasia.

Varennes L, et al. Fibromuscular dysplasia: What the radiologist should know: A pictorial review. *Insights Imaging*. 2015;6(3):295–307.

45. B.   Hypointense liver relative to spleen on T1 and T2

MR imaging is the best non-invasive method for measuring the level of iron in the liver for the purposes of confirming the diagnosis, determining the severity, and monitoring therapy with high sensitivity, specificity, and positive and negative predictive values. The accumulation of iron ions in the tissues, because of the super-paramagnetic properties of the ions, causes local distortion in the magnetic fields and relaxation of the spins, which results in shortening of the longitudinal relaxation time (T1), the transverse relaxation time (T2) and particularly the transverse relaxation time as affected by magnetic field inhomogeneity (T2*). This effect causes a loss of signal intensity in the affected organs that is proportional to the iron deposition. In the general protocol applied to an abdominal study, it is not possible to estimate the hepatic iron concentration, although most of the time it is possible to diagnose iron overload. This can be done by using 'dual sequence' (gradient in and out of phase) MR imaging, which demonstrates decreased signal intensity in the affected tissues on the in-phase images compared with the out-of-phase images. That effect is the opposite of the effect observed in patients with steatosis. This occurs because the echo time of the in-phase sequence is usually higher than that of the out-of-phase sequence; therefore, the in-phase pulse sequence is more sensitive to iron deposits because of the increased T2* effect.

Queiroz-Andrade M. MR imaging findings of iron overload. *RadioGraphics*. 2009;29:1575–89.

46. E. Thin hypointense pseudocapsule and fat content on T1W images

Fat necrosis appears as well circumscribed with translucent areas in the centre (homogenous fat density of the oil cyst). Occasionally, it shows curvilinear or eggshell calcification in the wall. On US, it appears as a hypoechoic or anechoic mass with ill- or well-defined margins, with or without acoustic shadowing or as a complex cyst. On MRI, even if the lesion appears irregular in both shape and margin, with a rim enhancement, the key to diagnosis is a fat internal signal on unenhanced sequences without fat suppression (high on T1-weighted images).

Dähnert W. *Radiology Review Manual*, 7th edn. Philadelphia, PA: Lippincott Williams & Wilkins, 2011:577–8.
Millet I, et al. Pearls and pitfalls in breast MRI. *Br J Radiol*. 2012;85(1011):197–207.

47. C. To assess for extra-articular fluid

The purpose of the T2-weighted fluid-sensitive sequence in MR shoulder arthrography is the identification of extra-articular fluid, for example, bursal fluid or paralabral cysts, which may not be visualised on the isolated T1-weighted post-contrast sequences, particularly if there is no intra-articular communication.

T2-weighted imaging also helps to identify abnormal fluid in the rotator cuff tendons by eliminating magic angle because of high TE.

Berquist TH. *MRI of the Musculoskeletal System*, 5th edn. New York: Lippincott Williams & Wilkins, 2006.

48. B. Lefort I involves the maxilla and medial wall of the orbit.

Lefort fractures always involve the pterygoid process/plates. Lefort I fractures are transverse maxillary fractures, involving the alveolar ridge and inferior wall of maxillary sinus. There is detachment of the teeth bearing alveolar process of maxilla. The orbits are not involved.

Lefort II fractures are also called *pyramidal fractures* and they involve the maxilla and the medial wall of the orbit. They can be unilateral. Lefort III fractures are also called *craniofacial disassociation* or *disjunction* and involves the maxilla and medial and lateral wall of the orbit (zygomatic arch).

Dähnert W. *Radiology Review Manual*, 7th edn. Philadelphia, PA: Lippincott Williams & Wilkins, 2011:212.

49. C. Mitral valve insufficiency

Dissection involving the ascending aorta can result in fatal complications, which include aortic rupture, cardiac tamponade, acute aortic regurgitation and acute myocardial infarction from dissection involving the coronary arteries. Involvement of the arch vessels results in morbidity from neurological complications.

Adam A, et al. *Grainger & Allison's Diagnostic Radiology: A Textbook of Medical Imaging*, 5th edn. New York: Churchill Livingstone, 2008:559.

50. B. Primary sclerosing cholangitis

Primary sclerosing cholangitis (PSC) is an idiopathic, chronic, fibrosing inflammatory disease of the bile ducts that eventually leads to bile duct obliteration, cholestasis and biliary cirrhosis. A strong association with inflammatory bowel disease, especially ulcerative colitis, is noted (70% of cases). Although the cause of PSC is unknown, most experts believe it to be an autoimmune process because PSC may be associated with other autoimmune diseases such as retroperitoneal fibrosis, mediastinal fibrosis and Sjögren syndrome. The rate of progression is unpredictable, with up to 49% of symptomatic patients eventually developing biliary cirrhosis and liver failure. Treatment is usually palliative and includes medical therapy with orally administered agents such as ursodiol (ursodeoxycholic acid) or endoscopic or percutaneous mechanical dilation of dominant strictures. Cholangiographic findings usually include multifocal, intrahepatic bile duct strictures alternating with normal-calibre ducts, which sometimes produce a beaded appearance.

Vitellas KM, et al. Radiologic manifestations of sclerosing cholangitis with emphasis on MR cholangiopancreatography 1. *RadioGraphics*. 2000;20:959–75.

51. D. Lactating adenoma

Lactating adenomas are newly discovered painless lumps that appear during the third trimester or lactation. They are a freely mobile, homogenous hypoechoic or isoechoic mass with posterior acoustic enhancement (most common) and septa. The lesion regresses after breastfeeding.

Dähnert W. *Radiology Review Manual*, 7th edn. Philadelphia, PA: Lippincott Williams & Wilkins, 2011:582.

52. E. Tumoural calcinosis

Tumoural calcinosis is a rare familial disease, typically presenting in young men of African origin, with progressive large nodular juxta-articular calcified soft-tissue masses. Patients have normal serum calcium and phosphorus and do not have any evidence of renal, metabolic or collagen–vascular disease. The hips are the most frequently affected, followed by the elbows, shoulders and feet, and the disease is usually along the extensor surface of the joints. The knees are almost never affected. Occasionally, fluid–fluid levels are seen with the calcium lying inferiorly, termed the *sedimentation sign*. The joints themselves are normal.

Dähnert W. *Radiology Review Manual*, 7th edn. Philadelphia, PA: Lippincott Williams & Wilkins, 2011.
Olsen KM, Chew FS. Tumoral calcinosis: Pearls, polemics, and alternative possibilities. *Radiographics*. 2006;26:871–85.
Sutton D. *Textbook of Radiology and Imaging*, 7th edn. Edinburgh: Churchill Livingstone, 2003.

53. D. Ependymoma

Radiographs of patients with ependymomas may reveal scoliosis, canal widening with vertebral body scalloping, pedicle erosion or laminar thinning.

Ependymomas enhance intensely after intravenous administration of iodinated contrast material.

Most spinal cord ependymomas are iso- or hypointense on T1-weighted images. Any hyperintensity suggests haemorrhage. They are hyperintense to the cord on T2-weighted images. About 20%–33% of ependymomas demonstrate the cap sign, a rim of extreme hypointensity (hemosiderin) seen at the poles of the tumour on T2-weighted images. This finding is secondary to haemorrhage, which is common in ependymomas and other highly vascular tumours (e.g., paraganglioma, haemangioblastoma) Most cases (60%) also show evidence of cord oedema around the masses. The average number of vertebral segments involved with abnormal signal intensity is 3.6. Cysts are a common feature, with 78%–84% of ependymomas having at least one cyst.

Subependymomas represent a variant of central nervous system (CNS) ependymomas. MR imaging findings are not sufficiently unique to enable the differentiation of ependymomas from subependymomas; however subependymomas are eccentric, may not enhance and may not have surrounding oedema.

Koeller KK, et al. Neoplasms of the spinal cord and filum terminale: Radiologic-pathologic correlation. *Radiographics*. 2000;20(6):1721–49.

54. B. Scimitar syndrome

Hypogenetic lung syndrome, also known as *congenital venolobar syndrome* or *scimitar syndrome*, is primarily a complex developmental lung abnormality with anomalous venous return. The most common features are lung hypoplasia, anomalous pulmonary venous return to IVC, pulmonary artery hypoplasia, bronchial anomalies and systemic arterial supply to hypoplastic lung. It almost always occurs on the right side and is slightly more common in women.

One constant component of this syndrome is an anomalous pulmonary vein or veins draining at least a part or the entire affected lung most commonly to the inferior vena cava just above or below the diaphragm. Uncommonly, the anomalous vein may drain into hepatic, portal, azygos veins; the coronary sinus; or the right atrium. A scimitar vein is a vertical curvilinear opacity in the right mid-lower lung, running along the right heart border inferomedially towards the diaphragm to join the IVC. A scimitar vein present on a frontal chest radiograph is called the *scimitar sign*.

Ahamed MF, Al Hameed F. Hypogenetic lung syndrome in an adolescent: Imaging findings with short review. *Ann Thorac Med*. 2008;3(2):60–3.

55. D. Flow characteristic at the aneurysm neck

An aneurysm occurs when a vessel diameter exceeds 1.5 times its normal size. In the abdomen this corresponds to 3 cm. These aneurysms should be repaired when the diameter exceeds 5–5.5 cm or the aneurysm expands more than 1 cm per year.

The greatest benefit of 3D volume-rendered imaging is the depiction and precise measurement of angulation in aneurysms with marked tortuosity.

The proximal landing zone consists of the region from the inferior-most renal artery to the beginning of the aneurysm. The maximal acceptable neck diameter is 32 mm. The length of the neck should be at least 15 mm (although one device allows a 7 mm neck). The angle between the superior portion of the aneurysm neck and the suprarenal aorta is preferably less than 60°.

Study results suggest higher complications for aneurysms larger than 5.5–6.5 cm. The shape can be described as saccular or fusiform. The residual lumen through the aneurysm should measure approximately 18 mm to allow passage and proper deployment of the device. The preferred distal landing zone is the common iliac artery. Evaluation is similar to that of the proximal neck with assessment of diameter, length, tortuosity and degree of calcification and thrombus. The common iliac artery diameter should not be larger than 25 mm, and at least 10 mm of length is required for an adequate seal.

Picel AC, Kansal N. Essentials of endovascular abdominal aortic aneurysm repair imaging: Preprocedural assessment. *AJR Am J Roentgenol*. 2014;203(4):347–57.

56. D. Crohn's disease

In Crohn's disease involving either the small bowel or colon, broad linear ulcers that crisscross in longitudinal and transverse directions can produce a pseudopolypoid appearance usually termed *cobblestoning*.

Buck JL, et al. Polypoid and pseudopolypoid manifestations of inflammatory bowel disease. *Radiographics*. 1991;11:293–304.

57. E.   Needs IV contrast   Does not need IV contrast

The advantages of mammograms include their reliable detection of calcification, lower cost than MRI, wide availability and their imaging speed, which is faster than MRI. The disadvantages include difficulty in presence of implants, discomfort caused by compression, difficulty in imaging dense breasts and the need to reposition the breast for different views. The advantages of MRI are its higher sensitivity, ability to be used with implants, good performance with dense breasts, not requiring compression, ability to image both breasts simultaneously and improved tissue resolution. The disadvantages of MRI are that it may not show calcification, is not good for DCIS, leads to many false-positive findings and is expensive.

Adam A, et al. *Grainger & Allison's Diagnostic Radiology: A Textbook of Medical Imaging*, 5th edn. New York: Churchill Livingstone, 2008.

58. B. Diffuse idiopathic skeletal hyperostosis (DISH)

DISH is not a cause of acro-osteolysis.

Other causes of acro-osteolysis include leprosy, frost bite, electrical and thermal burns, PVC workers, sarcoidosis, rheumatoid arthritis, Reiter syndrome, pyknodysostosis, syringomyelia and hyperparathyroidism.

Dähnert W. *Radiology Review Manual*, 6th edn. Philadelphia, PA: Lippincott Williams & Wilkins, 2007:20.
Zayas VM, Monu JUV. Imaging of psoriatic arthritis. *Contemp Diagn Radiol.* 2008;31(10):1–7.

59. C. Haemangioblastoma

Haemangioblastomas manifest with diffuse cord expansion and variable signal intensity on T1-weighted images, most commonly isointense (50%) or hyperintense (25%) relative to the cord. On T2-weighted images, they have high signal intensity with intermixed focal flow voids. Surrounding oedema and a cap sign may be seen. Although up to 25% of haemangioblastomas may appear to be solid, cyst formation or syringohydromyelia is very common (up to 100% in some series). In fact, some cases may have the classic appearance of a cystic mass with an enhancing mural nodule characteristic of cerebellar haemangioblastomas. Contrast-enhanced imaging typically shows an intensely homogeneous enhancing tumour nodule.

Koeller KK, et al. Neoplasms of the spinal cord and filum terminale: Radiologic-pathologic correlation. *Radiographics.* 2000;20(6):1721–49.

60. E. Langerhans cell histiocytosis

The vast majority of *vertebra plana* lesions in relatively healthy children are caused by an eosinophilic granuloma of Langerhans cell histiocytosis. The other available options are all possible, but less common, differential diagnoses. There is usually preservation of the disc space and no kyphosis. The posterior elements are rarely involved.

Platyspondyly (multiple flat vertebral bodies, as opposed to vertebra plana) specially affecting lumbar vertebra by 2–3 years of age is a typical feature of Morquio syndrome.

Dähnert W. *Radiology Review Manual*, 7th edn. Philadelphia, PA: Lippincott Williams & Wilkins, 2011.
Weissleder J, Weissleder R. *Primer of Diagnostic Imaging*, 5th edn. St. Louis, MO: Elsevier Mosby, 2011:618.

61. A. Size of aorta at the level of the renal artery

Several important characteristics of the aneurysm must be accurately described for standard stent-graft sizing. The aneurysm is described in terms of the proximal landing zone, the aneurysm sac, the distal landing zone and the vascular access. Reported diameters should include the aorta at the level of the most inferior renal artery, the aortic neck 15 mm distal to the lowest renal artery, aorta at the bifurcation, the largest aneurysm sac diameter and the size of the common iliac arteries. Additional measurements include the length of the aneurysm neck, the length from the lowest renal artery to the aortic bifurcation and the length of the aneurysm sac. The length of the distal landing zone is described as the distance from the aortic bifurcation to the common iliac artery bifurcation. Minimal diameters should be recorded in the distal landing zone and external iliac artery access vessels.

Unfavourable findings on CT

Proximal aneurysmal neck

- Length >32 mm
- Diameter <7–15 mm
- Angulation >60°

Aneurysm sac

- Residual lumen <18 mm
- Distal aorta diameter <20 mm
- Extension – involvement of common iliac arteries

Iliofemoral vessels

- Common iliac artery diameter >25 mm
- Landing zone length <10 mm
- External iliac artery diameter <6 mm

Picel AC, Kansal N. Essentials of endovascular abdominal aortic aneurysm repair imaging: Preprocedural assessment. *AJR Am J Roentgenol.* 2014;203(4):347–57.

62. D. Pyogenic liver abscess

Pyogenic abscesses, particularly when multiple, may be caused by haematogenous dissemination of either gastrointestinal infection via the portal vein or disseminated sepsis via the hepatic artery, ascending cholangitis or superinfection of necrotic tissue. Over one-half of liver abscesses are polymicrobic. *Escherichia coli* is the most common bacterium, but other anaerobic and aerobic organisms can be involved. Pyogenic abscesses demonstrate no sex predilection but most commonly involve middle-aged patients.

On US, pyogenic micro-abscesses may manifest as either discrete hypoechoic nodules or ill-defined areas of distorted hepatic echogenicity. There may be little or no enhanced through transmission.

At contrast-enhanced CT, they appear as multiple small, well-defined hypoattenuating lesions. Faint rim enhancement and perilesional oedema can be observed, findings that help differentiate them from hepatic cysts.

Mortelé KJ. The infected liver: Radiologic-pathologic correlation. *RadioGraphics.* 2004;24:937–55.

63. B. Pleomorphic

Calcifications are likely to be malignant if they are clustered rather than scattered throughout the breast and vary in size and shape (pleomorphic) and if they are found in a linear or ductal distribution. Benign calcifications could be coarse, 'popcorn' (fibroadenoma); 'eggshell' and curvilinear as in fat necrosis; 'tramline' (vascular), 'broken needle' or 'lead pipe' as in duct ectasia; punctate, stellate, and 'teacup' as in fibrocystic change.

Adam A, et al. *Grainger & Allison's Diagnostic Radiology: A Textbook of Medical Imaging,* 5th edn. New York: Churchill Livingstone, 2008:1186–7.

64. B. The blood supply of the proximal pole enters at the waist.

The blood supply to the proximal pole of the scaphoid enters at the waist and courses proximally. A waist fracture can therefore interrupt this tenuous blood supply, leading to avascular necrosis of the proximal pole or delayed/non-union. Non-displaced fractures are often treated conservatively, whereas displaced fractures usually require reduction and internal fixation. The scaphoid bone is the most commonly fractured carpal bone and tends to result from a fall on outstretched hand in a younger population rather than the common dorsally angulated distal radial fractures (Colles fracture). A high index of suspicion should be used when reporting trauma plain films of the wrist, and follow-up imaging following a period of conservative management should be employed when there is clinical concern but unremarkable presentation radiographs.

Manaster BJ, et al. *Musculoskeletal Imaging: The Requisites*, 4th edn. Philadelphia, PA: Mosby Elsevier, 2013:143–4.

65. B. Paraspinal mass is useful in differentiating metastatic from benign fracture.

Distinction between metastatic and acute osteoporotic compression fractures could be made on the basis of MR imaging findings.

A convex posterior border of the vertebral body is more frequent in metastatic compression fractures than acute osteoporotic compression fractures. A higher frequency of abnormal signal intensity of the pedicle or posterior element has been observed in metastatic compression fractures. Epidural soft-tissue mass is suggestive of malignant vertebral collapse.

A paraspinal mass is not helpful in differentiation of the cause of vertebral collapse but is more commonly encountered in the setting of metastatic compression, where it is typically focal rather than diffuse. Signal intensity abnormalities in the marrow of vertebrae other than the collapsed vertebrae are more frequently seen in metastatic compression fractures than acute osteoporotic compression fractures.

Enhancement on post-contrast T1-weighted FS images is not useful in differentiation of acute osteoporotic fractures from malignant compression fracture, but it may be useful for old or chronic fractures, which will not show intense enhancement.

Moreover, on diffusion-weighted imaging (DWI) vertebral metastases with compression fractures can be safely distinguished from vertebra with benign compression fractures based on significantly different ADC values.

Jung HS, et al. Discrimination of metastatic from acute osteoporotic compression spinal fractures with MR imaging. *Radiographics*. 2003;23(1):179–87.
Herneth AM, et al. Vertebral metastases: Assessment with apparent diffusion coefficient. *Radiology*. 2002; 225(3):889–94.

66. A. Pyknodysostosis

Pyknodysostosis is a congenital abnormality that should be considered in the differential diagnosis of osteosclerosis. The patients are typically short, have hypoplastic mandibles, widened cranial sutures, Wormian bones, brachycephaly, clavicular dysplasia, thick skull base and hypoplasia or non-pneumatisation of the paranasal sinuses. The distinguishing feature is acro-osteolysis with sclerosis. The distal phalanges appear as if they have been put in a pencil sharpener – they are pointed and dense.

Brant WE, Helms CA. *Fundamentals of Diagnostic Radiology*, 3rd edn. Philadelphia, PA: Lippincott Williams & Wilkins, 2006.
Dähnert W. *Radiology Review Manual*, 7th edn. Philadelphia, PA: Lippincott Williams & Wilkins, 2011.

67. C. The tip of the electrode is placed in the centre of the lesion.

In RFA, a high-frequency, alternating current with a wavelength of 460–500 kHz is emitted through an electrode placed within the targeted tissue. Grounding pads applied to the patient's thighs complete the electrical circuit. Cell death starts at 49 degrees. Temperature above 60 degrees causes immediate cell death, and tissue charring occurs at 105 degrees. Cell death is induced by the denaturation of proteins.

For percutaneous imaging-guided RFA, the energy is delivered into the target tissue by means of needle-like electrodes. Unlike in a typical biopsy, the electrode tip should be advanced to the deep margin of the tumour.

On follow-up CT, ablated tumours often have internal areas of increased attenuation or increased signal intensity at CT and MRI. Areas of contrast enhancement (>10 HU or >15% with CT and MRI, respectively) are indicative of residual viable RCC. Residual viable tumour can be treated with additional ablation sessions.

Heat-sink phenomena refers to the reduction in tissue temperature due to the conductive effects of adjacent vessels or airways. It is an explanation for distortion of the ablation zone and poor outcome in larger lesions. The heat-sink effect can be overcome by pharmacologically reducing blood flow, intra-arterial embolisation, intravascular balloon occlusion, Pringle manoeuvre or reducing treatment zone.

Kee ST, et al. Tumour response for image guided interventions: Assessment and validation. In: *Clinical Interventional Oncology*. Philadelphia, PA: Elsevier Saunders, 2013:48.
Zagoria RJ. Imaging-guided radiofrequency ablation of renal masses. *Radiographics*. 2004;24(Suppl 1):S59–71.

68. B. Cholangiocarcinoma

Intrahepatic cholangiocarcinoma is the second most common primary hepatic tumour. Various risk factors have been reported for intrahepatic cholangiocarcinoma, and the radiologic and pathologic findings of this disease entity may differ depending on the underlying risk factors. Intrahepatic cholangiocarcinoma can be classified into three types on the basis of gross morphologic features: mass-forming (the most common), periductal infiltrating and intraductal growth.

There are a number of recognised risk factors for cholangiocarcinoma that all share the common feature of chronic biliary inflammation: liver flukes (*Opisthorchis viverrini*, *Clonorchis sinensis*), hepatolithiasis (recurrent pyogenic cholangitis), PSC, viral infection (human immunodeficiency virus, hepatitis B virus, hepatitis C virus, Epstein–Barr virus), anomalies and malformations (anomalous pancreaticobiliary junction and choledochal cyst, fibrocystic liver diseases, such as Caroli disease), environmental or occupational toxins (Thorotrast, dioxin, polyvinyl chloride), biliary tract–enteric drainage procedures and heavy alcohol consumption.

Chung YN, et al. Varying appearances of cholangiocarcinoma: Radiologic-pathologic correlation. *Radiographics*. 2009;29:683–700.

69. D. Suspicious masses need biopsy.

Although the use of contrast-enhanced MRI of the breast has increased both the sensitivity and the specificity of breast cancer detection, common causes of false-positive and rarer causes of false-negative diagnoses still occur. Irregular heterogeneous enhancement is not typical of a benign lesion, hence biopsy is required. In addition, note that cancers can present with smooth well-defined margins, hence an apparent benign appearance in a patient with BRCA1 mutation should with be regarded with caution and may need biopsy.

Millet I, et al. Pearls and pitfalls in breast MRI. *Br J Radiol*. 2012;85(1011):197–207.

70. B. Calcaneonavicular coalition

Tarsal coalition is best confirmed with CT. CT and MRI can show direct bony continuity (osseous coalition) or fluid/cartilage intensity on MR/irregular serrated articular surface in case of cartilaginous coalition.

A calcaneonavicular coalition shows the classic anteater's nose appearance on lateral radiograph.

The C sign is seen on a lateral radiograph in a patient with talocalcaneal coalition. Prominent talar beak is also associated with talocalcaneal coalition. Both calcaneonavicular and talocalcaneal coalition are equally common.

Dähnert W. *Radiology Review Manual*, 6th edn. Philadelphia, PA: Lippincott Williams & Wilkins, 2007:167.

71. D. Melanoma

Drop metastasis refers to CSF seeding of intracranial neoplasm. Post-contrast images show 'sugar coating' of the brain and spinal cord in patients with leptomeningeal drop metastases or leptomeningeal carcinomatosis.

It can occur secondary to CNS involvement by distant primary tumours as well as primary CNS neoplasms.

CNS tumours with drop metastasis include PNET, medulloblastoma, anaplastic glioma, ependymoma, germinoma, pineoblastoma, pineocytoma and rarely choroid plexus carcinoma and angioblastic meningioma. Non-CNS primaries include breast, lung, melanoma and lymphoma.

Dähnert W. *Radiology Review Manual*, 7th edn. Philadelphia, PA: Lippincott Williams & Wilkins, 2011:221.

72. B. Osteogenesis imperfecta

Osteogenesis imperfecta is an inherited disorder that results from mutations in either the *COL1A1* or *COL1A2* gene of Type 1 collagen. The disease is usually apparent at birth or in childhood, but more mild forms of the disease may not be apparent until adulthood. The disease is classified into Types I–IV, with Type I, the mildest form, being described above. The presenile hearing loss is caused by otosclerosis. The differential diagnosis can be resolved by the extra-skeletal manifestations (blue sclerae and dentinogenesis imperfecta). The other types are Type II (lethal perinatal), Type III (severe progressive) and Type IV (moderately severe).

Adam A, et al. *Grainger & Allison's Diagnostic Radiology: A Textbook of Medical Imaging*, 5th edn. New York: Churchill Livingstone, 2008.

73. A. TACE is useful in patients with Child–Pugh Class C cirrhosis.

TACE combines the effect of targeted chemotherapy with the effect of ischaemic necrosis induced by arterial embolisation. TACE provides a survival benefit in primary hepatocellular carcinoma (HCC) based on randomised controlled studies. The normal parenchyma of the liver receives two-thirds of its necessary blood supply from the portal vein and the remaining one-third from the hepatic artery. However, it is well known that vascularisation of HCC is mostly dependent on the hepatic artery. TACE is not done for patients with a severely compromised liver function such as Child–Pugh classification C or late B. Though superselective TACE may be attempted in a patient with compromised liver function, if the patient has a diffuse or massive HCC or an HCC involving the major portal veins, this precludes the practice of safe TACE.

The underlying factors associated with increased procedural complication include compromised liver function, main portal vein obstruction, biliary tract obstruction and a previous history of bile duct surgery.

Shin SW. The current practice of transarterial chemoembolization for the treatment of hepatocellular carcinoma. *Korean J Radiol*. 2009;10(5):425–34.

74. E. Pneumatosis coli

Pneumatosis is the presence of gas bubbles within the wall of the involved segment of bowel. It is seen in a wide variety of conditions. It is widely divided into two groups: primary (idiopathic) and secondary. Conditions associated with secondary pneumatosis include obstruction, pulmonary disease such as COPD and asthma, vascular conditions such as ischaemia and infarction, inflammatory conditions such as Crohn's and UC, necrotising enterocolitis, drugs such as steroids and chemotherapy, collagen vascular diseases such as scleroderma, SLE and dermatomyositis.

Feczko PJ, et al. Clinical significance of pneumatosis of the bowel wall. *Radiographics*. 1992;12:1069–78.

75. E.   Renal papillary necrosis

Urographic findings during this period of early ischaemic change are usually normal. On CT, the early ischaemic changes are best depicted on nephrographic phase scans as small, poorly marginated areas of diminished enhancement at the tip of the medullary pyramid. Calyceal deformities in renal papillary necrosis occur in three forms: medullary (round or oval cavity, calyceal blunting), papillary (triangular cavity, 'lobster claw' appearance) and *in situ*. If the papilla detaches completely, a typical ring-like shadow is produced by the necrotic papilla in a contrast material–filled cavity; if the sloughed papillae remain *in situ* there is a 'signet ring' appearance.

Jung DC, et al. Renal papillary necrosis: Review and comparison of findings at multi-detector row CT and intravenous urography. *Radiographics*. 2006;26(6):1827–36.

76. C.   Secondary synovial osteochondromatosis

Primary synovial osteochondromatosis is a benign self-limiting monoarticular disorder characterised by proliferation and metaplastic transformation of the synovium with formation of multiple intra-articular cartilaginous or osteocartilaginous loose bodies. The form is not associated with OA, whereas the secondary form is associated with articular surface disintegration.

Classic radiographic features include multiple loose intra-articular bodies in varying grades of mineralisation. MRI shows varying grades of intermediate to high T1 signal to the loose bodies depending on the amount of mature osseous element (cf. pigmented villonodular synovitis, which shows low signal debris/areas on T2-weighted images; lipoma arborescens, which shows metaplastic frond-like synovial fat with high signal on T1-weighted images; and synovial haemangioma with mixed features).

Dähnert W. *Radiology Review Manual*, 6th edn. Philadelphia, PA: Lippincott Williams & Wilkins, 2007:166.

77. D.   Congenital short pedicles

Spinal stenosis is defined as encroachment of the spinal canal or lateral recess by bone or soft-tissue components.

Congenital short pedicles are idiopathic or developmental, secondary to achondroplasia, hypochondroplasia, Down's syndrome and Morquio disease. Acquired causes include hypertrophy of ligamentum flavum, facet joint OA, disc protrusion, spondylolysis or spondylolisthesis, surgical fusion, fracture (benign or metastatic), Paget's disease, epidural lipomatosis and ossification of the posterior longitudinal ligament.

Dähnert W. *Radiology Review Manual*, 7th edn. Philadelphia, PA: Lippincott Williams & Wilkins, 2011:227.

78. D.   Gaucher disease

Although the Ashkenazi Jews are particularly predisposed to this hereditary condition, Gaucher disease is not confined to any particular ethnic group or sex. Splenic enlargement is detected in up to 95% of cases. There is abnormal modelling of the distal femur and proximal tibia secondary to marrow infiltration, leading to an 'Erlenmeyer flask' deformity. However, this feature is not diagnostic for Gaucher disease and may be seen in all the other answer options. Diffuse medullary osteoporosis, bone infarcts and sharply circumscribed endosteal lytic lesions (owing to marrow replacement) can also be seen. The combination of Jewish ancestry, the radiographic features described and splenomegaly makes Gaucher disease the most likely diagnosis.

Dähnert W. *Radiology Review Manual*, 7th edn. Philadelphia, PA: Lippincott Williams & Wilkins, 2011.

79. A.   It depends on the histology of the tumour being treated.

The most common complication of TACE is post-embolisation syndrome, which consists of transient abdominal pain and fever occurring in 60%–80% of patients after TACE. Elevation of the level of hepatic transaminases typically accompanies post-embolisation syndrome. Whether post-embolisation syndrome reflects damage to the normal liver parenchyma or tumour necrosis is uncertain. Though prolonged hospitalisation may be required to monitor a patient and to control abdominal pain, vomiting and/or malaise, post-embolisation syndrome is self-limiting within 3–4 days, and the use of antibiotics is not necessary to treat the fever.

Hepatic failure after TACE is related to TACE-induced ischaemic damage to the non-tumorous liver tissue. Several risk factors have been identified, including portal vein obstruction, use of a high dose of anticancer drugs and Lipiodol, a high level of bilirubin, prolonged prothrombin time and advanced Child–Pugh class.

Other TACE-related complications occur in less than 10% of treatment sessions and include ischaemic cholecystitis, hepatic abscesses and biliary strictures. Development of a liver abscess has been linked to previous intervention in the biliary system being prone to an ascending biliary infection. Upper gastrointestinal complications such as gastritis, ulceration and bleeding can occur by the regurgitation of embolic agents into the gastric arteries (anatomical variants), which should be recognised on pretreatment imaging.

Shin SW. The current practice of transarterial chemoembolization for the treatment of hepatocellular carcinoma. *Korean J Radiol.* 2009;10(5):425–34.

Wigmore SJ, et al. Postchemoembolisation syndrome-tumour necrosis or hepatocyte injury? *Br J Cancer.* 2003;89:1423–7.

80. A. Desmoid tumour–Gardner's syndrome

Aggressive fibromatosis, or intra-abdominal Desmoid tumour, represents a benign proliferative process that has a tendency to locally recur. Mesenteric involvement is more often seen in cases related to typical familial adenomatous polyposis syndrome (FAPS) (Gardner syndrome).

At CT, the margins of these lesions may appear irregular or smooth. The specific diagnosis of a mesenteric Desmoid tumour would be strongly suggested by a known diagnosis of FAPS or its associated CT findings, such as colonic polyps or masses, previous total colectomy, and polyps or masses involving the duodenum, stomach or periampullary region.

Pickhardt PJ. Unusual non-neoplastic peritoneal and subperitoneal conditions: CT findings. *RadioGraphics.* 2005;25:719–30.

81. C. Diuretic administration reduces the time during which images can be obtained.

T2-weighted techniques were the first clinically relevant means of visualising the urinary tract with MRI. Static-fluid MR urography does not require the excretion of contrast material and is therefore useful for demonstrating the collecting system of an obstructed, poorly excreting kidney. Static-fluid MR urograms can be obtained in 1–2 seconds, which allows multiple images to be obtained sequentially in a short period of time and played as a cine loop. Cine MR urography is particularly helpful in confirming the existence of urinary tract stenosis. For patients with non-dilated systems, the use of hydration, diuretics or compression may enhance the quality of MR urography. In case of excretory MR urogram, a gadolinium-based contrast agent is administered intravenously, and the collecting systems are imaged during the excretory phase. Gadolinium shortens the T1 relaxation time of the urine, allowing the urine to initially appear bright on T1-weighted images. Diuretic administration can improve the quality of excretory MR urography by enhancing urine flow, resulting in dilution and uniform distribution of gadolinium-based contrast material throughout the urinary tract; it also expands the temporal window during which images can be obtained. The primary imaging sequence for excretory MR urography is the 3D gradient-echo sequence. Fat suppression enhances the conspicuity of the ureters and is recommended. Motion suppression is critical for MR urographic sequences, and breath-hold acquisitions have been shown to better demonstrate the pelvicaliceal systems compared with respiratory triggering. IV hydration is preferred to oral hydration because fluid-filled structures can interfere with imaging on T2 sequences.

MR urography is more sensitive and specific for non-calculous urinary tract obstruction than unenhanced CT. CT is more sensitive for stone disease. MRU is also used for evaluation of congenital urinary tract anomalies and haematuria, whereas the role of MRU for screening patients at risk for urothelial malignancy has yet to be defined.

Leyendecker JR, et al. MR urography: Techniques and clinical applications. *Radiographics*. 2008;28(1):23–46.

82. C. 2.0 mmol/L

It is important when performing MR arthrography that the correct concentration of gadolinium is used in order to achieve the best arthrographic result. Too concentrated or too dilute a solution will result in a suboptimal study. A dose of 2 mmol/L is the recognised concentration of Gd-DTPA; this can be achieved by adding 0.8 mL of neat Gd-DTPA to 100 mL of normal saline. An alternative method would be to inject 4 mL of Gd-DTPA into a 500-mL bag of normal saline to achieve the same 2 mmol/L concentration. It is also important to avoid inadvertent intra-articular injection of air, as this will result in susceptibility artefact at the subsequent MRI that may limit its diagnostic accuracy.

Zlatkin MB. *MRI of Shoulder*, 2nd edn. Philadelphia, PA: Lippincott, 2002:279–80.

83. B. Sacrococcygeal teratoma

Sacrococcygeal teratoma is the most common presacral germ cell tumour in children and the most common solid tumour in neonates. The benign form accounts for 60% of all sacrococcygeal teratomas.

Benign teratomas are predominantly cystic; have attenuation similar to fluid on CT; and may include bone, fat and calcification. Cystic areas appear low on T1-weighted and high on T2-weighted MRI. Fatty tissue demonstrates high signal intensity on T1-weighted images, whereas calcification is depicted as a signal void. The coccyx is always involved, even in benign sacrococcygeal teratoma, and must be resected with the tumour. Malignant teratomas are more solid, and haemorrhage and necrosis are common. Approximately 50% of benign teratomas contain calcification, whereas it is seldom seen in malignant tumours. Malignant teratomas may metastasise.

Anterior sacral meningocoele is a congenital abnormality that arises from herniation of the CSF-filled dura mater through a sacral foramen or a defect in the sacral bone. Eccentric defect in sacrum results in a scimitar appearance on plain film.

Kocaoglu M, Frush DP. Pediatric presacral masses. *Radiographics*. 2006;26(3):833–57.

84. C. Morquio syndrome

The mucopolysaccharidoses are a group of inherited diseases characterised by abnormal storage and excretion in the urine of various mucopolysaccharides. Patients with these diseases have short stature and characteristic plain film findings. A characteristic finding in the hands is a pointed proximal fifth metacarpal base that has a notched appearance to the ulnar aspect. There is generalised flattening of the vertebral bodies (platyspondyly). Hunter and Hurler syndromes demonstrate an anterior vertebral beak that is inferiorly positioned, whereas Morquio syndrome demonstrates an anterior vertebral beak that is centrally positioned. Although achondroplasia can cause rounded anterior beaking in vertebra of the upper lumbar spine, the findings described within the hands are more typical of the mucopolysaccharidoses.

Brant WE, Helms CA. *Fundamentals of Diagnostic Radiology*, 3rd edn. Philadelphia, PA: Lippincott Williams & Wilkins, 2006.
Dähnert W. *Radiology Review Manual*, 7th edn. Philadelphia, PA: Lippincott Williams & Wilkins, 2011.

85. E. Fibroids with high T1 signal pretreatment respond better to UFE.

UFE is a minimally invasive treatment for uterine fibroids. MRI should be used to evaluate patients before and after UFE to accurately assess fibroid location within the uterus, fibroid number and size, and the presence or absence of fibroid enhancement on contrast material–enhanced images.

Absolute contraindications include pregnancy, known or suspected gynaecologic malignancy, and current uterine or adnexal infection; relative contraindications include contrast material allergy, coagulopathy and renal failure. Pedunculated subserosal fibroids with a narrow stalk (<2–3 cm) are a relative contraindication to UFE because of the potential risk of detachment. Cervical fibroids tend to respond less favourably. The maximum size threshold for embolisation is 13–15 cm. Above this, the post-embolisation volume may still result in bulk symptoms, and the necrosis from a large fibroid may result in a protracted post-embolisation syndrome.

Fibroids with increased cellular content and degenerate fibroids may demonstrate a high signal on T2-weighted MRI; however, a heterogeneous or markedly hyperintense T2 signal suggests degeneration. Completely hyalinised fibroids have low T2. T1 hyperintensity pre-MRI suggests fatty or haemorrhagic/red degeneration and is a negative predictor of success with a lower reduction in vascularity compared to fibroids with a low T1 signal.

After successful embolisation, fibroids may undergo progressive liquefaction with increasing T2 signal. Volume reduction is greater in T2 hyperintense fibroids and hypervascular fibroids compared to hypovascular ones. Persistent enhancement post-embolisation is sign of incomplete fibroid infarction. An increase in signal on T1-weighted images is typically observed immediately after embolisation.

Bulman JC, et al. Current concepts in uterine fibroid embolization. *RadioGraphics*. 2012;32:1735–50.
Kirby JM, et al. Utility of MRI before and after uterine fibroid embolization: Why to do it and what to look for. *Cardiovasc Intervent Radiol*. 2011;34(4):705–16.

86. E. Ulcerative colitis

Gallbladder carcinoma is highly lethal, as anatomic factors promote early local spread. The ease with which this tumour invades the liver and surrounding structures, including the biliary tree, contributes to its high mortality. The median survival is 6 months, indicating that the majority of patients present with advanced disease.

Epidemiologic studies have shown that female sex, age, postmenopausal status and cigarette smoking are risk factors. Ethnic origin, increased body mass and physician-diagnosed typhoid are risk factors in the high-incidence populations of La Paz, Bolivia, and Mexico City, Mexico. Exposure to chemicals used in the rubber, automobile, wood finishing and metal fabricating industries has been associated with an increased risk of gallbladder carcinoma. Cholelithiasis is a well-established risk factor for the development of gallbladder carcinoma, and gallstones are present in 74%–92% of affected patients. Gallstones cause chronic irritation and inflammation of the gallbladder, which leads to mucosal dysplasia and subsequent carcinoma. Porcelain gallbladder is an uncommon condition in which there is diffuse calcification of the gallbladder wall, and 10%–25% of patients with this condition have gallbladder carcinoma.

Several pathologic and congenital anatomic anomalies are associated with a higher prevalence of gallbladder carcinoma, compared with that in the general population. These conditions include congenital cystic dilatation of the biliary tree, choledochal cyst, anomalous junction of the pancreaticobiliary ducts (with or without a coexistent choledochal cyst) and low insertion of the cystic duct.

The cross-sectional imaging patterns of gallbladder carcinoma have been described as a mass replacing the gallbladder in 40%–65% of cases, focal or diffuse gallbladder wall thickening in 20%–30% and an intraluminal polypoid mass in 15%–25%.

Angela D. Levy gallbladder carcinoma: Radiologic-pathology correlation. *Radiographics*. 2001;21:2.

87. B. Von Hippel–Lindau syndrome

Von Hippel–Lindau (VHL) disease is a rare, inherited, multisystem disorder that is characterised by development of a variety of benign and malignant tumours. The spectrum of clinical manifestations of the disease is broad. These include retinal and CNS haemangioblastomas (mostly affecting cerebellum/posterior fossa), endolymphatic sac tumours, renal cysts and tumours (renal cell carcinoma), pancreatic cysts and tumours (serous cystadenoma, adenocarcinoma and neuroendocrine tumours), pheochromocytomas, and epididymal cystadenomas.

Retinal haemangioblastomas are among the most frequently and earliest detected VHL disease lesions.

Leung RS, et al. Imaging features of von Hippel-Lindau disease. *Radiographics*. 2008;28(1):65–79.

88. C. Plantar fibromatosis

Plantar fibromas are benign fibrous nodules commonly affecting the medial plantar fascia, with typical anatomical location, ultrasound and MRI findings. Plantar fibromas are well defined and hypoechoic, appearing along the plantar fascia on ultrasound; some are vascular on Doppler. On MRI they are mainly low on T1-weighted and T2-weighted sequences, although sometimes T2-weighted signal is high secondary to an increased cellular component. Variable enhancement post-gadolinium is noted. They are bilateral in 10%–25%, and association with Dupuytren's contracture, palmar fibromatosis and Peyronie's disease has been described.

Ganguly A, et al. Lumps and bumps around the foot and ankle: An assessment of frequency with ultrasound and MRI. *Skeletal Radiol*. 2013;42:1051–60.

89. E. PICA

The location of blood in cases of subarachnoid haemorrhage from a ruptured aneurysm can pinpoint the site of aneurysm in 70% of cases.

Anterior chiasmatic cistern	ACOM
Septum pellucidum	ACOM
Anterior interhemispheric fissure	ACOM
Prepontine cistern	Basilar artery
Foramen magnum	PICA
Anterior pericallosal cistern	ACA, ACOM
Sylvian fissure	MCA, ICA, PCOM
Intraventricular	MCA, ICA, ACOM

Dähnert W. *Radiology Review Manual*, 7th edn. Philadelphia, PA: Lippincott Williams & Wilkins, 2011:271.

90. A. Klippel–Trénaunay syndrome

Klippel–Trénaunay syndrome is a sporadic, rare, mesodermal abnormality that usually affects a single lower limb. It is characterised by a triad of a port-wine naevus (unilateral cutaneous capillary haemangioma often in a dermatomal distribution on the affected limb), overgrowth of distal digits/entire extremity (involving soft tissue and bone) and varicose veins on the lateral aspect of the affected limb. Although the other options can produce limb hypertrophy, they would not be expected to show all the features of the triad described.

Auyeung KM, et al. Klippel–Trénaunay syndrome presenting in a child with vascular malformation. *J Hong Kong Coll Radiol*. 2002;5:227–9.
Dähnert W. *Radiology Review Manual*, 7th edn. Philadelphia, PA: Lippincott Williams & Wilkins, 2011.

91. E. Ovarian dysfunction after UAE is more common in women under 45 years.

MRI with contrast is required to delineate uterine and ovarian artery anatomy prior to treatment. In most cases, bilateral UAE is needed, because most uterine fibroids, whether single or multiple, receive blood supply from both uterine arteries. Women over 45 years of age have been shown to have a higher prevalence of uterine–ovarian arterial anastomoses and are at increased risk for ovarian dysfunction after UAE.

Although infrequent, major adverse events can occur and include ovarian failure or amenorrhea, fibroid expulsion and rarely venous thromboembolism. Intracavitary fibroids are more likely to be expelled. Ischaemia leading to uterine necrosis, arterial dissection, endometritis and fibroid infarction are other complications. On MRI, endometritis may manifest as uterine enlargement with T1 hyperintense intracavitary haematoma; gas appears as a signal void on all sequences. Contrast enhancement may increase the conspicuity of intracavitary fluid collections.

Embolic agents used for fibroids include PVA (300–350 microns) or embospheres, whereas agents used for post-partum haemorrhage are gel foam particles, coils (occasionally) or *n*-butyl-cyanoacrylate (glue).

Bulman JC, et al. Current concepts in uterine fibroid embolization. *RadioGraphics*. 2012;32:1735–50.

Kirby JM, et al. Utility of MRI before and after uterine fibroid embolization: Why to do it and what to look for. *Cardiovasc Intervent Radiol*. 2011;34(4):705–16.

92. E. Child–Pugh Class C cirrhosis

Absolute and relative contraindications for conventional TACE in patients with HCC are as follows.

Absolute contraindications:

- Decompensated cirrhosis (Childs–Pugh C or higher)
- Jaundice
- Clinical encephalopathy
- Refractory ascites
- Extensive tumour with massive replacement of both lobes
- Severely reduced portal vein flow
- Technical contraindications to hepatic intra-arterial treatment
- Renal insufficiency (creatinine clearance <30 mL/min)

Relative contraindications:

- Tumour size >10 cm.
- Co-morbidities involving compromised organ function such as cardiovascular and lung disease.
- Untreated varices present a high risk of bleeding.
- Bile duct occlusion or incompetent papilla due to stent or surgery.

Raoul JL, et al. Evolving strategies for the management of intermediate-stage hepatocellular carcinoma: Available evidence and expert opinion on the use of transarterial chemoembolization. *Cancer Treat Rev*. 2011;37(3):212–20.

93. D. Bilateral involvement in 75%

The GU tract is the second most common site after lungs. A single kidney is involved in 75% of cases. Radiological features include TB pyonephrosis (putty kidney), small shrunken kidney with dystrophic or amorphous calcification (autonephrectomy), irregular eroded calyx (moth-eaten appearance), cavities connected to the collecting system, hydrocalicosis and infundibular strictures, phantom and amputated calyces, kink of renal pelvis, and renal stones. Strictures in the ureter result in sawtooth, corkscrew, beaded and pipestem ureter. Calcification is seen in the distal ureter, whereas bladder wall calcification is rare. Bladder TB results in thick-walled small volume 'thimble' or shrunken bladder. Prostate TB causes radiating, streaky, low-signal areas on T2-weighted images (watermelon sign).

Dähnert W. *Radiology Review Manual*, 7th edn. Philadelphia, PA: Lippincott Williams & Wilkins, 2011:999–1000.

94. A. Diffuse bone metastasis

The findings of the bone scan are those of a so-called super scan. This is when a bone scan reveals a strikingly high radiotracer uptake within bone, compared with soft tissues, and diminished to absent renal uptake. A variety of diseases that cause diffusely increased bone turnover can demonstrate this picture. Widespread bone lesions, such as diffuse skeletal metastases, are the most frequent cause, but other causes include myelofibrosis, aplastic anaemia, leukaemia and widespread Paget disease. Metabolic causes include renal osteodystrophy, osteomalacia, hyperparathyroidism and hypothyroidism. Unlike in metastatic disease, the uptake in metabolic bone disease is more uniform in appearance and extends to the distal appendicular skeleton.

Dähnert W. *Radiology Review Manual*, 7th edn. Philadelphia, PA: Lippincott Williams & Wilkins, 2011:1.
Love C, et al. Radionuclide bone imaging: An illustrative review. *Radiographics*. 2003;23:341–58.

95. B. Arachnoid cyst

Arachnoid cysts are CSF-containing intra-arachnoid cysts with ventricular communication or brain maldevelopment. They can be congenital or acquired (leptomeningeal cyst). Most are asymptomatic, but they can present with weakness, mass effect, seizure, headache, developmental delay or craniomegaly. The most common site is the middle cranial fossa anteriorly. On MRI, they are CSF density, well defined, low on T1-weighted and high on T2-weighted images, without enhancement or calcification. They can erode the inner table of the calvarium.

Dähnert W. *Radiology Review Manual*, 7th edn. Philadelphia, PA: Lippincott Williams & Wilkins, 2011:272.

96. D. Brainstem glioma

Ring enhancement is seen in the most aggressive necrotic/cystic tumours. Displacement of the fourth ventricle is typical of brainstem glioma. Most diffuse brainstem gliomas do not enhance and do not show restricted diffusion.

Classic medulloblastoma typically arises from the roof of the fourth ventricle and is midline in location in 75%–90% of cases. They are hyperdense on CT; show contrast enhancement in >90% and show restricted diffusion. Atypical teratoid-rhabdoid tumour mimics medulloblastomas radiologically and histologically and have been often misdiagnosed in the past.

Dähnert W. *Radiology Review Manual*, 7th edn. Philadelphia, PA: Lippincott Williams & Wilkins, 2011.
Plaza MJ, et al. Conventional and advanced MRI features of pediatric intracranial tumors: Posterior fossa and suprasellar tumors. *AJR Am J Roentgenol*. 2013;200(5):1115–24.

97. A. Right heart failure

The TIPS procedure is effective in achieving portal decompression and in managing some of the major complications of portal hypertension.

Indications for TIPS include variceal bleeding, secondary prevention, acute bleeding refractory to medical and endoscopic treatments, refractory ascites, hepatorenal syndrome, Budd–Chiari syndrome, hepatic veno-occlusive disease, hepatic hydrothorax and portal hypertensive gastropathy.

Copelan A, et al. Transjugular intrahepatic portosystemic shunt: Indications, contraindications, and patient work-up. *Semin Intervent Radiol*. 2014;31:235–42.

98. E. T4 N2 M0

TNM Guidelines for Staging of Rectal Cancer

Tx: Determination of tumour extent is not possible because of incomplete information.
Tis: Tumour *in situ* involves only the mucosa and has not grown beyond the muscularis mucosa (inner muscle layer).
T1:   Tumour grows through the muscularis mucosa and extends into the submucosal.
T2:   Tumour grows through the submucosal and extends into the muscularis propria.
T3:   Tumour grows through the muscularis propria into the mesorectum.

T3a: Tumour extends <5 mm beyond the muscularis propria.

T3b: Tumour extends 5–10 mm beyond the muscularis propria.

T3c: Tumour extends >10 mm beyond the muscularis propria.

T4a: Tumour penetrates the visceral peritoneum.

T4b: Tumour directly invades or is adherent to other organs or structures.

Nx: Nodal staging is not possible because of incomplete information.

N0:   No cancer in regional nodes.

N1a: Tumour in one regional node.

N1b: Tumour in two or three regional nodes.

N1c: Tumour deposits in the subserosa, mesentery, or non-peritonealised or perirectal tissues without regional nodal metastasis.

N2a: Tumour in four to six regional nodes.

N2b: Tumour in seven or more regional nodes.

M0:   No distant spread.

M1a: Tumour is confined to one distant organ site (e.g., liver, lung, ovary, non-regional node)

M1b: Tumour has spread to more than one organ or site or the peritoneum.

Source: Adapted from the American Joint Committee on Cancer, *Lung Cancer Staging*, 7th ed, Springer, New York, 2010.

99. A.   Xanthogranulomatous pyelonephritis

Xanthogranulomatous pyelonephritis (XGP) is a chronic suppurative infection in chronic renal obstruction, that is, associated with staghorn calculus. MDCT often shows an enlarged kidney, associated staghorn calculus (75%), perirenal inflammatory stranding or fluid and, low-attenuation fatty masses replacing renal parenchyma. US shows hypoechoic dilated calyces with echogenic rim or with low-level internal echoes replacing the normal renal parenchyma.

Dähnert W. *Radiology Review Manual*, 7th edn. Philadelphia, PA: Lippincott Williams & Wilkins, 2011:971–2.

100. A.   Still disease

Still disease is a clinical manifestation of polyarticular juvenile rheumatoid arthritis characterised by fever, rash, hepatosplenomegaly and pericarditis. There is periosteal reaction of the hand phalanges and broadening of bones with cortical thickening. The presence of advance arthropathy in the hands at such a young age along with the other clinical findings would be compatible with this condition. Lyme disease tends to follow a monoarticular pattern with involvement of the large joints, usually the knee, with the radiological findings not as profound as that of juvenile rheumatoid arthritis.

Dähnert W. *Radiology Review Manual*, 6th edn. Philadelphia, PA: Lippincott Williams & Wilkins, 2007:156.

101. A.   Haemangioblastoma

Haemangioblastoma (HB) is a vascular tumour of the CNS. It occurs most often in the cerebellum, where it is the most common primary neoplasm in adults. Single tumours may be sporadic, but multiple tumours are almost always associated with VHL disease. The most common MR pattern of HB is an enhancing solid mural nodule with an adjacent non-enhancing cyst. The cyst is typically low on T1-weighted and high on T2-weighted images, but it can have areas of high T1 signal from fat or haemorrhage. HB can also look purely cystic, solid or a mural nodule with enhancing cystic wall. HB almost never calcifies.

Pilocytic astrocytoma are cystic, with larger mural nodule, calcification, thick walls and no contrast blush to the mural nodule on angiography.

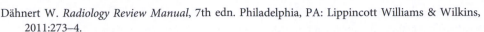

Dähnert W. *Radiology Review Manual*, 7th edn. Philadelphia, PA: Lippincott Williams & Wilkins, 2011:273–4.

Ho VB, et al. Radiologic-pathologic correlation: Hemangioblastoma. *AJNR Am J Neuroradiol.* 1992; 13(5):1343–52.

102. D. Craniopharyngioma

The differential diagnosis would include Rathke cleft cyst, but that is usually intrasellar and thin-walled in appearance. Craniopharyngioma contains calcification and is heterogeneous on MR. Medulloblastoma is usually infratentorial and within the posterior fossa arising in the roof of the fourth ventricle, appears hyperdense on CT, and shows contrast enhancement. Macroadenoma is typically seen in an older age group, whereas microadenoma is hypointense on T1 and non-enhancing post-gadolinium.

Dähnert W. *Radiology Review Manual*, 6th edn. Philadelphia, PA: Lippincott Williams & Wilkins, 2007:278.

103. D. Severe portal hypertension

Contraindications to placement of a TIPS	
Absolute	**Relative**
Primary prevention of variceal bleeding	Hepatoma, particularly if central
Severe congestive heart failure	Obstruction of all hepatic veins
Tricuspid regurgitation	Hepatic encephalopathy
Multiple hepatic cysts	Significant portal vein thrombosis
Uncontrolled systemic infection or sepsis	Severe uncorrectable coagulopathy (INR >5)
Unrelieved biliary obstruction	Thrombocytopenia (<20,000 platelets/mm^3)
Severe pulmonary hypertension	Moderate pulmonary hypertension

The main risk factors for developing HE include age >65 years, child score >12, prior HE, placement of a large diameter stent (>10 mm) and low PPG (<5 mm Hg).

Copelan A, et al. Transjugular intrahepatic portosystemic shunt: Indications, contraindications, and patient work-up. *Semin Intervent Radiol.* 2014;31:235–42.

104. B. Inability to identify T4 tumour.

In the setting of primary rectal cancer, MRI is used to assist in staging, in identifying patients who may benefit from preoperative chemotherapy–radiation therapy, and in surgical planning.

Currently, surgical resection with stage-appropriate neoadjuvant combined-modality therapy is the mainstay in the treatment of rectal cancer. In the past decade, the increasingly widespread adoption of total mesorectal excision (TME) has resulted in a dramatic decline in the prevalence of local recurrence from 38% to less than 10%. TME is a surgical technique that entails *en bloc* resection of the primary tumour and the mesorectum by means of dissection along the mesorectal fascial plane or the circumferential resection margin (CRM). The evolution of surgical techniques and the shift to neoadjuvant chemotherapy–radiation therapy, along with the prognostic heterogeneity of stage T3 tumours, necessitate accurate preoperative staging – primarily in terms of tumour (T) and nodal (N) staging, depth of tumour invasion outside the muscularis propria (early versus advanced stage T3 tumours) and the relationship of the tumour to the potential CRM. Accurate assessment of these factors allows the triage of patients to up-front surgical resection or short- or long-course preoperative radiation therapy or chemotherapy–radiation therapy with appropriate modification of the CRM. Recent studies have shown that high-resolution MRI is a reliable and reproducible technique with high specificity (92%) for predicting a negative CRM, the relationship of the tumour to the CRM and the depth of tumour invasion outside the muscularis propria.

Kaur H, et al. MR imaging for preoperative evaluation of primary rectal cancer: Practical considerations. *RadioGraphics.* 2012;32:389–409.

105. E.   Retrocaval ureter

Retrocaval ureter classically shows medial deviation at L3/4, returning to a more normal position anterior to the iliac vessels. Malakoplaki are rare plaque-like intramural lesions related to chronic UTI, affecting the bladder, ureter, collecting system and even renal parenchyma. They are not premalignant. Schistosomiasis and endometriosis typically cause multiple strictures, which can resemble multiple filling defects. Ureteritis cystica and pyeloureteritis cystica are fairly common post-inflammatory conditions resulting in ureteric filling defects. Other causes include multiple calculi (Steinstrasse), blood clots or multiple vascular collaterals.

Zagoria R. Urteral filling defects. In: *Genitourinary Radiology: The Requisites*, 2nd edn. Philadelphia, PA: Mosby, 2004:191–7.

106. C.   Reflex sympathetic dystrophy

Reflex sympathetic dystrophy, a syndrome that causes significant discomfort, is thought to be due to 'sympathetic overflow', which may explain the pain, warmth and swelling of the involved extremity. At bone scintigraphy, reflex sympathetic dystrophy usually manifests as diffuse, uniformly increased uptake throughout the affected region. Occasionally, reflex sympathetic dystrophy may manifest as a focal abnormality limited to, for example, the hand or knee. Decreased radiotracer accumulation has also been described, especially in children.

Three-phase bone scanning has an accuracy of over 90% and is the radionuclide procedure of choice for diagnosing osteomyelitis in bone not affected by underlying conditions. The first (dynamic) phase reflects the relative amount of blood flow to the area of interest, whereas the second (blood pool) phase reflects the amount of activity that has extravasated into the tissues around the area of interest. The third (delayed [bone]) phase reflects the rate of bone turnover. The classic appearance of osteomyelitis on three-phase bone scans consists of focal hyperperfusion, focal hyperaemia and focally increased bone uptake. Abnormalities at radionuclide bone imaging reflect increased bone mineral turnover in general, not infection specifically. Therefore, conditions associated with increased bone mineral turnover (e.g., tumours, fractures, joint neuropathy) may mimic osteomyelitis at three-phase bone scintigraphy. Under these circumstances, three-phase bone imaging is less useful, primarily because of diminished specificity.

Love C, et al. Radionuclide bone imaging: An illustrative review. *Radiographics*. 2003;23(2):341–58.

107. B.   Cavernous angioma

A cavernous angioma is a 'mulberry-like' vascular malformation. MRI is the most sensitive modality for the diagnosis. With T2-weighted sequences, the lesion is typically characterised by an area of mixed signal intensity, with a central reticulated core and a peripheral rim of decreased signal intensity related to deposition of hemosiderin.

Diffuse axonal injury shows multifocal microbleeds as low signal on GRE or SWI sequences. AVM are identified by serpiginous filling defects with large draining veins and feeding arteries. Haematomas will have mixed signal and will have surrounding oedema and mass effect, unless they are very small.

Brunereau L, et al. Familial form of intracranial cavernous angioma: MR imaging findings in 51 families. French Society of Neurosurgery. *Radiology*. 2000;214(1):209–16.

108. B.   Astrocytoma

About 50%–70% of all primary intracranial tumours are astrocytoma; it is also the most common paediatric brain neoplasm, accounting for 40%–50%.

Dähnert W. *Radiology Review Manual*, 6th edn. Philadelphia, PA: Lippincott Williams & Wilkins, 2007:270.

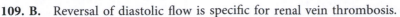
109. B. Reversal of diastolic flow is specific for renal vein thrombosis.

Acute tubular necrosis is the most common cause of 'delayed graft function', whereas chronic rejection is the most common cause of late graft loss.

US findings of diminished renal function include renal enlargement, increased cortical thickness, increased or decreased echogenicity of the renal cortex, loss of corticomedullary differentiation, prominent pyramids, collecting system thickening and effacement of the central sinus echo complex. Elevated resistive index (>0.8) is a non-specific parameter of renal transplant dysfunction; reversal of diastolic flow may also be seen. Renal artery stenosis is the most common vascular complication of transplantation. Doppler criteria include (1) velocities of greater than 2 m/sec, (2) a velocity gradient between stenotic and prestenotic segments of more than 2:1 and (3) marked distal turbulence. Although reversal of diastolic flow is non-specific, the combination with absent venous flow is virtually diagnostic of renal vein thrombosis. Renal artery thrombosis is diagnosed by lack of intrarenal venous and arterial flow. Renal vein stenosis results in three- to fourfold increase in flow velocity. Intrarenal arteriovenous fistulas and pseudoaneurysms are the result of vascular trauma during percutaneous biopsy. Extrarenal arteriovenous fistulas and pseudoaneurysms are extremely uncommon. They typically occur as a result of surgical technique rather than percutaneous biopsy.

Small crescentic peritransplant fluid collections seen immediately after transplantation are most likely haematomas or seromas and are not significant. More complex collections identified later in the post-operative period with clinical evidence of infection may represent abscesses. Although the appearance of urinomas is non-specific, internal septations are seen less often than in haematomas. Lymphocele results in a rounded collection along the mid-ureter, associated with hydronephrosis.

Viazzi F, et al. Ultrasound Doppler renal resistive index: A useful tool for the management of the hypertensive patient. *J Hypertens.* 2014;32(1):149–53.

110. E. All of the above

High-spatial-resolution MRI has already been established as an accurate tool for the preoperative staging of rectal cancer and has resulted in marked improvements in staging accuracy compared with historic studies.

MRI also defines the relationship between a tumour and the mesorectal fascia, which denotes the CRM at TME. The potential CRM is considered involved if the tumour extends to within 1 mm of this fascia.

Patients with locally advanced T3 or T4 disease or disease involving the potential CRM on baseline MRI are offered chemoradiation therapy (CRT). This approach has been shown to decrease the post-operative tumour recurrence rate.

The Magnetic Resonance Imaging and Rectal Cancer European Equivalence (MERCURY) study evaluated consecutive patients undergoing both primary surgery and preoperative therapy with histopathologic correlation and analysed survival outcomes.

The results of the study showed that post-CRT MRI assessment of tumour regression grade correlated with disease-free survival and overall survival and, thus, with patient prognosis. Furthermore, post-treatment MRI prediction of potential CRM involvement also gave prognostic information regarding the risk of local recurrence.

Patel UB. MRI after treatment of locally advanced rectal cancer: How to report tumor response – The MERCURY experience. *AJR Am J Roentgenol.* 2012;199:W486–95.

111. D. Enlarged prostate

Causes of reduced bladder volume include interstitial cystitis, TB cystitis (thimble bladder), cystitis cystica, schistosomiasis, surgical resection and radiation therapy. Prostate enlargement, urethral strictures and Marion's disease (primary bladder neck obstruction) result in increased bladder volume.

Dähnert W. *Radiology Review Manual*, 7th edn. Philadelphia, PA: Lippincott Williams & Wilkins, 2011:917.

112. B. Scapholunate ligament tear

Single-compartment and three-compartment injection techniques have been described for wrist magnetic resonance arthrography. In the three-compartment technique, the mid-carpal and distal radio ulnar joints are initially injected with approximately 1–1.5 mL of iodinated contrast under fluoroscopic guidance. About 3 mL of dilute gadolinium is then injected into the radiocarpal compartment after confirmation of the needle-tip position with the injection of a small volume of iodinated contrast. Contrast should normally be confined to the radiocarpal joint with no leak of contrast into the DRUJ proximally or the mid-carpal joint distally. If contrast extends lateral to the lunate, between it and the scaphoid this is diagnostic of a full-thickness scapholunate ligament tear.

Manaster BJ, et al. *The Requisites: MSK Imaging*, 3rd edn. Philadelphia, PA: Mosby, 2007:141–2.

113. B. Osmotic myelinolysis

Patients with osmotic demyelination syndrome typically present with severe electrolyte disturbances, which lead to seizures or encephalopathy.

A symmetric trident-shaped area in the central pons is a characteristic finding on T2-weighted and FLAIR MRI. The ventrolateral pons and the pontine portion of the corticospinal tracts are typically spared. Decreased signal intensity, with no mass effect, is a classic finding on T1-weighted images. Less commonly, lesions appear isointense relative to surrounding brain tissue on T1 and do not enhance after the administration of contrast material. Case reports have suggested that restricted diffusion may be seen earlier than the classic T2 changes.

It has been noted that myelinolysis can occur outside the pons, a condition that is referred to as *extrapontine myelinolysis*. Sites of extrapontine myelinolysis include the basal ganglia and cerebral white matter and, less commonly, the peripheral cortex, hippocampi and lateral geniculate bodies. Extrapontine myelinolysis occurs in conjunction with central pontine myelinolysis; however, it may also be seen in isolation.

Howard SA, et al. Best cases from the AFIP: Osmotic demyelination syndrome. *Radiographics*. 2009; 29(3):933–8.

114. D. Ependymoma

Medulloblastoma is the most common neoplasm of the posterior fossa in childhood and is the most malignant infratentorial tumour; however, it arises from the roof of the fourth ventricle. Calcification is an atypical feature of medulloblastoma. Brainstem gliomas displace the fourth ventricle. Pilocytic astrocytoma commonly occurs in the cerebellar hemispheres, not in the fourth ventricle.

Ependymoma is the third most common posterior fossa tumour in children. The point of origin is the floor of the fourth ventricle in ependymoma, versus the roof in medulloblastoma. Calcification is a common feature seen in 50% of ependymoma cases, and contrast enhancement is heterogeneous. Although not pathognomonic, the plastic nature of ependymoma results in the classic presentation of a fourth ventricle mass extending through the foramen of Luschka (15%) or foramen of Magendie (60%).

Dähnert W. *Radiology Review Manual*, 6th edn. Philadelphia, PA: Lippincott Williams & Wilkins, 2007:285.
Plaza MJ, et al. Conventional and advanced MRI features of pediatric intracranial tumors: Posterior fossa and suprasellar tumors. *AJR Am J Roentgenol.* 2013;200(5):1115–24.

115. A. Infection

There is a general agreement that 0.70 should be considered the upper limit of normality in adults but not in children, in whom resistive index values are typically higher, especially within the first year of life.

Renal resistive index (RRI) is used for assessment of chronic renal allograft rejection, detection and management of renal artery stenosis, evaluation of progression of risk in chronic kidney disease, differential diagnosis in acute and chronic obstructive renal disease, and more recently as a predictor of renal and overall outcome in the critically ill patient.

Viazzi F, et al. Ultrasound Doppler renal resistive index: A useful tool for the management of the hypertensive patient. *J Hypertens.* 2014;32(1):149–53.

116. D. Findings that might be seen in active long-standing Crohn's disease include submucosal fat deposition, pseudosacculation, surrounding fibro-fatty proliferation and fibrotic strictures.

The main diagnostic purpose of CT enterography in the setting of Crohn's disease is to differentiate active inflammatory strictures from fibrotic strictures in order to guide therapy.

CT features of active Crohn's disease include mucosal hyperenhancement, wall thickening (thickness >3 mm), mural stratification with a prominent vasa recta (comb sign) and mesenteric fat stranding, all of which are exquisitely demonstrated at CT enterography. The capability of CT enterography for depicting extra-enteric disease allows the simultaneous diagnosis of complications associated with Crohn's disease, such as obstruction, sinus tract, fistula and abscess formation.

Mural enhancement is the most sensitive indicator of active Crohn's disease. Care should be taken to compare bowel loops with similar distention, since both the jejunum and normal collapsed loops may demonstrate regions of higher attenuation simulating enhancement. Inadequately distended bowel loops may be difficult to assess, and secondary signs of active disease, such as mesenteric fat stranding, vasa recta prominence or complications such as fistulas and abscesses should be sought to maximise the accuracy of a diagnosis of active disease.

Prominence of the vasa recta adjacent to the inflamed loop of bowel (comb sign), along with increased mesenteric fat attenuation, is the most specific CT feature of active Crohn's disease. Findings that might be seen in inactive long-standing Crohn's disease include submucosal fat deposition, pseudosacculation, surrounding fibro-fatty proliferation and fibrotic strictures.

Elsayes KM, et al. CT enterography: Principles, trends, and interpretation findings. *RadioGraphics.* 2010;30:1955–197.

117. C. Risk of death is high in renal artery aneurysm rupture in non-pregnant patients.

The decision to repair a renal artery aneurysm (RAA) should be based on several factors, including patient age, gender, anticipated pregnancy in female patients and anatomic features including its size. An isolated aneurysm smaller than 2 cm is unlikely to rupture.

Rupture of RAAs is unlikely in most patients. Although some consider calcification to be protective of rupture, no correlation between calcification and risk of rupture is evident. Rupture has historically been associated with a high death rate, especially during pregnancy, and pregnancy is associated with an increased risk of aneurysm rupture. In non-pregnant patients, RAA rupture is likely to be associated with death in less than 10% of cases. Reports suggest that nephrectomy is not always a certain outcome of a RAA rupture, and attempts at kidney salvage in properly selected patients can be justified.

Henke PK, et al. Renal artery aneurysms. A 35-year clinical experience with 252 aneurysms in 168 patients. *Ann Surg.* 2001;234(4):454–63.

118. B. Baker's cyst

A Baker's cyst, or popliteal cyst, is essentially a communicating synovial cyst from the posterior joint capsule. The location of the cyst, which tracks between the medial head of the gastrocnemius and semimembranosus tendon, is characteristic. *Pes anserinus bursitis* refers to inflammation of the bursa around the conjoined tendon insertions of the gracilis, sartorius and semitendinosus muscles at the anteromedial aspect of the proximal tibia. A large parameniscal cyst is a differential, but this requires a meniscal horizontal tear and no mention of this is made.

Dähnert W. *Radiology Review Manual*, 6th edn. Philadelphia, PA: Lippincott Williams & Wilkins, 2007:147.

119. D. Myelomeningocele

Chiari I malformation, also called *cerebellar tonsillar ectopia*, is often an abnormality affecting the hind brain in isolation. Associations of Chiari I malformation include syringohydromyelia, hydrocephalus, basilar impression or basilar invagination, occipitalisation of the atlas, unfused posterior arch of C1, platybasia and Klippel-Feil anomaly. Myelomeningocele are not associated with Chiari I but Chiari II malformation.

Dähnert W. *Radiology Review Manual*, 7th edn. Philadelphia, PA: Lippincott Williams & Wilkins, 2011:278–9.

120. B. Cerebellar pilocytic astrocytoma

The classic imaging appearance of a JPA, which is observed in 30%–60% of cases, is of a large cyst with a solid mural nodule within one of the cerebellar hemispheres; less commonly, JPA may present on imaging as a predominantly solid mass with little to no cyst-like component. Enhancement patterns may vary, but JPA most commonly (46%) appears as a cyst with an enhancing wall and an intensely enhancing mural nodule. DWI of JPAs shows no restricted diffusion, which is consistent with the characteristics of a low-grade tumour.

Although both haemangioblastoma and pilocytic astrocytoma appear similar, the latter is more common within the first two decades, with peak between birth and 9 years of age. Medulloblastoma and ependymoma occur in the fourth ventricle. Arachnoid cyst does not enhance post-contrast.

Dähnert W. *Radiology Review Manual*, 6th edn. Philadelphia, PA: Lippincott Williams & Wilkins, 2007:271.

Plaza MJ, et al. Conventional and advanced MRI features of pediatric intracranial tumors: Posterior fossa and suprasellar tumors. *AJR Am J Roentgenol.* 2013;200(5):1115–24.

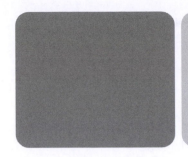

CHAPTER 5
TEST PAPER 3

Questions

Time: 3 hours

1. A 77-year-old man presents with a progressively enlarging pulsatile mass in the left groin corresponding to the puncture site of a previous coronary angiography.
   Urgent outpatient ultrasound shows a large anechoic lesion with peripheral filling defect and arterial pattern intraluminal flow. What is most appropriate management plan?
   A. Covered stent
   B. Ultrasound-guided compression
   C. Ultrasound-guided thrombin injection
   D. Open surgery
   E. CT angiogram first for treatment planning

2. All of the following are associations of Chiari II malformation, except
   A. Dysgenesis of corpus callosum
   B. Klippel–Feil deformity
   C. Syringomyelia
   D. Meningomyelocele
   E. Tectal beaking

3. A 17-year-old girl is newly diagnosed with Crohn's disease and an MR enterography has been requested for evaluation of the disease extent and distribution. All of the following are late findings of Crohn's disease on MRE, except
   A. Fistulae
   B. Skip lesions
   C. Strictures
   D. Small bowel obstruction
   E. Ulcers

4. A 76-year-old woman with one previous history of admission in the medical ward with acute renal failure 6 years ago has now been referred to the radiology department for a CT angiography of the lower limb arteries subject to symptoms of claudication. The renal team were again involved when she developed acute worsening of renal function after the CT study. All the following are features of contrast-induced nephropathy, except
   A. Alternative major insults to kidneys ruled out.
   B. Increase in serum level of creatinine of 0.5 mg/dL.
   C. Rise in serum creatinine level by >50% above baseline.
   D. Increase in serum creatinine occurs 48–72 hours after administration of contrast.
   E. Raised serum creatinine persists for 2–5 days.

5. Skeletal survey is indicated as an investigation for all of the following, except
   A. Eosinophilic granuloma
   B. Multiple myeloma
   C. Non-accidental injury
   D. Skeletal metastasis
   E. Suspected skeletal dysplasia

6. A central mass with homogeneous signal intensity is identified on MRI in the fourth ventricle of a 4-year-old child. Which of the following is the most likely diagnosis?
   A. Astrocytoma
   B. Medulloblastoma
   C. Ependymoma
   D. Pontine glioma
   E. Tectal plate glioma

7. A young woman with positional headache shows a well-defined round mass at the anterior margin of the third ventricle with high signal on both T1W and T2W images. Asymmetrical lateral ventricular enlargement is evident. What is the diagnosis?
   A. Colloid cyst
   B. Choroid plexus cyst
   C. Porencephalic cyst
   D. ACA aneurysm
   E. Haemorrhagic contusion

8. A CT scan of a 25-year-old woman on OCP shows a focal area of low attenuation that demonstrates homogenous enhancement in the arterial phase with rapid washout on the portal venous and delayed phases. She presents a week later with an acute abdomen and hemodynamic instability. What is the most appropriate management?
   A. Gel foam embolisation
   B. Liver resection
   C. Conservative management
   D. Coil embolisation
   E. Radiofrequency ablation

9. A 43-year-old woman currently on treatment for Crohn's disease needs to have her medication reviewed following the recommendation of the MDT. The gastroenterologist wants to perform a CT enterography to assess her disease status and response to treatment prior to the medication review. Which one of the following CT signs suggests inactive Crohn's disease?
   A. Increased mesenteric fat attenuation
   B. Mesenteric fibro-fatty proliferation
   C. Target sign
   D. A non-enhancing thickened bowel wall
   E. Comb sign

10. A 36-year-old woman with small cystic lesions identified in the liver when she had an ultrasound assessment a year ago underwent a CT urogram for renal colic. The CT urogram revealed speckled calcification in the medulla of both kidneys. Review of an old IVU showed a striated nephrogram and filling defects in the proximal right ureter. What is the most likely diagnosis?
    A. Hyperparathyroidism
    B. Medullary sponge kidney
    C. Medullary cystic disease
    D. Acquired renal cystic disease
    E. PCKD

11. A 30-year-old woman is struck over the right cheek during an altercation with another woman. There is bruising and swelling, and a fracture is suspected. What view is the best for demonstrating a zygomatic arch fracture?
    A. Townes view
    B. Submentovertex view
    C. Swimmer's view
    D. Occipito-mental view 45 degrees
    E. Occipito-mental view 30 degrees

12. A 1-year-old infant is admitted with acute stridor. A viral cause is suspected. On AP chest radiography no foreign body is identified, but there is an inverted V appearance of the subglottic trachea. Which of the following is the most likely diagnosis?
    A. Foreign body
    B. Acute laryngotracheobronchitis
    C. Whooping cough
    D. Tracheobronchomalacia
    E. Epiglottitis

13. When can you see the radiographic changes of fat embolism on a chest X-ray?

	<24 hours	48–72 hours	>1 week
A.	No	Yes	No
B.	Yes	No	No
C.	Yes	Yes	No
D.	No	Yes	Yes
E.	Yes	Yes	Yes

14. A 46-year-old woman with constant headache undergoes a CT brain for preliminary evaluation. CT brain reveals a suprasellar solid cystic lesion with some calcification. MRI confirms the suprasellar mass with high signal in both T1W and T2W images. Marginal enhancement of the peripheral solid rim portion of the lesion is also noted. What is the diagnosis?
    A. Craniopharyngioma
    B. Pituitary adenoma
    C. Pineaoblastoma
    D. Meningioma
    E. Dermoid cyst

15. A 53-year-old woman with a long-standing history of known Crohn's disease is referred for a CT enterography for assessment of disease status. Which one of the following statements regarding the CT evaluation of Crohn's disease is true?
    A. Perianal disease is uncommon
    B. A thickened hyperenhancing bowel wall is a sign of active disease
    C. Mural stratification implies perforation in the bowel wall
    D. The comb sign is a specific sign
    E. Perienteric stranding is a specific sign

16. A young woman with polycystic ovarian disease is currently under the transplant team, being reviewed and worked up for potential renal transplantation. Regarding renal transplantation, all of the following are true, except
    A. US kidney, CT angiography and plain abdominal film provide similar information to MR angiography and MR urography.
    B. Pelvicalyceal duplication precludes kidney donation.

C. Twenty percent of kidneys have accessory arterial supply.

D. Right kidney is placed in the left iliac fossa because it is easier technically.

E. Carrel patch is used only for cadaveric kidney.

17. A 25-year-old man presents with progressive increase in knee pain. Plain films show features of osteoarthrosis with increased soft-tissue swelling and density. An MRI shows diffuse low signal on T2W images to the synovium of the knee on the background of large joint effusion. What is the likely diagnosis?

   A. Amyloid arthropathy

   B. Haemophilic arthropathy

   C. PVNS

   D. Primary synovial osteochondromatosis

   E. Rapidly destructive articular disease

18. A 10-year old girl is diagnosed with pilocytic astrocytoma. Which of the following are the most likely findings on MRI?

   A. Hyperintense to brain on T1WI and hypointense on T2WI

   B. Isointense to brain on T1WI and hypointense on T2WI

   C. Isointense to brain on T1WI and isointense on T2WI

   D. Hypointense to brain on T1WI and hyperintense on T2WI

   E. Hyperintense to brain on T1WI and hyperintense on T2WI

19. A 53-year-old woman with chronic renal failure and polycystic renal disease had renal transplantation surgery 5 weeks ago. Initial recovery was uneventful and she is regularly being followed up by the transplant and the renal team. A follow-up graft ultrasound done at 5 weeks post-surgery reveals a large simple fluid collection in relation to the graft. What is the most likely explanation?

   A. Abscess

   B. Resolving haematoma

   C. Lymphocele

   D. Urinoma

   E. Seroma

20. All of the following are causes of lower zone fibrosis, except

   A. Amiodarone

   B. Idiopathic pulmonary fibrosis

   C. Asbestosis

   D. Ankylosing spondylitis

   E. Neurofibromatosis I

21. All of the following are true for neurocysticercosis, except

   A. There are four recognised stages on CT/MR.

   B. The granular nodular stage is not associated with oedema.

   C. The vesicular stage does not show any oedema.

   D. The vesicular stage shows a nodule with a 'hole with dot' appearance.

   E. Colloidal stage shows an avid ring–enhancing capsule.

22. A 43-year-old woman currently on treatment for known Crohn's disease has recently been unwell again with a mildly raised CRP. MRI could not be performed because she was claustrophobic, so a CT was done instead. Which one of the following statements concerning CT enterography for evaluation of small bowel Crohn's disease is not true?

   A. Patients should ideally ingest 1 L of positive oral contrast medium before the start of the examination.

   B. Small bowel distension is a key factor in the examination.

C. Patients should ideally ingest 1 L of negative oral contrast medium before the start of the examination.

D. In CT enterography, CT scanning should start 65 seconds after the start of IV administration of contrast infusion.

E. Patients should fast for 4 hours before the exam.

23. A 5-year-old boy with a large head has widened sutures and Wormian bones on a skull radiograph. Review of other examinations performed earlier shows bilateral hypoplastic clavicles and delayed ossification of symphysis pubis. A chest radiograph shows supernumerary ribs. What is your diagnosis?
    A. Hypothyroidism
    B. Primary hyperparathyroidism
    C. Cleidocranial dysostosis
    D. Ehler–Danlos syndrome
    E. Down's syndrome

24. A child presents following a witnessed first seizure. An MRI scan is arranged. This shows a well-demarcated, T1 hypointense, T2 hyperintense supratentorial mass with a bright rim on FLAIR. There was no enhancement post-contrast. Which of the following is the most likely diagnosis?
    A. Ependymoma
    B. Dysembryoplastic neuroepithelial tumour
    C. Pilocytic astrocytoma
    D. Oligodendroglioma
    E. Ganglioglioma

25. A 2-year-old girl with headache shows a large cyst in the posterior fossa with communicating hydrocephalus; bone windows reveal scalloping of the petrous pyramids. What is the likely diagnosis?
    A. Dandy–Walker malformation
    B. Dandy–Walker variant
    C. Astrocytoma
    D. Haemangioblastoma
    E. Chiari malformation

26. HRCT shows numerous, randomly scattered thin-walled cysts surrounded by normal lung parenchyma. There is interlobular septal thickening and a left pleural effusion. What is the likeliest diagnosis?
    A. Neurofibromatosis
    B. Langerhans's cell histiocytosis
    C. Lymphangiomyomatosis
    D. Alfa-1 antitrypsin deficiency
    E. Lymphocytic interstitial pneumonia

27. A 23-year-old woman with recent diagnosis of Crohn's disease is referred for cross-sectional imaging to assess disease status by the gastroenterology team. She has been booked for MR enterography and will be followed up with MRI. Which of the following statement is false?
    A. MR enterography has less sensitivity and specificity compared to MR enteroclysis for established disease.
    B. MR enteroclysis is better than MR enterography for demonstrating mucosal abnormalities.

C. MR imaging provides superior soft-tissue contrast and excellent depiction of fluid and oedema.

D. MR enterography is more acceptable to the patient than MR enteroclysis.

E. Jejunal distension is better with MR enteroclysis.

28. An adolescent with growth disturbance presents with a visual difficulty. A non-calcified, thin-walled cyst with no enhancement is seen in the intrasellar region on MRI. Which of the following is the most likely diagnosis?

A. Craniopharyngioma

B. Macroadenoma

C. Epidermoid

D. Rathke cleft cyst

E. Metastasis

29. A 56-year-old woman shows an 8-cm solid enhancing mass in the left kidney with a central area of low attenuation on contrast-enhanced CT scan. US study performed earlier showed a large heterogeneous solid mass in the left kidney with a central stellate hypoechoic area. The most likely diagnosis based on the imaging finding would be

A. Renal cell carcinoma

B. Clear cell carcinoma

C. Rhabdomyoma

D. Adenoma

E. Oncocytoma

30. A 25-year-old man has injured his knee. Sagittal T2W MRI sequences show a double posterior cruciate ligament (PCL) sign. Which of the following is the most likely injury?

A. Ruptured PCL

B. Bucket-handle tear of meniscus

C. Osteochondral fragmentation

D. Radial tear of meniscus

E. Anterior cruciate ligament (ACL)

31. A 40-year-old man presents with shortness of breath. Chest X-ray shows a diffuse bilateral reticulonodular pattern within the middle and upper zones. There are multiple small cysts in keeping with honeycomb lung. The lung volumes are preserved. What is the most likely diagnosis?

A. Langerhans cell histiocytosis

B. Lymphangiomyomatosis

C. Centrilobular emphysema

D. Idiopathic pulmonary fibrosis

E. Allergic bronchopulmonary aspergillosis

32. A 67-year-old woman with systemic amyloidosis diagnosed on rectal biopsy presents to her GP with progressive central abdominal pain, bloating, and abdominal distension. All of the following are abnormalities due to amyloid infiltration in the gastrointestinal tract, except

A. 'Jejunisation' of the ileum

B. Macroglossia

C. Gastroesophageal reflux

D. Diffuse nodular wall thickening in small bowel

E. Colonic dilatation due to adynamic ileus

33. A 44-year-old man with a painful right index finger and positive Love's test undergoes a plain film study, which shows extrinsic erosion involving the terminal phalanx with a preserved sclerotic rim. There is no definite history of previous injury to the index finger. MRI is

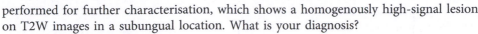

performed for further characterisation, which shows a homogenously high-signal lesion on T2W images in a subungual location. What is your diagnosis?

A. Epidermoid inclusion cyst
B. Glomus tumour
C. Implantation dermoid cyst
D. Soft-tissue component of osteosarcoma
E. Giant cell tumour of the tendon sheath

34. A 66-year-old man with a palpable mass in the left loin and painless haematuria undergoes a staging CT of the abdomen for renal cell carcinoma. The staging CT shows a 6 cm heterogeneous, solid left renal mass with direct extension into the perinephric fat. Tumour mass is seen in the left renal vein extending into the IVC, but this is confined to below the level of the diaphragm. What is the T stage?

A. T1
B. T2
C. T3a
D. T3b
E. T3c

35. A 25-year-old man with headache shows a heterogeneous mass on T2W MRI, in the fourth ventricle. No contrast enhancement is evident, but closer inspection reveals subarachnoid fat droplets in the ambient cisterns and a fat fluid level in the ventricles. What is the diagnosis?

A. Epidermoid cyst
B. Uncomplicated dermoid cyst
C. Ruptured dermoid cyst
D. Arachnoid cyst
E. Infected arachnoid cyst

36. An 11-day-old child presents with duct-dependant cyanosis and congestive cardiac failure. Chest X-ray shows an enlarged heart with a figure of eight pattern and prominent veins. What is the likely diagnosis?

A. Transposition of the great vessels (TGA)
B. Truncus arteriosus
C. Tetralogy of Fallot
D. Vein of Galen aneurysm
E. Total anomalous pulmonary venous return (TAPVR)

37. A middle-aged man presents with easy fatigability. CT shows an anterior mediastinal mass with areas of calcifications, invading the mediastinal structures. There are multiple small pleural masses. What is the most likely diagnosis?

A. Thymoma
B. Thymic lipoma
C. Lymphoma
D. Teratoma
E. Asbestosis

38. A 27-year-old man is complaining of central umbilical pain, which has gradually settled in the right iliac fossa with local guarding and rebound tenderness suggesting local peritonitis. Clinical features suggest acute appendicitis; however, an apparent mass is felt in the right iliac fossa, which prompts a CT scan.

Which one of the following CT findings has the highest specificity and sensitivity for perforated appendicitis?

A. Free intra-abdominal fluid
B. Enlarged periappendiceal lymph nodes

C. Periappendiceal abscess

    D. Periappendiceal fluid

    E. Focal appendiceal wall enhancement defect

39. A 22-year-old man involved in an RTA is admitted to ITU with multiorgan injury in an obtunded state. Initial CT is thought to be normal and an MRI is organised. Limited sequence MR scan reveals several round foci of low T1, high T2 signal change bilaterally at the grey–white interface with further areas in the splenium of the corpus callosum. What is the diagnosis?
    A. Multiple sclerosis
    B. Vasculitis
    C. Diffuse axonal injury
    D. Infection
    E. Neurosarcoid

40. A 42-year-old woman with hereditary non-polyposis colon cancer syndrome (HNPCC) shows a suspicious filling defect in the left renal pelvis on IVU, which is subsequently confirmed on CT urography. She is currently being investigated for haematuria and left loin pain. What is the most likely diagnosis, given her genetic background?
    A. Renal lymphoma
    B. TCC of the renal pelvis
    C. Squamous cell cancer of the renal pelvis
    D. Renal metastasis
    E. Endometriosis

41. A 15-year-old boy with haemophilia presents to his GP with progressive worsening of right knee pain. Plain films exclude the presence of a fracture. All of the following are features of haemophilic arthropathy affecting the knee, except
    A. Epiphyseal enlargement
    B. Widened intercondylar notch
    C. Squared patella
    D. Flattening of femoral condyles
    E. Erlenmeyer flask deformity

42. A 7-year-old boy presents with acute scrotum. Which one of the following features on ultrasound is more suggestive of a diagnosis other than testicular torsion?
    A. Abnormal testicular texture
    B. Testicular swelling
    C. Coiled spermatic cord
    D. Scrotal wall oedema
    E. Decreased or absent blood flow

43. All of the following are true of herpes simplex encephalitis, except
    A. It mostly affects the limbic system.
    B. CT may be negative in the first few days.
    C. There is a tendency for haemorrhage.
    D. Increased signal is seen on T2W images in the temporal lobe.
    E. DWI shows low signal in the affected area.

44. CXR demonstrates a mediastinal mass. The heart borders are not obscured and the hilar vessels are visible. Which of the following is in keeping with the CXR findings?
    A. Lymphoma
    B. Teratoma
    C. Retrosternal goiter
    D. Nerve sheath tumour
    E. Left ventricular aneurysm

45. A 27-year-old woman is complaining of lower abdominal pain localised to the left iliac fossa. A CT scan raises a suspicion of epiploic appendagitis. All of the following statements about epiploic appendagitis are true, except
    A. Treatment is usually medical.
    B. It can mimic acute appendicitis or diverticulitis.
    C. It is usually associated with change in bowel habits.
    D. Most patients have normal inflammatory markers.
    E. The most common site of appendagitis is adjacent to the sigmoid colon.

46. A 35-year-old man undergoing a plain abdominal X-ray in the A&E department reveals multiple punctuate areas of calcification over both renal areas. Review of the notes reveals a history of upper GI endoscopy and previous psychiatric consultations. Which of the following are you going to suggest in your report?
    A. Urology referral and check of serum TSH levels
    B. Urology referral and check of serum parathyroid hormone levels
    C. Urology referral and check of serum alkaline phosphatase
    D. Urology referral and check of serum LDH
    E. Urology referral and check of serum calcitonin levels

47. A previously well 29-year-old presents with inversion injury. An X-ray demonstrates no fracture. However, there is a well-circumscribed lesion in the tibia with a ground-glass matrix and a narrow zone of transition. There is no periosteal reaction or associated soft-tissue mass. Which of the following is the most likely diagnosis?
    A. Polyostotic fibrous dysplasia
    B. Osteosarcoma
    C. Osteoid osteoma
    D. Adamantinoma
    E. Monostotic fibrous dysplasia

48. A 2-year-old boy presents with bowing of the left leg. There is no history of trauma and the right leg appears normal. Standing anteroposterior radiography is performed. This shows a varus deformity of the left knee with fragmentation of the posteromedial tibial metaphysis and absence of the medial epiphysis. The right leg appears radiographically normal and bony density is preserved throughout. Which of the following is the most likely cause?
    A. Neurofibromatosis
    B. Blount disease
    C. Congenital bowing
    D. Developmental bowing
    E. Osteogenesis imperfecta

49. Barium swallow shows anterior indentation of the oesophagus and posterior indentation of the trachea. The cause for this is
    A. Aberrant right subclavian artery
    B. Double aortic arch
    C. Right-sided aortic arch
    D. Aberrant left pulmonary artery
    E. Aberrant left subclavian artery

50. A 34-year-old woman has been complaining of acute right upper-quadrant pain for the last 2 days. Her inflammatory markers are raised and she looks unwell. She is known to have gallstones from a previous US study. All of the following are MR findings consistent with the diagnosis of acute cholecystitis, except
    A. Gallbladder wall thickening greater than 3 mm
    B. Gallbladder wall oedema

C. Contracted gallbladder

    D. Pericholecystic fluid

    E. Echogenic bile

51. A 65-year-old man with three months' history of painless haematuria was diagnosed as having a primary bladder cancer on cystoscopy. An MRI of the pelvis is scheduled for staging. With regard to MRI for staging of bladder cancer, which of the following is incorrect?

    A. Papillary tumour is best seen on T1W images.

    B. Infiltrating component is better assessed with post-contrast T1W than T2W images.

    C. Endorectal coil improves visualisation of bladder wall layers.

    D. T2W helps in differentiating T2b and T3 tumours.

    E. Involved seminal vesicles show high signal on T2W images.

52. The following are true regarding hyperparathyroidism, except

    A. Brown tumours are more common in the primary form.

    B. Soft-tissue calcification is typically associated with the secondary form.

    C. Chondrocalcinosis is more common in the primary form.

    D. Osteosclerosis is more common in the primary form.

    E. Bone resorption is equally seen in both primary and secondary conditions.

53. All of the following are associated with multiple focal hyper intensities in both cerebral hemispheres, except

    A. CADASIL

    B. ADEM

    C. MS

    D. Epidermoid

    E. Sarcoidosis

54. A 12-year-old girl with known thalassaemia major undergoes skull radiography. Which area of the skull is least affected by this condition?

    A. Facial bones

    B. Frontal bone

    C. Occipital bone

    D. Temporal bone

    E. Parietal bone

55. A 30-year-old man recently treated with bone marrow transplant for acute myeloid leukaemia 12 weeks ago presents with cough and fever. HRCT demonstrates multiple micronodules with areas of consolidation and ground-glass attenuation. What is the likeliest diagnosis?

    A. Pneumocystis carinii pneumonia

    B. Cytomegalovirus pneumonitis

    C. Drug toxicity

    D. Acute rejection

    E. Graft versus host disease

56. A 49-year-old man patient previously fit and well has been admitted with acute epigastric pain and raised amylase. A diagnosis of pancreatitis is made. What is the most appropriate imaging examination for assessment of acute pancreatitis?

    A. Abdominal radiography

    B. Ultrasound

    C. Magnetic resonance cholangiopancreatography (MRCP)

    D. Contrast-enhanced CT

    E. EUS

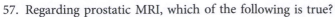

57. Regarding prostatic MRI, which of the following is true?
   A. Zonal anatomy is best seen on T1.
   B. The central and transition zones show similar low signal.
   C. The transition zone is heterogeneous in the young.
   D. The peripheral zone maintains a uniform shape throughout the length of the gland.
   E. US is better than MRI for assessing prostate volume.

58. A 25-year-old woman presents to the A&E department with an acutely painful right hip and difficulty in weight-bearing. A radiograph is obtained in casualty. No fractures are identified but the radiograph reveals a subluxed femoral head on the right with a shallow acetabulum and a centre-edge angle of 18 degrees. What is your diagnosis?
   A. Perthes disease
   B. Ollier's disease
   C. Developmental dysplasia of the hip
   D. Traumatic subluxation
   E. Congenital coxa vara with subluxation

59. A 53-year-old woman with facial pain shows a lobulated, homogenous CSF density mass in the left CP angle on CT. No contrast enhancement is evident and the differentials considered are either an arachnoid cyst or an epidermoid cyst. Which of the following investigations will you consider to confirm your diagnosis?
   A. MR angiogram of the circle of Willis
   B. Diffusion-weighted MRI
   C. PET CT
   D. Post-gadolinium MR brain
   E. MR spectroscopy

60. A 15-year-old girl presents with acute pelvic pain. Beta-human chorionic gonadotrophin (β-hCG) is normal. US demonstrates a thin-walled 5 cm echogenic adnexal mass with posterior acoustic enhancement. There is no colour internal Doppler signal. Follow-up imaging after 3 months fails to demonstrate the mass. What is the most likely cause?
   A. Appendix abscess
   B. Haemorrhagic ovarian cyst
   C. Ovarian dermoid
   D. Ectopic pregnancy
   E. Ovarian torsion

61. A truck driver has been involved in an RTA. He has sustained head injuries and lower limb fractures. A CT performed 3 hours after injury shows small patches of consolidation within the posterior aspect of the lungs. What are these most likely to represent?
   A. Fat embolism
   B. Pulmonary contusion
   C. ARDS
   D. Traumatic lung cysts
   E. Pulmonary embolism

62. A 27-year-old woman who is 26 weeks pregnant has been complaining of lower abdominal pain, which has gradually settled in the right iliac fossa. On surgical review, she is suspected to have acute appendicitis. An MRI of the abdomen is organised. All of the following features are expected features of acute appendicitis on MRI, except
   A. Calibre of greater than 7 mm
   B. Thick wall (>2 mm)
   C. High-signal-intensity luminal contents

D. Periappendiceal fat stranding

E. Low luminal signal intensity on T1 and T2-weighted images.

63. A 75-year-old man undergoing MRI of the prostate for known malignancy reveals low signal intensity in the peripheral zone of the prostate on T2W images extending from the 3 o'clock position to the 8 o'clock position. Further note is also made of bulky low-signal seminal vesicles bilaterally. What is the T stage of the tumour?

A. T2b

B. T2c

C. T3a

D. T3b

E. T4

64. A 52-year-old woman is involved in a RTA. Trauma series radiographs reveal a complex pelvic fracture. There are no other appreciable injuries. She is haemodynamically unstable, and fluid resuscitation is commenced. Which of the following steps is the next most important?

A. Trauma protocol CT scan with angiographic sequences

B. Immediate surgery under the orthopaedic surgeons

C. Discussion with interventional radiologists with view to catheter angiography and possible intervention

D. Placement of a pelvic wrap device

E. Blood transfusion

65. CT brain of a 10 year old girl shows a large cyst in the posterior fossa. All of the following favour pilocystic astrocytoma over haemangioblastoma, except

A. Size greater than 5 cm

B. Calcifications

C. Smaller nodule

D. Thicker-walled lesion

E. No angiographic contrast blush of the mural nodule

66. An 8-year-old girl is admitted with sudden onset acute pelvic pain, and ovarian torsion is suspected. Which of the following statements regarding ovarian torsion is least accurate?

A. Benign cystic teratoma is the most common neoplastic cause.

B. It most commonly occurs on the left.

C. The 'whirlpool sign' is a feature on ultrasound.

D. The most common finding is asymmetric ovarian volumes.

E. An urgent referral to gynaecology should be made.

67. A 20-year-old man with a history of thrombophlebitis and recurrent mouth and genital ulcers undergoes a CXR. A well-defined opacity in the right hilum is noted. Contrast-enhanced CT confirms that the opacity has sharp borders, with intense enhancement in the arterial phase. What is the most likely diagnosis?

A. Pulmonary artery aneurysm

B. Pulmonary vein varix

C. Necrotic hilar node

D. Endobronchial carcinoid

E. Pulmonary AVM

68. A 39-year-old woman weighing 22 stone is referred for weight loss surgery. With regard to bariatric surgical procedures, which one of the following statements concerning complications of the laparoscopic adjustable gastric banding procedure (LAGBP) is false?

A. Lap band misplacement is usually due to inexperience on the part of the surgeon.

B. Stomal stenosis is a rare complication.

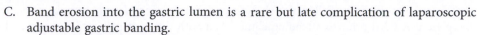

C. Band erosion into the gastric lumen is a rare but late complication of laparoscopic adjustable gastric banding.

D. Acute pouch dilation usually results from marked stomal narrowing secondary to overfilling of the band or from distal band slippage and obstruction.

E. Distal band slippage is thought to result from recurrent vomiting, overinflation of the band or faulty surgical technique.

69. A 31-year-old man involved in an RTA has sustained a pelvic fracture and is investigated with retrograde urethrography to assess urethral injury. There is no opacification of the urinary bladder and contrast is seen to extravasate into the perineum. What is the most likely grade of urethral injury?
    A. Grade I – stretching without tear
    B. Incomplete tear Grade II – above the urogenital diaphragm
    C. Complete tear Grade II – above the urogenital diaphragm
    D. Incomplete tear Grade III – at the level of the urogenital diaphragm
    E. Complete tear Grade III – at the level of the urogenital diaphragm

70. A 66-year-old woman presents with progressive worsening of right shoulder pain and limitation of movement. X-ray and MRI show a combination of rotator cuff tear and established arthropathy described as Milwaukee shoulder. All of the following are recognised features, except
    A. Large osteophytes
    B. Multiple loose bodies
    C. Subacromial abutment of humeral head
    D. Large subchondral cysts
    E. Subchondral collapse and deformed humeral head

71. MRI brain on a patient with head injury shows a 3 × 3 cm haematoma in the right occipital lobe, which retuns high signals on both T1W and T2W images. What is the phase of the intracerebral haematoma?
    A. Hyperacute
    B. Acute
    C. Early subacute
    D. Late subacute
    E. Chronic

72. A 3-month-old infant with abdominal distension is seen to have enlarged adrenal glands on ultrasound along with hepatosplenomegaly. CT confirms the enlarged liver and spleen and demonstrates bilateral enlarged adrenal glands, which are of normal triangular morphology but contain widespread punctate calcification. What is the most likely diagnosis?
    A. Bilateral neuroblastomas
    B. Non-traumatic adrenal haemorrhage
    C. Wolman disease
    D. Adrenocortical hyperplasia
    E. Bilateral adrenocortical carcinoma

73. A 3-year-old boy presenting with gross haematuria is found to have a renal mass on ultrasound, thought to represent a Wilms tumour. Which of the following statements regarding Wilms tumour is inaccurate?
    A. Beckwith–Wiedemann syndrome is a recognised association.
    B. The majority present with an asymptomatic palpable mass.
    C. Horseshoe kidney is a recognised association.
    D. Stage IV disease refers to bilateral renal involvement at diagnosis.
    E. Nephroblastomatosis is a recognised precursor.

74. A 60-year-old man has a CXR, which shows a peripheral opacity forming an obtuse angle with the pleura. A CXR prior to attending clinic taken with different inspiration shows a slight change in position and shape of this lesion. A wrist X-ray performed previously following trauma showed periosteal reaction in the radius and ulna. What is the likeliest cause for the above presentation?
    A. Mesothelioma
    B. Primary lung cancer
    C. Pleural fibroma
    D. Pleural lipoma
    E. Asbestosis

75. A 56-year-old woman weighing 22 stone is referred to the bariatric surgeon for a bypass procedure for weight loss. An Roux-en-Y gastric bypass surgery (RYGBP) is performed after discussion about the advantages and disadvantages of the procedure. Regarding complications of this procedure, the following are all true, except
    A. Extraluminal leak is the most serious early complication of RYGBP.
    B. Transient anastomotic narrowing and obstruction may occur during the early post-operative period.
    C. Strictures at the gastrojejunal anastomosis may be caused by post-surgical scarring at the anastomosis or by chronic ischaemia resulting from tension on the gastrojejunostomy.
    D. Anastomotic strictures usually appear on upper GI studies as an irregular long segment narrowing at the gastrojejunal anastomosis.
    E. Anastomotic leak.

76. A 36-year-old man notices a hard, non-tender lump in his right testes. He cannot convincingly recollect a history of recent or past trauma to the scrotum. US reveals a well-defined, hyporeflective homogenous mass without internal calcification or cystic spaces in the right testes. What is the most likely diagnosis?
    A. Seminoma
    B. Teratoma
    C. Sertoli cell tumour
    D. Lymphoma
    E. Embryonal cell tumour

77. A 76-year-old man with progressive hind- and midfoot pain is referred to the radiology department for a plain film of his foot. Advanced neuropathic type arthropathy involving the mid-tarsal joints of the foot is noted. All of the following are acquired peripheral causes of neuropathic osteoarthropathy, except
    A. Diabetes mellitus
    B. Leprosy
    C. Syringomyelia
    D. Repeated intra-articular corticosteroid injections
    E. Peripheral nerve injury

78. Antenatal ultrasound shows an abnormal facial contour with a large cyst without any cortical mantle of cerebral tissue anteriorly. Septum pellucidum, falx cerebri and optic tracts are not identified with evidence of a fused midline thalamus. A single large ventricle is identified. Normal brain stem, midbrain and cerebellum are noted. What is the diagnosis?
    A. Alobar holoprosencephaly
    B. Lobar holoprosencephaly
    C. Hydranencephaly
    D. Anencephaly
    E. Congenital hydrocephalous

79. Causes of 'tree in bud' appearance include all, except
    A. Tuberculosis
    B. Allergic bronchopulmonary aspergillosis
    C. Cystic fibrosis
    D. Tumour emboli
    E. Chronic pulmonary embolism

80. Following a motorcycle accident a patient notices wasting of the small muscles of his left hand. Neurologist diagnoses brachial plexus injury and arranges a MRI to determine whether it is preganglionic or postganglionic. Which of the following findings would suggest a preganglionic brachial plexus injury?
    A. Pseudomeningocele
    B. Thickened nerves
    C. Increased T2 signal in the peripheral nerve
    D. Discontinuity of the peripheral nerve with distal nerve contraction
    E. Direct compression of the brachial plexus by haematoma

81. A 3-year-old girl presents with isosexual precocious puberty, gelastic seizures, and a soft-tissue density round mass at the region of the hypothalamus on MR brain. No contrast enhancement is evident and the lesion returns signal similar to grey matter on all sequences. What is the diagnosis?
    A. Pituitary macroadenoma
    B. Cyst of the Rathke's pouch
    C. Hamartoma of tuber cinereum
    D. Meningioma
    E. Aneurysm of ACA

82. A 60-year-old man presents with a long-standing, painless mass in his left thigh, which has been increasing in size over recent months. Plain film demonstrates a soft-tissue mass with poorly defined curvilinear calcification and cortical erosion of the underlying femur. MRI demonstrates an inhomogeneous, poorly defined lesion that is isointense to muscle on T1W images and hyperintense on T2W images. Which of the following is the most likely diagnosis?
    A. Liposarcoma
    B. Pleomorphic undifferentiated sarcoma
    C. Rhabdomyosarcoma
    D. Lipoma
    E. Osteomyelitis

83. A 77-year-old woman is sent for a staging scan following a diagnosis of melanoma. All are true for melanoma involving the abdomen, except
    A. The small bowel is the most common site of gastrointestinal tract involvement by melanoma.
    B. Metastatic disease to the liver is always calcified.
    C. Omental and peritoneal deposits occur early in disease.
    D. Large bowel lesions are uncommon.
    E. Mesenteric involvement could mimic lymphoma.

84. All the following statements regarding testicular tumour are correct, except
    A. Testicular lymphoma commonly involves the epididymis and spermatic cord.
    B. Testicular microlithiasis is associated with alveolar microlithiasis.
    C. Sertoli cell tumour is associated with Peutz–Jeghers syndrome.
    D. Primary extragonadal germ cell tumours commonly affect the testes.
    E. The testis is a common site of leukaemia recurrence.

85. An 18-month-old child is suspected of having sustained non-accidental head injury (NAHI). He has a CT scan on admission, which was normal but has ongoing focal neurology. Which one of the following is the most appropriate next step?
    A. Repeat non-contrast CT of head
    B. Repeat CT of head with contrast
    C. MRI of cervical spine
    D. MRI of head with T2* GE and DWI
    E. MRI head with gadolinium

86. A 53-year-old man with painful haematuria and left loin to groin pain progressing over the last 5 days has been scheduled for a CT urogram to look for a left ureteric calculus. Regarding CT evaluation of uretric calculi, all of the following are true, except
    A. Indinavir stones are often missed on CT.
    B. Ureteric stones tend to lodge at PUJ, VUJ and where the ureter crosses the iliac vessels.
    C. Periureteric stranding is a secondary sign of ureteric obstruction.
    D. Stones less than 10 mm can pass spontaneously without intervention.
    E. Comet tail sign is specific for distal ureteric calculus.

87. A middle-aged woman presents to casualty with progressive increase in right hip pain and inability to weight-bear. Plain films performed in the A&E department reveal a stress fracture involving the neck of the femur, which accounts for her clinical state. However, there is no history of acute trauma. Which one of the following statements concerning fatigue and insufficiency fractures is true?
    A. A fatigue fracture is due to abnormal stress on an abnormal bone.
    B. A fatigue fracture is due to normal stress on a normal bone.
    C. An insufficiency fracture is due to abnormal stress on a normal bone.
    D. A fatigue fracture is due to abnormal stress on a normal bone.
    E. The cause of these two fractures is essentially the same.

88. All the following are true of Creutzfeldt Jacob disease, except
    A. No contrast enhancement
    B. No white matter involvement
    C. Bilateral high T2 signal change in the caudate and putamen
    D. Associated with dementia and myoclonus
    E. Self-limiting disease of good prognosis

89. A 42-year-old woman with right upper abdominal pain and worsening LFTs is referred for an US. The scan shows heterogeneous echotexture to the liver without any definite focal lesions and no Doppler flow within the hepatic veins.
    A dual phase CT liver shows hepatomegaly and a hyperenhancement of the caudate lobe with hypoenhancement to the rest of the liver. Ascites is present. A diagnosis of Budd–Chiari syndrome is made. All of the following are predisposing factors, except
    A. Pregnancy
    B. Antiphospholipid syndrome
    C. Alcohol abuse
    D. Membranous web-like obstruction of HV or IVC
    E. Tumour invasion of the hepatic veins

90. A 10-year-old boy with history of Down's syndrome, recurrent chest infection and dyspnoea on exertion presents to the paediatrician. Chest X-ray shows mild cardiomegaly and prominent pulmonary venous markings. What is the most likely diagnosis?
    A. Hypertrophic cardiomyopathy
    B. Ostium primum ASD

C. Ostium secundum ASD
D. VSD
E. PDA

91. A 10-year-old boy undergoes a contrast-enhanced CT abdomen following blunt abdominal trauma. Anaphylactic shock is suspected. What is the treatment?
    A. 0.5 ml of 1:1000 IM adrenaline
    B. 0.5 ml of 1:10,000 IM adrenaline
    C. 0.15 ml of 1:1000 IM adrenaline
    D. 0.3 ml of 1:1000 IM adrenaline
    E. 0.3 ml of 1:1000 IV adrenaline

92. A middle-aged woman with a history of right-sided breast cancer underwent adjuvant radiotherapy following surgery several years ago. She has been symptom free with no features to suggest local recurrence. Over the last few weeks she has developed worsening right-sided chest pain. Chest radiograph shows a partially destroyed right rib with a large eccentric soft-tissue component. Which one of the following is the most likely histology of the lesion?
    A. Osteosarcoma
    B. Chondrosarcoma
    C. Ewing's sarcoma
    D. Angiosarcoma
    E. Fibrosarcoma

93. A 60-year-old man with sepsis and moderate left hydronephrosis secondary to an obstructing left mid-ureteric calculus has been referred to the interventional team for a percutaneous nephrostomy. All of the following statements regarding percutaneous nephrostomy are true, except
    A. The Brodel bloodless zone lies just anterior to the lateral convex border of the kidney.
    B. The posterior calix of the upper/middle collecting system is best for ureteral negotiation.
    C. Large bore drains are used in procedures complicated by gross haematuria.
    D. Nephrostomogram and over-distension can cause bacteraemia.
    E. Renal arteriovenous fistula are a recognised complication.

94. A 43-year-old man with a known diagnosis of AIDS presents with headache, personality change and seizure. Unenhanced CT brain shows a 5 cm, slightly hyperdense lesion in the right frontal lobe with significant peritumoural oedema with little mass effect. Contrast-enhanced MRI brain shows an irregular ring-enhancing lesion in the corresponding location in a sea of oedema. What is your diagnosis?
    A. Primary CNS lymphoma
    B. Systemic NHL
    C. PML
    D. Toxoplasmosis
    E. CMV encephalitis

95. A 5-year-old girl presents with left-sided abdominal pain. On examination, there is a palpable mass in the left flank. CT demonstrates a well-circumscribed multiseptated cystic renal mass replacing the lower pole of the left kidney. The intervening septae are thick and enhanced post-contrast, and the cysts appear to be herniating into the renal pelvis. What is the most likely diagnosis?
    A. Multicystic dysplastic kidney
    B. Multilocular cystic nephroma
    C. Nephroblastomatosis
    D. Polycystic kidney disease
    E. Mesoblastic nephroma

96. CXR shows a large mass in the right lower lobe. Staging CT shows it to be 8 cm invading the right mediastinal pleura with ipsilateral mediastinal and subcarinal nodes. There is also a contralateral 3 cm mass in the left upper lobe. This would be staged:
    A. T3 N2 M1a
    B. T4 N2 M1a
    C. T3 N3 M1b
    D. T4 N3 M1b
    E. T3 N2 M1b

97. A 74-year-old man with orthopnoea, ankle swelling and paroxysmal nocturnal dyspnoea has had US to evaluate right upper-quadrant pain. The scan shows hepatomegaly with a coarse liver. He subsequently has CT of the liver. All of the following are CT findings of hepatic congestion secondary to congestive heart failure, except
    A. Late enhancement of the IVC and central hepatic veins.
    B. Heterogeneous mottled mosaic pattern of enhancement on the portal phase.
    C. Hepatomegaly and ascites may be present.
    D. Dilated hepatic veins.
    E. Periportal oedema.

98. A 56-year-old man undergoes US of the scrotum to investigate painless swelling of both testes. He does not recall any previous trauma and has been systemically well apart from chronic anaemia, for which he is being investigated by the haematologists. US reveals bilateral solid testicular masses. What is the most likely diagnosis?
    A. Metastases from renal cell carcinoma
    B. Leukaemia
    C. Seminoma
    D. Fractures
    E. Lymphoma

99. A 23-year-old woman with multiple skin lesions presents to the ophthalmologist with worsening of vision. MRI brain and orbits reveal a thickened enhancing right optic nerve with further focal areas of T2W hyperintensities in the brainstem and basal ganglia. What is the diagnosis?
    A. NF2 – optic tract meningioma
    B. TS – optic neuritis
    C. MS – optic neuritis
    D. NF1 – optic glioma
    E. VHL – optic haemangioblastoma

100. A 17-year-old man presents with new onset back and loin pain. A low-dose CT KUB reveals a sclerotic lesion in the lamina of one of the thoracic vertebra. Which one of the following statements concerning osteoid osteomas of the spine is true?
    A. They can cause painful scoliosis.
    B. Involvement of the lumbar vertebrae is atypical.
    C. Lesions of more than 2 cm in diameter are more common on presentation.
    D. The 'nidus' within the lesion is osteosclerotic.
    E. They rarely enhance on MRI after intravenous administration of contrast material.

101. A 50-year-old woman recently returned from holiday complaining of fever and malaise. CXR showed bilateral non-segmental bronchopneumonic pattern. CT showed multiple small nodules in the lungs with enlarged mediastinal and hilar nodes, which show popcorn calcification. What is the most likely diagnosis?
    A. Histoplasmosis
    B. Tuberculosis

C. Lymphoma
D. Legionnaire's disease
E. Blastomycosis

102. A 7-month-old baby is seen at the general paediatric clinic with failure to thrive and irritability. Few clinical signs are present on examination, although the child cries on manipulation of his lower limbs. A plain radiograph of the left leg was performed a few weeks ago for a suspected fracture, but no acute bony injury was identified. The doctor reviews this radiograph again. It shows generalised osteopaenia of the distal femur and proximal tibia and fibula. A sclerotic rim surrounds the distal femoral epiphysis, which itself is abnormally lucent. A bony spur can be seen arising from the distal femoral metaphysis. What is the most likely diagnosis?
   A. Hypoparathyroidism
   B. Scurvy
   C. Rickets
   D. Hypothyroidism
   E. Hypophosphatasia

103. A 37-year-old man has recently returned from a holiday and has been feeling unwell. Blood tests carried out by the GP show raised inflammatory markers and abnormal liver function test results. A provisional diagnosis of viral hepatitis is made. All of the following are MR features of acute hepatitis, except
   A. Heterogeneous liver enhancement.
   B. Irregular outline to liver with caudate lobe hypertrophy.
   C. Extrahepatic findings in patients with severe acute hepatitis include gallbladder wall thickening due to oedema and, infrequently, ascites.
   D. Involved areas may be normal or demonstrate decreased signal intensity on T1W images and increased signal intensity on T2W images.
   E. Periportal oedema appears as high-signal-intensity areas on T2W images.

104. A 26-year-old man presents to his GP with progressive swelling of the right hemi-scrotum, pain, and sick sensation, following an impact during a recent cricket match played 4 days ago. Which of the following statements regarding scrotal trauma is incorrect?
   A. The tunica albuginea is intact in testicular fracture.
   B. The tunica albuginea is disrupted in testicular rupture.
   C. Intratesticular hematomas can be multifocal.
   D. Testicular fracture requires urgent surgical exploration.
   E. Epididymal injuries are generally associated with testicular injuries.

105. A 15-year-old man patient presents with pain on the medial aspect of the right elbow. MRI shows no joint effusion or signal change. The medial collateral ligament is lax, ill-defined, and irregular in appearance. Which of the following is the most likely diagnosis?
   A. Acute partial ulnar collateral ligament tear
   B. Acute partial radial collateral tear
   C. Chronic ulnar collateral ligament injury
   D. Chronic radial collateral ligament injury
   E. Chronic lateral ulnar collateral ligament injury

106. A 66-year-old man with a chronic skin condition and progressive painful small joints of the hand has been referred for an X-ray. Plain radiograph reveals extensive arthropathy involving the DIPJs mainly, with some joints showing a pencil-in-cup deformity. Which one of the following statements regarding the condition is false?
   A. In 15%–20% of cases, arthropathy precedes the onset of skin rash.
   B. Involvement of the sacroiliac joints is often bilateral.

C. The severity of the skin rash correlates with the degree of articular abnormalities.

D. It affects both synovial and cartilaginous joints.

E. Marginal erosions around the joints of the fingers and toes are common.

107. All of the following are features of NF2, except
A. Bilateral vestibular neuroma
B. Multiple meningioma
C. Skeletal dysplasia
D. Spinal cord ependymoma
E. Meningiomatosis

108. A 9-year-old boy on antibiotics from the GP for presumed throat infection presents with abdominal pain. Movement aggravates the pain and the child prefers to lie with a flexed hip. What is the next investigation to help ascertain the diagnosis?
A. Urine test
B. Throat swab
C. US abdomen
D. CT abdomen
E. MRI abdomen

109. A middle-aged Caucasian man presents with haemoptysis. CXR shows multiple round, well-defined pulmonary nodules >5 mm. The most likely cause is
A. Rheumatoid nodules
B. Wegener's granulomatosis
C. Metastasis
D. Miliary nodules
E. Staphylococcal abscess

110. A 66-year-old woman with biopsy-proven hepatic cirrhosis is scheduled to have an MRI for further evaluation of her disease status. Which one of the following MR features is seen earliest in chronic liver disease?
A. Ascites
B. Nodular liver contour
C. Fine reticular pattern of hepatic fibrosis
D. Splenomegaly
E. Oesophageal varices

111. A 26-year-old man presents with a lump in the right scrotum; US reveals a 1.5 cm simple cyst in the head of the epididymis. Incidentally, the US also shows multiple non-shadowing echogenic foci in both testes, consistent with testicular microlithiasis. Which one of the following statements regarding testicular microlithiasis is false?
A. It usually is an incidental finding on US.
B. The calcifications develop in the seminiferous tubules.
C. It is typically unilateral.
D. The calcifications are non-shadowing on US.
E. It is variably associated with an increased incidence of testicular tumours.

112. A 17-year-old man with reduced upward gaze on clinical examination reveals a moderate-sized heterogeneous mass in the region of the pineal gland in sagittal MRI of the brain. T1W images reveal areas of fat in the tumour, whereas calcification is best seen on CT. What is the diagnosis?
A. Pineoblastoma
B. Pineal teratoma

C. Pineal cyst

D. Pineal teratocarcinoma

E. Pineocytoma

113. A man with previous episodes of PE presents with acute shortness of breath and chest pain. Recurrent PE is suspected. On CTPA, which is the most common finding of chronic PE?

A. Complete occlusion of a vessel

B. Acute angle between the thrombus and the vessel wall

C. Right ventricular dilatation

D. Contrast flowing in an apparently thickened vessel wall

E. Polo mint sign

114. A 12-year-old girl presents to her GP with mild fever persistent over a month, myalgia, arthralgia, headache and night sweats. On examination, the GP notes tender nodules in the finger. Blood test shows raised WCC, raised ESR, and raised CRP. What is the primary investigation to confirm the diagnosis?

A. Chest X-ray and blood culture

B. CT of the chest and blood culture

C. MRI of the heart and blood culture

D. Echocardiography and blood culture

E. US of the neck and blood culture

115. A 65-year-old man with known alcoholic liver cirrhosis presents to casualty with an acute episode of GI bleed. This is managed medically, and a CT is requested to assess for complications of cirrhosis. Which of the following statements regarding cirrhosis-associated hepatocellular nodules is false?

A. Regenerative nodules are premalignant.

B. Accurate characterisation of cirrhosis-associated nodules may be difficult even on histology.

C. Features such as size and vascularity on imaging may help in characterisation.

D. MRI is better than contrast CT for characterising cirrhotic nodules.

E. Regenerative nodules are benign.

116. A 16-year-old presents to the A&E department with an acutely painful testicle and is evaluated for possible torsion. US reveals swollen right testes with reduced vascularity on Doppler imaging. What degree of torsion of the spermatic cord is needed to completely occlude the testicular artery?

A. 120

B. 240

C. 480

D. 600

E. 720

117. A 27-year-old man presents with back pain. Anteroposterior pelvis radiograph shows bilateral symmetric bone erosions, sclerosis and widening of the sacroiliac joints. All of the following are expected radiographic findings, except

A. Bilateral hip joint involvement

B. Vertebral anterosuperior corner osteitis

C. Discovertebral erosions

D. Large flowing osteophytes

E. Fusion of facet joints

118. A 43-year-old woman on bromocriptine for pituitary adenoma presents to the A&E department with severe headache, stiff neck, visual symptoms and obtundation. CT shows increased

density in the sella, but it is not diagnostic. MRI of the brain shows significant enlargement of the pituitary with high signal on T1W images. What is the diagnosis?

A. Pituitary adenoma
B. Pituitary carcinoma
C. Pituitary apoplexy
D. Conversion of micro- to macroadenoma
E. Metastasis involving the pituitary gland

119. A 4-year-old boy is brought to the A&E department following a motor vehicle accident in which he was a restrained back-seat passenger. He is in respiratory distress with circulatory collapse. Chest X-ray demonstrates lack of definition of the left hemidiaphragm with multiple cystic-appearing structures projected over the left hemithorax. What is the most likely diagnosis?

A. Morgagni hernia
B. Traumatic diaphragmatic rupture
C. Aspiration pneumonia
D. Bochdalek hernia
E. Congenital lobar emphysema

120. The differential diagnosis for diseases affecting the bowel in paediatric patients can be narrowed by paying attention to specific radiologic signs and the patient's clinical history. Which of the following findings are incorrectly matched to the underlying pathology?

A. Hyperattenuating wall is seen with haemorrhage.
B. The halo sign is seen in graft versus host disease.
C. The accordion sign is classic in Crohn's disease.
D. The comb sign suggests active inflammation.
E. The toothpaste sign is seen in chronic bowel disease.

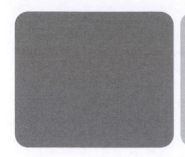

CHAPTER 6
TEST PAPER 3

Answers

1. C. Ultrasound-guided thrombin injection

Pseudoaneurysms are common vascular abnormalities that represent a disruption in arterial wall continuity.

Surgical repair was the treatment of choice for superficial extremity pseudoaneurysms until US-guided compression was introduced. US-guided percutaneous thrombin injection has replaced US-guided compression as the therapeutic method of choice for treatment of post-catheterisation pseudoaneurysms. Endovascular techniques like stent placement (indispensable artery) or embolisation (dispensable artery) have a lower complication rate in the treatment of visceral pseudoaneurysms than does surgical management.

Saad NE, et al. Pseudoaneurysms and the role of minimally invasive techniques in their management. *Radiographics*. 2005;25 Suppl 1: S173–89.

2. B. Klippel–Feil deformity

The hallmarks of Chiari II malformation include caudally displaced fourth ventricle (the fourth ventricle is in normal position in Chiari I malformation), caudally displaced brain stem, and tonsillar or vermian herniation through the foramen magnum.

Associations include lumbar myelomeningocele, syringohydromyelia, dysgenesis of the corpus callosum, obstructive hydrocephalous, absent septum pellucidum and excess cortical gyration.

It is not associated with any of the bony abnormalities described in Chiari I malformation, like basilar impression, occipitalisation of the atlas, platybasia and Klippel–Feil anomaly.

Dähnert W. *Radiology Review Manual*, 7th edn. Philadelphia, PA: Lippincott Williams & Wilkins, 2011:278–9.

3. E. Ulcers

At pathologic analysis, active inflammation is characterised by varying degrees of neutrophilic crypt injury. In mildly active Crohn's disease, a small fraction of crypts are infiltrated by neutrophils (cryptitis), with associated crypt destruction and mucin depletion.

As the degree of activity increases, there is a corresponding increase in the proportion of involved crypts and the severity of crypt injury, including crypt epithelial necrosis, intraluminal exudates (crypt abscess), and eventual ulcer formation. Two types of ulcers are seen in Crohn's disease: superficial aphthous ulcers and deep fissuring ulcers. Deep fissuring ulcers are more problematic than superficial aphthous ulcers; they break through the mucosa and into the deeper layers of the bowel wall, initially resulting in submucosal inflammation and oedema. Some investigators have reported that deep ulcers may be seen in MR enterography, whereas superficial ulcers defy detection.

Leyendecker JR, et al. MR enterography in the management of patients with Crohn's disease. *RadioGraphics*. 2009;29:1827–46.

4. C. Rise in serum creatinine level by >50% above baseline.

Diagnosis of CIN (contrast-induced nephropathy) is most often based on an increase in the serum level of creatinine after exposure to a contrast agent. Diagnostic criteria for CIN include exposure to contrast agent, increase in serum level of creatinine of 0.5 mg/dL or 25% greater than baseline, increase in serum level of creatinine occurring 48–72 hours after administration of contrast agent and persisting for 2–5 days, and alternative major injuries being ruled out.

Jorgensen AL. Contrast-induced nephropathy: Pathophysiology and preventive strategies. *Crit Care Nurse.* 2013;33 (1): 37–46.

5. D. Skeletal metastasis

Eosinophilic granuloma is associated with Langerhans cell histiocytosis and is an indication for a skeletal survey, along with multiple myeloma and non-accidental injury. Skeletal surveys are never performed for skeletal metastasis.

Radiological evaluation of skeletal dysplasia often starts with a skeletal survey for several non-lethal skeletal dysplasia.

Panda A, et al. Skeletal dysplasias: A radiographic approach and review of common non-lethal skeletal dysplasias. *World J Radiol.* 2014;6(10):808–25.

6. B. Medulloblastoma

Medulloblastoma is the most common infratentorial paediatric brain tumour. It typically presents as a midline, non-calcified solid vermal mass, obstructing the fourth ventricle.

Classic medulloblastoma typically arises from the roof of the fourth ventricle and is midline in location in 75%–90% of cases. Classic medulloblastoma is a highly cellular, densely packed tumour, which is reflected on imaging; it appears hyperdense relative to brain on CT (89% of cases) and shows restricted diffusion on DWI. This feature of medulloblastoma allows differentiation from JPA, ependymoma and brainstem glioma. Almost all medulloblastomas enhance post-contrast; the degree of enhancement varies from diffuse homogenous to heterogeneous.

Dähnert W. *Radiology Review Manual*, 6th edn. Philadelphia, PA: Lippincott Williams & Wilkins, 2007:305.
Plaza MJ, et al. Conventional and advanced MRI features of pediatric intracranial tumors: Posterior fossa and suprasellar tumors. *AJR Am J Roentgenol.* 2013;200(5):1115–24.

7. A. Colloid cyst

The most common true mass of the foramen of Monro is a colloid cyst, a benign lesion that occurs in adult patients. This well-defined round cyst may be from several millimeters to 3 cm in size and attaches to the anterior superior aspect of the third ventricle roof. Often hyperattenuating at non-enhanced CT, it has variable signal intensity at MR imaging and is often hyperintense on T1-weighted and FLAIR images. Peripheral gadolinium enhancement is rarely seen. Ninety percent of colloid cysts are asymptomatic and stable, whereas 10% are reported to enlarge or cause hydrocephalus. Rapid enlargement has been associated with coma and death.

Glastonbury CM, et al. Masses and malformations of the third ventricle: Normal anatomic relationships and differential diagnoses. *Radiographics.* 2011;31(7):1889–905.

8. D. Coil embolisation

Ruptured hepatic adenoma is a clinical emergency. Many adenomas are first diagnosed in symptomatic patients presenting with acute abdominal pain, hemodynamic instability, or other signs of rupture, most of whom are on OCP. The gold standard has been to perform emergency laparotomy with gauze packing or partial liver resection. Laparoscopic resection is also possible in theory, but it is technically difficult. Recently, less invasive procedures such as transarterial embolisation have been developed that may also lead to adequate haemostasis without the need for urgent laparotomy, and they are considered the first treatment option. RFA is used in non-ruptured adenomas and its use after haemorrhage may be irrelevant.

Large-Vessel Permanent Occlusion	Coils and Amplatzer Plugs
• GI bleed, pulmonary AVM, traumatic pseudoaneurysms, carotid or vertebral artery sacrifice, and visceral artery aneurysms	
Large-Vessel Temporary Occlusion	Gel foam
• Haemorrhage following pelvic trauma	
Small-Vessel Permanent Occlusion (Tissue Viability Retained)	PVA particles (>300 μ)
• Uterine fibroid embolisation	
• Bronchial artery or small-vessel GI bleed	
Small-Vessel Permanent Occlusion (Tissue Death Desired)	Absolute alcohol
• Renal ablation	Sodium tetradecyl sulphate
• Peripheral AVM	PVA particles (<300 μ)
Small-Vessel Temporary Occlusion	Gel foam
• Repeat tumour embolisation	

Huurman VAL, Schaapherder AF. Management of ruptured hepatocellular adenoma. *Dig Surg*. 2010;27:56–60
Lubarsky M, et al. Embolization agents – Which one should be used when? part 1: Large-vessel embolization. *Semin Intervent Radiol*. 2009;26(4):352–7.
Vaidya S, et al. An overview of embolic agents. *Semin Intervent Radiol*. 2008;25(3):204–15.

9. B. Mesenteric fibro-fatty proliferation

The main diagnostic purpose of CT enterography in the setting of Crohn's disease is to differentiate active inflammatory strictures from fibrotic strictures in order to guide therapy.

CT features of active Crohn's disease include mucosal hyperenhancement, wall thickening (thickness >3 mm), mural stratification with a prominent vasa recta (comb sign) and mesenteric fat stranding, all of which are exquisitely demonstrated at CT enterography. The capability of CT enterography to depict extra-enteric disease allows the simultaneous diagnosis of complications associated with Crohn's disease, such as obstruction, sinus tract, fistula and abscess formation.

Mural enhancement is the most sensitive indicator of active Crohn's disease. Care should be taken to compare bowel loops with similar distention, since both the jejunum and normal collapsed loops may demonstrate regions of higher attenuation, simulating enhancement. Inadequately distended bowel loops may be difficult to assess, and secondary signs of active disease, such as mesenteric fat stranding, vasa recta prominence or complications such as fistulas and abscesses should be sought to maximise the accuracy of a diagnosis of active disease.

Prominence of the vasa recta adjacent to the inflamed loop of bowel (comb sign), along with increased mesenteric fat attenuation, is the most specific CT feature of active Crohn's disease. Findings that might be seen in inactive long-standing Crohn's disease include submucosal fat deposition, pseudosacculation, surrounding fibro-fatty proliferation and fibrotic strictures.

Elsayes KM, et al. CT enterography: Principles, trends, and interpretation findings. *RadioGraphics*. 2010;30:1955–70.

10. B. Medullary sponge kidney

Medullary sponge kidney involves dysplastic dilatation of medullary and papillary collecting ducts. It is known to be associated with Ehlers–Danlos syndrome, parathyroid adenoma and Caroli's disease. Recognised features include medullary nephrocalcinosis, 'bunch of flower appearance' and dense, striated nephrogram; it can affect a single kidney (25%) or single pyramids.

Note that papillary blush on IVU without dense streaks is a normal variant, especially when not associated with nephrocalcinosis.

Dähnert W. *Radiology Review Manual*, 7th edn. Philadelphia, PA: Lippincott Williams & Wilkins, 2011:954.

11. B. Submentovertex view

The submentovertex (SMV) view, also called the *bucket-handle view*, shows fractures of the zygomatic arch best. Townes and occipitomental views are for skull and facial bone fractures. Swimmer's view is for viewing the cervico-thoracic junction.

Raby N, et al. *Accident and Emergency Radiology: A Survival Guide*. Philadelphia, PA: Elsevier Saunders, 2005.
Siemionow MZ, Eisenmann-Klein M (eds.). *Plastic and Reconstructive Surgery*, 1st edn. London: Springer, 2010:278.

12. B. Acute laryngotracheobronchitis

Croup (laryngotracheobronchitis) most commonly affects children between 6 months and 3 years and presents with acute stridor, usually following viral infection. A subglottic inverted V sign is seen on plain film, but the epiglottis and aryepiglottic folds are usually normal.

In contrast, epiglottitis is a life-threatening condition affecting 3–6-year-olds, with a lateral soft-tissue neck radiograph showing thickening of the epiglottis and aryepiglottic folds described as the 'thumb sign'.

Dähnert W. *Radiology Review Manual*, 7th edn. Philadelphia, PA: Lippincott Williams & Wilkins, 2011.

13. A. No   Yes   No

The chest radiographic appearance of fat embolism syndrome is non-specific. Normal radiographs can also be seen. Most patients presenting with a normal initial radiograph develop radiographic-evident abnormalities within 72 hours of injury, and most cases show radiographic resolution within 2 weeks of hospitalisation.

Muangman N, et al. Chest radiographic evolution in fat embolism syndrome. *J Med Assoc Thai.* 2005;88(12):1854–60.

14. A. Craniopharyngioma

Craniopharyngiomas account for about 3% of all primary intracranial tumours. Two types of craniopharyngiomas have been described: a childhood type, with frequent occurrence of cyst formation and calcifications and generally a poor prognosis, and an adult type, generally without calcifications or cyst formation and generally a good prognosis.

The cystic areas may be iso-, hyper- or hypointense relative to brain tissue with T1-weighted sequences. The short T1 relaxation times are the result of very high protein content. With T2-weighted sequences, both the cystic and solid components tend to have high signal intensity. After the administration of contrast material, the solid portions enhance heterogeneously. The thin walls of the cystic areas nearly always enhance. The characteristic calcifications in paediatric craniopharyngiomas may not be discernible, although gradient-echo images may show susceptibility effects from calcified components. Occasionally, craniopharyngiomas are predominantly solid, typically without calcification.

Saleem SN, et al. Lesions of the hypothalamus: MR imaging diagnostic features. *Radiographics.* 2007;27(4):1087–108.

15. B. A thickened hyperenhancing bowel wall is a sign of active disease.

The main diagnostic purpose of CT enterography in the setting of Crohn's disease is to differentiate active inflammatory strictures from fibrotic strictures in order to guide therapy.

CT features of active Crohn's disease include mucosal hyperenhancement, wall thickening (thickness >3 mm), mural stratification with a prominent vasa recta (comb sign) and mesenteric fat stranding, all of which are exquisitely demonstrated at CT enterography. The capability of

CT enterography to depict extra-enteric disease allows the simultaneous diagnosis of complications associated with Crohn's disease, such as obstruction, sinus tract, fistula and abscess formation.

Mural enhancement is the most sensitive indicator of active Crohn's disease. The term *mural stratification* denotes the visualisation of bowel wall layers at CT. At CT enterography, the oedematous bowel wall has a trilaminar appearance, with enhanced outer serosal and inner mucosal layers and an interposed submucosal layer of lower attenuation. However, this feature is not specific to Crohn's disease; it is seen also in other inflammatory bowel diseases and even in some cases of bowel ischaemia. Prominence of the vasa recta adjacent to the inflamed loop of bowel (comb sign) along with increased mesenteric fat attenuation, is the most specific CT feature of active Crohn's disease. Findings that might be seen in inactive long-standing Crohn's disease include submucosal fat deposition, pseudosacculation, surrounding fibro-fatty proliferation and fibrotic strictures.

Perianal disease is common in Crohn's disease.

Elsayes KM, et al. CT enterography: Principles, trends, and interpretation findings. *RadioGraphics*. 2010;30:1955–70.

16. B. Pelvicalyceal duplication precludes kidney donation.

The aims of preoperative evaluation of living related donors are to show that the donor will retain a normal kidney after unilateral nephrectomy, to demonstrate that the kidney to be transplanted has no major abnormality, and to outline the vascular anatomy. US assesses the parenchyma, CT angiogram shows the arterial and venous anatomy, and the plain film demonstrates the pelvicalyceal system. MR angiography and MR urography provide similar information.

Conditions that do not preclude donation include pelvicalyceal duplication, solitary renal cyst, unilateral mild reflux nephropathy and only one scar. In the case of unilateral duplication, the contralateral kidney is donated. Twenty percent of kidneys have accessory arterial supply. Kidneys with multiple arterial supply are more likely to have vascular complications. The transplanted kidney is placed extraperitonealy in the iliac fossa; usually the right kidney is placed in the left iliac fossa because the vascular anastomosis is easier. When a cadaveric kidney is used, an aortic patch (Carrel patch) is removed with the renal artery.

Adam A, et al. *Grainger & Allison's Diagnostic Radiology: A Textbook of Medical Imaging*, 5th edn. New York: Churchill Livingstone, 2008:851.

17. B. Haemophilic arthropathy

Radiographic findings vary greatly with the different stages of haemophilic arthropathy (acute, subacute or chronic haemarthrosis) and reflect the presence of haemarthrosis (joint effusion), synovial inflammation and hyperaemia (osteoporosis and epiphyseal overgrowth), chondral erosions and subchondral resorption (osseous erosions and cysts), cartilaginous denudation (joint space narrowing), intraosseous or subperiosteal haemorrhage (pseudotumours) and osseous proliferation (sclerosis and osteophytosis). Some abnormalities of osseous shape, such as widening of the intercondylar notch, flattening of the condylar surface or squaring of the patella, are very characteristic of chronic haemarthrosis of the knee. At MR imaging, hypertrophied synovial membrane resulting from repetitive haemarthrosis has characteristic low signal intensity with all pulse sequences, especially with gradient-echo sequences, due to the magnetic susceptibility effect caused by haemosiderin. As in pigmented villonodular synovitis, the signal intensity of the subarticular defects varies and may indicate the presence of fluid (high signal intensity on T2-weighted images), soft tissue (intermediate signal intensity) or synovial tissue with haemosiderin (low signal intensity).

Rapidly destructive articular disease is an unusual form of osteoarthritis that typically involves the hip. The disease is almost always unilateral, but bilateral lesions and involvement of shoulder have also been reported. Serial radiographs show progressive loss of joint space and loss of subchondral bone in the femoral head and acetabulum, resulting in marked flattening and deformity of the femoral head ('hatchet' deformity). Superolateral subluxation of the femoral head or intrusion deformity within the ilium can be observed. Most cases demonstrate subchondral defects and mild sclerosis. However, osteophytes are small or absent.

Llauger J, et al. Nonseptic monoarthritis: Imaging features with clinical and histopathologic correlation. *Radiographics*. 2000;20:S263–78.

18. D. Hypointense to brain on T1WI and hyperintense on T2WI

Pilocytic astrocytoma typically presents in first two decades, with peak age from birth to 9 years of age. It is the most common paediatric glioma, with the majority located in the cerebellum. Pilocytic astrocytomas are predominantly cystic with an intensely enhancing mural nodule; half show enhancement of the cyst wall. The magnetic resonance signal pattern is as for cysts: hypointense on T1-weighted images and hyperintense on T2-weighted images. Post-contrast T1-weighted images shows enhancement of the mural nodule.

Dähnert W. *Radiology Review Manual*, 7th edn. Philadelphia, PA: Lippincott Williams & Wilkins, 2011.

19. C. Lymphocele

Urine leaks and urinomas are relatively rare complications and are usually found in the first 2 weeks post-operative between the transplanted kidney and the bladder. They appear as a well-defined, anechoic fluid collection with no septations that increases in size rapidly. Antegrade pyelography is necessary to provide detailed information about the site of origin of the urinoma and in planning appropriate intervention. Haematomas are common in the immediate post-operative period, but they may also develop spontaneously or as a consequence of trauma or biopsy. At US, haematomas demonstrate a complex appearance. Acute haematomas are echogenic and become less echogenic with time. Older haematomas even appear anechoic, more closely resembling fluid, and septations may develop. Lymphoceles are the most common peritransplant fluid collections that may develop at any time, from weeks to years after transplantation. However, they usually occur within 1–2 months after transplantation. At US, lymphoceles are anechoic and may have septations. Similar to other peritransplant fluid collections, they can become infected and can develop a more complex appearance. Abscesses have a complex, cystic, non-specific appearance at US. Peritransplant abscesses are an uncommon complication and usually develop within the first few weeks after transplantation.

Akbar SA, et al. Complications of renal transplantation. *Radiographics*. 2005;25(5):1335–56.

20. D. Ankylosing spondylitis

Causes of lower zone fibrosis include asbestosis, aspiration, cryptogenic alveolitis (IPF), neurofibromatosis I and tuberous sclerosis; connective tissue diseases like RA, scleroderma and SLE; and drug toxicity to substances like amiodarone and nitrofurantoin.

Dähnert W. *Radiology Review Manual*, 7th edn. Philadelphia, PA: Lippincott Williams & Wilkins, 2011:414–25.

21. B. The granular nodular stage is not associated with oedema.

Neurocysticercosis has been classified into active and non-active forms on the basis of clinical presentation, results of CSF analysis and imaging findings. The active forms include arachnoiditis with or without ventricular obstruction and vasculitis with or without infarction. On the basis of radiologic findings, neurocysticercosis is divided into five stages: non-cystic, vesicular, colloidal vesicular, granular nodular and calcified nodular. Of these, all the stages apart from the first (non-cystic stage) are visible on CT/MRI.

Vesicular stage: Cyst signal intensity similar to that of CSF on T1-weighted and T2-weighted images; cyst wall is well defined and thin, with little or no enhancement on gadolinium-enhanced images; scolex (hole with dot appearance); iso- or hypointense relative to white matter on T1-weighted images; iso- to hyperintense relative to white matter on T2-weighted images; best seen on PD-weighted images.

Colloidal vesicular stage: Cyst contents are hyperintense on T1-weighted and T2-weighted images (proteinaceous fluid), cyst wall is thick and hypointense, pericystic oedema (best seen on FLAIR), pericystic enhancement on gadolinium-enhanced images.

Granular nodular stage: Similar to the colloidal vesicular stage but with more oedema, thicker ring enhancement.

Calcified nodular stage: Hypointense nodules, no oedema, no enhancement.

Kimura-Hayama ET, et al. Neurocysticercosis: Radiologic-pathologic correlation. *Radiographics*. 2010;30(6):1705–19.

22. A. Patients should ideally ingest 1 L of positive oral contrast medium before the start of the examination.

Patients undergoing CT enterography are asked to withhold all oral intake, starting 4 hours before the examination. To improve visualisation of the mucosa and achieve better bowel distension, a negative oral contrast agent is administered. A typical regimen with regard to the timing of administration of oral contrast agents involves the ingestion of a total of 1.35 L over 1 hour: 450 mL at 60 minutes, 450 mL at 40 minutes, 225 mL at 20 minutes and 225 mL at 10 minutes before scanning. After the oral contrast agent is ingested, a bolus of intravenous contrast material followed by 50 mL of saline solution is administered with a power injector at a rate of 4 mL/sec.

Helical scanning is performed from the diaphragm to the symphysis pubis, beginning 65 seconds after the administration of intravenous contrast material; it includes a single (venous) phase for the evaluation of known or suspected Crohn's disease or dual (arterial and venous) phases for the evaluation of mesenteric vessels, GI tract bleeding and suspected tumours. Scanning parameters include a section thickness of 0.625 mm and interval of 0.625 mm.

Elsayes KM, et al. CT enterography: Principles, trends, and interpretation findings. *RadioGraphics*. 2010;30:1955–70.

23. C. Cleidocranial dysostosis

Cleidocranial dysplasia (CCD) is characterised by aplasia or hypoplasia of the clavicles, characteristic craniofacial malformations, and the presence of numerous supernumerary and unerupted teeth. Cranial abnormalities include wide-open sutures, patent fontanelles and the presence of Wormian bones. Delayed closure of cranial sutures and fontanelles leads to frontal, parietal and occipital bossing. Additionally, there may be poor or absent pneumatisation of paranasal, frontal and mastoid, and sphenoid sinuses.

Pelvic features include delayed ossification with wide pubic symphysis, hypoplastic iliac wings, widened sacroiliac joints and a large femoral neck resulting in coxa vara.

The differential diagnosis of CCD includes Crane–Heise syndrome (CCD with cleft lip and agenesis of cervical vertebra), mandibuloacral dysplasia (CCD plus hypoplastic mandible), pyknodysostosis (CCD and osteopetrosis), Yunis–Varon syndrome (CCD with hypoplastic thumb and big toe), CDAGS syndrome (craniosynostosis, anal anomalies and genital hyplasia).

Patil PP, et al. Cleidocranial dysplasia: A clinico-radiographic spectrum with differential diagnosis. *J Orthop Case Rep.* 2015;5(2):21–4.

24. B. Dysembryoplastic neuroepithelial tumour

History of seizure that may be medically refractory makes dysembryoplastic neuroepithelial tumour (DNET) more likely.

DNET is a benign, supratentorial and predominantly cortical intra-axial lesion, characterised by a multinodular architecture. Although DNETs are usually located in the temporal lobe, any lobe within the brain lobes may be involved. They have a cortical base and an apex pointing towards the lateral ventricle. They are homogeneously hyperintense on T2-weighted images and hypointense on T1-weighted images. Some delicate septa-like structures are visible within the lesions. Despite their size, neither mass effect nor surrounding parenchymal oedema is present. On FLAIR images, the lesions show a hyperintense ring. Susceptibility-weighted images do not depict any hypointense signal in the lesion, which indicates the absence of calcium or blood products. Very high ADC values are measured inside the mass. No contrast enhancement is noted and there is scalloping of overlying bone.

The differential diagnosis includes other brain tumours, such as ganglioglioma (cyst with a strongly enhancing mural nodule, frequent calcification), angiocentric glioma (hyperintense on T1 and star-like extension to ventricle), low-grade astrocytoma (similar to DNET but no scalloping of bone or rim of FLAIR) and pleomorphic xanthoastrocytoma (cyst with mural nodule, enhancement and dural tail).

Raz E, et al. Case 186: Dysembrioplastic neuroepithelial tumour. *Radiology*. 2012;265(1):317–20.

25. A. Dandy–Walker malformation

The characteristic triad of the Dandy–Walker malformation includes (1) complete or partial agenesis of the vermis, (2) cystic dilatation of the fourth ventricle and (3) an enlarged posterior fossa with upward displacement of the lateral sinuses, tentorium and torcula. The triad is usually associated with hydrocephalus (most common presentation 80%), but this condition should be considered a common complication and not as part of the malformation itself. Depending on the degree of hydrocephalus, the age at diagnosis varies from the neonatal period to later childhood.

The skull is enlarged, with characteristic thinning and bulging of the occiput. Pressure from the massively dilated fourth ventricle, along with cerebrospinal fluid pulsations, causes erosive scalloping of the occiput and petrous temporal bones.

The cerebellar hemispheres are typically hypoplastic, and in extreme cases only a small nubbin of compressed cerebellar tissue is identified contiguous laterally with the wall of the posterior fossa cyst. Anomalies of the posterior inferior cerebellar arteries, especially absence of the inferior vermian branches and absence of the inferior vermian vein, help in the angiographic differentiation of a Dandy–Walker cyst from an arachnoid cyst, in which the vessels are displaced but present.

The Dandy–Walker variant is used to describe a cystic posterior fossa malformation with varying degrees of agenesis of the vermis associated with expansion (often considerable) of the fourth ventricle, which communicates freely with the perimedullary subarachnoid space.

Kollias SS, et al. Cystic malformations of the posterior fossa: Differential diagnosis clarified through embryologic analysis. *Radiographics*. 1993;13(6):1211–31.

26. C. Lymphangioleiomyomatosis

Lymphangioleiomyomatosis (LAM) is a rare disorder occurring almost exclusively in women of childbearing age. LAM associated with tuberous sclerosis is 5–10 times more common than sporadic LAM. Lymphatic obstruction may result in chylous pleural effusion, chylous ascites or both. Spontaneous or recurrent pneumothorax may be the presenting finding in up to 50% of patients.

Characteristic HRCT features of LAM are diffuse thin-walled cysts surrounded by normal lung without regional sparing. Cysts are usually 2–5 mm but can be as large as 25–30 mm. Cysts are typically round or ovoid, but they may become polygonal with severe parenchymal involvement. Small centrilobular nodules and focal ground-glass opacities have been reported. Lymphatic obstruction may cause septal thickening.

Seaman DM, et al. Diffuse cystic lung disease at high-resolution CT. *AJR Am J Roentgenol*. 2011;196:1305–11.

27. A. MR enterography has less sensitivity and specificity compared to MR enteroclysis for established disease.

The benefits of using enteric contrast material to achieve bowel distension for cross-sectional imaging are not disputed, although the optimal type of contrast material and method of administration remain somewhat controversial.

Current data suggest that although bowel distension achieved with the enteric intubation technique generally is superior to that achieved with enterography, the improved distension does not necessarily translate into a clinically significant improvement in diagnostic effectiveness. A recent study confirmed the benefit of enteric intubation for bowel distension but reported equivalent diagnostic performances with the enteric and oral techniques in identifying stenoses and fistulas. However, MR enteroclysis was superior to MR enterography in demonstrating mucosal abnormalities. The importance of detecting mucosal disease in patients without bowel obstruction has diminished in the era of capsule endoscopy. Patient acceptance, which favours MR enterography over MR enteroclysis, also must be considered, because many patients need multiple examinations.

Leyendecker JR, et al. MR enterography in the management of patients with Crohn's disease. *RadioGraphics*. 2009;29:1827–46.

28. D. Rathke cleft cyst

Rathke cleft cysts are benign cystic sellar lesions that are generally asymptomatic, but they may be associated with hypopituitarism, visual disturbance and headache. At MR imaging, Rathke cleft cysts have a variable T1 signal, depending on the protein concentration. Cysts with high protein content demonstrate high T1 signal and usually low intracystic water content that leads to T2 signal decrease. Thus, typical Rathke cleft cysts appear as non-enhancing well-demarcated intrasellar rounded lesions located exactly at the midline between the anterior and posterior pituitary lobes. The cysts have a homogeneously hyperintense T1 signal and, often, a hypointense T2 signal. Axial images are crucial for identifying the specific location and characteristic kidney shape of a Rathke cleft cyst.

The presence of fluid–fluid level or haemorrhagic debris in an intrasellar lesion suggests a pituitary adenoma, because a Rathke cleft cyst almost never bleeds.

Craniopharyngioma typically appears as intrasellar or suprasellar heterogeneously enhancing lesions with a tripartite structure of solid, calcified and cystic components. They are difficult to distinguish from pituitary adenoma, although the fluid–fluid level is more likely to suggest a pituitary adenoma.

Bonneville F, et al. T1 signal hyperintensity in the sellar region: Spectrum of findings. *Radiographics*. 2006; 26(1): 93–113.

29. E. Oncocytoma

Oncocytomas are tubular adenomas with a specific histological appearance. They were previously considered benign but have now been recognised to metastasise. They vary from 1 to 20 cm in diameter and tend to be large. They are usually solitary and unilateral. US shows a solid mass with internal echoes, which occasionally have a stellate hypoechoic centre. CECT demonstrates a well-defined solid mass, with a low-attenuation central scar, when large. Large lesions can extend into and engulf perinephric fat. RCC and oncocytoma look similar on MRI.

Adam A, et al. *Grainger & Allison's Diagnostic Radiology: A Textbook of Medical Imaging*, 5th edn. New York: Churchill Livingstone, 2008:865.

30. B. Bucket-handle tear of meniscus

Bucket-handle tears of the meniscus involve displacement of the free edge of the meniscus into the intercondylar notch. The free edge can be seen adjacent to the PCL on sagittal images giving a double PCL sign. On coronal imaging, the meniscal fragment is displaced medially. A radial meniscal tear manifests as a linear collection of high signal in the meniscus that extends to the superior or inferior articular surfaces. Rupture of the ACL or PCL results in the ligament losing the normal position and morphology but not a double PCL sign. When assessing the PCL, be aware that the ligaments of Humphrey and Wrisberg can give the impression of a tear to the inexperienced eye. These ligaments are extensions of the meniscofemoral ligament; the ligament of Humphrey passes anterior to the PCL and the ligament of Wrisberg posteriorly.

Helms CA. *Fundamentals of Skeletal Radiology*, 3rd edn. Philadelphia, PA: Elsevier Saunders, 2005:169–75.

31. A. Langerhans cell histiocytosis

Pulmonary LCH is a smoking-related lung disease. Peribronchiolar nodules are found; they may subsequently cavitate and form thick- and thin-walled cysts. Frequently, both nodules and cysts are seen. Cysts may be round but are often irregular, cloverleaf or bizarre shapes. Irregular cysts, cysts with nodules and upper zone predominance with sparing of the costophrenic angles are features that distinguish LCH from lymphangioleiomyomatosis.

Centrilobular emphysema represents the permanent destruction of bronchiolar walls with resultant enlargement of the airspaces distal to the terminal bronchiole. The distinguishing features of centrilobular emphysema include the lack of a perceptible cyst wall and the central location of the vascular structures (central dot sign).

Seaman DM, et al. Diffuse cystic lung disease at high-resolution CT. *AJR Am J Roentgenol.* 2011;196:1305–11.

32. A. 'Jejunisation' of the ileum

In both primary and secondary amyloidosis, the most commonly involved organ system is the gastrointestinal system, with the colon being the most frequently involved organ. Oesophageal and gastric involvement usually manifests as dysmotility, wall thickening and gastroesophageal reflux disease. This results from amyloid infiltration of the muscularis and/or destruction of the Auerbach plexus. When the small intestine is involved, the most common finding is diffuse or nodular wall thickening. Abdominal pain, malabsorption and haemorrhage are rare complications. Colonic biopsy specimens are positive in 80% of patients with systemic amyloidosis.

Contrary to the high pathologic specificity, radiologic findings are rare and non-specific. The most common finding is colonic dilatation owing to adynamic ileus and more rarely bowel wall thickening. Even more rarely, intramural bowel haemorrhage or perforation can occur.

Splenomegaly is the only finding associated with splenic involvement. This causes increased fragility, and spontaneous rupture can ensue with life-threatening consequences. The liver is also commonly involved, but radiologic signs are also non-specific. Diffuse infiltration is the rule, which causes decreased attenuation at CT and hepatomegaly.

Macroglossia can also result from amyloid infiltration of the intrinsic muscles. Jejunisation of the ileum can be seen with coeliac disease.

Georgiades CS, et al. Amyloidosis: Review and CT manifestations. *RadioGraphics.* 2004;24:405–16.

33. B. Glomus tumour

A glomus tumour is a hamartoma arising from the glomus body within the dermis of the finger. The subungual position is characteristic of the lesion, which results in extrinsic erosion of the adjacent terminal phalanx. The tumour can also occur entirely within bone, although this is less common. It exhibits intense high T2 signal with avid contrast enhancement as it is a highly vascular lesion. Epidermoid inclusion cysts, otherwise known as *implantation dermoid cysts*, are associated with a history of penetrating trauma. A giant cell tumour of the tendon sheath lies in close relation to the tendon and does not exhibit such intense T2 signal. The description is not compatible with a soft-tissue osteosarcoma.

Dähnert W. *Radiology Review Manual*, 6th edn. Philadelphia, PA: Lippincott Williams & Wilkins, 2007:174.

34. D. T3b

T-stage

T1a: Limited to kidney, <4 cm

T1b: Limited to kidney, >4 cm but <7 cm

T2a: Limited to kidney, >7 cm but not more than 10 cm

T2b: Limited to kidney, >10 cm

T3a: Spread to perinephric fat

T3b: Spread to renal vein or IVC below diaphragm

T3c: Spread to supra diaphragmatic IVC or invades the wall of the IVC

T4: Involves ipsilateral adrenal gland or invades beyond Gerota's fascia

N-stage

N0: No nodal involvement

N1: Metastasis to one regional lymph node(s)

M-stage

M0: No distant metastases

M1: Distant metastases

Edge SB, et al. *AJCC Cancer Staging Manual*, 7th edn. New York: Springer-Verlag; 2010.

35. C. Ruptured dermoid cyst

Dermoid cysts are congenital ectodermal inclusion cysts. They tend to occur in the midline sellar, parasellar, or frontonasal regions or in the posterior fossa, where they occur either as vermian lesions or within the fourth ventricle.

Imaging findings vary, depending on whether the cyst has ruptured. Unruptured cysts have the same imaging characteristics as fat because they contain liquid cholesterol. All are hyperintense on T1-weighted images and do not enhance. The masses have heterogeneous signal intensity on T2-weighted images and vary from hypo- to hyperintense. The best diagnostic clue of a ruptured dermoid cyst is fatlike droplets in the subarachnoid cisterns, sulci and ventricles. Extensive pial enhancement can be seen from chemical meningitis caused by ruptured cysts.

Dermoid cysts may be confused with an epidermoid cyst, craniopharyngioma, teratoma or lipoma. Epidermoid cysts typically resemble CSF (not fat), lack dermal appendages, and are usually located off-midline. Like dermoid cysts, craniopharyngiomas are suprasellar, with a midline location, and demonstrate nodular calcification. However, most craniopharyngiomas are strikingly hyperintense on T2-weighted images and enhance strongly. Teratomas may also have a similar location but usually occur in the pineal region. Lipomas demonstrate homogeneous fat attenuation and/or signal intensity and show a chemical shift artefact, which typically does not occur with dermoid cysts.

Osborn AG, Preece MT. Intracranial cysts: Radiologic-pathologic correlation and imaging approach. *Radiology*. 2006;239(3):650–64.

36. E. Total anomalous pulmonary venous return (TAPVR)

TAPVR occurs when the pulmonary veins fail to drain into the left atrium and instead form an aberrant connection with some other cardiovascular structure.

On chest radiographs, this cardiovascular anomaly resembles a snowman (figure of eight appearance). In infants affected by TAPVR, cyanosis and congestive heart failure typically develop in the early neonatal period.

TA, TGA typically does not present with heart failure. Vein of Galen aneurysm presents with features of heart failure on a chest X-ray but without any specific pattern.

Ferguson EC, et al. Classic imaging signs of congenital cardiovascular abnormalities. *Radiographics*. 2007; 27(5): 1323–34.

37. A. Thymoma

Thymomas are classified as encapsulated, infiltrative and metastasising, with pulmonary and pleural deposits and thymic carcinoma. Half the thymomas are asymptomatic and 30% are associated with myasthenia gravis.

At CT a benign thymoma appears round, oval or lobulated. Focal calcification is seen in 25%, which may be dense, irregular or coarse. Benign thymomas show mild homogenous enhancement; cystic changes are also described. Invasive thymoma are heterogeneous in appearance; pericardial and pleural nodules suggest malignancy. Egg-shell calcification is described in invasive thymoma. Absent fat planes between thymoma and mediastinum does not necessarily reflect invasion.

Tecce PM, et al. CT evaluation of the anterior mediastinum: Spectrum of disease. *Radiographics*. 1994; 14(5):973–90.

38. E. Focal appendiceal wall-enhancement defect

Defect in enhancing appendiceal wall has the highest specificity (100%) and sensitivity (64.3%) for indicating perforated appendicitis.

Horrow MM, et al. Differentiation of perforated from nonperforated appendicitis at CT1. *Radiology*. 2003;227:46–51.

39. C. Diffuse axonal injury

Diffuse axonal injury (DAI) is a type of brain damage that is secondary to rotational acceleration/deceleration. MR can identify DAI lesions, whereas CT scan often fails to do so. T2-weighted images show high signal with blooming artefact. SWI (or GRE) sequences, exquisitely sensitive to blood products, may demonstrate small regions of susceptibility artefact at the grey–white matter junction, in the corpus callosum or the brain stem.

DAI is classified into three stages: the involvement of the grey–white matter junction indicates Stage I; corpus callosum involvement, particularly the splenium, indicates Stage II; and brainstem involvement indicates Stage III. Clinical studies demonstrate that the prognosis becomes poorer as deeper structures are involved.

Beretta L, et al. The value of MR imaging in posttraumatic diffuse axonal injury. *J Emerg Trauma Shock*. 2008;1(2):126–7.

40. B. TCC of the renal pelvis

Hereditary non-polyposis colon cancer syndrome (HNPCC) is an autosomal dominant condition that is associated with a high incidence of tumours of the renal pelvis, colorectal cancer, and tumours of the ovaries and small bowel. Squamous cell carcinoma of the renal pelvis is rare and is a highly aggressive tumour with a poor prognosis. Chronic infection and calculi play an important aetiological role in this malignancy, and stones are present in 57% of patients.

Renal lymphomas typically demonstrate sheet-like diffuse infiltration of the perirenal tissues or multiple low-attenuation focal lesions. Renal metastases are usually small (<3 cm), multiple and confined to the cortex. They are associated with metastases elsewhere, are of low attenuation, do not calcify, and do not invade the renal vein; they are also more infiltrative than exophytic compared to renal cell carcinoma.

Adam A, et al. *Grainger & Allison's Diagnostic Radiology: A Textbook of Medical Imaging*, 5th edn. New York: Churchill Livingstone, 2008:866–7.

41. E. Erlenmeyer flask deformity

Erlenmeyer flask deformity is associated with thalassaemia.

Non-specific findings of haemophilic arthropathy include joint effusion and periarticular osteopaenia from hyperaemia. Classical features include epiphyseal enlargement with associated gracile diaphysis (differentials are juvenile rheumatoid arthritis). Secondary degenerative disease with symmetrical loss of joint cartilage involving all compartments equally with periarticular erosions, subchondral cysts, osteophytes and sclerosis is seen in end-stage arthropathy.

Specific findings at the knee include widened intercondylar notch, squared margins of the patella, expanded femoral condyles and flattened surface of femoral condyles.

Specific findings at the elbow include enlargement of the radial head and widening of the trochlear notch.

Dähnert W. *Radiology Review Manual.* Philadelphia, PA: Lippincott Williams & Wilkins, 2007.
Weissleder R, et al. *Primer of Diagnostic Imaging.* Maryland Heights, MO: Mosby Inc., 2003.

42. D. Scrotal wall oedema

Differential diagnosis of acute scrotum includes testicular torsion (the most important differential) along with torsion of the testicular appendix, epididymitis and epididymo-orchitis. US (including the use of Doppler imaging) plays a vital role in distinguishing between these diagnoses. All of the above features can be seen in testicular torsion, along with such findings as epididymal enlargement and hydrocoele. However, scrotal wall oedema is the only one of these findings that is more commonly seen with alternative causes of acute scrotum than it is with acute testicular torsion. Decreased or absent blood flow is considered the most important finding, although torsion is not excluded if there is normal or increased blood flow, which may occur after spontaneous detorsion.

Dähnert W. *Radiology Review Manual*, 6th edn. Philadelphia, PA: Lippincott Williams & Wilkins, 2007:975.
Karmazyn B, et al. Clinical and sonographic criteria of acute scrotum in children: A retrospective study of 172 boys. *Pediatr Radiol.* 2005;35:302–10.

43. E. DWI shows low signal in the affected area.

In the immunocompetent adult patient, the pattern is quite typical and manifests as a bilateral asymmetrical involvement of the limbic system, medial temporal lobes, insular cortices and inferolateral frontal lobes. The basal ganglia are typically spared. Extralimbic involvement is more prevalent in children than in adults, seen most commonly in the parietal lobe, with sparing of the basal ganglia. Eventually, it results in marked cystic encephalomalacia and volume loss in affected areas.

In immunocompromised patients, involvement can be more diffuse and is more likely to involve the brainstem. Early diagnosis is difficult and a 'normal' CT is often seen. Affected areas appear low on T1-weighted MRI due to oedema. High T1 signal suggests areas of haemorrhage. Post-contrast enhancement is usually late and can be gyral, leptomeningeal, ring or diffuse enhancement. Affected white matter and cortex appears high signal on T2-weighted and FLAIR images. Areas of haemorrhage show low T2 signal and blooming artefact. DWI is more sensitive than T2-weighted images. Cytotoxic oedema is seen as high signal on DWI with corresponding low signal on ADC map. Vasogenic oedema is bright on both (T2 shine-through).

Bulakbasi N, Kocaoglu M. Central nervous system infections of herpesvirus family. *Neuroimaging Clin N Am.* 2008; 18(1): 53–84.

44. D. Nerve sheath tumour

Anatomical and radiological division of the mediastinum into anterior, middle and posterior varies. Anatomically, structures in the pericardial space including great vessels constitute the middle mediastinum; structures anterior to the pericardial sac constitute the anterior mediastinum, and structures behind the sac constitute the posterior mediastinum. The Felson method of radiological division is based on lateral chest radiography. A line extending from the diaphragm to the thoracic inlet along the back of the heart and anterior to the trachea separates the anterior and middle mediastinum, whereas a line that connects points 1 cm behind the anterior margins of the vertebral bodies separates the middle and posterior mediastinal compartments.

The hilum overlay sign is present when the normal hilar structures project through a mass, meaning that the mass is either anterior or posterior to the hilum. Loss of anterior junction line and cardiac contours would suggest anterior location; preservation of these lines and the loss or widening of the posterior junction lines, paraspinal lines, would suggest posterior location.

Lymphoma, teratoma and goitre are anterior mediastinal masses. Nerve sheath tumours are the only true posterior mediastinal structures amongst the examples.

Whitten CR, et al. A diagnostic approach to mediastinal abnormalities. *Radiographics*. 2007;27(3):657–71.

45. C. It is usually associated with change in bowel habits

The condition most commonly manifests in the fourth to fifth decades of life, predominantly in men. With diagnosis based on clinical manifestations alone, acute epiploic appendagitis is misdiagnosed in the majority of patients. Clinically, acute epiploic appendagitis manifests with acute onset of pain, most often in the left lower quadrant, and this symptom often leads to its being mistaken for acute diverticulitis. Unlike acute epiploic appendagitis, acute diverticulitis is more likely to manifest with evenly distributed lower abdominal pain and to be associated with nausea, fever and leucocytosis. Although most patients with acute epiploic appendagitis do not report any change in their bowel habits, a minority experience constipation or diarrhoea.

Most patients with acute epiploic appendagitis have a normal white blood cell count and body temperature. CT images from less than 8% of patients evaluated for exclusion of sigmoid diverticulitis or appendicitis show features of primary acute epiploic appendagitis. When acute epiploic appendagitis involves the cecum or ascending colon, it may be mistaken clinically for acute appendicitis. The most common sites of acute epiploic appendagitis, in order of decreasing frequency, are areas adjacent to the sigmoid colon, the descending colon and the right hemicolon.

Singh AK, et al. Acute epiploic appendagitis and its mimics. *Radiographics*. 2005;25:1521–34.

46. B. Urology referral and check of serum parathyroid hormone levels.

The most common clinical manifestations of hyperparathyroidism include renal stones and nephrocalcinosis, high blood pressure, acute arthropathy (CPPD), osteoporosis, peptic ulcer, acute pancreatitis, proximal muscle weakness, depression and confusional state (often described in medical text books as 'stones, groans and moans'). It is diagnosed by raised serum parathormone levels. Serum TSH levels are related to hyper- and hypothyroidism. Calcitonin is typically raised in medullary carcinoma of the thyroid. Serum alkaline phosphatase is a non-specific enzyme marker, which is raised, in several inflammatory, metabolic and malignant conditions. LDH is also a non-specific enzyme marker, raised in heart disease and myositis.

Adam A, et al. *Grainger & Allison's Diagnostic Radiology: A Textbook of Medical Imaging*, 5th edn. New York: Churchill Livingstone, 2008:1099–1100.

47. E. Monostotic fibrous dysplasia

Fibrous dysplasia is an uncommon, benign disorder characterised by a tumour-like proliferation of fibro-osseous tissue. It may either present as monostotic (affecting one bone) or polyostotic (affecting many bones). Fibrous dysplasia is usually found in the proximal femur, tibia, humerus, ribs and craniofacial bones in decreasing order of incidence. Polyostotic cases can affect multiple adjacent bones or multiple extremities. Men and women are equally affected by the disorder.

Fibrous dysplasia is usually asymptomatic, although pain and swelling may accompany the lesion. Radiographically, fibrous dysplasia appears as a well-circumscribed lesion in a long bone with a ground-glass or hazy appearance of the matrix. There is a narrow zone of transition and no periosteal reaction or soft-tissue mass. The lesions are normally located in the metaphysis or diaphysis. There is sometimes focal thinning of the overlying cortex, called 'scalloping from within'. The radiological appearance can also be cystic, pagetoid, or dense and sclerotic. Repeated fractures through lesions in the proximal femur can result in the formation of a so-called shepherd's crook deformity. The Tc-99m bone scan uptake may be normal or increased. Bone scans are not helpful in diagnosing these lesions but can be useful in identifying asymptomatic lesions. MRI or CT scans can be helpful in delineating the extent of the lesion and identifying possible pathological fractures. Sarcomatous change within the lesion can be identified by MRI or CT.

Kransdorf ML, et al. Fibrous dysplasia. *Radiographics*. 1990;10(3):519–37.

48. B.   Blount disease

All of the answers can lead to leg bowing in paediatric groups. However, the description is that of Blount disease, otherwise known as *tibia vara*. This is a common condition that is unilateral or asymmetrical and is thought to arise as a result of abnormal stress (such as obesity and walking at an early age) on the posteromedial proximal tibial physis. There are three types: infantile (the most common), juvenile and adolescent. Anteroposterior radiography of both legs is necessary. Neurofibromatosis may cause anterolateral tibial bowing, possibly with fibular hypoplasia, and one or both bones may fracture to give a pseudarthrosis. Developmental or physiological bowing is where there is exaggeration of varus angulation between the ages of 12 and 24 months, which again may be caused by obesity or early walking. There is metaphyseal beaking but no fragmentation, and it is usually symmetrical and bilateral. Congenital bowing is usually convex posteromedially (unlike neurofibromatosis). Marked dorsiflexion of the foot is evident at birth, as this condition is thought to arise from an abnormal intrauterine position. Radiography shows thickening of the cortex of the concavity of the curvature. Osteogenesis imperfecta causes bowing of multiple long bones as a result of osteoporotic softening and fractures; hence bone density reduction and bilateral bowing would be more likely.

Cheema JI, et al. Radiographic characteristics of lower-extremity bowing in children. *Radiographics*. 2003;23:871–80.

49. D.   Aberrant left pulmonary artery

Vascular anomalies of the aortic arch and the pulmonary artery can cause vascular impression on the barium-filled oesophagus. The most common is a right-sided aortic arch, which results in an indentation on the right and absence of normal aortic impression on the left. Bilateral indentation is caused by a double aortic arch; the right arch is normally higher and larger than the left.

Aberrant right subclavian artery from a normal arch or an aberrant left subclavian artery from a right-sided arch traverses behind the oesophagus as it crosses the mediastinum and results in a posterior impression on the oesophagus seen on a lateral view. An aberrant left pulmonary artery traverses between the trachea and oesophagus above the carina, resulting in a posterior indentation on the trachea and an anterior indentation on the oesophagus on lateral view. Coarctation of the aorta results in a reverse-3 impression on the left of the oesophagus on an AP image. Type-3 anomalous pulmonary veins traverse the diaphragm with the oesophagus and drain into a systemic vein, causing an impression on the anterior wall of the oesophagus, low down close to the diaphragm.

Eisenberg RL. Extrinsic impressions on the thoracic oesophagus. In: *Gastrointestinal Radiology: A Pattern Approach*, 4th edn. Eisenberg RL (ed.). Philadelphia, PA: Lippincott Williams & Wilkins, 2003: 27–42.

50. C. Contracted gallbladder

Features of acute cholecystitis include thickened GB wall >4–5 mm, echogenic bile/sludge, gallbladder distention, pericholecystic fluid in the absence of ascites and subserosal oedema.

Contracted GB is generally a feature of chronic cholecystitis.

Dähnert W. *Radiology Review Manual*, 7th edn. Philadelphia, PA: Lippincott Williams & Wilkins, 2011:713–4.

51. E. Involved seminal vesicles show a high signal on T2W images.

MR tumour staging criteria follow the TNM system. A papillary tumour is best seen on T1-weighted images, where it is seen as higher signal than the urine. It appears similar in signal intensity on T2-weighted sequences. Tumour demonstration (especially a small one) is facilitated by use of contrast. To evaluate infiltration, T2-weighted or post-contrast T1-weighted sequences are required. Use of surface coils (endorectal coils) improves visualisation of layers of the bladder wall, improving staging of T2–T3b tumours. Visualisation of low-intensity bladder wall on T2-weighted sequence between the tumour and perivesical fat helps in differentiating a T2b tumour from a T3 tumour. Disruption of low-signal bladder wall, perivesical fat stranding and irregularity of the outer bladder wall suggests T3b disease. Dynamic contrast-induced MRI improves bladder cancer staging accuracy by helping differentiation of tumour (enhances earlier) from inflammatory post-biopsy changes in the bladder wall or perivesical fat (slower rate of enhancement). It is also useful in staging nodes, because abnormal nodes (normal or abnormal by size) enhance earlier than non-metastatic lymph nodes.

Involvement of the seminal vesicle is evident as an increase in size of the vesicle, reduced T2 signal, and obliteration of the angle between the seminal vesicle and posterior bladder wall. In contrast, invasion of the prostate and rectum is seen as direct tumour extension and an increase in signal intensity on T2-weighted images.

T staging of bladder tumours

Ta: Non-invasive papillary tumour
Tis: In situ (non-invasive flat)
T1: Through lamina propria into subepithelial connective tissues
T2a: Only invades the inner half of the muscle
T2b: Invades into the outer half of the muscle
T3a: Microscopic extravesical invasion
T3b: Macroscopic extravesical invasion
T4: Direct invasion into adjacent structures (prostate, uterus, vaginal vault)
T4b: Direct involvement of pelvic side wall and/or abdominal wall

Adam A, et al. *Grainger & Allison's Diagnostic Radiology: A Textbook of Medical Imaging*, 5th edn. New York: Churchill Livingstone, 2008:892–3.

52. D. Osteosclerosis is more common in the primary form.

Osteosclerosis, as seen in the rugger jersey spine, is associated with the secondary form of hyperparathyroidism from chronic renal failure. The rest of the statements are true. In summary, the radiological findings, which are more associated with the primary form, include Brown tumours, subperiosteal bone resorption, soft-tissue calcification (although less common than in the secondary forms), and chondrocalcinosis. The findings for secondary hyperparathyroidism include subperiosteal bone resorption, osteosclerosis and soft-tissue calcification.

Dähnert W. *Radiology Review Manual*, 6th edn. Philadelphia, PA: Lippincott Williams & Wilkins, 2007:105.

53. D. Epidermoid

Causes of white matter hyperintensities are protean; however certain categories are recognised. These include the following:

Hypoxic/ischaemic aetiology secondary to hereditary conditions (Fabry's disease, PKU, MELAS, amyloid deposition, CADASIL, moyamoya, Rendu–Weber–Osler syndrome, etc.) or acquired conditions (hypertension, hypotension, atherosclerosis, NPH, embolic events, Wallerian degeneration, etc.).

Inflammatory conditions like MS and its variants, ADEM, SSPE, vasculitis (Behcet's disease, GCA, PAN, etc.), sarcoid, bacterial, protozoal, viral (HSV, HIV, PML), spirochetal (Lyme disease) and fugal.

Toxic or metabolic causes like CPM, CO intoxication, methotrexate treatment, Marchiafava–Bignami syndrome and B12 deficiency. Other conditions include radiation, contusion, hystiocytosis and Erdheim–Chester disease.

Epidermoid cysts are extraparenchymal, mimic CSF, do not enhance and show restricted diffusion.

Barkhof F, Scheltens P. Imaging of white matter lesions. *Cerebrovasc Dis.* 2002;13 Suppl 2: 21–30.

54. C. Occipital bone

Thalassaemia major, as with other causes of chronic anaemia, causes widening of the diploic space in the skull as a result of marrow hyperplasia, with thinning of the outer table and thickening of the inner table. A 'hair on end' appearance is seen, with periosteal bony spicules extending beyond the outer table. The occipital bone normally has a lower bone marrow content and is therefore not affected to the same extent by these changes. Occasionally, solitary or multiple lytic lesions may be seen in the skull. Paranasal sinuses and mastoids are often absent or underpneumatised owing to frontal, temporal and facial bone marrow hyperplasia. The ethmoid sinuses are the exception because there is minimal marrow content in the surrounding bones.

Tyler PA, et al. The radiological appearances of thalassemia. *Clinical Radiol.* 2006;61:40–52.

55. B. Cytomegalovirus pneumonitis

Early complications include interstitial pneumonitis (infective and non-infective types), infection, oedema, haemorrhage, thromboembolism and calcification. COP is a rare complication that may occur early or late. Cytomegalovirus (CMV) is the most important viral pathogen that causes pneumonia in transplant recipients. RSV, HHV6, pneumocystis jiroveci and adenovirus are less common. Idiopathic interstitial pneumonia has various causes including acute graft-versus-host disease.

Unfortunately, CT appearances of both infectious and non-infectious interstitial pneumonitis are non-specific. Notable features include increased interstitial markings, multilobar infiltrates, areas of ground-glass opacity and nodules. Biopsy is frequently undertaken to identify the cause.

Levine DS, et al. Imaging the complications of bone marrow transplantation in children. *Radiographics.* 2007;27(2):307–24.

56. D. Contrast-enhanced CT

Contrast-enhanced CT is the imaging modality of choice for the diagnosis and staging of acute pancreatitis. The pancreas enhances uniformly in mild acute pancreatitis and may be normal or enlarged with a variable amount of increased attenuation in the adjacent fat, termed 'stranding'. Local oedema is a common finding and may extend along the mesentery, mesocolon and hepatoduodenal ligament and into the peritoneal spaces. Extension of oedematous fluid into the anterior perirenal space may create a mass effect and a halo sign with sparing of the perinephric fat.

Abnormal ultrasound findings are seen in 33%–90% of patients with acute pancreatitis. Interstitial oedema in acute pancreatitis is depicted on ultrasound as an enlarged hypoechoic gland. Although ultrasound may be used to identify peripancreatic acute fluid collections, it is not useful for the detection of necrosis. Thus its main role in the imaging of acute pancreatitis is limited to the detection of cholelithiasis and choledocholithiasis and identification of fluid collections in the peritoneum, retroperitoneum and pleural spaces.

O'Connor OJ, et al. Imaging of acute pancreatitis. *AJR Am J Roentgenol*. 2011;197:W221–5.

57. B. The central and transition zones show similar low signal.

On T1-weighted images, the prostate shows homogenous intermediate signal intensity, and the zones cannot be differentiated. The zonal anatomy is best seen on T2-weighted images with the peripheral zone showing a high signal compared to both the central and the transitional zones. The central and transitional zones have similar low signal. At a young age, the transitional zone is homogenous low signal; it gets increasingly heterogeneous with age and BPH changes. On T2-weighted images, the shape of the peripheral zone changes from the base to apex. At the base, the peripheral zone surrounds the posterolateral aspect of the central zone, while at the apex it concentrically surrounds the central zone. The prostatic capsule separates the peripheral zone from the periprostatic tissue, whereas the surgical pseudocapsule separates the peripheral zone from the transitional zone in the older population. MRI is recognised to be more accurate than US and CT in assessment of prostate volume.

Adam A, et al. *Grainger & Allison's Diagnostic Radiology: A Textbook of Medical Imaging*, 5th edn. New York: Churchill Livingstone, 2008:899–900.

58. C. Developmental dysplasia of the hip

The patient has developmental dysplasia of the hip, which has resulted in subluxation of the femoral head. The centre edge angle is useful in older toddlers up to adulthood to estimate the degree of acetabular over or under coverage. It is the angle between a vertical line drawn up from the centre of the femoral head and the outer edge of the acetabular roof. In an adult, an angle less than 20 degrees indicates underlying dysplasia. Perthes disease is a paediatric condition characterised by avascular necrosis of the femoral head. Ollier's disease is the condition of multiple enchondromas (enchondromatosis). Isolated traumatic subluxation requires significant trauma in the absence of an underlying dysplasia.

Dähnert W. *Radiology Review Manual*, 6th edn. Philadelphia, PA: Lippincott Williams & Wilkins, 2007:65–6.

59. B. Diffusion-weighted MR imaging

Epidermoid cysts are characteristically well demarcated and have a homogeneous low density, similar to CSF on CT scan, showing no contrast enhancement. On MRI, epidermoid cysts are hypointense on T1-weighted images and hyperintense on T2-weighted images. On FLAIR, epidermoid cysts become hyperintense or appear more heterogeneous compared to an arachnoid cyst. There are occasions when an epidermoid may appear as a low-intensity lesion on FLAIR. However, on diffusion-weighted imaging, epidermoid cysts show restriction and remain bright (due to a combination of true restricted diffusion and T2 shine-through).The latter helps with definitive differentiation of an epidermoid cyst from an arachnoid cyst.

Dutt SN, et al. Radiologic differentiation of intracranial epidermoids from arachnoid cysts. *Otol Neurotol*. 2002;23(1):84–92.

60. B. Haemorrhagic ovarian cyst

All of the above may present as a right hemipelvic mass. Haemorrhage into an ovarian follicular cyst is the most common of these, and it usually resolves after one or two menstrual cycles. Several patterns of ultrasound findings have been described, including an echogenic mass, a ground-glass pattern (diffuse low-level echoes), a whirled pattern of mixed echogenicity and a 'fishnet weave' pattern (fine septations or reticular echoes). Appendix abscess would be thick-walled. Ovarian dermoid may present as an echogenic mass, although acoustic shadowing would be more typical owing to internal calcifications and would not resolve in this fashion. Ectopic pregnancy may present as an echogenic 'tubal mass', although elevated β-hCG would be a feature. Ovarian torsion may appear as an enlarged echogenic ovary (owing to oedema) and, like haemorrhagic cyst, often lacks internal colour Doppler flow, although it is less common than haemorrhagic cyst. It would also necessitate urgent surgery rather than follow-up imaging.

Dähnert W. *Radiology Review Manual*, 6th edn. Philadelphia, PA: Lippincott Williams & Wilkins, 2007:1054–6.

Donnelly LF. *Pediatric Imaging: The Fundamentals*. Philadelphia, PA: Saunders Elsevier, 2009:151–3.

61. B.   Pulmonary contusion

Lung contusion is the most common type of lung injury in blunt chest trauma. It occurs at the time of injury, but it may be undetectable on chest radiography for the first 6 hours after trauma; however, CT may show it immediately. The pooling of haemorrhage and oedema will blossom at 24 hours, rendering the contusion more evident. The appearance of consolidation on CXR after the first 24 hours should raise the suspicion of other pathological conditions such as aspiration, pneumonia and fat embolism. Clearance of an uncomplicated contusion begins at 24–48 hours with complete resolution after 3–14 days. Lack of resolution within the expected time frame should raise the suspicion of complications such as pneumonia, abscess or ARDS.

Lung laceration results in ground-glass change or consolidation with pneumatocoele, haematocele or pneumothorax. Rib fractures may be associated with peripheral lacerations.

Oikonomou A, Prassopoulos P. CT imaging of blunt chest trauma. *Insights Imaging*. 2011;2(3):281–95.

62. E.   Low luminal signal intensity on T1- and T2-weighted images

MR imaging features of a normal appendix include a diameter less than 6 mm, an appendiceal wall thickness less than 2 mm, low luminal signal intensity on T1- and T2-weighted images and no periappendiceal fat stranding or fluid. MRI features of appendicitis include an appendiceal diameter greater than 7 mm, an appendiceal wall thickness greater than 2 mm, high-signal-intensity luminal contents on T2-weighted images due to fluid or oedema and hyperintense periappendiceal fat stranding and fluid.

An appendix with high-signal-intensity luminal contents on T2-weighted images and a diameter between 6 and 7 mm without associated wall thickening or periappendiceal fat stranding or fluid is considered indeterminate for appendicitis and warrants close clinical follow-up. MRI has been described as an effective modality for the diagnosis of appendicitis during pregnancy, with 100% sensitivity and 94% specificity reported.

Spalluto LB. MR imaging evaluation of abdominal pain during pregnancy: Appendicitis and other nonobstetric causes. *RadioGraphics*. 2012;32:317–34.

63. D.   T3b

T staging of prostate cancer

T1: Not palpable via DRE or seen using TRUS.
T1a: Cancer found incidentally during TURP, less than 5% of the gland.
T1b: Cancer found incidentally but over 5% of the gland is involved.
T1c: Found by needle biopsy for a raised PSA.

T2: Palpable on DRE, but confined to the prostate.
T2a: Less than half of one lobe.
T2b: More than half of one lobe.
T2c: Cancer in both lobes of the prostate.

T3: Spread outside the prostate.

T3a: Extracapsular extension (one or both sides).

T3b: Tumour invades the seminal vesicles.

T4: Spread into the adjacent tissues (other than seminal vesicles).

Claus FG, et al. Pretreatment evaluation of prostate cancer: Role of MR imaging and 1H MR spectroscopy. *Radiographics*. 2004;24 Suppl 1:S167–80.

64. D. Placement of a pelvic wrap device

All of these steps may be required, but the most important is to place a pelvic wrap device. The purpose of this device is to stabilise the pelvis. If the patient is hypotensive as a result of venous bleeding, a pelvic wrap should stabilise the pelvis sufficiently to cause significant reduction or cessation in the venous haemorrhage and thus avoid unnecessary endovascular intervention.

If this fails to achieve sufficiently prompt haemodynamic stability, there is a significant chance that there is arterial haemorrhage; hence endovascular intervention is likely to be necessary. Many centres use angiographic sequences as part of the trauma CT scan to identify such a bleeding point as part of planning stage of endovascular management. CT would be the next step once the pelvic binder is *in situ*.

Zealley IA, Chakraverty S. The role of interventional radiology in trauma. *Brit Med J*. 2010;340:356–60.

65. C. Smaller nodule

Pilocytic astrocytoma is the most common paediatric cerebellar neoplasm and the most common paediatric glioma. They can be differentiated from haemangioblastoma on the following basis: astrocytomas are more likely to be larger than 5 cm, contain calcification, have a larger mural nodule, are thick-walled lesions, do not show angiographic contrast blush to the mural nodule and are not associated with erythrocythaemia.

Dähnert W. *Radiology Review Manual*, 7th edn. Philadelphia, PA: Lippincott Williams & Wilkins, 2011:273–4.

66. B. It most commonly occurs on the left.

Ovarian torsion is most common in prepubertal girls and may be caused by ovarian enlargement (for example owing to neoplastic causes, of which benign cystic teratoma is the most common) or abnormally increased adnexal mobility. It is more common on the right than the left, which is postulated to occur because of a protective effect of the sigmoid colon on the left side. On ultrasound, the most reliable positive finding is asymmetry between the volumes of the right and left ovaries. Arterial Doppler waveform is usually but not always absent, as there is blood supply from both the ovarian and uterine arteries.

A whirlpool sign may be seen because of twisting of the ovarian pedicle. Treatment is with emergency surgery; hence immediate referral to gynaecology is required.

Dähnert W. *Radiology Review Manual*, 6th edn. Philadelphia, PA: Lippincott Williams & Wilkins, 2007:1064–5.

Donnelly LF. *Pediatric Imaging: The Fundamentals*. Philadelphia, PA: Saunders Elsevier, 2009:1064–5.

67. A. Pulmonary artery aneurysm

One of the most common findings of Behcet's disease at chest radiography is a lung mass attributed to a pulmonary artery aneurysm. The pulmonary artery is the second most common site of arterial involvement, with the aorta being the most common, and aneurysms are more common than thromboembolism. Behcet's disease is the most common cause of pulmonary artery aneurysms.

Hughes–Stovin syndrome is a rare disorder of unknown aetiology that is characterised by the combination of multiple pulmonary artery aneurysms with mural thrombi and deep venous thrombosis.

Another well-known finding is the mediastinal widening caused by thrombosis of the SVC and accompanying mediastinal oedema. Thrombosis of the brachiocephalic, subclavian and axillary veins may also accompany SVC occlusion.

Arterial involvement may occur in the ascending thoracic aorta and the aortic arch, as well as in the coronary artery and subclavian artery in the thorax. Aneurysm formation occurs more frequently than arterial occlusion.

Chae EJ, et al. Radiologic and clinical findings of Behçet disease: Comprehensive review of multisystemic involvement. *Radiographics*. 2008;28(5):e31.

68. B.   Stomal stenosis is a rare complication.

The most common complication after gastric banding is stomal stenosis. This complication occurs when the band is too tight, causing excessive luminal narrowing and obstruction.

Affected individuals usually present with nausea and vomiting, regurgitation, dysphagia or upper abdominal pain. When stomal stenosis is found on barium studies in patients with obstructive symptoms, the band should be deflated to increase luminal calibre and relieve the patient's symptoms.

Acute pouch dilation usually results from marked stomal narrowing secondary to overfilling of the band or from distal band slippage and obstruction. In this setting, the band should be deflated to prevent further complications, including irreversible pouch dilation and progressive band slippage.

Distal band slippage is thought to result from recurrent vomiting, overinflation of the band or faulty surgical technique.

Malpositioning of the band is an unusual complication that occurs at the time of surgical placement, most often when this procedure is performed by an inexperienced surgeon.

Band erosion into the gastric lumen is a rare but late complication of laparoscopic adjustable gastric banding and results from high pressures generated by the inflated band, with pressure necrosis of the adjacent gastric wall and subsequent erosion of the band into the lumen.

Levine MS. Imaging of bariatric surgery: Normal anatomy and postoperative complications. *Radiology*. 2014;270(2):327–41.

69. E.   Complete tear Grade III – at the level of the urogenital diaphragm

Urethral injuries associated with a pelvic fracture were classified into five types by Goldman and Sandler and into three types by Colapinto and McCallum, with Types IV and V being exclusive to Goldman and Sandler: Type I, posterior urethra stretched but intact (no extravasation of contrast); Type II, urethra disrupted at the membrano-prostatic junction above the urogenital diaphragm (contrast in pelvis); Type III, membranous urethra disrupted, with extension to the proximal bulbous urethra and/or disruption of the urogenital diaphragm (most common – contrast in pelvis and perineum); Type IV, bladder neck injury with extension into the urethra; and Type V, partial or complete pure anterior urethral injury. Grades II and III are subdivided into complete and incomplete tear depending on the absence or presence of bladder filling.

Adam A, et al. *Grainger & Allison's Diagnostic Radiology: A Textbook of Medical Imaging*, 5th edn. New York: Churchill Livingstone, 2008.

70. A.   Large osteophytes

Milwaukee shoulder consists of the association of complete tear of the rotator cuff, osteoarthritic changes, non-inflammatory joint effusion containing calcium hydroxyapatite and calcium pyrophosphate dihydrate crystals, hyperplasia of the synovium, destruction of cartilage and subchondral bone, and multiple osteochondral loose bodies. This entity most frequently affects older women and manifests clinically as a rapidly progressive and destructive arthritis of the shoulder.

It manifests as joint space narrowing, subchondral sclerosis with cyst formation, destruction of subchondral bone, soft-tissue swelling, capsular calcifications and intra-articular loose bodies. MR imaging demonstrates a large effusion, a complete rotator cuff tear, narrowing of the glenohumeral joint, thinning of cartilage and destruction of subchondral bone.

Llauger J, et al. Nonseptic monoarthritis: Imaging features with clinical and histopathologic correlation. *Radiographics*. 2000;20:S263–78.

71. D.   Late subacute

Phase	Age	Compartment	T1W	T2W
Hyperacute	4–6 hours	Intracellular oxyHb	Iso	Hyper
Acute	12–48 hours	Intracellular deoxyHb	Hypo	Hypo
		Extracellular deoxyHb	Iso	Iso
Early subacute	3–7 days	Intracellular methHb	Hyper	Hypo
Late subacute	>7 days	Extracellular methHb	Hyper	Hyper
Chronic	>30 days	Hemosiderin rim	Hypo rim	Hypo rim

Dähnert W. *Radiology Review Manual*, 7th edn. Philadelphia, PA: Lippincott Williams & Wilkins, 2011:295.

72. C.   Wolman disease

Wolman disease is an uncommon autosomal recessive disorder characterised by accumulation of fat within such tissues as the liver, spleen, lymph nodes and adrenal glands. Accordingly, these tissues will increase in size. The adrenal findings are diagnostic of the condition, with glands that are of normal shape but increased size, with diffuse punctate calcification throughout both glands. It is usually fatal by the age of 6 months. Neuroblastomas may be seen in both adrenal glands simultaneously and are often calcified, although they will usually be large irregular masses. Non-traumatic haemorrhage of both adrenals may be seen, often caused by perinatal stressors, although this also takes the form of a mass and calcification is usually peripheral (initially) or dense (chronic stage). Adrenal glands may be thickened in adrenocortical hyperplasia but calcification is not a typical feature. Adrenocortical carcinoma is typically unilateral and is not usually seen until after the age of 6 months.

Hindman N, Israel GM. Adrenal gland and adrenal mass calcification. *Eur J Radiol*. 2005;15:1163–7.

73. D.   Stage IV disease refers to bilateral renal involvement at diagnosis.

Wilms tumour has multiple associations. One-third of patients with sporadic aniridia develop Wilms tumour; it also occurs in up to 20% of Beckwith–Wiedemann syndrome sufferers (otherwise known as EMG syndrome – exomphalos, macroglossia, gigantism – with hepatomegaly also a feature). Other associations include hemihypertrophy and a variety of genitourinary disorders including Drash syndrome, renal anomalies (including horseshoe kidney) and genital anomalies. Nephroblastomatosis is a recognised precursor and is seen in 99% of cases of bilateral Wilms tumour. Presentation of Wilms tumour is most commonly as an asymptomatic palpable abdominal mass, although other presentations include hypertension, pain and fever. Stage IV disease refers to the presence of haematogenous or extra-abdominopelvic lymph nodes.

Dähnert W. *Radiology Review Manual*, 6th edn. Philadelphia, PA: Lippincott Williams & Wilkins, 2007:992–3.

74. C.   Pleural fibroma

Chest radiographs of patients with pleural fibroma typically demonstrate a well-defined, lobular, solitary nodule or mass, which may appear to be in the lung periphery and typically abuts a pleural surface or is located within a fissure. Pedunculated tumours may show mobility within the pleural space or changes in shape and orientation on fluoroscopy or with changes in the patient's position.

Hypertrophic osteoarthropathy is characterised by periosteal reaction without an underlying bone lesion; causes include bronchogenic carcinoma (squamous cell cancer being the most common), pulmonary lymphoma, lung abscess, bronchiectasis, pulmonary metastases, pleural fibroma and mesothelioma.

Dähnert W. *Radiology Review Manual*, 7th edn. Philadelphia, PA: Lippincott Williams & Wilkins, 2011:110–524.

Rosado-de-Christenson ML. From the archives of the AFIP: Localized fibrous tumour of the pleura. *Radiographics*. 2003;23(3):759–83.

75. D. Anastomotic strictures usually appear on upper GI studies as irregular long segment narrowing at the gastrojejunal anastomosis.

Extraluminal leak is the most serious early complication of Roux-en-Y gastric bypass, occurring in up to 5% of patients. Between 69% and 77% of leaks involve the gastrojejunal anastomosis, but other less common sites of perforation include the gastric pouch, blind-ending jejunal stump and jejunojejunostomy. Leaks usually occur within 10 days of surgery; early detection is critical because of the risk of abscess formation, peritonitis and sepsis, with a mortality rate of more than 5%. Affected individuals may present with leucocytosis, fever, abdominal pain and tachycardia.

Transient anastomotic narrowing and obstruction may occur during the early post-operative period secondary to residual oedema and spasm in this region. Upper GI examinations may reveal focal narrowing of the gastrojejunal anastomosis and thickened, irregular folds in the Roux limb abutting the anastomosis. These findings usually resolve within several days.

Strictures at the gastrojejunal anastomosis have been reported in 3%–9% of patients. These strictures typically develop 4 weeks or more after surgery; they may be caused by post-surgical scarring at the anastomosis or by chronic ischaemia resulting from tension on the gastrojejunostomy.

Anastomotic strictures usually appear on upper GI studies as short segments of smooth narrowing at the gastrojejunal anastomosis.

Though adhesions are the most common cause of SBO after open Roux-en-Y gastric bypass, internal hernias are the most common cause after the laparoscopic form of surgery.

Marc S. Levine. Imaging of bariatric surgery: Normal anatomy and postoperative complications. *Radiology*. 2014;270(2).

76. A. Seminoma

Seminoma is the most common pure germ cell tumour. The imaging characteristics of seminomas reflect their uniform cellular nature. On US images, these tumours are generally uniformly hypoechoic. Embryonal carcinoma is the second most common histologic type of testicular tumour after seminoma. The tunica albuginea may be invaded, and the borders of the tumour are less distinct, as expected; they are more heterogeneous and ill-defined than seminomas on US image. Yolk sac tumours account for 80% of childhood testicular tumours, with most cases occurring before the age of 2 years. Imaging findings are non-specific, especially in children, in whom the only finding may be testicular enlargement without a defined mass. After yolk sac tumour, teratoma is the second most common testicular tumour in children. The complex nature of teratoma is reflected in its sonographic appearance. Teratomas generally form well-circumscribed complex masses. Cysts are a common feature and may be anechoic or complex, depending on the cyst contents (i.e., serous, mucoid or keratinous fluid). Cartilage, calcification, fibrosis and scar formation result in echogenic foci that may or may not produce posterior accoustic shadow. Testicular tumours from the sex cords (Sertoli cells) and interstitial stroma (Leydig cells) constitute 4% of tumours. Their sonographic appearance is variable and is indistinguishable from that of germ cell tumours. Sertoli cell tumours are typically well-circumscribed, unilateral, round to lobulated masses. The sonographic appearance of testicular lymphoma is variable and indistinguishable from that of germ cell tumours.

Testicular lymphoma generally appears as discrete hypoechoic lesions, which may completely infiltrate the testicle.

Woodward PJ, et al. From the archives of the AFIP: Tumors and tumorlike lesions of the testis: Radiologic-pathologic correlation. *Radiographics*. 2002;22(1):189–216.

77. C. Syringomyelia

Neuropathic osteoarthropathy can be categorised as originating from a congenital or acquired cause. The acquired causes include a central origin (e.g., syringomyelia, spinal cord tumours and multiple sclerosis) or a peripheral origin (e.g., poliomyelitis, leprosy, diabetes mellitus and peripheral nerve injury).

Dähnert W. *Radiology Review Manual*, 6th edn. Philadelphia, PA: Lippincott Williams & Wilkins, 2007:128.

78. A. Alobar holoprosencephaly

Holoprosencephaly (HPE) is considered the most common malformation of the brain and face in humans. In alobar HPE, prosencephalic cleavage fails, resulting in a single midline forebrain with a primitive monoventricle often associated with a large dorsal cyst. The olfactory bulbs and tracts, the corpus callosum and anterior commissure, the cavum septum pellucidum and the interhemispheric fissure are absent, whereas the optic nerves may be normal, fused or absent. The basal ganglia, hypothalamic and thalamic nuclei are typically fused in the midline, resulting in absence of the third ventricle.

In lobar HPE, the interhemispheric fissure is present along nearly the entire midline, and the thalami are completely or almost completely separated. The corpus callosum may be normal or incomplete, but the cavum septum pellucidum is always absent.

Hydranencephaly is the result of a vascular insult (anterior circulation) with the cerebral hemispheres variably replaced by fluid covered with leptomeninges and dura. Falx cerebri is present. The cerebellum, midbrain, thalami, basal ganglia, choroid plexus and portions of the occipital lobes, all fed by the posterior circulation, are typically preserved. It is differentiated from hydrocephalus by absence of an intact rim of cortex (seen with even the most severe hydrocephalus).

Kurtz AB, Johnson PT. Diagnosis please. Case 7: Hydranencephaly. *Radiology*. 1999;210(2):419–22.
Winter TC, et al. Holoprosencephaly: A survey of the entity, with embryology and fetal imaging. *Radiographics*. 2015;35(1):275–90.

79. E. Chronic pulmonary embolism

The tree-in-bud pattern on HRCT is characterised by small centrilobular nodules of soft-tissue attenuation connected to multiple branching linear structures of similar calibre originating from a single stalk. Initially described in cases of endobronchial *Mycobacterium tuberculosis*, it has subsequently been reported in peripheral airways diseases such as infection (bacterial, fungal, viral or parasitic), congenital disorders (like cystic fibrosis and Kartagener's syndrome), idiopathic disorders (obliterative bronchiolitis, panbronchiolitis), aspiration, inhalation, immunologic disorders (like ABPA), connective tissue disorders and peripheral pulmonary vascular diseases such as neoplastic pulmonary emboli.

Rossi SE. Tree-in-bud pattern at thin-section CT of the lungs: Radiologic-pathologic overview. *Radiographics*. 2005;25(3):789–801.

80. A. Pseudomeningocele

The prognosis is better in postganglionic injuries, where surgical repair in the form of nerve grafting is possible. In preganglionic injuries, usually nerve root avulsions, direct surgical repair cannot be performed. A MRI scan of postganglionic injuries can show thickened nerves with a low signal intensity on T1-weighted images and an increased signal intensity on T2-weighted images. Nerve may be in contiguity, or there can be discontinuity with distal nerve contraction. Direct brachial plexus compression by a haematoma, fracture fragment or callus formation can also cause brachial plexopathy. A MRI scan of preganglionic injuries can show nerve root avulsions with or without pseudomeningoceles. Pseudomeningoceles are cerebrospinal fluid collections resulting from a dural tear. The presence of a pseudomeningocele is a valuable sign. Spinal cord abnormalities occur in 20% of those with preganglionic injuries, such as oedema, haemorrhage and myelomalacia. An uncommon but useful finding is the enhancement of intradural nerve roots or root.

Sureka J, Cherian RA, Alexander M, Thomas BP. MRI of brachial plexopathies. *Clinical Radiology* 2009;64: 208–18.

van Es HW, Bollen TL, van Heesewijk HP. MRI of the brachial plexus: a pictorial review. *European Journal of Radiology* 74:391–402.

81. C. Hamartoma of tuber cinereum

Hypothalamic hamartomas are developmental malformations consisting of tumour-like masses located in the tuber cinereum of the hypothalamus. Most patients present in the first or second decade of life, with boys being more commonly affected than girls. These lesions have been divided into parahypothalamic hamartomas and intrahypothalamic hamartomas. Parahypothalamic hamartomas are pedunculated masses attached to the floor of the hypothalamus. These lesions seem more likely to be associated with precocious puberty than with gelastic seizures. Intrahypothalamic hamartomas are sessile masses with a broad attachment to the hypothalamus. They lie within the hypothalamus and may distort the contour of the third ventricle. In addition, they seem to be associated more often with gelastic seizures than with precocious puberty. At MR imaging, they are seen as well-defined pedunculated or sessile lesions at the tuber cinereum and are isointense or mildly hypointense on T1-weighted images and iso- to hyperintense on T2-weighted images, with no contrast enhancement or calcification. The absence of any long-term change in the size, shape or signal intensity of the lesion strongly supports the diagnosis of hypothalamic hamartoma.

Saleem SN, et al. Lesions of the hypothalamus: MR imaging diagnostic features. *Radiographics.* 2007;27(4):1087–108.

82. B. Pleomorphic undifferentiated sarcoma

Pleomorphic undifferentiated sarcoma was previously known as *malignant fibrous histiocytoma*. Malignant fibrous histiocytoma is the most common soft-tissue sarcoma of late adult life.
It typically presents as a painless, soft-tissue mass, which is often located in the thigh and measures 5–10 cm. X-ray demonstrates a non-specific soft-tissue mass with calcification/ossification detected in 5%–20% of patients. Secondary osseous involvement is uncommon. It can be identified as periosteal reaction, cortical erosion and pathological fracture.

CT findings include a non-specific, large, lobulated, soft-tissue mass of predominantly muscle density with nodular and peripheral enhancement of solid portions. There are often central areas of low attenuation, which represent myxoid change, old haemorrhage or necrosis. The lesion does not contain fat.

MRI typically reveals an intramuscular mass with heterogeneous signal intensity on all pulse sequences. As with other soft-tissue neoplasms, the signal intensity pattern is non-specific, usually low to intermediate on T1-weighted images and intermediate to high on T2-weighted images. Regions of prominent fibrous tissue (high collagen content) may demonstrate low signal intensity on both T1-weighted and T2-weighted images and calcification may present as foci of low signal on both T1-weighted and T2-weighted sequences.

Manaster BJ, et al. *Musculoskeletal Imaging: The Requisites.* Maryland Heights, MO: Mosby Inc., 2002.

Meyers SP. *MRI of Bone and Soft Tissue Tumors and Tumorlike Lesions, Differential Diagnosis and Atlas.* New York: Thieme Publishing Group, 2008.

Yip D, et al. Malignant fibrous histiocytoma imaging. emedicine.medscape.com/article/391453-overview [accessed on 16 February 2017].

83. B. Metastatic disease to the liver is always calcified.

The small bowel is the most common site of the gastrointestinal tract involved by melanoma. Appearance can be indistinguishable from that of primary or metastatic adenocarcinoma, lymphoma or other metastasis. Tumour masses may occur as infiltrating lesions with or without ulceration. Mesenteric involvement by melanoma can mimic lymphoma. Involvement of the large bowel is uncommon but can occur as large ulcerating lesions. Lesions in the liver can be single or multiple and may be partly calcified. Larger lesions are often necrotic.

Fishman EK. Melanoma in the chest, abdomen and musculoskeletal system. *Radiographics*. 1990;10:603–20.

84. D. Primary extragonadal germ cell tumours commonly affect the testes.

Lymphoma can occur in the testis in one of three ways: as the primary site, as the initial manifestation of occult disease or as the site of recurrence. It is the most common bilateral tumour and epididymis and spermatic cord are commonly involved. Primary leukaemia of the testis is rare. However, the testis is a common site of leukaemia recurrence in children.

Testicular microlithiasis is an uncommon condition but several associations are known, including cryptorchidism, infertility, Klinefelter syndrome, Down's syndrome, atrophy, alveolar microlithiasis and testicular carcinoma.

There is a calcifying subgroup of Sertoli cell tumours that can be multiple and bilateral with large areas of calcification and is known to be associated with Peutz–Jeghers syndrome and Carney syndrome.

Primary germ cell tumours can occur outside the gonads and should be differentiated from regressed germ cell tumours with metastasis. Primary extragonadal germ cell tumours occur in extratesticular locations like the retroperitoneum, mediastinum, sacrococcygeal area and pineal gland. Regressed germ cell tumour may present with widespread metastases even though the primary tumour has involuted. US plays a vital role in the search for the primary regressed tumour. They have a variable appearance, are generally small, and can be hypoechoic, hyperechoic or merely an area of focal calcification.

Woodward PJ, et al. From the archives of the AFIP: Tumors and tumorlike lesions of the testis: Radiologic-pathologic correlation. *Radiographics*. 2002;22(1):189–216.

85. D. MRI of head with T2* GE and DWI

When a child is admitted acutely with suspected NAHI, the primary neuroimaging performed on Day 1 is non-contrast CT of the brain. This has the advantage over MRI in the acute setting of being fast to acquire in a potentially unstable patient and is highly sensitive to hyperacute blood. The main aim at this stage is to diagnose/exclude any acute haemorrhage amenable to neurosurgical treatment.

If the child has ongoing neurological signs/symptoms or an abnormal initial CT brain, then an MRI should be performed. This is normally done at 3–5 days.

Contrast is not necessary but DWI – for ischaemia and T2* GE or similar sequence (for the detection of blood products) – should be considered. If there is abnormal imaging during the patient's acute admission or persistent neurological signs or symptoms, then a repeat MRI brain at 3–6 months should be considered.

If the first presentation is non-acute, then MRI is the appropriate initial imaging modality.

Royal Colleges of Radiologists and Paediatrics and Child Health. *Standards for Radiological Investigation of Suspected Non-accidental Injury*. Royal Colleges of Radiologists and Paediatrics and Child Health, 2008. www.rcr.ac.uk/docs/radiology/pdf/RCPCH_RCR_final.pdf [accessed on 16 February 2017].

86. E. Comet tail sign is specific for distal ureteric calculus.

Most textbooks of anatomy describe the ureter as having three anatomical narrowest points. These are the pelvi-ureteric junction (PUJ), the point where the ureter crosses anterior to the iliac vessels, and the uretero-vesical junction (UVJ); however, contrary to previous teaching there is debate whether these are the most common places for stones to be lodged. Indinavir stones have soft-tissue attenuation (15–30 HU) and are likely to be missed at unenhanced CT. However, renal colic in a patient receiving indinavir therapy for HIV infection, along with the presence of obstructive features at CT, usually helps clinch the diagnosis. The most reliable signs of ureteric obstruction include hydroureter, hydronephrosis, perinephric stranding, periureteral oedema, and unilateral renal enlargement. Stones less than 5 mm have a 68% chance of passing spontaneously, and stones between 5 and 10 mm have a 47% chance. The soft-tissue rim sign consists of a halo of soft-tissue attenuation around a calcific focus and is very specific for ureteric calculi. The comet tail sign is created by an eccentric tapering soft-tissue area adjacent to a phlebolith. These two signs are used to differentiate ureteric and pelvic calcification.

Kambadakone AR, et al. New and evolving concepts in the imaging and management of urolithiasis: Urologists' perspective. *Radiographics*. 2010;30(3):603–23.

87. D. A fatigue fracture is due to abnormal stress on a normal bone.

A fatigue fracture occurs from excessive and repeated stress on normal bone. An insufficiency fracture occurs from normal physiological stresses on abnormal bone. Both entities are part of the larger group of fractures known as *stress fractures*, which is the term used to describe fractures occurring from a mismatch of bone strength and chronic mechanical stress.

Manaster BJ, et al. *The Requisites: MSK Imaging*, 4th edn. Philadelphia, PA: Mosby, 2013:9.

88. E. Self-limiting disease of good prognosis

Creutzfeldt–Jakob disease (CJD), a fatal neurodegenerative disorder, is diagnosed by the detection of an accumulation of an abnormal form of the human prion protein PrPSc in the brain. It is characterised by rapidly progressive dementia, cerebral atrophy, myoclonus and death.

The T2-weighted MRI of sCJD (sporadic CJD) patients often shows high signal in the head of the caudate nucleus and in the putamen as compared with the thalamus and the cerebral cortex. Hyperintense signal changes can also occur in the thalamus, but in sCJD they are usually less prominent than those in the putamen or the caudate nucleus. In addition, there is high signal in the cerebral cortex in some cases. With the introduction of the new sequences FLAIR and DWI, these signal changes are more easily identified. Patients with the new variant of CJD (vCJD) show bilateral increased signal on MRI in the pulvinar thalami (relative to the grey matter of other basal ganglia and the cerebral cortex). There is currently no curative treatment and the disease is invariably fatal.

Tschampa HJ, et al. MRI in the diagnosis of sporadic Creutzfeldt-Jakob disease: A study on inter-observer agreement. *Brain*. 2005;128(Pt 9): 2026–33.

89. C. Alcohol abuse

In approximately 75% of patients, a haematologic abnormality or a cause of thrombotic diathesis can be identified that predisposes the patient to the occurrence of Budd–Chiari syndrome.

The presence of multiple causes in the same patient has been reported. Haematologic diseases, especially myeloproliferative disorders, are the most common cause, and it has been suggested that patients with idiopathic Budd–Chiari syndrome may have an underlying myeloproliferative disorder. Causes of thrombotic diathesis that have been associated with Budd–Chiari syndrome include paroxysmal nocturnal haemoglobinuria, antiphospholipid syndrome, inherited deficiencies of proteins C and S and antithrombin III, factor V Leiden mutation, prothrombin gene mutation, methylene tetrahydrofolate reductase mutation, use of oral contraceptives, pregnancy and immediate post-partum status.

Metastatic invasion of the hepatic vein, IVC or right atrium and primary tumour occurrence in the kidney, liver, adrenal gland, IVC or heart are less frequent causes of Budd–Chiari syndrome. Membranous web-like obstruction of the hepatic vein or IVC is a more prevalent cause of hepatic venous outflow obstruction in the Asian population. Membranous webs of the hepatic vein or IVC may be congenital or represent sequelae of thrombosis.

Cura M. Diagnostic and interventional radiology for Budd-Chiari Syndrome. *RadioGraphics*. 2009;29:669–81.

90. B. Ostium primum ASD

Ostium primum defects are often seen in Down's syndrome and are part of endocardial cushion defects, which also include atrioventricular canal defects (ASD + VSD + abnormal AV valves). Most children with small defects are asymptomatic. Those with larger defects are predisposed to recurrent chest infection and heart failure.

Ostium secundum type ASD are well tolerated, and symptoms and complications usually only present in the third decade or later.

VSD can be asymptomatic or present at various age with recurrent chest infection or heart failure and cyanosis at a later stage subject to progressive pulmonary hypertension.

HOCM shows cardiomegaly without plethoric lungs. HOCM presents with tiredness, fatigability and is a recognised cause of sudden death.

Tasker RC, et al. *Oxford Handbook of Paediatrics*. Oxford: Oxford University Press, 2008.

91. D. 0.3 ml of 1:1000 IM adrenaline

Adrenaline IM dose – adults
0.5 mg IM (= 500 micrograms = 0.5 mL of 1:1000) adrenaline

Adrenaline IM dose – children
>12 years: 500 micrograms IM (0.5 mL) – i.e., same as adult dose; (300 micrograms (0.3 mL) if child is small or prepubertal)
>6–12 years: 300 micrograms IM (0.3 mL)
>6 months–6 years: 150 micrograms IM (0.15 mL)
<6 months: 150 micrograms IM (0.15 mL)

Emergency treatment of anaphylactic reactions: Guidelines for healthcare providers. Working Group of the Resuscitation Council (UK), 2008:22.

92. A. Osteosarcoma

The most common radiation-induced sarcoma is pleomorphic undifferentiated sarcoma, previously described as malignant fibrous histiocytoma (which is a soft-tissue sarcoma), followed by osteosarcoma and lastly by fibrosarcoma. In this case, the pathology is centred on the bone, making osteosarcoma the most probable diagnosis.

Dähnert W. *Radiology Review Manual*, 6th edn. Philadelphia, PA: Lippincott Williams & Wilkins, 2007:144.

93. A. Brodel bloodless zone lies just anterior to the lateral convex border of the kidney.

Percutaneous access to the urinary tract is used to relive urinary tract obstruction and also allows the urologists to perform endourological procedures (e.g., stone removal), which is less invasive and associated with fewer complications than open surgery. The renal artery divides into the ventral and dorsal branches, which creates a zone of relative avascularity between the divisions known as the *Brödel bloodless line of incision*, which lies just posterior to the lateral convex border of the kidney. A lower pole posterior calix access via a subcostal approach is usually best for simple urinary drainage. A posterior calix of the upper or middle collecting system offers the easiest access to the pelviureteric junction for potential ureteral negotiation. Tubes with self-retaining properties should always be used to lessen the risk of inadvertent dislodgment. Tubes of 8–10 F are usually sufficient for drainage of non-infected urine. Larger tubes (12–14 F) may be necessary for drainage of infected urine or to ensure appropriate urine flow in procedures complicated by gross haematuria. Formal nephrostography should be delayed for 24–48 hours following tube placement in case of infected urine to reduce the chance of bacteraemia.

Transient haematuria occurs in all patients post-nephrostomy. Hydrothorax and pneumothorax can also occur particularly with supracostal entries. Renal arteriovenous fistula, pseudoaneurysm or vessel laceration are recognised vascular complications during nephrostomy.

Dyer RB, et al. Percutaneous nephrostomy with extensions of the technique: Step by step. *Radiographics*. 2002;22(3):503–25.

94. A. Primary CNS lymphoma

Toxoplasmosis typically manifests on CT scans and MRIs as nodular (small encephalitis) and/or ring-enhancing (large abscess) lesions within the brain parenchyma. The enhancing ring, when present, may be somewhat thicker and more ill-defined than that seen in association with a typical bacterial abscess.

The lesions are associated with surrounding oedema and tend to be multiple at presentation. However, a significant percentage of patients present with solitary lesions. Toxoplasmic lesions are most often seen in the basal ganglia and cerebral hemispheres. On non-enhanced T1-weighted MR images, the lesions are of low signal intensity. On T2-weighted MR images, the lesions are mildly to moderately hyperintense in relation to the brain parenchyma and can be difficult to separate from the surrounding oedema. The presence of small haemorrhages may be a sign of toxoplasmosis, and calcifications can occasionally be seen in treated lesions.

On CT scans and MR images, lymphoma most commonly manifests as an enhancing, space-occupying mass with surrounding oedema. However, much of the time the lesions undergo central necrosis and present as ring-enhancing masses; on non-contrast-enhanced T1-weighted images, typical lesions are isointense in relation to brain parenchyma, whereas on T2-weighted images the lesions are isointense to hyperintense. On non-enhanced CT, a small percentage of the lesions are of increased attenuation with respect to the brain parenchyma (as is commonly observed in cases of primary CNS lymphoma in patients who do not have AIDS).

The imaging characteristics of lymphoma and toxoplasmosis overlap to such a significant degree that it is nearly impossible to differentiate the lesions on the basis of their appearance on CT scans or MR images alone. Patients with a few solid lesions or ring-enhancing subependymal or periventricular lesions (particularly those with subependymal extension) tend to have lymphomas, whereas patients with multiple ring-enhancing lesions (particularly those that are haemorrhagic) in the basal ganglia and cerebral hemispheres are more likely to have toxoplasmosis.

Walot I, et al. Neuroimaging findings in patients with AIDS. *Clin Infect Dis*. 1996;22(6):906–19.

95. B. Multilocular cystic nephroma

Multilocular cystic nephroma is a benign renal tumour that occurs in children and, less commonly, adult women. There is no known association with Wilms tumour. It is usually a unilateral abnormality that replaces an entire renal pole and presents as a large mass, often around 8–10 cm in diameter. Radiological appearances, while not entirely specific, can help to differentiate this lesion from other renal mass lesions. A sharply well-circumscribed, multiseptated cystic mass is typical with a thick surrounding capsule. The cysts appear to herniate into the renal pelvis – an appearance that is relatively specific for mesoblastic nephroma. Unsurprisingly, these lesions are excised, as definitive radiological differentiation from malignancy is often not possible. Multilocular cystic nephroma can be differentiated from multicystic dysplastic kidney by the presence of normal functioning renal parenchyma and symmetrical renal excretion. Polycystic kidney disease involves the entire kidney, unlike multilocular cystic nephroma, which tends to be localised around a renal pole.

Multicystic dysplastic kidney is the most common cystic renal disease affecting infants and is twice as common in boys. It is a common cause for abdominal masses in this age group and typically involves one kidney. There are strong associations with a range of genitourinary abnormalities, including vesico-ureteric reflux, horseshoe kidney and ureteric anomalies. The classical ultrasound features are as described above, with near total replacement of the normal renal parenchyma by cysts of varying size and shape. The presence of thin septations can help to differentiate this condition from multilocular cystic nephroma, in which thick septations are typical. Wilms tumour typically presents in children of 3–4 years of age.

Dähnert W. *Radiology Review Manual*, 6th edn. Philadelphia, PA: Lippincott Williams & Wilkins, 2007:937–8.

96. A. T3 N2 M1a

Primary tumour (T)

Tx: No tumour found on bronchoscopy or imaging.

Tis: Carcinoma *in situ*.

T1: Tumour size equal to or less than 3 cm not involving the main bronchus

   T1a: Smaller than 2 cm in longest dimension.

   T1b: Larger than 2 cm but smaller than or equal to 3 cm.

T2: Tumour size more than 3 cm but less than/equal to 7 cm or involving the main bronchus but >2 cm from carina or visceral pleural involvement or lobar atelectasis extending to the hilum but not collapse of the entire lung.

   T2a: Larger than 3 cm but smaller than 5 cm.

   T2b: Larger than 5 cm but smaller than 7 cm.

T3: Tumour size larger than 7 cm or tumour <2 cm from carina but not involving trachea or carina or involvement of the chest wall, including Pancoast tumour, diaphragm, phrenic nerve, mediastinal pleura or parietal pericardium, or separate tumour nodule(s) in the same lobe or atelectasis or post-obstructive pneumonitis of entire lung.

T4: Any size tumour with involvement of the trachea, oesophagus, recurrent laryngeal nerve vertebra, great vessels or heart or separate tumour nodules in the same lung but not in the same lobe.

Nodal status (N)

Nx: Regional nodes cannot be assessed.

N0: No regional nodal metastases.

N1: Ipsilateral peribronchial, hilar or intrapulmonary nodes, including direct invasion

N2: Ipsilateral mediastinal or subcarinal nodes.

N3: Contralateral nodal involvement; ipsilateral or contralateral scalene or supraclavicular nodal involvement.

Distant metastasis (M)

Mx: Distant metastases cannot be assessed.

M0: No distant metastases.

M1: Distant metastases present.

   M1a: Presence of a malignant pleural or pericardial effusion, pleural dissemination, or pericardial disease, and metastasis in opposite lung.

   M1b: Extrathoracic metastases.

American Joint Committee on Cancer. *Lung Cancer staging*, 7th ed. New York, NY: Springer, 2010.

97. A. Late enhancement of the IVC and central hepatic veins.

Passive congestion occurs with the stasis of blood within liver parenchyma as a result of impaired hepatic venous drainage secondary to cardiac disease. Elevated central venous pressure is directly transmitted from the right atrium to the hepatic veins. Passive hepatic congestion may occur with congestive heart failure, constrictive pericarditis, pericardial effusion, cardiomyopathy or right-sided valvular disease involving the tricuspid or pulmonary valve.

Symptoms of congestive heart failure mask gastrointestinal symptoms. Patients may present with asymptomatic elevation of liver enzymes, jaundice, right upper-quadrant pain, hepatomegaly and increased abdominal girth.

In the arterial phase, there is early enhancement of a dilated IVC and central hepatic veins because of the reflux of contrast material from the right atrium into the IVC.

Parenchymal phase images show a heterogeneous, mottled mosaic pattern of enhancement, with linear and curvilinear areas of poor enhancement due to delayed enhancement of small and medium-sized hepatic veins.

There may be peripheral large patchy areas of poor delayed enhancement due to stagnant flow within the periphery of the liver.

Perivascular lymphedema may be seen as linear low-attenuation regions encircling the intrahepatic IVC or portal veins and should not be confused with venous thrombosis. Hepatomegaly and ascites may be present. Chest images may show cardiomegaly, congestive heart failure and pericardial and pleural effusion.

Torabi M. CT of nonneoplastic hepatic vascular and perfusion disorders. *RadioGraphics*. 2008;28: 1967–82.

98. E. Lymphoma

Lymphoma can occur in the testis in one of three ways: as the primary site, as the initial manifestation of occult disease or as the site of recurrence. It is the most common bilateral tumour, and the epididymis and spermatic cord are commonly involved. The sonographic appearance of testicular lymphoma is variable and indistinguishable from that of germ cell tumours. Testicular lymphoma generally appears as discrete hypoechoic lesions, which may completely infiltrate the testicle. Primary leukaemia of the testis is rare. However, the testis is a common site of leukaemia recurrence in children. Seminoma is the most common pure germ cell tumour but affects unilateral testis. Metastases are rare but are reported most commonly in cases of primary prostate and lung cancer. Testicular fracture usually appears as a linear hypoechoic band extending across the testicular parenchyma.

Woodward PJ, et al. From the archives of the AFIP: Tumors and tumorlike lesions of the testis: Radiologic-pathologic correlation. *Radiographics*. 2002;22(1):189–216.

99. D. NF1 – Optic glioma

NF1 is also called *peripheral neurofibromatosis* or von Recklinghausen disease. The classic triad includes cutaneous lesions, skeletal abnormalities and mental deficiency.

CNS lesions include optic pathway glioma (thickened enhancing optic nerve), cerebral gliomas, hydrocephalus due to aqueduct stenosis, vascular dysplasia including Moyamoya disease, cranial nerve neurofibromas or craniofacial plexiform neurofibromatosis, CNS hamartomas (unidentified bright objects on T2-weighted MRI) and vacuolar/spongiotic myelinopathy. Spinal lesions include cord neurofibroma or neurofibroma of peripheral nerves.

Optic nerve meningioma, seen as ring enhancement in cross section, would be suggestive of NF2 or central neurofibromatosis, classically associated with bilateral vestibular/acoustic schwannomas and ependymomas.

Optic neuritis would also show nerve swelling, high signal on T2 and enhancement post-contrast on T1-weighted FS images; however, enlargement of the nerve on imaging may not be as pronounced as in glioma, and MS is not associated with skin lesions. Note that tuberous sclerosis can cause skin lesions but is associated with optic nerve hamartoma rather than glioma or optic neuritis.

Dähnert W. *Radiology Review Manual*, 7th edn. Philadelphia, PA: Lippincott Williams & Wilkins, 2011:319–21.

100. A. They can cause painful scoliosis.

When osteoid osteomas occur in the spine, they typically involve the posterior elements of lumbar vertebrae and are less than 2 cm in diameter. A painful scoliosis is a common presentation. The 'nidus' within the lesion is osteolytic. Both the nidus and soft-tissue components enhance on MRI after intravenous administration of contrast material.

Dähnert W. *Radiology Review Manual*, 6th edn. Philadelphia, PA: Lippincott Williams & Wilkins, 2007:136–7.

101. A. Histoplasmosis

Histoplasmosis is only seen frequently in North America. Radiograph may reveal multiple poorly defined nodules in the acute phase. Segmental or lobar pneumonia is less common. Chronic histoplasmosis resembles post-primary TB, with upper lobe cavitation, calcification and fibrosis. Hilar and mediastinal nodes show calcification. Occasionally a solitary well-defined nodule may form, a so-called histoplasma. When the centre of this lesion calcifies, it forms a target lesion, which is very specific. In some cases, fibrosing mediastinitis can develop and lead to constriction of mediastinal structures, including airways, SVC, and pulmonary arteries and veins.

Adam A, et al. *Grainger & Allison's Diagnostic Radiology: A Textbook of Medical Imaging*, 5th edn. New York: Churchill Livingstone, 2008:279–80.

102. B. Scurvy

Scurvy is a dietary deficiency of vitamin C. It typically affects babies from 6 to 9 months and is characterised by non-specific symptoms of irritability, lower limb tenderness and reluctance to move legs normally. Bleeding gums can also occur. The condition usually manifests at the distal femur and proximal and distal ends of the tibia and fibula, and it can also affect the upper limb bones and the ribs. There are several key radiographic findings: bony spurs arising from the metaphysis of long bones are eponymously termed *Pelkan spurs*. Wimberger line refers to the appearance of a sclerotic line running around the perimeter of the epiphyses, which reflects osteopaenic change. Ground-glass osteoporosis and cortical thinning are also recognised findings. In contrast, rickets manifests as cupping and fraying of the metaphyses, periosteal reaction, bowing of the long bones and widening of the growth plates. Hypophosphatasia is often indistinguishable from rickets on imaging. Hypothyroidism in infancy also results in osteopaenia, with fragmentation of the epiphyses.

Dähnert W. *Radiology Review Manual*, 6th edn. Philadelphia, PA: Lippincott Williams & Wilkins, 2007:160.

103. B. Irregular outline to liver with caudate lobe hypertrophy.

In acute viral hepatitis, the major histologic findings are necrosis of random isolated liver cells or small cell clusters, diffuse liver cell injury, reactive changes in Kupffer cells and sinusoidal lining cells and an inflammatory infiltrate in portal tracts, and evidence of hepatocytic regeneration during the recovery phase. Confluent necrosis may lead to bridging necrosis connecting portal, central or portal-to-central regions of adjacent lobules, signifying a more severe form of acute hepatitis.

The imaging features of acute hepatitis are non-specific and the diagnosis is usually based on serologic, virologic and clinical findings. Probably the most important role of radiology in patients with suspected hepatitis is to help rule out other diseases that produce similar clinical and biochemical abnormalities, such as extrahepatic cholestasis, diffuse metastatic disease and cirrhosis.

At US, in acute hepatitis, the liver is often enlarged and may demonstrate a diffuse decrease in parenchymal echogenicity, which causes a relative increase in the echogenicity of the portal vein walls ('starry night' pattern). A normal liver echotexture does not exclude the diagnosis of acute hepatitis.

At CT and MR imaging, findings in acute viral hepatitis are non-specific and include hepatomegaly and periportal oedema. At CT, heterogeneous enhancement and well-defined regions of low attenuation may be present. At MR imaging, periportal oedema appears as high-signal-intensity areas on T2-weighted images. Involved areas may be normal or demonstrate decreased signal intensity on T1-weighted images and increased signal intensity on T2-weighted images. Extrahepatic findings in patients with severe acute hepatitis include gallbladder wall thickening due to oedema and, infrequently, ascites.

Mortelé KJ. The Infected liver: Radiologic-pathologic correlation. *RadioGraphics*. 2004;24:937–55.

104. D. Testicular fracture requires urgent surgical exploration.

Testicular fracture usually appears as a linear hypoechoic band extending across the testicular parenchyma. The contour remains smooth and the shape of the testicle is maintained. The tunica albuginea is intact. An associated haematocele or testicular haematoma may be seen. The fracture line may not be visible if filled with isoechoic haematoma. Testicular fractures are treated conservatively if normal flow is identified in the surrounding testicular parenchyma. In testicular rupture there is discontinuity of the echogenic tunica albuginea with haemorrhage and extrusion of testicular contents into the scrotal sac. This is an indication for emergency scrotal exploration to salvage the testis. US shows poorly defined testicular margins and heterogeneous echotexture, with areas of haemorrhage or infarction. Intratesticular haematomas are usually focal and fairly well defined and may be multiple. They are usually hyperechoic in the acute phase or hypoechoic (as the haemorrhage evolves) and lack vascularity. Isolated epididymal injuries are not very common, and these are usually associated with testicular injuries. Contusion or traumatic epididymitis appears as an enlarged and heterogeneous epididymis on US with increased vascularity, sometimes associated with haematocele. The appearance is indistinguishable from infective epididymitis. Hydrocele or scrotal haematoma can occur in isolation or be associated with other injuries.

Rao MS, Arjun K. Sonography of scrotal trauma. *Indian J Radiol Imag*. 2012;22(4):293–7.

105. C. Chronic ulnar collateral ligament injury

Injury to the ulnar collateral ligament (UCL), also known as the *medial collateral ligament* or medial ulnar collateral ligament, is a common cause of medial elbow pain and valgus instability in athletes. The UCL is made of anterior, transverse and posterior bundles, and is most often injured following acute or recurrent valgus stress of the elbow.

MRI may demonstrate increased T2-weighted signal within the ligament (commonly within the anterior band) or hyperintensity within the sublime tubercle. Intra-articular contrast may result in a 'T sign' when contrast extends in the interval between the sublime tubercle and stripped ligamentous attachment; complete rupture will show extravasation of contrast through the ligamentous defect.

Chronic valgus stress, often secondary to throwing or pitching sports, can result in chronic damage to the UCL, with appearances similar to those described and the UCL often appearing lax, irregular and with poor definition. Plain radiograph findings may include heterotopic new bone formation around the medial epicondyle and local subchondral cysts, sclerosis and osteophyte formation.

The differential diagnosis includes medial epicondylitis and a sublime tubercle fracture. Lateral ulnar collateral ligament forms part of the lateral ligament complex and presents with symptoms of lateral or postero-lateral elbow pain/instability.

Hackl M, et al. Reliability of magnetic resonance imaging signs of posterolateral rotatory instability of the elbow. *J Hand Surg Am*. 2015;40(7):1428–33.
Magee T. Accuracy of 3-T MR arthrography versus conventional 3-T MRI of elbow tendons and ligaments compared with surgery. *AJR Am J Roentgenol*. 2015;204(1):W70-5.
O'Dell MC, et al. Imaging sports-related elbow injuries. *Appl Radiol*. 2015.

106. C. The severity of the skin rash correlates with the degree of articular abnormalities.

If there is joint space narrowing, signs of inflammation, multiple joint involvement and distal involvement in the hands and feet with added features of bone proliferation, a seronegative spondyloarthropathy is suggested. Approximately 10%–15% of patients with skin manifestations of psoriasis will develop psoriatic arthritis. Usually such manifestations will precede the development of arthritis. The hallmarks of psoriatic arthritis, similar to those of the other seronegative spondyloarthropathies, are signs of inflammatory arthritis combined with bone proliferation, periostitis, enthesitis and a distal joint distribution in the extremities.

Involvement of several joints in a single digit, with soft-tissue swelling, produces what appears clinically as a 'sausage digit'. The bone proliferation produces an irregular and indistinct appearance to the marginal bone about the involved joint, characterised as a 'fuzzy' appearance or 'whiskering'. Periostitis may take several forms. It may appear as a thin periosteal layer of new bone adjacent to the cortex, a thick irregular layer or irregular thickening of the cortex itself. Because of the degree of bone destruction, an involved joint may take the appearance of a 'pencil and cup', with one end of the joint forming a cup and the other a pencil that projects into this cup. One characteristic feature of psoriatic arthritis in the foot is the 'ivory phalanx', which classically involves the distal phalanges (especially in the first digit).

Sacroiliac joint involvement in psoriatic arthritis is usually bilateral, either symmetric or asymmetric in distribution. The thoracolumbar spine may show large comma-shaped paravertebral ossifications.

There is no association between the dermatological extent of psoriasis and the musculoskeletal manifestations.

Jacobson JA, et al. Radiographic evaluation of arthritis: Inflammatory conditions. *Radiology*. 2008;248(2):378–89.

107. C. Skeletal dysplasia

NF2 or central neurofibromatosis is associated with bilateral acoustic neuromas (*sine qua non*), schwannoma of other cranial nerves, multiple meningiomas, meningiomatosis, paraspinal neurofibromas and spinal cord ependymomas.

Unlike NF1, NF2 is not associated with Lisch nodules, skeletal dysplasia, optic pathway glioma, vascular dysplasia or mental deficiency.

Dähnert W. *Radiology Review Manual*, 7th edn. Philadelphia, PA: Lippincott Williams & Wilkins, 2011:322.

108. C. US abdomen

Be aware of a child who is presumed to have throat or upper respiratory infection, on treatment by GP, who presents with atypical abdominal pain. Younger children cannot describe their symptoms, and up to one-third have atypical clinical findings for appendicitis. Lower abdominal pain and flexed leg should raise strong suspicion of a serious pathology. Urine test is abnormal in 30% of acute appendicitis; hence it doesn't help to confirm or refute the diagnosis.

CT involves ionisation radiation, and MRI is not the primary modality of investigation. US is the primary modality for assessment of the abdomen in children.

The most accurate US finding for acute appendicitis is an outer-wall diameter greater than 6 mm under compression. Less sensitive and specific US findings for appendicitis include hyperaemia within the appendiceal wall on colour Doppler images, echogenic inflamed periappendiceal fat and the presence of an appendicolith. Enlarged, reactive mesenteric lymph nodes may be seen with

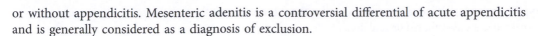

or without appendicitis. Mesenteric adenitis is a controversial differential of acute appendicitis and is generally considered as a diagnosis of exclusion.

Cogley JR, et al. Emergent paediatric US: What every radiologist should know. *Radiographics*. 2012;32(3):651–65.

109. C. Metastasis

The causes of multiple macronodules (>5 mm) include metastasis (the first thing that needs to be excluded unless there is a pre-existent explanation), granuloma, eosinophilic lung disease (eosinophilia, asthma or typical reverse batwing pattern radiograph), abscesses, AVM (history of Osler–Rendu–Weber disease), Wegner's disease (associated sinus disease, renal dysfunction), rheumatoid lungs (symptoms of connective tissue disease or arthropathy), amyloidosis (chronic disease), parasites and sarcoidosis (uveitis, parotitis or features of Lofgren syndrome).

Dähnert W. *Radiology Review Manual*, 7th edn. Philadelphia, PA: Lippincott Williams & Wilkins, 2011:427.

110. B. Nodular liver contour

Cirrhosis is most commonly caused by chronic hepatitis infection or alcohol abuse, although a number of other diseases causing hepatic injury can lead to cirrhosis. It is pathologically defined by three main characteristics: fibrosis, nodular transformation and distortion of hepatic architecture.

Subtle morphologic changes of the liver may be among the earliest detectable with imaging, including enlargement of the hilar periportal space, enlargement of the major interlobar fissure and expansion of pericholecystic space or gallbladder fossa. Typically, the anterior segment of the right lobe and medial segment of the left lobe atrophy, whereas the caudate lobe and left lateral segment hypertrophy.

The nodular changes in cirrhosis yield characteristic radiologic findings. The nodularity is best seen affecting the liver margin, especially on the left lateral segment. Micronodular cirrhosis, common in alcoholic liver disease, gives rise to a fine cobblestone appearance resulting from nodules typically smaller than 3 mm. A grossly nodular liver margin with 3–15-mm regenerative nodules is characteristic of macronodular cirrhosis, more commonly associated with viral hepatitis. Other changes in cirrhosis include diffuse heterogeneity of the organ on CT and T1- and T2-weighted MRI. Fibrosis is the predominant cause for hepatic heterogeneity and appears high in signal intensity on T2-weighted MRI.

Gupta AA. CT and MRI of Cirrhosis and its Mimics. *AJR Am J Roentgenol*. 2004;183:1595–601.

111. C. It is typically unilateral.

Testicular microlithiasis is a relatively uncommon finding in the general population. It is usually an incidental finding, which was initially thought to be innocuous. However known association include cryptorchidism, infertility, Klinefelter syndrome, Down's syndrome, atrophy, alveolar microlithiasis and, most importantly, testicular carcinoma. The prevalence of carcinoma in patients with testicular microlithiasis has been reported to be as high as 40%, and follow-up US was routine. However, recent articles and guidelines do not recommend regular US follow-up.

At histopathologic analysis, the microcalcifications appear as laminated concretions within the seminiferous tubules, secondary to defective Leydig cells.

On sonograms, microlithiasis appears as punctate, non-shadowing, hyperechoic foci within the usually homogeneous testicle. Five or more calcifications/image should be present to make the diagnosis.

Typically, they are bilateral, symmetric and scattered throughout the testicle; however, they can be asymmetrically distributed or unilateral.

Woodward PJ, et al. From the archives of the AFIP: Tumors and tumorlike lesions of the testis: Radiologic-pathologic correlation. *Radiographics*. 2002;22(1):189–216.

112. B. Pineal teratoma

Pineal teratomas reveal a multiloculated, lobulated lesion with foci of fat attenuation, calcification and cystic regions on CT scan. T1-weighted MR images may show foci of T1 shortening due to fat and variable signal intensity related to calcification. On T2-weighted images, the soft-tissue component is iso- to hypointense. The soft-tissue component demonstrates enhancement on post-contrast images.

Pineocytomas are slow-growing pineal parenchymal neoplasms. At CT they are well demarcated, usually less than 3 cm, and iso- to hyperattenuating. At MR imaging, pineocytomas are well-circumscribed lesions that are hypo- to isointense on T1-weighted images and hyperintense on T2-weighted images. On post-contrast images, they typically demonstrate avid, homogeneous enhancement. Cystic or partially cystic changes may occur, occasionally making differentiation from a pineal cyst difficult. However, at immediate post-contrast imaging, cystic-appearing pineocytomas demonstrate internal or nodular wall enhancement.

Pineoblastomas are highly malignant pineal parenchymal neoplasms. CT reveals a large (typically ≥3 cm), lobulated, typically hyperattenuating mass, an appearance that reflects its highly cellular histologic features. Nearly 100% of patients have obstructive hydrocephalus. At MR imaging, pineoblastomas are heterogeneous in appearance, with the solid portion appearing hypo- to isointense on T1-weighted images and iso- to mildly hyperintense to the cortex on T2-weighted images. Pineoblastomas demonstrate heterogeneous enhancement on post-contrast images. Necrotic regions and haemorrhage may be present. CSF dissemination is a common finding and necessitates imaging of the entire craniospinal axis.

Ninety percent of patients with pineal germinomas are less than 20 years old. CT demonstrates a sharply circumscribed, hyperattenuating mass that engulfs the pineal calcifications. Hydrocephalus may be present. MR imaging typically reveals a solid mass that may have cystic components. Germinomas are iso- to hyperintense to grey matter on T1- and T2-weighted images and demonstrate avid, homogeneous enhancement on post-contrast images.

Smith AB, et al. From the archives of the AFIP: Lesions of the pineal region: Radiologic-pathologic correlation. *Radiographics*. 2010;30(7):2001–20.

113. D. Contrast flowing in an apparently thickened vessel wall

Direct signs of chronic PE include complete occlusion with decrease in the diameter of the vessel distal to the complete obstruction; intimal irregularities, as broad-based, smooth, margined abnormalities that create obtuse angles with the vessel wall; and intraluminal bands or webs. Indirect signs of chronic PE include post-stenotic dilatation, tortuous vessels, enlargement of the main pulmonary artery, enlarged bronchial artery and differential perfusion of lung parenchyma (mosaic pattern). The polo mint sign of acute PE refers to the well-defined central thrombus, which is completely surrounded by contrast material.

Wittram C, et al. Acute and chronic pulmonary emboli: Angiography–CT correlation. *AMJ Am J Roentgenol*. 2006;186: S421–9.

114. D. Echocardiography and blood culture

Children with turbulent blood flow through the heart or where prosthetic material has been inserted following surgery for PDA, VSD, coarctation and so on are at particular risk of acute and subacute forms of infective endocarditis.

In the early stage symptoms are mild. Children can present with prolonged fever over months accompanied by non-specific symptoms like malaise, myalgia, arthralgia, headache, weight loss, night sweats or an acute episode of fever. Tender nodules in finger suggest Osler's node. Clubbing, retinal haemorrhage (Roth spots), nail bed haemorrhage and splenomegaly could be other features of infective endocarditis.

Blood culture and echocardiography to demonstrate vegetations is the main modality of investigation. Although MRI and CT would show vegetations, they are not the primary modality for investigation.

Tasker RC, et al. *Handbook of Paediatrics*. Oxford: Oxford University Press, 2008.

115. A.   Regenerative nodules are premalignant.

Cirrhotic livers are characterised by advanced fibrosis and the formation of hepatocellular nodules, which are classified histologically as either (1) regenerative lesions (e.g., regenerative nodules, lobar or segmental hyperplasia, focal nodular hyperplasia) or (2) dysplastic or neoplastic lesions (e.g., dysplastic foci and nodules, hepatocellular carcinomas).

The differentiation of these lesions is important because regenerative nodules are benign, whereas dysplastic and neoplastic nodules are premalignant and malignant, respectively. However, their accurate characterisation may be difficult even at histopathologic analysis.

Comparing the clinical and pathologic findings with radiologic imaging features may facilitate differential diagnosis; in particular, nodule size, vascularity, hepatocellular function and Kupffer cell density assessed at MRI are suggestive of the correct diagnosis.

MRI is more useful than CT for such assessments because it provides better soft-tissue contrast and a more nuanced depiction of different tissue properties. Moreover, a wider variety of contrast agents is available for use in MR imaging. Familiarity with the MR imaging characteristics of cirrhosis-associated hepatocellular nodules is therefore important for optimal diagnosis and management of cirrhotic disease.

Hanna RF, et al. Hepatocellular nodules: Correlation of histopathologic and MR imaging features. *Radiographics*. 2008;28:747–69.

116. E.   720

Testicular torsion causes venous engorgement that results in oedema, haemorrhage and subsequent arterial compromise. The degree of torsion ranges from 180 to 720 degrees. Experimental studies indicate that 720-degree torsion is required to completely occlude the testicular artery. When torsion is 180 degrees or less, diminished blood flow is seen. A nearly 100% salvage rate exists within first 6 hours after onset of symptoms, which drops to 20% within 12–24 hours.

Buttaravoli P, Leffler S. *Minor Emergencies*, 3rd edn. Philadelphia, PA: Elsevier Saunders, 301–5.
Dogra VS, et al. Sonography of the scrotum. *Radiology*. 2003;227(1):18–36.

117. D.   Large flowing osteophytes

Sacroiliac involvement is typically bilateral and symmetric, and it usually precedes spinal involvement in ankylosing spondylitis. Initially, there is indistinctness and discontinuity of the thin white subchondral bone plate about the sacroiliac joints. These changes can progress to gross bone erosions. Early erosions of the subchondral bone are often best seen in the inferior aspect of the joints. Along with the bone erosions, the adjacent bone is often sclerotic and joint space narrowing and bone fusion eventually occur. The differential diagnosis of bilateral sacroiliac joint erosions includes inflammatory bowel disease and hyperparathyroidism; however, in hyperparathyroidism, sacroiliac joint space widening is more dramatic.

Early radiographic findings are erosions at the anterior margins of the vertebral body at the discovertebral junction. These focal areas of osteitis become increasingly sclerotic, a finding termed the 'shiny corner sign'. More extensive discovertebral erosions may also occur (Anderson lesion).

Associated bone proliferation leads to a squared appearance of the vertebral body. Thin and slender syndesmophytes are generally evident, representing ossification of the outer layer of the annulus fibrosis. The differential diagnosis for bone production at the vertebral margins includes diffuse idiopathic skeletal hyperostosis, or DISH, although this latter condition more commonly reveals a flowing and undulating appearance.

As the syndesmophytes thicken and become continuous, the term *bamboo spine* is used on anteroposterior lumbar spine radiographs. Facet joint inflammation leads to indistinctness and narrowing of the involved joint, and bone fusion of the joints appears later. Ossification of the posterior interspinous ligaments produces a dense radiopaque line, designated the 'dagger sign', on anteroposterior radiographs of the lumbar spine. The combination of the fused facets and ossification of the interspinous ligaments produces the 'trolley-track sign'. Disk calcification may also occur.

Other peripheral joints can be involved in ankylosing spondylitis. Hip involvement is usually bilateral in distribution.

Jacobson JA, et al. Radiographic evaluation of arthritis: Inflammatory conditions. *Radiology*. 2008;248(2):378–89.

118. C. Pituitary apoplexy

Pituitary apoplexy is a severe and potentially fatal medical condition characterised by the variable association of headache, vomiting, visual impairment, ophthalmoplegia, altered mental state and panhypopituitarism. The syndrome is often related to haemorrhagic infarction of the pituitary gland, usually in a condition of a pre-existing macroadenoma.

CT typically a heterogeneously hyperdense (haemorrhagic components) intrasellar lesion, with significant increase in size in comparison to previous imaging. MRI shows a similar finding, with the appearance of blood varying on T1-weighted and T2-weighted images, based on the interval between haemorrhage and imaging. In the subacute phase (7–21 days), methaemoglobin shortens the T1 relaxation time, and the haemorrhage will appear hyperintense on T1-weighted images as well as on T2-weighted images. In the chronic phase (>21 days), macrophages digest the clot and the presence of haemosiderin and ferritine causes a strong hypointensity on both T1-weighted and T2-weighted images.

Boellis A. Pituitary apoplexy: An update on clinical and imaging features. *Insights Imaging*. 2014;5(6):753–762.

119. B. Traumatic diaphragmatic rupture

The presenting features include respiratory distress, tracheal deviation and dullness to percussion on one side. Motor vehicle accidents are the cause of traumatic diaphragm rupture in 90% of cases, with falls from height and a kick to the abdomen or object falling on the abdomen as alternative aetiologies. The initial chest X-ray is abnormal in 40%–90% of cases. It may show irregularity or obscuring of the leaf of the diaphragm, fractured ribs, mediastinal shift, intrapleural fluid or detectable viscera within the thorax. The most important radiological sign is incomplete visualisation of the entire diaphragm.

Kadish HA. Thoracic Trauma. In Fleisher GR, Ludwig S eds. *Textbook of Pediatric Emergency Medicine*, 6th edn. Philadelphia, PA: Lippincott Williams & Wilkins, 2010:1471.

120. C. The accordion sign is classic in Crohn's disease.

Several patterns of wall attenuation have been described in association with specific diseases. A hyperattenuating wall is seen with haemorrhage as a result of trauma, purpura or vasculitis. A submucosal fatty halo has been described as a result of chronic inflammation, such as in inflammatory bowel disease and GVHD. Submucosal oedema is definitive evidence of a bowel wall injury (typically acute), often producing the target sign.

The accordion sign is caused by contrast material trapped between thickened oedematous haustral folds in the colon. Although the accordion sign is most commonly seen in pseudomembranous colitis, it is not pathognomonic. The comb sign represents hypervascular engorged vasa recta aligned like the teeth of a comb on the mesenteric site of the bowel. This finding is classically seen in inflammatory bowel disease, especially Crohn's disease, and suggests a clinically active disease. The comb sign can also be seen in vasculitis and purpura. The toothpaste or lead pipe sign has been associated with chronic diseases leading to a 'featureless' bowel. It is commonly seen with Crohn's disease or chronic GVHD or as the sequela of radiation therapy.

d'Almeida M, et al. Bowel wall thickening in children: CT findings. *Radiographics*. 2008;28(3):727–46.

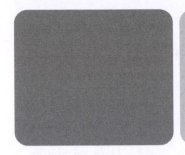

CHAPTER 7
TEST PAPER 4

Questions

Time: 3 hours

1. A 71-year-old man with a long history of alcohol-related liver cirrhosis showed a subtle but equivocal area of abnormality on a screening ultrasound. His AFP was raised at 2,000. An MRI of the liver with contrast is performed. All of the following are expected features of infiltrative HCC on MRI, except
   A. Hyperintense on MR images acquired during the hepatobiliary phase after injection of hepatocyte-specific contrast agent.
   B. A reticular appearance of the tumour can be seen during the venous and equilibrium phase.
   C. Washout appearance of the tumour is usually reported as irregular and heterogeneous.
   D. Infiltrative HCC may commonly appear as iso- or hypointense on images obtained during the arterial phase.
   E. Infiltrative HCC may be difficult to discern from underlying heterogeneous cirrhosis because of its permeative appearance.

2. Which of the following is false?
   A. NSIP   Scleroderma
   B. Sjogren's syndrome   Lymphocytic interstitial pneumonitis (LIP)
   C. Lofgren's syndrome   Systemic lupus erythematosus (SLE)
   D. Loeffler's syndrome   Acute eosinophilia
   E. Folded lungs   Asbestosis

3. Which one of the following statements regarding the testes is false?
   A. Tubular ectasia of the testis is a benign condition.
   B. Undescended testes are most commonly found in the inguinal canal.
   C. Metastases are most commonly from prostate and lung primary.
   D. Testicular cysts are mostly incidental and non-palpable.
   E. Sertoli cell tumour is the most common malignant testicular tumour.

4. A 21-year-old woman attends the A&E department with acute onset of pain in the right upper arm with limitation of mobility. The plain radiograph report describes a 'fallen fragment' sign. Which one of the following bony lesions does this finding refer to?
   A. Giant cell tumour
   B. Simple bone cyst
   C. Eosinophilic granuloma
   D. Aneurysmal bone cyst
   E. Benign cortical defect

5. A 43-year-old patient with known diagnosis of AIDS presented with ataxia and progressive neurological deficits. MRI brain revealed patchy high signal on T2W images in the parieto-occipital white matter. No mass effect or contrast enhancement was evident. What is the diagnosis?
   A. Primary CNS lymphoma
   B. AIDS dementia complex
   C. Progressive multifocal leukoencephalopathy
   D. Periventricular leukomalacia
   E. Encephalitis

6. A 6-year-old with spina bifida has a chest X-ray performed for possible lower respiratory tract infection. The lungs are clear but there is a well-defined, round paraspinal mass with an air–fluid level. What is the most likely diagnosis?
   A. Bronchogenic cyst
   B. Morgagni hernia
   C. Oesophageal duplication cyst
   D. Cystic teratoma
   E. Oesophageal tumour

7. A 77-year-old man with weight loss and deranged LFTs had an ultrasound scan that showed multiple liver lesions suspicious for metastases. Contrast-enhanced CT of the chest and abdomen was done in search of the primary. Which one of the following is the most common primary tumour that has hypovascular liver metastases?
   A. Pancreas
   B. Stomach
   C. Colon
   D. Kidney
   E. Melanoma

8. A 65-year-old woman is recovering from a double lung transplant. On the fourth day post-transplant, she starts complaining of shortness of breath. Clinical findings include some basal crackles; air entry seems satisfactory in the upper zones. An urgent chest X-ray is organised. Portable up-to-date chest X-ray shows evidence of pulmonary oedema. What is the most likely cause for this appearance?
   A. Barotrauma
   B. Acute graft failure
   C. Volume overload
   D. Response to antirejection treatment
   E. Reimplantation response

9. Cryptorchidism has an increased risk of development of all of the following testicular tumours, except
   A. Leydig cell tumour
   B. Seminoma
   C. Yolk sac tumour
   D. Embryonal cell tumour
   E. Choriocarcinoma

10. A 15-year-old teenager presents with a worsening pain in his right ankle. He is an active sports player and plays football for the school club. A radiograph reveals an undisplaced fragment in the medial aspect of the talar dome with a small lucent line around it.
    All of the following are well-recognised locations for osteochondral lesions or defects, except
    A. Lateral aspect of the medial femoral condyle
    B. Medial aspect of the talar dome
    C. Lateral aspect of the medial tibial plateau

D.   Anterior aspect of the capitellum

E.   Humeral head

11. A 35-year-old woman with pre-eclampsia underwent a CT of the brain to exclude intracranial haemorrhage. The CT revealed low attenuation in the white matter of the posterior aspect of both cerebral hemispheres. The abnormal area appeared low on T1W and high on T2W images and was isointense on DWI. No contrast enhancement was evident. What is the diagnosis?

A.   Periventricular leukomalacia

B.   Progressive multifocal leukoencephalopathy

C.   Encephalitis

D.   Reversible posterior leukoencephalopathy syndrome

E.   CNS lymphoma

12. A male infant is born at 39 + 3 weeks gestation. Prenatal ultrasound demonstrated a partly cystic, partly echogenic mass in the right upper lobe. Shortly after delivery the infant is in respiratory distress. Initial chest X-ray demonstrates dense lungs bilaterally with increased volume on the right. On Day 2, a repeat chest X-ray demonstrates multiple air-filled cystic masses of varying sizes within the right upper lobe with mediastinal shift to the left. What is the most likely diagnosis?

A.   Bronchogenic cyst

B.   Morgagni hernia

C.   Congenital cystic adenomatoid malformation

D.   Congenital lobar emphysema

E.   Hyaline membrane disease

13. A 78-year-old woman with worsening right upper-quadrant pain and worsening obstructive liver function test has a CT scan that shows a heterogeneous mass in the peripheral aspect of the liver with capsular retraction and segmental biliary duct dilatation proximal to the mass. There is no prior history of chronic liver disease. What is the most likely diagnosis?

A.   HCC

B.   Siderotic nodule

C.   Adenoma

D.   Cholangiocarcinoma

E.   Angiosarcoma

14. A 36-year-old immunocompromised woman with a known history of gestational trophoblastic disease showed bilateral bronchopneumonic infiltrates on chest X-ray. An HRCT was suggested for further characterisation. The HRCT showed several areas of ground glass change surrounded by a rim of consolidation. The differential diagnosis for these findings would include all of the following, except

A.   Wegner's granulomatosis

B.   Invasive pulmonary aspergillosis

C.   Choriocarcinoma metastasis

D.   Sarcoidosis

E.   Lymphangioleiomyomatosis

15. Enhanced CT scan of an otherwise healthy motor vehicle accident victim demonstrates no enhancement of the right kidney on Day 0. A repeat contrast-enhanced CT scan obtained on Day 3 demonstrates a thin marginal rim of subcapsular enhancement of uniform thickness, described as the rim sign. The collecting system was mildly prominent. What is the most likely explanation?

A.   Analgesic overuse

B.   Renovascular compromise

C.   Diabetes mellitus

D. Pyelonephritis

E. Developing hydronephrosis

16. A 44-year-old man presents with increasingly severe and disabling pain in the left inguinal and anterior thigh region. The pain is exacerbated by weight-bearing and relieved by rest. The patient mentions that the pain began 2 months ago, was acute in onset, and there was no preceding trauma. A radiograph of his left hip reveals a focal osteopaenic region within the left femoral head; this is no longer evident on a follow-up film 8 months later. Which of the following is the most likely diagnosis?

A. Osteomalacia

B. Avascular necrosis

C. Transient osteonecrosis

D. Transient osteoporosis

E. Occult fracture

17. A 35-year-old woman with bilateral facial nerve palsy showed extensive nodular deposits with diffuse enhancement of the meninges on CECT of the brain. Which of the following imaging investigation will likely confirm the diagnosis?

A. MR angiogram of the circle of Willis

B. Ultrasound of the liver

C. Intravenous urogram

D. Plain chest radiograph

E. Plain radiograph of both hands

18. A 10-month-old infant attends the local infectious diseases unit with his mother who recently emigrated from Zimbabwe. The child has shortness of breath, fever and bilateral inspiratory crackles. Chest X-ray demonstrates diffuse bilateral ground-glass opacification. What is the most likely diagnosis?

A. Varicella pneumonia

B. Round pneumonia

C. Pneumocystis pneumonia (PCP)

D. Bronchopulmonary dysplasia

E. Congestive cardiac failure

19. A 65-year-old hepatitis C–positive man is found to have a liver mass on screening ultrasound. A suspicion of HCC was raised. Which one of the following statements regarding HCC screening is false?

A. HCC is characteristically hyperechoic on ultrasound.

B. The majority of nodules that measure less than 1 cm are not HCC.

C. It develops in a background of preexisting liver parenchymal damage.

D. HCC is commonly diagnosed on the basis of imaging features alone, without histologic confirmation.

E. The nodules that are suspicious for HCC are new nodules that measure more than 1 cm or nodules that enlarge over a time interval.

20. A 42-year-old factory worker complains of chest tightness and shortness of breath during the early days of the week, settling down during the weekend over the last several months. Chest radiograph is normal. HRCT is requested for further evaluation. What do you expect the HRCT to show?

A. Crazy paving pattern

B. Patchy ground-glass opacities with centrilobular nodules

C. Perilymphatic nodules with beaded fissures

D. Central bronchiectasis

E. Extensive mediastinal and hilar lymphadenopathy

21. A CT scan, obtained in a patient with haematuria after minimal trauma, reveals a rim of enhancement surrounding a markedly dilated right renal pelvis and collecting system. Note is made of variable thickness to the enhancing rim and enhancing cortical strands. The report describes it as a rim sign. What is the likely diagnosis?
    A. Hydronephrosis
    B. Renovascular compromise
    C. Diabetes mellitus
    D. Pyelonephritis
    E. Fractured kidney

22. In the case of a vertebral compression fracture, all the statements regarding imaging findings suggests a malignant cause, except
    A. Involvement of the posterior elements
    B. Persistent loss of T1W bone marrow signal on sequential imaging
    C. Paravertebral soft-tissue component
    D. Post-contrast gadolinium enhancement
    E. Convex posterior border of the vertebral body

23. All of the following are true of toxoplasmosis of AIDS, except
    A. It is the most common focal CNS infection.
    B. Treatment is started empirically based on imaging.
    C. The basal ganglia and cerebral hemispheres are commonly involved.
    D. Haemorrhage and calcification are common post-therapy.
    E. A single lesion is the most common.

24. On newborn heel stick screening, a newborn infant is found to suffer from congenital hypothyroidism. On ultrasound, the thyroid gland is diffusely enlarged, and on Technetium 99m thyroid scintigraphy there is increased uptake of radioactive tracer within the gland. There is no evidence of ectopic thyroid tissue.
    What is the most likely cause for the congenital hypothyroidism?
    A. Thyroid hypoplasia
    B. Hypothalamic dysfunction
    C. Thyroid dyshormonogenesis
    D. Maternal antibody-induced hypothyroidism
    E. Hypopituitarism

25. An 8-year-old child with right upper-abdominal pain and a palpable mass was sent for US of the liver. The US showed a large heterogeneous mass occupying at least half of the right lobe of the liver. The rest of the liver was normal in appearance. Which one of the following is the most common benign primary liver tumour in children?
    A. Hepatocellular carcinoma
    B. Hepatoblastoma
    C. Angiosarcoma
    D. Infantile haemangioendothelioma
    E. Cholangiocarcinoma

26. A 43-year-old woman with history of proteinuria presented to the A&E department with shortness of breath and haemoptysis. Chest X-ray showed diffuse airspace opacities and an HRCT was organised. The HRCT showed diffuse airspace opacities, ground-glass change and confluent consolidation, which was reported as acute diffuse alveolar haemorrhage. Which of the following can be classically expected on CT sinus study?
    A. Bilateral frontal mucocoele
    B. Unilateral sinusitis involving all the sinuses on one side

C. Chronic destructive sinusitis with nasal perforation

D. Hypoplastic maxillary sinuses

E. Oro-antral fistula

27. A CT scan, obtained to exclude retroperitoneal hematoma in a patient with sustained hypotension for 1 hour after cardiac catheterisation and subsequent cardiac arrest, shows a hypoattenuating renal cortex compared with the medullary enhancement. No additional contrast material was given at the time of the CT. Which of the following signs is being described here?

A. Hydronephrotic rim sign

B. Comet tail sign

C. Crescent sign

D. Reverse rim sign

E. Soft-tissue rim sign

28. A report is issued stating that there is a periosteal reaction associated with what the radiologist believes is a benign bony lesion. What type of periosteal reaction is most likely to be associated with a benign lesion?

A. Codman

B. Sunburst

C. Hair-on-end

D. Lamination

E. Buttressing

29. All of the following are associated with tuberous scleoris, except

A. Giant cell astrocytoma

B. Subependymal hamartomas

C. Pheochromocytoma

D. Cardiac rhabdomyoma

E. Chylothorax

30. A 22-month-old boy presents with abdominal pain and is found on US to have an intussusception.

Which of the following statements is false with regard to his initial management and treatment?

A. The patient should be reviewed for signs of peritonitis by a paediatric surgeon.

B. Bowel infarct, peritonitis and perforation are potential complications if the intussusception is left untreated.

C. The patient should be fluid resuscitated prior to attempts at air enema reduction.

D. A plain abdominal radiograph should be obtained prior to air enema reduction to rule out signs of perforation.

E. A successful intussusception reduction is noted when air is seen to fill the small bowel loops.

31. An MRI of the liver with contrast was performed in a 50-year-old woman after a complex mass was identified on US. The mass was reported as suspicious for epithelioid haemangioendothelioma. All of the following are expected features of this lesion, except

A. Vascular origin

B. Female predominance

C. Typical presentation of multifocal nodules

D. Avid arterial phase enhancement

E. Capsular retraction

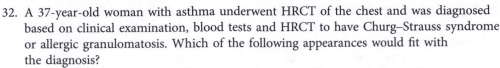

32. A 37-year-old woman with asthma underwent HRCT of the chest and was diagnosed based on clinical examination, blood tests and HRCT to have Churg–Strauss syndrome or allergic granulomatosis. Which of the following appearances would fit with the diagnosis?
    A. Peripheral predominant lobular consolidation with centrilobular nodules
    B. Peripheral predominant homogenous consolidation without centrilobular nodules
    C. Peripheral predominant interstitial reticular opacities with underlying traction bronchiectasis
    D. Central bronchiectasis and patchy airspace opacities with mucous plugs
    E. Upper lobe predominant interstitial pulmonary fibrosis with architectural distortion

33. Which of the following is incorrect?
    A. Spoke wheel sign   Renal oncocytoma
    B. Pear-shaped bladder sign   Pelvis lipomatosis
    C. Pie-in-the-sky bladder sign   Bilateral psoas hypertrophy
    D. Spaghetti sign   Haematuria
    E. Balloon-on-a-string sign   Hydronephrosis

34. A young adult man presents with a painful left wrist following a fall from height. A lateral view of the wrist shows loss of co-linearity of the radius/lunate/capitate axis with the capitate displaced dorsally. What injury is this constellation of findings compatible with?
    A. Midcarpal dislocation
    B. Perilunate dislocation
    C. Lunate dislocation
    D. Volar intercalated segmental instability
    E. Dorsal intercalated segmental instability

35. All the following are true of venous angioma, except
    A. It can be considered normal.
    B. It contains small arterial channels.
    C. It is associated with cavernomas.
    D. It shows a spoked wheel configuration on imaging.
    E. It normally has a large draining vein but no feeding arteries.

36. A 5-year-old boy, who underwent a bone marrow transplantation 1 week earlier for an underlying haematological malignancy, presents with shortness of breath, cough and chest tightness.
    Which of the following complications would be least likely?
    A. Lymphoid interstitial pneumonitis
    B. Pulmonary oedema
    C. Pulmonary embolism
    D. Infective interstitial pneumonitis from CMV
    E. Idiopathic interstitial pneumonitis

37. A 56-year-old woman presented to her GP with pain and palpable mass in the right upper quadrant. She was sent for US, which showed a large heterogeneous mass in the right lobe of the liver. A contrast-enhanced MRI of the liver is urgently organised for further characterisation. The lesion is reported as consistent with fibrolamellar carcinoma.
    All of the following are expected findings, except
    A. Central scar low on T1W and T2W images.
    B. Solitary mass is the usual presentation.
    C. Favorable prognosis.
    D. Rare pathological subtype of hepatocellular carcinoma.
    E. Background cirrhotic change to the liver parenchyma.

38. A 37-year-old woman involved in a frontal car collision and collapse at the scene of incident was brought to the A&E department and sent for an emergency whole-body CT. All of the following are correct regarding blunt cardiac trauma, except
    A. Cardiac concussion results in abnormal cardiac enzymes.
    B. Traumatic pericardial rupture resulting from blunt chest trauma is rare.
    C. Cardiac herniation is a serious complication of pericardial rupture.
    D. Traumatic ventricular septal defects affect the muscular portion.
    E. Myocardial contusion is associated with cardiac tamponade.

39. An 88-year-old man with obstructive uropathy and hard nodular prostate gland on digital rectal examination was being further investigated for his prostate cancer. Which one of the following magnetic resonance spectroscopic imaging metabolic peaks is expected in a patient with prostate cancer?
    A. High citrate peak, low choline/creatine peak
    B. High citrate peak, high choline/creatine peak
    C. Low citrate peak, high choline/creatine peak
    D. Low citrate peak, low choline/creatine peak
    E. Low citrate peak, normal choline/creatine peak

40. A 42-year-old woman with knee joint stiffness, pain and reduced mobility is investigated with a plain X-ray, which reveals extensive soft-tissue swelling around the joint with large periarticular erosions. There is no evidence of calcification and bone density is maintained. MRI shows low-signal foci within the soft-tissue mass. What is the likely diagnosis?
    A. Pigmented villonodular synovitis
    B. Haemophilia
    C. Synovial sarcoma
    D. Behcet's syndrome
    E. Psoriatic arthropathy

41. A 40-year-old woman with progressive difficulty in walking and difficulty in holding objects reveals a large burn over the dorsum of her right hand on clinical examination. Sagittal MRI of the cervical spine shows a long segment lesion in the cervical and upper thoracic spinal cord with low signal on T1W images and high signal on T2W images without any change on post-contrast images. What is the diagnosis?
    A. Ependymoma
    B. Syringomyelia
    C. Astrocytoma
    D. Haemangioblastoma
    E. AVM

42. A chest CT is performed on a 10-year-old boy with known underlying chronic lung changes. Current imaging demonstrates levocardia with areas of air trapping, bronchial dilatation and bronchial wall thickening, which were also present on previous imaging from 1 year earlier. There are no significantly enlarged mediastinal lymph nodes.
    Which of the following differential diagnoses would be least likely to account for the underlying changes?
    A. Cystic fibrosis
    B. IgA deficiency
    C. Juvenile dermatomyositis
    D. Primary ciliary dyskinesia
    E. Recurrent pneumonias

43. A 10-year-old boy falls while running for the school bus and hurts his arm. An X-ray demonstrates a fracture through the proximal humeral diaphysis through a 'bony lesion'. What is the most likely underlying predisposing bone pathology?
    A. Giant cell tumour
    B. Osteosarcoma
    C. Simple bone cyst
    D. Eosinophilic granuloma
    E. Ewing's sarcoma

44. A 43-year-old woman with known diagnosis of tuberous sclerosis presented to her GP with increasing right upper-abdominal pain. Although the LFT was normal, the GP organised a liver MR in search of angiomyolipomas in the liver. All of the following are MR features of angiomyolipomas of the liver, except
    A. A well-defined mass.
    B. Moderately hyperintense signal intensity on T1W images.
    C. Moderately hyperintense signal intensity on T2W images.
    D. Loss of signal on fat-suppressed sequences.
    E. Usually shows late arterial enhancement on the post-contrast sequence.

45. With regard to the progression of pulmonary consolidation on CXR, all of the following options are true except
    A. Lung contusion appears in 6 hours and clears in 3–7 days.
    B. Aspiration appears in minutes and clears in 24–48 hours unless infected.
    C. Lung infarction due to pulmonary embolism manifests after 3–5 days and clears in approximately 3 weeks.
    D. Fat embolism appears in 6 hours and clears in 7–10 days.
    E. ARDS with diffuse alveolar damage appears after 24–48 hours and clears in 4–6 weeks.

46. An 88-year-old man with obstructive uropathy and hard nodular prostate gland on digital rectal examination is being further investigated for his prostate cancer. He has been scheduled for a staging MRI of the prostate. Which one of the following is the characteristic imaging finding of prostate cancer on DWI?
    A. High on DWI, low on ADC and corresponding low signal intensity on T2W MRI
    B. Low on DWI, high on ADC and corresponding low signal intensity on T2W MRI
    C. High on DWI, low on ADC and corresponding high signal intensity on T2W MRI
    D. Low on DWI, high on ADC and corresponding high signal intensity on T2W MRI
    E. High on DWI, low on ADC and corresponding normal signal intensity on T2W MRI

47. A 50-year-old patient presents with shortness of breath to his GP. Following abnormalities on the chest radiograph, a CT is performed, demonstrating bilateral hilar and right paratracheal lymphadenopathy along with coarse reticulations and nodular thickening along the fissures and bronchovascular bundles. Elevated ACE serum levels are noted. What is not a typical musculoskeletal manifestation of this disease?
    A. Lacy lytic lesions in the phalanges of the hands
    B. Polyarthralgia with tenosynovitis
    C. Multiple bony lesions with high T2W and intermediate T1W signal characteristics
    D. Soft-tissue calcifications
    E. Dactylitis

48. An infant boy was investigated with MRI for seizures. The left side of the brain is smaller than the right and there is evidence of T2 hypointensity on the gyri. There is diffuse contrast enhancement adjacent to the gyri and sulci on the same side. Some enhancement is

also noted along the ipsilateral posterior globe. Which of the following is the most likely diagnosis?

A. Hypoxic ischaemic encephalopathy
B. Meningitis
C. Sturge–Weber syndrome
D. Gliomatosis cerebri
E. Tuberous sclerosis

49. A 36-year-old woman on oral contraceptives was sent for a liver US by her GP following complaints of right upper-quadrant pain. No gallstones were found and bile ducts were normal. However, a large lesion was discovered in the right lobe of the liver. Which one of the following would be the most likely diagnosis in this scenario?

A. Focal nodular hyperplasia
B. Hepatocellular adenoma
C. Angiomyolipoma
D. Haemangioma
E. Biliary hamartoma

50. A 73-year-old woman with a known splenic lesion underwent a CT of the chest, which demonstrated multiple pulmonary nodules with surrounding halos. A follow-up CT chest done a few weeks later showed cavitations developing in some of the nodules and a right pneumothorax. The most likely diagnosis is

A. Lymphoma
B. Hydatid disease
C. Metastatic angiosarcoma
D. Sarcoidosis
E. Bronchoalveolar carcinoma

51. A 77-year-old man with obstructive uropathy and TRUS biopsy–proven prostate cancer was scheduled to have an MRI for local staging of the known prostate cancer. Which one of the following statements regarding identification of prostate cancer by dynamic contrast enhancement (DCE) is true?

A. Fast enhancement and slow washout suggest prostate cancer.
B. Slow enhancement peak and slow washout suggest prostate cancer.
C. Slow enhancement and fast washout are highly suggestive of prostate cancer.
D. Small prostate tumours are detected easily.
E. The higher the tumour grade, the greater the grade of enhancement.

52. A 40-year-old man presents to his general practitioner with intermittent left leg pain and stiffness of 5 years duration. Plain radiograph reveals eccentric and irregular sclerosis along the medial aspect of the distal femur, crossing the joint into the adjacent tibia. Cortical new bone formation along the outer aspect of the cortex is also seen, with an appearance similar to flowing wax. In addition, there are adjacent ossified soft-tissue masses. Which of the following is the most likely diagnosis?

A. Melorheostosis
B. Osteopoikilosis
C. Fibrous dysplasia
D. Osteoarthritis
E. Osteopetrosis

53. A 37-year-old woman presented to the A&E department with acute worsening of arm weakness and pins and needles at the C4/5 levels. MRI of the spine revealed an elongated area of high T2W signal change, which showed variable contrast enhancement. There was no

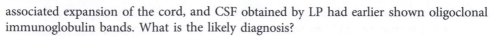

associated expansion of the cord, and CSF obtained by LP had earlier shown oligoclonal immunoglobulin bands. What is the likely diagnosis?

A. Lyme disease
B. Multiple sclerosis
C. Sarcoidosis
D. LCH
E. Lymphoma

54. A 9-year-old female patient is incidentally found to have a pelvic mass on US. The features are thought to represent those of a mature cystic teratoma (dermoid cyst).

Which of the following complications relating to this diagnosis is the least likely?

A. Malignant transformation
B. Associated ovarian torsion
C. Rupture of the lesion
D. Autoimmune haemolytic anaemia
E. Bleeding

55. An 11-year-old girl is currently under investigation for an adnexal mass recently found on a US scan. Which of the following statements regarding paediatric ovarian tumours is least accurate?

A. Gonadoblastomas are associated with dysgenetic gonads.
B. Sertoli–Leydig cell tumours may present with virilising symptoms.
C. Mature cystic teratomas are the most common ovarian tumours in children.
D. Immature teratomas are associated with elevated serum AFP levels.
E. Elevated CA-125 levels are commonly seen in children with germ cell tumours.

56. A 36-year-old woman on oral contraceptives was sent for a liver US by her GP with complaints of right upper-quadrant pain and fullness. No gallstones were found and bile ducts were normal. However, an incidental small hyperechoic lesion was discovered in the right lobe of the liver. The appearance was benign and the most likely diagnosis would be

A. Focal nodular hyperplasia
B. Hepatocellular adenoma
C. Biliary hamartoma
D. Angiomyolipoma
E. Haemangioma

57. A 43-year-old man with known history of arteriovenous malformation involving various organs had a chest X-ray following a recent bout of haemoptysis. The chest X-ray was abnormal and a CTPA was organised for clarification/confirmation and help in treatment planning. All of the following CT findings are true regarding treatment of pulmonary AVM, except

A. Surgery is preferred over embolisation.
B. Coils are the preferred embolisation material.
C. Intolerance to exercise is an indication for treatment.
D. Aneurysm size greater than 2 cm needs to be treated.
E. Large feeding arteries are associated with increased risk of brain abscess.

58. An 81-year-old man with progressive worsening hesitancy, dribbling, incomplete voiding and haematuria was found to have a hard nodular prostate gland on digital rectal examination. He is due to have a staging prostatic MRI, which will take place shortly after TRUS biopsy. Which one of the following is characteristic of post-biopsy haemorrhage of the prostate gland on MR imaging?

A. Hyperintense on T1W imaging and hypointense on T2W imaging
B. Hypointense on T1W imaging and hypointense on T2W imaging
C. Hypointense on T1W imaging and hyperintense on T2W imaging

D. Hyperintense on T1W imaging and hyperintense on T2W imaging

E. Hyperintense on T1W imaging and isointense on T2W imaging

59. A 52-year-old man has a lower-leg radiograph performed after a fall. No acute bony injury is identified, but the reviewing doctor notices a flame-shaped lucency involving the medulla of the tibia, extending superiorly from the distal subarticular into the diaphysis. He is unsure of the significance of this appearance and seeks the opinion of the radiologist. Which of the following is the most likely diagnosis?

A. Osteomyelitis

B. Giant cell tumour

C. Plasmacytoma

D. Paget disease (acute phase)

E. Paget disease (chronic phase)

60. A 40-year-old woman with history of severe diarrhoea following salmonella gastroenteritis presented with increasing headache. Clinically bilateral papilloedema was noted. Acute drop in GCS prompted an urgent CT of the brain, which showed suspicious high density in the superior sagittal sinus with bilateral subcortical haemorrhages in the parietal lobes. What is your diagnosis?

A. Acute haemorrhagic infarct

B. Encephalitis

C. Meningeal metastasis

D. Superior sagittal sinus thrombosis

E. Transverse sinus thrombosis

61. A 42-year-old woman was found to have a mass in the right lobe of the liver on US and sent for an MRI liver for further characterisation. All of the following are expected MR features of FNH, except

A. High signal intensity of the central scar on T2W images

B. Uniform enhancement of the mass in the arterial phase

C. Lack of capsular enhancement in the arterial phase

D. Hypointense to surrounding liver on the enhanced portal venous phase

E. Maximum intensity of central scar on enhanced delayed phase images

62. A 57-year-old woman with a personal and familial (father, brother and grandfather) history of epistaxis and multiple telangiectasia, presented with dyspnoea and weakness leading to performance of a chest and head CT scan which showed a peripheral lobulated enhancing mass in the thorax and areas of hypoattenuation in the brain.

A. Churg–Strauss disease

B. Wegener's granulomatosis

C. Osler–Rendu–Weber syndrome

D. Metastatic choriocarcinoma

E. Kaposi sarcoma

63. CT of the pelvis in a 37-year-old woman who was undergoing ovulation induction showed massive cysts in the pelvis surrounding a core of central ovarian stroma with relatively higher attenuation. More cephalad images demonstrated ascites. All of the following are features of ovarian hyperstimulation syndrome, except

A. Enlarged multicystic ovaries

B. Free intraperitoneal fluid

C. Low serum estradiol levels

D. Pleural or pericardial effusion

E. Risk of deep vein thrombosis

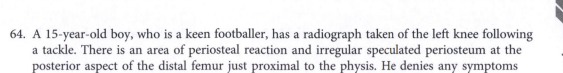

64. A 15-year-old boy, who is a keen footballer, has a radiograph taken of the left knee following a tackle. There is an area of periosteal reaction and irregular speculated periosteum at the posterior aspect of the distal femur just proximal to the physis. He denies any symptoms before the injury. The next imaging should be which one of the following?
   A. A comparison radiograph of the contralateral knee
   B. Non-contrast CT of the distal femur
   C. Contrast-enhanced CT of the distal femur
   D. MRI of the distal femur
   E. A nuclear medicine bone scan

65. A 16-year-old boy with learning difficulties presented to the A&E department with increasing frequency of epileptic fits, which he has had since childhood. Bilateral brisk reflexes were noted clinically. CT of the brain performed to exclude haemorrhage revealed a large heterogeneous lobulated mass replacing the third ventricle with further areas of subependymal calcification. What is the diagnosis?
   A. Sturge–Weber syndrome
   B. Tuberous sclerosis
   C. Arnold–Chiari malformation
   D. Neuroblastoma metastasis
   E. VHL

66. A previously fit and healthy 16-year-old presents with recurrent wheeze. Chest X-ray demonstrates tubular, branching structures of increased density relative to normal lung radiating from the left hilum. The surrounding lung is hyperlucent. What is the most likely diagnosis?
   A. Allergic bronchopulmonary aspergillosis
   B. Cystic fibrosis
   C. Bronchial atresia
   D. Kartagener syndrome
   E. Swyer–James syndrome

67. A 14-year-old female patient is found on US to have a large pelvic mass comprised of mainly cystic elements. The right ovary is not seen separate to the mass.
   With regard to adnexal masses in children, which of the following statements is true?
   A. Mature cystic teratomas tend to be bilateral when present.
   B. A raised serum AFP level is indicative of choriocarcinoma.
   C. The majority of mature cystic teratomas are malignant.
   D. The most common malignant germ cell tumour is a dysgerminoma.
   E. Yolk sac tumours tend to have a benign clinical course.

68. A 33-year-old lady with a history of right upper-quadrant pain and deranged LFTs is sent for an ultrasound, which shows a large cystic lesion in the right liver lobe. Blood tests also show eosinophilia. Which of the following statements regarding the imaging of Hydatid disease is false?
   A. US findings are variable and range from purely cystic to solid-appearing pseudotumours.
   B. Daughter cysts are frequently seen.
   C. Cysts usually appear well defined on CT.
   D. Coarse wall calcification may be present.
   E. CT imaging best demonstrates the pericyst, matrix and daughter cysts.

69. A 50-year-old man with known lung transplant presented with shortness of breath. Blood gases revealed Type 1 respiratory failure. A late post-transplant complication was suspected

and a baseline chest X-ray was organised as a start. All of the following are late complications of lung transplantation, except

A. Bronchial stenosis
B. Chronic rejection
C. Recurrence of primary disease
D. Cryptogenic organising pneumonia
E. Bronchial dehiscence

70. A 37-year-old woman in her third trimester presented to the labour ward with acute onset of pain in the lower central abdomen. She had had two previous caesarean sections and an appendectomy with unremarkable recovery. On clinical examination, there was definite tenderness at the site of a previous caesarean scar. The best imaging modality for evaluation of caesarean section scar dehiscence is

A. CT
B. Transabdominal US
C. MRI
D. Angiography
E. Transvaginal US

71. A 23-year-old man presents with an acute injury of his knee sustained during a friendly football match following a rough tackle. The patient reports having heard a pop and the knee started swelling immediately. He is unable to weight-bear and had to be carried off the field. An MRI is organised with high suspicion of ACL injury. All of the following are indirect signs of ACL injury, except

A. Bone bruising in lateral tibiofemoral compartment
B. Deep lateral femoral sulcus >1.5 mm
C. Uncovering of the posterior horn of the lateral meniscus
D. Posterior translation of the tibia
E. PCL bowing <105 degrees

72. MRI brain images of a 42-year-old man diagnosed with HIV showed areas of cloud-like high signal on T2W images in the periventricular area bilaterally. All of the following are true regarding CNS infections in HIV, except

A. High signal in the periventricular area suggest HIV subacute encephalitis.
B. Subacute encephalitis caused by HIV and CMV have similar appearances.
C. Basal meningitis suggests neurosyphilis.
D. Cerebral infarcts can occur with neurosyphilis in HIV patients.
E. CMV infection can manifest as ventriculoencephalitis.

73. A 74-year-old woman presented with post-operative gastric cancer, at 4 days after onset of fever, cough and sputum. CT was organised for characterisation. All of the following are true regarding MRSA and MSSA pneumonia on CT chest, except

A. Lung nodules are more common in MSSA.
B. Effusion is more common in MRSA.
C. There is no significant difference in zonal distribution between MSSA and MRSA pneumonia.
D. Hilar lymph nodes are more common in MRSA.
E. Consolidation is seen in both groups.

74. A 4-year-old girl presents with progressive enlargement of her right thigh, with episodes of unprovoked bleeding from pigmented lesions over her right thigh, which were present since birth. A lower-limb venogram of the right leg demonstrates absence of the deep

venous system, with varicose veins on the lateral aspect of the right leg. Which of the following is the most likely diagnosis?

A. Klippel–Trenaunay syndrome
B. Neurofibromatosis Type 1
C. Beckwith–Wiedemann syndrome
D. Macrodystrophia lipomatosis
E. Maffucci syndrome

75. A 42-year-old man with epigastric pain and upper-abdominal fullness was sent for US assessment. No gallstones were observed and bile ducts were normal. Multiple tiny liver lesions were noted and an MRI was advised for characterisation. MRI was reported as biliary hamartomas (von Meyenburg complexes, VMC) of the liver and the patient was reassured. Which one of the following statements concerning VMC is false?

A. They may be solitary or multiple.
B. They are benign cystic biliary malformations.
C. They are high signal intensity on T1W MRI.
D. They usually are smaller than 1 cm in diameter.
E. They do not show perilesional enhancement on MRI.

76. A previously hypertensive 34-year-old post-partum woman who presented with right upper-quadrant pain, pelvic pain and hypotension was sent for an urgent CT. The CT scan showed a large, subcapsular liver hematoma and hemiperitoneum within the abdomen and pelvis. No liver lesions were seen on a prepartum US. What is the diagnosis?

A. Haemorrhagic adenoma
B. HELLP syndrome
C. Iatrogenic injury at caesarean section
D. Acute hepatic steatosis of pregnancy
E. Fitz Hugh–Curtis syndrome

77. A 25-year-old woman presents with pain and swelling over the sternoclavicular joints. Clinical examination reveals small pustules in the palms and soles along with facial acne. As part of the series of investigations, a bone scan shows increased uptake around the sternoclavicular joints and anterior chest wall resulting in a bull's horn appearance. What is the diagnosis?

A. Osteomyelitis of sternoclavicular joint
B. Ankylosing spondylitis
C. SAPHO syndrome
D. POEMS syndrome
E. Soto syndrome

78. A 70-year-old woman came to the A&E department with a 4-day history of generalised malaise, fever and drowsiness. Blood, urine and sputum cultures were negative and an urgent CT of the brain was advised due to rapid drop in GCS and left lower-limb motor weakness. MRI showed diffuse high signal in the right temporal lobe, inferior frontal lobe and hippocampus with a small area of haemorrhage and mass effect.

A. Tuberous sclerosis
B. Lymphoma
C. Toxoplasmosis
D. HSV encephalitis
E. Gliomatosis cerebri

79. A suspected low-density lesion in the pancreas of a 59-year-old man seen on US was reassessed with CT, which confirmed the presence of a small central cyst in the proximal part of the body of the pancreas. All of the following are characteristic features of the

main duct subtype of intraductal papillary mucinous neoplasms (IPMNs) of the pancreas, except
A. Long or short segments of marked stricture in the main pancreatic duct
B. Excess drainage of thick mucin from a patulous papillary orifice on endoscopic retrograde cholangiopancreatography
C. A papillary intraductal mass
D. Malignant potential
E. A nodular intraductal mass

80. A 65-year-old man presents with shortness of breath, fever and cough. His blood results show leucocytosis and a raised CRP. His CXR shows a large right-sided effusion. Empyema was suspected clinically and a contrast-enhanced CT chest was organised urgently for further evaluation. All of the following features on a chest CT would suggest an empyema, except
A. Obtuse angle with the chest wall.
B. Gas locules in the fluid is most specific.
C. Lenticular-shaped pleural fluid collection.
D. Obvious septations.
E. Enhancing thickened pleura.

81. Urgent MRI done on a patient who had recently undergone caesarean delivery showed a large (>5 cm) intermediate- to high-signal-intensity haematoma at the lower uterine incision site that communicates with the endometrium on sagittal fat-saturated T2W images. The uterine serosa was intact. What is the diagnosis?
A. Uterine dehiscence
B. Uterine rupture
C. Bladder flap haematoma
D. Subfascial haematoma
E. Endometritis

82. All of the following are true regarding imaging of the sternum and sternoclavicular joint, except
A. Primary osteomyelitis may suggest immunodeficiency.
B. Primary osteomyelitis is more common than secondary osteomyelitis.
C. Internal mammary artery graft has a higher association with post-sternotomy infection.
D. Sternal fracture suggests high-energy trauma.
E. With regard to sternoclavicular joint dislocation, anterior is more common than posterior.

83. A 43-year-old man with a 2 × 2 cm lump below the ear lobule on the right. The lump has been there for 4 years and is slowly increasing in size without being painful or exhibiting any features to suggest local neural involvement. How would you investigate the lump further?
A. MRI of the neck
B. CT of the neck with contrast
C. US of the neck
D. US of the neck with FNA
E. Sialogram

84. While reporting plain films in a paediatric radiology setting, you look at the plain abdominal film of an 8-year-old child admitted with abdominal pain and vomiting. The film demonstrates multiple gas-filled bowel loops throughout the abdomen, with paucity of gas and a small calcific density in right lower quadrant. The right psoas outline is not clear. What is the likely diagnosis?
A. Acute appendicitis
B. Acute cholecystitis
C. Renal colic

D. Abdominal teratoma

E. Chronic peritonitis

85. A young girl presents with visual disturbance and headache. The paediatrician notices papilloedema on fundoscopy. CT demonstrates a posterior fossa tumour with cystic elements and obstructive hydrocephalus. The patient is referred to the neurosurgeons, who arrange an MRI of the brain and abdomen. The MRI of the brain confirms a posterior fossa tumour with a nodule and cystic components. The nodule shows strong enhancement with contrast. Multiple flow voids are demonstrated within the tumour. What is the diagnosis and what were the findings of the abdomen MRI?
    A. Neurofibromatosis Type 1 – multifocal RCC
    B. Neurofibromatosis Type 2 – renal AMLs
    C. Sturge–Weber syndrome – renal and pancreatic AVM
    D. VHL syndrome – renal and pancreatic cysts
    E. Li–Fraumeni syndrome – ovarian cysts

86. A 66-year-old woman with discomfort in the epigastric region was sent for US of the upper abdomen. GB and bile ducts were normal but an incidental mass was identified in the pancreas. A dual-phase CT was requested for further characterisation. The CT showed a large, lobulated, multicystic lesion with a central scar, enhancing septae and some stellate calcification. Which one of the following is the most likely diagnosis?
    A. Solid pseudopapillary tumour
    B. Intraductal papillary mucinous neoplasm
    C. Mucinous cystic neoplasm
    D. Serous cystadenoma
    E. Gastrinoma

87. A 50-year-old man with chronic dyspnoea showed unresolving consolidation in both lungs on chest X-ray. Following a course of steroids, the consolidations improved and a provisional diagnosis of cryptogenic organising pneumonia was made. An HRCT was organised at this point, which showed multiple nodules and masses. All of the following are expected appearance for masses seen in COP on CT, except:
    A. Sparing of subpleural region
    B. Cylindrical bronchial dilatation in consolidation
    C. Fissural and septal nodules
    D. Small lung nodules
    E. Peribronchial distribution

88. A middle-aged man undergoes CT of the abdomen for chronic low-grade abdominal pain, early satiety and weight loss; the CT reveals a large retroperitoneal mass. Which one of the following primary retroperitoneal tumours is most likely to appear on CT as a soft-tissue density mass with a large area of central necrosis?
    A. Liposarcoma
    B. Lymphoma
    C. Leiomyosarcoma
    D. Lymphangioma
    E. Paraganglioma

89. A 5-year-old girl known to the endocrinologists presented to the A&E department after a fall and had radiographs of her lower limb taken to exclude fractures. No fractures were identified, but there were several well-defined lytic lesions in the metaphysis and diaphysis

of the femur and tibia with an internal ground-glass matrix. Clinical examinations revealed several irregular areas of skin pigmentation. What is your diagnosis?
A. McCune–Albright syndrome
B. Mazabraud syndrome
C. NF1
D. NF2
E. Cherubism

90. A 37-year-old man with a lump behind the ramus of the right mandible showed a well-defined, isodense, homogenous nodule in the superficial part of the right lobe of the parotid gland; there was no involvement of the facial nerve or retromandibular vein. Previous sialogram performed for possible stones had shown displacement of the intraglandular ducts without occlusion. What is the diagnosis?
A. Pleomorphic adenoma
B. Warthin's tumour
C. Lymphoma
D. Mucoepidermoid tumour
E. Adenoid cystic tumour

91. A 50-year-old woman with palpable fullness in the epigastric region was sent for US of the upper abdomen. The GB and bile ducts were normal but a hypoechoic mass was identified in the pancreas. A dual-phase CT was requested for further characterisation, which showed a multicystic lesion in the pancreatic head and reported possible serous cystadenoma. All of the following are expected features, except
A. Multiple small cysts (usually <2 cm)
B. High glycogen content in aspirated fluid
C. Communication with the pancreatic duct
D. Thin enhancing internal septa on MRI
E. Central stellate fibrotic scar in large lesions

92. A 25-year-old immunocompromised patient presented with a long history of progressive exertional dyspnoea and was found to have an abnormal chest X-ray. An HRCT was organised for further characterisation of disease. HRCT suggested pulmonary *Mycobacterium avium* complex infection. Which one of the following features is a characteristic finding on CT?
A. Upper lobe bronchiectasis
B. Lower-lobe bronchiectasis
C. Thick-walled cavities
D. Right middle lobe and lingular bronchiectasis
E. Large pleural effusion

93. A child with a previous history of infantile spasms now presents with myoclonic seizures. She is noted to have a port wine stain on her face. An MRI scan of the brain is arranged to confirm the suspected diagnosis. What MRI findings would you expect in the suspected diagnosis?
A. Posterior fossa haemangioblastoma
B. Pial angioma demonstrated by leptomeningeal enhancement
C. Bilateral acoustic schwannomas
D. Multiple white matter T2 hyperintensities
E. Multiple T1W hyperintensities and cerebellar hypoplasia

94. Contrast-enhanced CT of the abdomen done on a middle-aged woman revealed a large heterogeneous retroperitoneal mass with distortion of regional anatomy and forward

displacement of the posterior abdominal structures. All of the following CT signs will help distinguish a tumour arising within a retroperitoneal organ from a primary retroperitoneal tumour, except
A. Beak sign
B. Phantom organ sign
C. Embedded organ sign
D. Prominent feeding artery sign
E. Soft-tissue rim sign

95. A 65-year-old woman currently under the care of rheumatologists complains of worsening morning stiffness and polyarthropathy with a positive rheumatoid factor. Over the recent months she has noticed progressive worsening of shoulder pain with increasing limitation of motion. A shoulder X-ray is requested. All of the following are expected in her shoulder radiograph, except
A. Marginal erosions
B. Soft-tissue swelling
C. Superior subluxation of humeral head
D. Osteophytes
E. Osteopaenia

96. A 30-year-old apyrexial, systemically well woman came to the ENT clinic with sudden appearance of a large swelling in the left side of her neck, which had been moderately painful over the past few weeks. The swelling was non-tender and fluctuant; US of the neck showed a large fluid-filled cavity and guided FNA from the wall of the cyst showed benign histology. What is the diagnosis?
A. Metastatic squamous cell carcinoma
B. Lymphoma
C. Abscess
D. Branchial cyst
E. Thyroglossal cyst

97. A 45-year-old man with shortness of breath and bronchiectatic changes in the basal lobes showed moderate to marked dilatation of trachea on axial CT images. Which one of the following conditions is most likely?
A. Cystic fibrosis
B. Mounier–Kuhn syndrome
C. Williams–Campbell syndrome
D. Pulmonary sarcoidosis
E. Allergic bronchopulmonary aspergillosis

98. A 65-year-old man with a cystic lesion of the pancreas detected on US was sent for a dual-phase pancreatic CT for further characterisation. The most commonly encountered cystic lesion of the pancreas is
A. Serous cystadenoma
B. Mucinous cystic neoplasm
C. Pancreatic pseudocyst
D. Main duct intraductal papillary mucinous neoplasm
E. Side branch intraductal papillary mucinous neoplasm

99. Which of the following MRI sequences is most sensitive to assess normal myelination in children less than 1 year of age?
A. Fluid-attenuated inversion recovery (FLAIR)
B. T1W TSE

C. T2W TSE

   D. Susceptibility-weighted imaging (SWI)

   E. T2W GRE

100. A 33-year-old woman was referred for a transabdominal pelvic ultrasound examination to investigate for congestive dysmenorrhoea and deep dyspareunia. US examination revealed a complex right adnexal mass lesion with internal fishnet appearance. A normal right ovary was not identified separately; hence the complex mass was thought to be ovarian in origin. What is the likely diagnosis?

   A. Endometrioma

   B. Simple follicular cyst

   C. Haemorrhagic cyst

   D. Corpus luteal cyst

   E. Cystadenocarcinoma

101. Owing to normal appearances on initial plain radiographs, MRI is increasingly requested in suspected stress fractures, particularly in professional athletes and keen sportspersons.
MRI performed in one such instance showed periosteal oedema and increased marrow signal on T2W fat-suppressed images with hardly any signal change on T1W images.
Considering the stages of the MR grading system for stress injuries, what would be the grade of this injury?

   A. 0

   B. 1

   C. 2

   D. 3

   E. 4

102. A 23-year-old man presents with a congenital swelling underneath the left jaw, which has not changed over the past few years. Clinical examination reveals a horizontal scar overlying the same area. US shows multiloculated fluid-filled spaces at the site of the swelling in the neck. What is the diagnosis?

   A. Cystic hygroma

   B. Abscess

   C. Thyroglossal cyst

   D. Branchial cyst

   E. Cystic metastasis

103. A 36-year-old man with productive cough and abnormal chest X-ray had an HRCT for further characterisation and diagnosis. HRCT showed changes of bronchiectasis. Which one of the following is a direct radiographic sign of bronchiectasis?

   A. Bronchial wall thickening

   B. Mucoid impaction

   C. Lack of tapering of a bronchus

   D. Bronchial artery hypertrophy

   E. Lobar atelectasis

104. A 76-year-old man came to the A&E department with abdominal pain. A plain radiograph of the abdomen done in casualty was reported as showing pneumatosis intestinalis without any complications. Which one of the following statements regarding the radiographic findings in adult pneumatosis intestinalis is true?

   A. Pneumatosis cystoides intestinalis is characterised by linear gas collections.

   B. Pneumatosis cystoides intestinalis occurs mainly in the rectum.

   C. Portal venous gas usually is located in the central portion of the liver.

D. The submucosal gas in pneumatosis cystoides intestinalis can mimic colonic polyps on a barium enema when viewed *en face*.

E. The linear form in the small bowel allows differentiation between the benign and life-threatening forms.

105. A 23-year-old woman with history of pelvic inflammatory disease, 2 months amenorrhea, left lower-abdominal pain, weakness and occasional spotting showed lower-than-expected levels of HCG for pregnancy on urine assay. As far as US of the pelvis is concerned, which one of the following sonographic findings definitively distinguishes ectopic pregnancy from corpus luteum?
    A. Visualisation of a yolk sac
    B. 'Ring of fire' appearance
    C. Low-impedance flow on Doppler to the ring of fire
    D. Visualisation of a heartbeat
    E. Presence of echogenic pelvic fluid

106. Which of the following areas of the brain is normally the last to myelinate?
    A. Anterior limb of the internal capsule
    B. Posterior limb of the internal capsule
    C. Cerebellum
    D. Peritrigonal region
    E. Brainstem

107. A 50-year-old woman presents with painful wrists and clubbing. An X-ray demonstrates bilateral symmetrical periostitis involving the radius. The differential diagnosis includes hypertrophic pulmonary osteoarthropathy (HPOA). Which of the following is not a known cause of HPOA?
    A. Mesothelioma
    B. Pleural fibroma
    C. Bronchogenic carcinoma
    D. Bronchiectasis
    E. Pleural plaque secondary to asbestos exposure

108. A 23-year-old man presented with a hard swelling of the left side of the jaw. Plain radiograph showed a well-defined oval lucent lesion in the left side of the mandible with the crown of a unerrupted lower third molar. What is the most likely diagnosis?
    A. Odontogenic keratocyst
    B. Dentigerous cyst
    C. Dental cyst
    D. Periapical cyst
    E. Adamantinoma

109. A 55-year-old man with progressive productive cough and copious sputum was referred for an HRCT for disease characterisation. Which one of the following radiographic features distinguishes the bronchiectasis of allergic bronchopulmonary aspergillosis from that of cystic fibrosis?
    A. High-density mucus plugging
    B. Upper lobe predominance
    C. Cylindrical-type predominance
    D. Presence of associated hilar adenopathy
    E. Presence of air trapping

110. A 69-year-old man came to the A&E department with abdominal pain, and a plain X-ray of the abdomen and chest was requested for further evaluation. The chest X-ray showed free gas

under the diaphragm; a plain radiograph of the abdomen showed pneumatosis intestinalis with free intraperitoneal air. All of the following are causes of the life-threatening form of adult pneumatosis intestinalis, except

A. Ingestion of corrosive agents
B. Toxic megacolon
C. Post-bone marrow transplantation
D. Surgical placement of a jejunostomy tube
E. Primary infarction of the bowel wall

111. A 33-year-old woman with progressive congestive dysmenorrhoea, deep dyspareunia and infertility was being evaluated for possible endometriosis. Transabdominal US was organised as the first point of investigation. All of the following are acceptable features of endometrioma, except

A. Multiloculated cyst
B. Diffuse low-level echoes within a cyst
C. Homogeneous hypoechoic mass
D. Homogenous hyperechoic mass
E. A solid component with intense enhancement on Doppler

112. A 28-year-old woman is referred for a CT KUB for loin pain. The study unexpectedly shows grossly enlarged and abnormal kidneys with areas of fat density tissue within it. Small cystic areas are noted within the scanned lung bases. Further investigations reveal small subependymal lesions. What is a common musculoskeletal manifestation of this disease?

A. Osteochondroma
B. Sclerotic bone lesions
C. Enostoses
D. Fibrous dysplasia
E. Enchondroma

113. A 38-year-old woman presented with night-time stridor for several months. No definite lumps were felt clinically on examination, but chest radiograph showed marked deviation of the trachea to the left and a large soft-tissue mass on the right. US showed background multinodular change, but it was difficult to identify the lower pole of the right lobe of the thyroid. On detailed questioning, the patient admitted to facial and hand swelling on raising both arms for a reasonable length of time. What is the diagnosis?

A. Multinodular goitre with dominant nodule
B. Retrosternal goitre
C. Papillary carcinoma thyroid
D. Medullary carcinoma thyroid
E. Thyroid cyst with haemorrhage

114. Which of the following is the correct order of normal myelination?

A. Peripheral to central, caudal to rostral, ventral to dorsal
B. Central to peripheral, caudal to rostral, ventral to dorsal
C. Central to peripheral, rostral to caudal, dorsal to ventral
D. Peripheral to central, rostral to caudal, dorsal to ventral
E. Central to peripheral, caudal to rostral, dorsal to ventral

115. A 24-year-old man with chronic productive cough, fever, shortness of breath and recurrent chest infections shows predominantly lower-lobe bronchiectasis on HRCT. All the following differentials should be considered, except

A. Kartagener's syndrome
B. Sarcoidosis

C. Common variable immunodeficiency

D. α$_1$-Antitrypsin deficiency

E. Chronic aspiration

116. Which one of the following statements concerning papillary and solid epithelial neoplasms of the pancreas is true?

A. They occur mainly in elderly men.

B. They are a high-grade malignant tumour.

C. Heterogeneous content is detected within the mass on CT.

D. They typically present as a small cystic mass in the pancreatic head.

E. Weight loss and jaundice are the usual presentation.

117. Sagittal transvaginal US scan demonstrates a tubular-shaped cystic mass with several incomplete septa and indentations on opposite sides of the mass, often described as the 'waist' sign. What is the likely diagnosis?

A. Paraovarian cyst

B. Hydrosalpinx

C. Tubal pregnancy

D. Salpingitis isthmica nodosa

E. Peritoneal inclusion cyst

118. A 29-year-old runner presents to his family doctor with progressive increase in forefoot pain, which is limiting his training. Initial X-rays in the A&E department were normal. A follow-up bone scan detects focal abnormality in one of the metatarsals. Which one of the following is the most likely location for a metatarsal stress fracture appearing as an area of focal linear sclerosis on radiographs?

A. Base of the first metatarsal

B. Mid-shaft of the second metatarsal

C. Head of the third metatarsal

D. Distal shaft of the fourth metatarsal

E. Base of the fifth metatarsal

119. A 35-year-old woman with a palpable nodule in the left lobe of the thyroid gland showed a corresponding area of low activity on nuclear medicine study consistent with a cold nodule. How would you investigate this patient further?

A. MRI neck

B. CT neck with contrast

C. US neck

D. US neck with FNA

E. Sialogram

120. A 3-month-old man is brought to the accident and emergency department following possible aspiration of a foreign body. The abdominal X-ray is normal, but CXR demonstrates a large mediastinal mass with wavy margins. No foreign body is identified. What is the most appropriate management?

A. Check full blood count

B. Discharge with reassurance

C. Repeat CXR in 6 weeks

D. List for bronchoscopy under anaesthetic

E. CT of chest

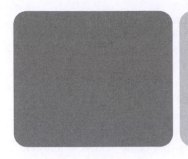

CHAPTER 8
TEST PAPER 4

Answers

1. A. Hyperintense on MR images acquired during the hepatobiliary phase after injection of hepatocyte-specific contrast agent

At contrast-enhanced CT and MR imaging, infiltrative HCC may be difficult to discern from underlying heterogeneous cirrhosis because of its permeative appearance, its minimal and inconsistent arterial enhancement and the heterogeneous washout appearance that occurs during the venous phase. The enhancement pattern of infiltrative HCC seen on images obtained during the hepatic arterial phase has been reported as minimal, patchy or miliary.

Although arterial hyperenhancement is a key diagnostic feature of nodular and massive HCC, infiltrative HCC may commonly appear as iso- or hypointense on images obtained during the arterial phase. Washout appearance is a specific CT and MR imaging feature of typical nodular HCC. Hypointensity relative to the surrounding liver parenchyma during the venous phase of enhancement remains a valid sign for the detection of infiltrative HCC. However, washout appearance of the tumour is usually reported as irregular and heterogeneous and is less frequently seen in infiltrative HCC than in other HCC subtypes.

Moreover, a reticular appearance of the tumour has been seen on images obtained during the venous and equilibrium phases, possibly related to fibrosis. Finally, the tumour generally appears as hypointense on MR images acquired during the hepatobiliary phase after injection of hepatocyte-specific contrast agent because of the lack of contrast agent uptake.

Reynolds AR. Infiltrative hepatocellular carcinoma: What radiologists need to know. *Radiographics*. 2015;35: 371–86.

2. C. Lofgren's syndrome Systemic lupus erythematosus (SLE)

NSIP is more common than UIP. Although NSIP is defined as idiopathic, the morphologic pattern is seen with connective-tissue diseases, hypersensitivity pneumonitis or drug exposure. LIP is exceedingly rare. It is seen as a secondary disease in association with Sjögren syndrome, HIV infection and variable immunodeficiency syndromes.

Loffler's syndrome refers to simple pulmonary eosinophilia, with high eosinophil count in peripheral blood and fleeting air space opacities. Round atelectasis or folded lung is a recognised asbestos-related lung abnormality. Lofgren's syndrome is an acute form of sarcoidosis characterised by erythema nodosum, bilateral hilar lymphadenopathy and polyarthralgia or polyarthritis.

Adam A, et al. *Grainger & Allison's Diagnostic Radiology: A Textbook of Medical Imaging*. 5th edn. New York: Churchill Livingstone, 2008:372, 412.
Dähnert W. *Radiology Review Manual*. 7th edn. Philadelphia, PA: Lippincott Williams & Wilkins, 2011:540.
Mueller-Mang C, et al. What every radiologist should know about idiopathic interstitial pneumonias. *Radiographics*. 2007;27(3):595–615.

3. E. Sertoli cell tumour is the most common malignant testicular tumour.

Cryptorchidism is defined as complete or partial failure of the intra-abdominal testes to descend into the scrotal sac. The undescended testis may be positioned anywhere along the normal path of descent. The most common location is in the inguinal canal (72%), followed by prescrotal (20%). Simple testicular cysts are mostly found incidentally, non-palpable, in men above 40 years, located at the mediastinum testis. Testicular metastases are rare and a sign of advanced primary disease, mostly from the prostate (35%), lung (20%), melanoma, colon or kidney. They may appear discrete or diffusely infiltrate the parenchyma. Tubular ectasia of the rete testis is a benign condition resulting from partial or complete obliteration of the efferent ducts that cause ectasia of the rete testis. Germ cell tumours are the most common testicular malignancy.

Dogra VS, et al. Sonography of the scrotum. *Radiology*. 2003;227(1):18–36.

4. B. Simple bone cyst

The fallen fragment sign comprises a small fragment that lies in the dependant portion of a radiolucent skeletal lesion. It is mostly recognised in radiograph, but analogous findings can be seen on CT or MRI.

A dependant bone fragment can result from a pathologic fracture through thin cortical wall of a simple bone cyst. After minor trauma periosteum and surrounding muscle prevents centrifugal displacement of fracture fragment. However, a fractured fragment can become dislodged and fall centrally. The fluid content of the lesion allows the fragment to drop to the dependant portion of the cyst.

Killeen, KL. The fallen fragment sign. *Radiology*. 1998;207:261–2.

5. C. Progressive multifocal leukoencephalopathy

The most common imaging manifestation of HIV infection is global atrophy that is out of proportion to age. The finding of diffuse cerebral atrophy can be accompanied by diffuse, confluent, ill-defined areas of abnormally increased signal intensity on T2-weighted MRI of the periventricular white matter. No enhancement is noted. The findings may be accompanied by encephalopathy (AIDS dementia complex). These global abnormalities were previously attributed to a subacute encephalitis caused by HIV. It now seems likely that both HIV and CMV can cause subacute encephalitis and encephalopathy; these conditions have an identical non-specific imaging appearance. CMV encephalopathy appears to manifest itself late in the illness, whereas HIV dementia (although usually presenting late) can occasionally be the AIDS-defining illness.

Progressive multifocal leukoencephalopathy is the most serious focal lesion without significant mass effect. It is caused by the JC virus. On CT, the lesions have low attenuation. On MRI, they are of low signal intensity on TI-weighted images and high signal intensity on T2-weighted images. They exhibit little or no mass effect. Although ring enhancement has been reported, these lesions generally do not enhance on CT or MRI. They often occur at the interface between the grey matter and the white matter and have a scalloped contour secondary to involvement of peripheral U-fibres. The parietal lobe is predominantly affected, but these lesions also occur in the periventricular white matter, posterior fossa, brainstem, spinal cord and even the basal ganglia.

Walot I, et al. Neuroimaging findings in patients with AIDS. *Clin Infect Dis*. 1996;22(6):906–19.

6. C. Oesophageal duplication cyst

Oesophageal duplication cysts are rare congenital anomalies. They are associated with vertebral anomalies (spina bifida, hemivertebrae, fusion defects). There is also an association with oesophageal atresia and small bowel duplication. Most cysts develop in the right posteroinferior mediastinum.

CT demonstrates a well-marginated round, oval or tubular-shaped fluid-filled cystic structure that has a well-defined, thin wall. The cyst is of water attenuation with no enhancement of contents and no infiltration of surrounding structures. Malignant degeneration is rare.

Bronchogenic cyst is the most common cystic mediastinal mass that typically lies in the middle mediastinum, not in a paraspinal location; in addition, you would not expect an air–fluid level. Cystic teratoma is an anterior mediastinal mass. Morgagni hernia would be unlikely to cause a solitary round lesion; multiple structures would be expected.

Dähnert W. *Radiology Review Manual.* 7th edn. Philadelphia, PA: Lippincott Williams & Wilkins, 2011:840. Rattan KN, et al. Mediastinal foregut duplication cysts. *Indian J Pediatr.* 2004;71;103–5.

7. C. Colon

Liver metastases may be hypovascular or hypervascular. Colon, lung, breast and gastric carcinomas are the most common tumours causing hypovascular liver metastases, and they typically show perilesional enhancement. Neuroendocrine tumours (including carcinoid and islet cell tumours) renal cell carcinoma, breast, melanoma and thyroid carcinoma are the tumours most commonly causing hypervascular hepatic metastases, which may develop early enhancement with variable degrees of washout and peripheral rim enhancement.

Statistically, colonic metastases are more common than gastric carcinoma metastasis to the liver.

Namasivayam S, et al. Imaging of liver metastases: MRI. *Cancer Imaging.* 2007;7(1):2–9.

8. E. Reimplantation response

Ischaemia–reperfusion injury or reimplantation response is a non-cardiogenic pulmonary oedema that typically occurs more than 24 hours after transplantation, peaks in severity on post-operative Day 4, and generally improves by the end of the first week. The oedema may continue up to 6 months post-operative; however, in most lung transplant recipients, it has cleared completely by 2 months. The radiographic and HRCT features are non-specific and may include perihilar ground-glass opacities, peribronchial and perivascular thickening, and reticular interstitial or airspace opacities located predominantly in the middle and lower lung lobes.

Acute rejection due to a cell-mediated immune response commonly occurs in the second week post-operative. HRCT features are also relatively non-specific and may include ground-glass opacities (often with basal distribution), peribronchial cuffing, septal thickening and pleural effusion.

Krishnam MS. Post-operative complications of lung transplantation: Radiologic findings along a time continuum. *Radiographics.* 2007;27(4):957–74.

9. A. Leydig cell tumour

Cryptorchidism is associated with an increased risk of testicular germ cell tumours, more so with bilateral undescended testes. Germ cell tumours are seminomatous or non-seminomatous, which are embryonal cell tumour, yolk sac tumour, choriocarcinoma and teratoma. Sertoli cell and Leydig cell tumours are non-germ cell tumours.

Dogra VS, et al. Sonography of the scrotum. *Radiology.* 2003;227(1):18–36.

10. C. Lateral aspect of the medial tibial plateau

Osteochondral defect (OCD) (previously called *osteochondritis dissecans*) may result directly from trauma or secondarily from loss of blood supply to an area of subchondral bone, resulting in avascular necrosis. The overlying cartilage, which is nourished by synovial fluid, remains intact to variable degrees. As the necrotic bone is resorbed, the overlying cartilage loses its support. Without its cartilage cover, the bony fragment may become dislodged into the joint.

Common sites of involvement include the lateral aspect of the medial femoral condyle, followed by the talar dome (posteromedial more than anteromedial), anterolateral aspect of the capitellum and the tibial plafond. Rarer sites include navicular, femoral head, humeral head, glenoid and scaphoid.

MRI Grading of OCD

I.   Marrow oedema (stable).
II. Articular cartilage breached. Low-signal rim surrounding fragment indicates fibrous attachment (stable).

III. Pockets of fluid (high signal on T2-weighted images) around undetached and undisplaced osteochondral fragment (unstable).

IV. Displaced osteochondral fragment (unstable).

MSK Residents Project. University of Washington, UWMC Roosevelt Clinic, Musculoskeletal Radiology.

11. D. Reversible posterior leukoencephalopathy syndrome

Reversible posterior leukoencephalopathy syndrome also known as posterior reversible encephalopathy syndrome (PRES), is most commonly encountered in association with acute hypertension, preeclampsia or eclampsia, renal disease, sepsis and exposure to immunosuppressants. At CT or MR imaging, the brain typically demonstrates focal regions of symmetric hemispheric oedema. The parietal and occipital lobes are most commonly affected, followed by the frontal lobes, the inferior temporal–occipital junction and the cerebellum. Lesion confluence may develop as the extent of oedema increases. MR DWI was instrumental in establishing and consistently demonstrating that the areas of abnormality represent vasogenic oedema. The oedema usually completely reverses. Focal or patchy areas of PRES vasogenic oedema may also be seen in the basal ganglia, brainstem and deep white matter (external/internal capsule). When they accompany hemispheric or cerebellar PRES, it is easy to recognise these. Present in isolation or when the hemispheric pattern is incompletely expressed (partial/asymmetric), diagnosis of PRES can be challenging. If cerebellar or brainstem involvement are extensive, hydrocephalus and brainstem compression may occur. Focal areas of restricted diffusion (likely representing infarction or tissue injury with cytotoxic oedema) are uncommon (11%–26%) and may be associated with an adverse outcome. Haemorrhage (focal haematoma, isolated sulcal/subarachnoid blood or protein) is seen in approximately 15% of patients.

Bartynski WS. Posterior reversible encephalopathy syndrome, part 1: Fundamental imaging and clinical features. *AJNR Am J Neuroradiol.* 2008;29(6):1036–42.

Fugate JE, et al. Posterior reversible encephalopathy syndrome: Associated clinical and radiologic findings. *Mayo Clin Proc.* 2010;85(5):427–32.

12. C. Congenital cystic adenomatoid malformation

Congenital cystic adenomatoid malformation is a developmental hamartomatous abnormality of lung with adenomatoid proliferation of cysts resembling bronchioles. It is thought to be caused by focal arrest in foetal lung development before the seventh week of gestation. Congenital cystic adenomatoid malformation represents 25% of all congenital lung lesions.

A CXR on Day 1 of life usually demonstrates dense lungs with increased volume on the affected side. On Day 2, a CXR usually demonstrates resorption of fluid from affected areas of lung, which are then replaced with air-containing spaces.

Communication with the tracheobronchial tree is maintained and the vascular supply and drainage are to the pulmonary circulation. There is a slight predilection for the upper lobes.

Newborns often present with respiratory distress secondary to mass effect and pulmonary compression or hypoplasia. The chest is dull to percussion with decreased air entry. Prenatal ultrasound shows a partly cystic, partly echogenic mass.

Mandel G. *Imaging in Congenital Cystic Adenomatoid Malformation.* emedicine.medscape.com/article/407407-overview [accessed on 18 February 2017].

13. D. Cholangiocarcinoma

Intrahepatic cholangiocarcinoma is the second most common primary hepatic tumour. Various risk factors have been reported for intrahepatic cholangiocarcinoma, and the radiologic and pathologic findings of this disease entity may differ depending on the underlying risk factors.

Intrahepatic cholangiocarcinoma can be classified into three types on the basis of gross morphologic features: mass forming (the most common), periductal infiltrating and intraductal growth. At CT, mass-forming intrahepatic cholangiocarcinoma usually appears as a homogeneous low-attenuation mass with irregular peripheral enhancement; it can be accompanied by capsular retraction, satellite nodules and peripheral intrahepatic duct dilatation. Periductal infiltrating cholangiocarcinoma is characterised by growth along the dilated or narrowed bile duct without mass formation. On CT and MRI, diffuse periductal thickening and increased enhancement can be seen with a dilated or irregularly narrowed intrahepatic duct. Intraductal cholangiocarcinoma may manifest with various imaging patterns, including diffuse and marked duct ectasia either with or without a grossly visible papillary mass, an intraductal polypoid mass within localised ductal dilatation, intraductal cast-like lesions within a mildly dilated duct and a focal stricture-like lesion with mild proximal ductal dilatation.

Chung YE, et al. Varying appearances of cholangiocarcinoma: Radiologic-pathologic correlation. *Radiographics*. 2009;29:683–700.

14. E. Lymphangioleiomyomatosis

The reversed halo sign is characterised by a central ground-glass opacity surrounded by denser air–space consolidation in the shape of a crescent or a ring. Causes include opportunistic and endemic fungal infection, with invasive pulmonary aspergillosis being the most common type. Other infectious causes include TB, bacterial infection, Legionnaires' pneumonia and pneumocystis jiroveci pneumonia. Non-infectious causes include COP, sarcoidosis, lipoid pneumonia, Wegner's granulomatosis and pulmonary embolism. Neoplastic causes include lymphomatoid granulomatosis, pulmonary adenocarcinoma and haemorrhagic metastasis like renal or choriocarcinoma. RFA and radiation therapy are other causes. Lymphangioleiomyomatosis typically manifests as multiple thin walled cysts uniformly distributed throughout the lungs.

Godoy MCB, et al. The reversed halo sign: Update and differential diagnosis. *Br J Radiol*. 2012;85(1017): 1226–35.

15. B. Renovascular compromise

The rim sign is associated with major vascular compromise in the kidney. This sign is most commonly seen with renal artery obstruction from thrombosis, embolus or dissection. On contrast-enhanced CT or MRI, a 1- to 3-mm rim of subcapsular enhancement, paralleling the renal margin, can be seen as a result of preserved perfusion of the outer renal cortex by capsular perforating vessels. The finding may be accompanied by an abrupt termination of contrast material in the renal artery, referred to as the *arterial cut-off sign*. The rim sign of vascular compromise has also been described with renal vein thrombosis and acute tubular necrosis.

Dyer RB, et al. Classic signs in uroradiology. *Radiographics*. 2004;24 Suppl 1:S247–80.

16. D. Transient osteoporosis

Transient osteoporosis is a rare, self-limiting condition that usually affects the hip. Classically, it is characterised by disabling pain in the hip without preceding trauma, and there is radiographic evidence of a focal region of osteopenia isolated to the hip. Although avascular necrosis can also present with a focal region of osteopenia in the early stages of the disease, transient osteoporosis resolves in 6–8 months, whereas avascular necrosis is usually progressive. It is thought that transient osteoporosis could represent a non-traumatic form of Sudeck atrophy or reflex sympathetic dystrophy.

Guerra JJ, Steinberg ME. Distinguishing transient osteoporosis from avascular necrosis of the hip. *J Bone Joint Surg Am*. 1995;77:616–24.
Sutton D. *Textbook of Radiology and Imaging*. 7th edn. Edinburgh: Churchill Livingstone, 2003.

17. D. Plain chest radiograph

Central nervous system involvement is seen in 5% of patients with systemic sarcoidosis (neurosarcoidosis). The most common parenchymal abnormality described in some series is multiple non-enhancing periventricular white matter lesions, seen as high signal intensity on T2-weighted images.

Enhancing parenchymal mass lesions are also commonly reported. These lesions may be mistaken for primary or metastatic tumour or tumefactive demyelination. Enhancing mass lesions are frequently associated with nearby leptomeningeal involvement. Leptomeningeal involvement is perhaps the most typical manifestation of central nervous system sarcoidosis, seen in about 40% of cases. This is usually seen as thickening and enhancement of the leptomeninges on contrast-enhanced T1-weighted images. The enhancement may be diffuse or nodular. Leptomeningeal involvement around the hypothalamus and pituitary infundibulum may be seen with basilar leptomeningeal involvement or as an isolated finding. Cranial nerve involvement is also described. Any cranial nerve can be affected, but the most common cranial nerve deficit involves the facial nerve (VII), whereas radiographically the optic nerves (II) are most commonly abnormal.

Smith JK, et al. Imaging manifestations of neurosarcoidosis. *AJR Am J Roentgenol.* 2004;182(2):289–95.

18. C. Pneumocystis pneumonia (PCP)

PCP is the most common opportunistic infection in immunosuppressed children, occurring in up to 90% of HIV-positive patients. A clinico-pathological and radiological continuum has been reported since the earliest documented cases of PCP. At one end of the spectrum are children with a florid clinical course, who progress from health to death in days. They show marked hypoxia and rapid radiographic evolution of parahilar granular infiltrates to extensive bilateral airspace opacification. Pathologically, an extensive foamy alveolar exudate is seen. Conversely, there are those with an insidious presentation, less profound hypoxia and a slower recovery. These patients tend not to progress to alveolar opacification but show persistent bilateral granular or ground-glass opacification, representing relative prominence of interstitial pulmonary involvement.

Pitchera RD, Zar HJ. Radiographic features of paediatric pneumocystis pneumonia – A historical perspective. *Clin Radiol.* 2008;63:666–72.

19. A. HCC is characteristically hyperechoic on ultrasound.

HCC does not have a characteristic appearance at US. The lesions are typically hypoechoic, but they can be hyperechoic or have mixed echogenicity. The majority of nodules that measure less than 1 cm are not HCC. Detected nodules that measure less than 1 cm should be rescanned at a 3-month interval with the modality by which the lesions were first identified. If the nodules remain stable for a 2-year period, regular 6-month follow-up examinations can be resumed for routine surveillance. The nodules that are suspicious for HCC are new nodules that measure more than 1 cm or nodules that enlarge over a time interval. These suspicious nodules require immediate further investigation with multiphasic CT or MRI.

The radiologic diagnosis of HCC can be made at either CT or MR imaging, provided that a multiphasic contrast material–enhanced study is used. Characteristically, HCC enhances during the arterial phase because of its blood supply from abnormal hepatic arteries. Contrast medium in the surrounding liver parenchyma is diluted during this phase, because the parenchymal blood supply arises mostly from the portal veins, which are not yet opacified. In the portal venous phase, the surrounding liver parenchyma becomes relatively hyperattenuated and the lesion is perceived to be hypoattenuated because of its lack of portal venous supply. This appearance is the so-called washout effect. Occasionally, washout is evident only during a delayed-phase sequence.

HCC differs from most malignancies because it is commonly diagnosed on the basis of imaging features alone, without histologic confirmation.

McEvoy SH, et al. Hepatocellular carcinoma: Illustrated guide to systematic radiologic diagnosis and staging according to guidelines of the American Association for the Study of Liver Diseases. *Radiographics.* 2013;33:1653–68.

20. B. Patchy ground-glass opacities with centrilobular nodules

In acute hypersensitive pneumonitis, symptoms may begin after patients return to an environment from which they have been absent for a while (e.g., resuming work following weekends or holidays). Chest radiographs obtained in many patients with hypersensitivity pneumonitis are normal. HRCT typically shows patchy ground-glass opacities and centrilobular nodules. Respiratory bronchiolitis–interstitial lung disease is a smoking-related lung disease that has similar imaging features.

Perilymphatic nodules and beaded features are features of sarcoidosis, while central bronchiectasis is a typical feature of ABPA. The crazy paving pattern is seen in pulmonary alveolar proteinosis but can also be seen in mucinous broncho-alveolar carcinoma, exogenous lipoid pneumonia, sarcoidosis, NSIP, pneumocystis pneumonia and several other diffuse acute conditions.

Elicker B, et al. High-resolution computed tomography patterns of diffuse interstitial lung disease with clinical and pathological correlation. *J Bras Pneumol*. 2008;34(9):715–44.

21. A. Hydronephrosis

A different type of rim sign is seen in association with chronic hydronephrosis. After contrast material is administered, enhancement occurs in the residual, but markedly atrophic, renal parenchyma, surrounding the dilated calices and renal pelvis. Unlike vascular compromise, the thickness of the enhancing rim varies along its length. The inner margin of this hydronephrotic rim is concave towards the renal hilum, and enhancement of the cortical columns between the dilated collecting system elements may be seen. Unopacified urine in the dilated collecting system may produce a negative pyelogram.

Dyer RB, et al. Classic signs in uroradiology. *Radiographics*. 2004;24 Suppl 1:S247–80.

22. D. Post-contrast gadolinium enhancement

A convex posterior border of the vertebral body is more frequent in metastatic compression fractures than acute osteoporotic compression fractures. A higher frequency of abnormal signal intensity of the pedicle of metastatic fractures is seen in comparison to acute osteoporotic fractures; posterior element involvement is observed more commonly in metastatic compression fractures in comparison to benign fractures. Although epidural mass was suggestive of metastatic fractures, a paraspinal mass is more commonly associated with metastatic compression fracture. Metastatic involvement of other vertebra is also more likely to suggest malignant compression fracture.

Spared normal bone marrow signal intensity of the vertebral body is highly suggestive of acute osteoporotic compression fractures. Band-like low signal intensity on T1-weighted and T2-weighted images is more common in acute osteoporotic compression fractures than metastatic compression fractures. Retropulsion of a posterior bone fragment is more frequent in osteoporotic compression fractures than metastatic compression fractures, although multiple fractures are more commonly benign. Post-contrast enhancement is seen in both malignant and benign causes.

Jung et al. Discrimination of metastatic from acute osteoporotic compression spinal fractures with MR imaging. *Radiographics*. 2003;23:179–87.

23. E. A single lesion is the most common.

Toxoplasmosis is the most common opportunistic CNS infection in patients with AIDS. Toxoplasmosis typically manifests on CT scans and MRIs as nodular (small-encephalitis) and/or ring-enhancing (large-abscess) lesions within the brain parenchyma. The enhancing ring, when present, may be somewhat thicker and more ill-defined than that seen in association with a typical bacterial abscess.

The lesions are associated with surrounding oedema and tend to be multiple at presentation. However, a significant percentage of patients present with solitary lesions. Toxoplasmic lesions are most often seen in the basal ganglia and grey–white interface of the cerebral hemispheres. On non-enhanced T1-weighted MR images, the lesions are of low signal intensity; on T2-weighted MR images, the lesions are mildly to moderately hyperintense in relation to the brain parenchyma and can be difficult to separate from the surrounding oedema. Therapy is often begun empirically as soon as CT scans or MR images show focal parenchymal lesions of any sort because the infection is so common in this population. The presence of small haemorrhages may be a sign of toxoplasmosis, and calcifications can occasionally be seen in treated lesions.

Walot I, et al. Neuroimaging findings in patients with AIDS. *Clin Infect Dis.* 1996;22(6):906–19.

24. C.   Thyroid dyshormonogenesis

Thyroid dysgenesis is the most common cause for congenital hypothyroidism, accounting for up to 85% of cases (causes include ectopy, aplasia and hypoplasia); however in this case, the ultrasound and scintigraphy findings do not suggest this as a cause.

The second most common reason is therefore thyroid dyshormonogenesis, accounting for 10%–15% of cases (also described as *thyroid hormone biosynthetic defect*, e.g., hereditary Pendred's syndrome). The remainder of the causes listed are extremely rare.

Tasker RC, et al. *Oxford Handbook of Paediatrics.* Oxford. Oxford University Press, 2008.

25. D.   Infantile haemangioendothelioma

Although primary hepatic neoplasms represent only a small percentage of solid tumours that occur in children, the finding of focal hepatic lesions in a child is not an uncommon event in a busy radiology practice. The most common neoplasm involving the liver in children, as in adults, is metastatic disease. Most primary liver tumours in children are malignant, but one-third are benign; benign lesions may be of mesenchymal or epithelial origin. The most common benign tumours are, in decreasing order of frequency, infantile haemangioendothelioma, FNH, mesenchymal hamartoma, nodular regenerative hyperplasia (NRH) and hepatocellular adenoma.

Chung EM, et al. Pediatric liver masses: Radiologic-pathologic correlation part 1. Benign tumors. *Radiographics.* 2010;30:801–26.

26. C.   Chronic destructive sinusitis with nasal perforation

Wegener's granulomatosis is a probable autoimmune disease characterised by systemic necrotising granulomatous destructive angitis, with a classic triad of respiratory tract inflammation, systemic small vessel vasculitis and necrotising glomerulonephritis.

Sinus disease classically includes destructive sinusitis, nasal septal ulceration, septal perforation and saddle nose deformity.

Dähnert W. *Radiology Review Manual.* 7th edn. Philadelphia, PA: Lippincott Williams & Wilkins, 2011: 551–2.

27. D.   Reverse rim sign

The reverse rim sign refers to a hypoattenuating renal cortex visualised at CT, seen against a background of intact medullary perfusion after contrast material is given. This sign also implies severe derangement of cortical blood flow with development of cortical necrosis. Cortical necrosis may develop as a consequence of obstetric complications, shock from numerous causes, transfusion reaction or other causes of intravascular haemolysis, toxins and rejection in the transplanted kidney. The comet tail sign refers to pelvic phleboliths and the soft-tissue rim sign is related to distal ureteric calculus. The crescent sign refers to the appearance of concentrated contrast material in collecting tubules, arranged parallel to the margin of a dilated calix, which produces a thin line of contrast material at the edge of the calices, resembling a crescent.

Dyer RB, et al. Classic signs in uroradiology. *Radiographics.* 2004;24 Suppl 1:S247–80.

28. E. Buttressing

Periosteal reaction is a sign of new bone formation. Buttressing indicates a slow-growing process with a single, thick layer of periosteum (i.e., a solid periosteal reaction). It is found in conditions such as hypertrophic pulmonary osteoarthropathy, atherosclerosis and benign tumours.

More aggressive, faster-growing lesions can cause an interrupted periosteal reaction; lamination (layering) of the periosteum, Codman's triangles where new bone formation only occurs at the margins of the tumour, sunburst pattern and hair-on-end (this is seen in lesions that invade bone marrow).

Periosteal reaction is, however, only one of a list of many characteristics of a bone lesion that help determine whether the lesion is biologically active or not.

Dähnert W. *Radiology Review Manual*. 6th edn. Philadelphia, PA: Lippincott Williams & Wilkins, 2007:12.

29. C. Pheochromocytoma

Tuberous sclerosis is a neuroectodermal disorder, characterised by the classic triad of adenoma sebaceum, seizures and mental retardation. CNS findings include subependymal hamartomas, giant cell astrocytoma (at the foramen of Monro), cortical tubers and heterotopic islands of grey in white matter. Pulmonary involvement include interstitial fibrosis at lung bases, LAM, multiple lung cysts and chylothorax. Cardiac involvement includes rhabdomyoma, aortic aneurysm and congenital cardiomyopathy. Renal involvement includes AML, cysts and RCCs. Ocular lesions include optic nerve glioma and hamartoma. Other visceral abnormalities include splenic tumour, pancreatic and hepatic adenomas.

Dähnert W. *Radiology Review Manual*. 7th edn. Philadelphia, PA: Lippincott Williams & Wilkins, 2011: 333–5.

30. D. A plain abdominal radiograph should be obtained prior to air enema reduction to rule out signs of perforation.

The traditional role of plain radiography in the evaluation of children suspected to have intussusception is threefold:

1. When the clinical suspicion is low, the role of plain radiography is to allow exclusion of intussusception and diagnosis of other pathologic processes that are responsible for the patient's symptoms.
2. When the clinical suspicion is high, the role of plain radiography is to allow confirmation of intussusception.
3. If intussusception is present, the role of plain radiography is to allow exclusion of intestinal obstruction or perforation.

del Pozo G, et al. Intussusception in children: Current concepts in diagnosis and enema reduction. *Radiographics*. 1999;19:299–319.

31. D. Avid arterial-phase enhancement

HEH is a low-grade primary malignancy of the hepatic vasculature with an incidence of less than 0.1 per 100,000 in the general population per year. Because its occurrence is so rare, the patient demographics cannot be accurately assessed.

However, demographic data from case review studies indicate an age range of 25–58 years (average 43.5 years) and a slight female predominance (male to female ratio 2:3). Typical manifestations of HEH include non-focal abdominal pain, jaundice and hepatosplenomegaly, but HEH has also been discovered incidentally in asymptomatic patients. Budd–Chiari syndrome can develop if the tumour invades the hepatic veins.

Alternating high- and low-signal-intensity rings on T2-weighted and contrast-enhanced T1-weighted images have been characterised as a 'target' sign. The tumours typically exhibit central signal hypointensity on unenhanced T1-weighted images and a multilayered target-like appearance with prominent rim-like enhancement on contrast-enhanced T1-weighted images.

The presence of capsular retraction in subcapsular hepatic tumours, along with a target-like appearance of the tumours on contrast-enhanced CT and MR images, is suggestive but not necessarily indicative of HEH. This constellation of findings can be found in peripheral cholangiocarcinoma, confluent foci of hepatic fibrosis (usually in the setting of advanced cirrhosis), previously treated primary or metastatic HCCs and large atypical cavernous haemangiomas. However, the absence of cirrhosis in a patient with multiple liver masses that coalesce over time to form larger masses, in combination with other characteristic imaging findings of HEH, increases the likelihood of this diagnosis.

Azzam RI. Hepatic epithelioid hemangioendothelioma. *Radiographics*. 2012;32:789–94.

32. A.   Peripheral predominant lobular consolidation with centrilobular nodules.

On thin-section CT, the parenchymal abnormal findings of CSS could be classified into three patterns. The first pattern is subpleural consolidation with lobular distribution. The second pattern is centrilobular perivascular densities, diffusely scattered centrilobular nodules <5 mm in diameter, especially within the ground-glass opacity lesion. The third pattern is multiple larger nodules. Bronchial wall thickening, with or without bronchial dilatation, and hyperinflation are likely to be related to asthma. Interlobular septal thickening may reflect the interstitial pulmonary oedema attributed to the cardiac and pericardial involvement.

Peripheral predominant homogenous consolidation is a feature of chronic pulmonary eosinophilia. Nodules are not a feature of chronic pulmonary eosinophilia. Central bronchiectasis and mucous plugs are a feature of ABPA.

Choi YH, et al. Thoracic manifestation of Churg-Strauss syndrome: Radiologic and clinical findings. *Chest*. 2000;117(1):117–24.

33. C.   Pie-in-the-sky bladder sign   Bilateral psoas hypertrophy

The spoked wheel description was applied to the angiographic appearance of the vascular pattern seen in some oncocytomas. Centripetal 'spoke' vessels arising from a peripheral 'rim' vessel were initially thought to be characteristic of this tumour. However, the pattern is now known to be non-specific, and a similar vascular arrangement has been described with renal cell carcinoma.

The normal round shape of the opacified bladder may assume a pear or tear drop shape when it is symmetrically compressed in the pelvis by an extrinsic process. The differential diagnosis includes pelvic fluid (haematoma, lymphocele, urinoma or abscess), pelvic lipomatosis, vascular dilatation (aneurysm or collateral vessel development), symmetric lymph node enlargement and psoas muscle hypertrophy. A pie-in-the-sky bladder may be seen with pelvic trauma. The sign refers to the high position of the opacified bladder within the pelvis at imaging and implies the presence of a large pelvic haematoma; it should raise concern for an associated urethral injury.

A linear filling defect within the bladder may result from extrusion of a blood clot from the ureter, which has acted as a mould, in gross haematuria. This spaghetti sign implies that the bleeding source is above the bladder.

Balloon-on-a-string sign refers to the appearance of a high and somewhat eccentric exit point of the ureter from a dilated renal pelvis and is a typical finding of ureteropelvic junction obstruction.

Dyer RB, et al. Classic signs in uroradiology. *Radiographics*. 2004;24 Suppl 1:S247–80.

34. B.   Perilunate dislocation

Lunate and perilunate dislocations and fracture dislocations may be easily overlooked on plain films and should be actively sought and excluded given an appropriate clinical history. On the AP view, the lines along the proximal poles of both the proximal and distal carpal rows should be

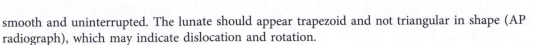

smooth and uninterrupted. The lunate should appear trapezoid and not triangular in shape (AP radiograph), which may indicate dislocation and rotation.

On the lateral view, the distal radius, lunate and capitate should be in alignment. Volar loss of lunate alignment is seen in lunate dislocation, and dorsal loss of capitate alignment is seen in perilunate dislocation. In addition, the scapholunate (normal 30–60 degrees) and the capitolunate (normal 0–30 degrees) should be assessed for evidence of intercalated segmental instability.

Murray PM. Perilunate fracture dislocations. http://emedicine.medscape.com/article/1240108-overview [accessed on 18 February 2017].

35. B. It contains small arterial channels

Developmental venous anomalies (DVAs), also called *venous angiomas*, are variations of the normal veins that are necessary for the drainage of white and grey matter. They are associated with other vascular malformations like cavernoma. On contrast-enhanced CT, the venous collector of the DVA is readily detectable as a linear or curvilinear focus of enhancement, typically coursing from the deep white matter to a cortical or a deep vein or to the dural sinus. On MRI, DVAs typically have a transhemispheric flow void, on both T1-weighted and T2-weighted images. The collector vein is detected as a linear or small, round, signal-void structure on all sequences and is shown most clearly on T2-weighted imaging. On contrast-enhanced MRI, the cluster of veins in DVAs has a spoked wheel appearance; the veins are small at the periphery and gradually enlarge as they approach a central draining vein. This appearance has been referred to as *caput medusae* (or the 'head of Medusa').

Lee M, Kim MS. Image findings in brain developmental venous anomalies. *J Cerebrovasc Endovasc Neurosurg.* 2012;14(1):37–43.

36. A. Lymphoid interstitial pneumonitis

Early complications – complications that occur at any point from the time of transplantation to the end of the early post-engraftment period – include interstitial pneumonitis (infective and non-infective types), infection, oedema, haemorrhage, thromboembolism and calcification.
Bronchiolitis obliterans with organising pneumonia (BOOP) is a rare complication that may occur during the early or late post-engraftment period.

Late pulmonary complications – complications that occur more than 100 days after engraftment – include chronic GVH disease, infections, bronchiolitis obliterans, fibrosis and lymphoid interstitial pneumonitis.

Levine DS, et al. Imaging the complications of bone marrow transplantation in children. *Radiographics.* 2007;27:307–24.

37. E. Background cirrhotic change to the liver parenchyma

Fibrolamellar HCC is a rare hepatic neoplasm that accounts for less than 1% of HCC in the United States. This tumour has unique clinicopathologic features that are significantly different compared with conventional HCC. Fibrolamellar HCC predominantly occurs in young individuals.

On MRI, fibrolamellar HCC is usually hypointense on T1-weighted images and hyperintense on T2-weighted images. The fibrous central scar is typically hypointense on both T1-weighted and T2-weighted images. This feature can help to distinguish fibrolamellar HCC from FNH because the central scar in the latter is predominantly T2 hyperintense. The presence of intralesional fat has not been reported in fibrolamellar HCC. Calcification may be difficult to identify on MRI. Gadolinium contrast enhancement characteristics of fibrolamellar HCC mimic the patterns seen on CT showing marked heterogeneous contrast enhancement on the arterial phase and becoming isointense or hypointense on the portal venous and delayed phase. Some authors have reported that fibrolamellar HCC does not retain hepatobiliary-specific contrast agents, such as gadoxetate disodium and gadobenate dimeglumine, on the hepatobiliary phase, which potentially may be useful in differentiating fibrolamellar HCC from FNH.

Ghaneshan D, et al. Imaging Features of Fibrolamellar Hepatocellular Carcinoma. *AJR Am J Roentgenol.* 2014;202:544–52.

38. A. Cardiac concussion results in abnormal cardiac enzymes.

Blunt cardiac injury (BCI) is the most common type of cardiac injury after blunt thoracic trauma. In cardiac concussion, the mildest form of cardiac injury, there is no myocardial cell damage or elevated enzyme levels. Cardiac contusion can present as bilateral cardiogenic pulmonary oedema and elevated cardiac enzymes. Echocardiography shows increased myocardial echogenicity and focal systolic hypokinesia, and it is useful in diagnosing other traumatic cardiac injuries that are commonly associated with myocardial contusion, such as pericardial effusion, tamponade, traumatic ventricular septal defect and valvular injury. Typically, traumatic ventricular septal defects occur in the muscular portion of the interventricular septum, near the cardiac apex.

Haemopericardium is commonly associated with cardiac rupture. Tamponade resulting from ventricular rupture is often fatal; however, bleeding from lower pressure atria may be survivable. Besides cardiac chamber rupture, traumatic haemopericardium may also result from aortic root injury, myocardial contusion and coronary artery laceration.

Traumatic pericardial rupture resulting from blunt chest trauma is rare. Tearing may involve either the pleuropericardium or the diaphragmatic pericardium. Cardiac herniation is a serious complication of pericardial rupture.

Restrepo CS. Imaging patients with cardiac trauma. *Radiographics.* 2012;32(3):633–49.

39. C. Low citrate peak, high choline/creatine peak

MRS is a modality that provides information about the cellular metabolites within the prostate gland; it displays the relative concentrations of key chemical constituents, such as citrate, choline and creatine. The normal prostate gland contains low levels of choline and high levels of citrate, whereas prostate cancers have increased levels of choline and decreased levels of citrate. The high choline levels in prostate tumours are related to increased cell turnover. In prostate cancers, the levels of zinc in secretary epithelial cells are lower, which eventually leads to diminished amounts of citrate. Thus, the ratio of choline to citrate is an index of malignancy. The ratio of choline (Cho) plus creatine (Cr) to citrate (Cit) ([Cho + Cr]/Cit) has been widely studied and cut-off values have been suggested for detection of cancer.

Besides analysis of choline, citrate and creatine content, newer image acquisition and analysis software may enable evaluation of other metabolites, such as polyamine peaks, which have also been associated with prostate cancers. MR spectroscopy of tissue samples revealed that levels of polyamines (putrescine and spermine) were reduced in prostate cancer compared with the levels in benign tissue.

Shukla-Dave A, et al. Detection of prostate cancer with MR spectroscopic imaging: An expanded paradigm incorporating polyamines. *Radiology.* 2007;245:499–506.

Turkbey B, et al. Imaging techniques for prostate cancer: Implications for focal therapy. *Nat Rev Urol.* 2009;6(4): 191–203.

40. A. Pigmented villonodular synovitis.

Radiographs may be normal or may reveal periarticular soft-tissue swelling. Visible calcifications are extremely unusual. The joint space is normal in width until late in the course of the disease, and juxta-articular osteoporosis is absent or mild. Bone erosions with sclerotic margins may be present on both sides of the affected joints, particularly in joints with a tight capsule, such as the hip. On MRI, the synovial lesions have low to intermediate signal intensity relative to that of muscle on T1-weighted images and low signal intensity on T2-weighted images, caused by the magnetic susceptibility effect produced by haemosiderin at the periphery of the lesions. The 'black synovium' appearance can also be seen with amyloid deposition or recurrent intra-articular bleeding (e.g., in haemophiliac arthropathy).

Synovial sarcoma presents as a solitary calcified mass outside the joint.

Llauger J, et al. Nonseptic monoarthritis: Imaging features with clinical and histopathologic correlation. *Radiographics*. 2000;20 Spec No:S263–78.

41. B. Syringomyelia

Syringomyelia refers to any cavity within the substance of the spinal cord that may communicate with the central canal, usually extending over several vertebral segments. MRI shows a cystic area with low signal on T1-weighted and increased signal intensity on T2-weighted images. CSF flow void (low signal on T2-weighted images) is often seen in the cavity from pulsation. The cord may show enlargement.

Post-traumatic, post-inflammatory or idiopathic syringomyelia show no abnormal contrast enhancement post-administration of gadolinium. Tumour-associated syrinx may show abnormal enhancement.

Dähnert W. *Radiology Review Manual*. 7th edn. Philadelphia, PA: Lippincott Williams & Wilkins, 2011:229.

42. C. Juvenile dermatomyositis

All other options would cause bronchiectasis, apart from juvenile dermatomyositis (JDM).

JDM is a multisystem autoimmune disease of unknown aetiology that results from inflammation of the small vessels of the muscles, skin, gastrointestinal tract and other organs. It accounts for 85% of cases of paediatric inflammatory myopathy. JDM affects children with an incidence of two or three cases per million children per year. Clinical characteristics of JDM include symmetric proximal muscle weakness, inflammatory cutaneous lesions and Gottron papules (erythematous scaly lesions over the metacarpophalangeal and/or interphalangeal joints), heliotrope (violaceous hue over the eyelids), periorbital oedema, malar erythema, periungual telangiectasia and erythematous scaly rashes over the neck, upper back and extensor surfaces of the extremities.

Agarwal V, et al. Calcinosis in juvenile dermatomyositis. *Radiology*. 2007;242:307–11.

43. C. Simple bone cyst

Simple bone cysts constitute 5% of primary bone lesions with unknown aetiology and consist of cysts filled with yellowish fluid lined by fibrous tissue (rather than epithelial cells; hence some dispute the term *true cyst*).

They are most commonly seen at the proximal humerus and femur; other sites include the fibula, calcaneus, talus and rarer sites like the ribs, hands and feet. They are metaphyseal, intramedullary and central in location (rather than eccentric like ABC). They are close to the epiphysis in the growth phase and migrate to the diaphysis with growth. They do not cross the epiphyseal plate, have a thin sclerotic rim, can cause endosteal scalloping and demonstrate the 'fallen fragment sign' when complicated by pathological fracture.

Dähnert W. *Radiology Review Manual*. 7th edn. Philadelphia, PA: Lippincott Williams & Wilkins, 2011.

44. E. Usually shows late arterial enhancement on the post-contrast sequence.

Angiomyolipoma (AML) is a benign, unencapsulated mesenchymal tumour that is composed of varying proportions of three elements: smooth muscle cells, thick-walled blood vessels and mature adipose tissue. AML occurs more commonly in the kidneys; hepatic involvement is rare. In contrast to renal AML, which is associated with tuberous sclerosis in 20% of patients, hepatic AML is associated with tuberous sclerosis in only 6%. AML can be histologically classified on the basis of fat content into mixed, lipomatous (70% fat), myomatous (10% fat) and angiomatous types. US, CT and MR imaging typically demonstrate the fat component and prominent central vessels. At US, AML may be highly echogenic and is then indistinguishable from haemangiomas.

Frequently, AML has a high fat content, with high signal intensity on T1-weighted images and a significant drop in signal intensity on fat-suppressed images. AML demonstrates early intense contrast enhancement that peaks later than that of a HCC. Dynamic contrast-enhanced CT or MR images obtained during the early phase of enhancement may be useful in discriminating between AML and fat-containing HCC. The fatty areas of AMLs are well vascularised and enhance early, whereas steatotic foci in HCC are relatively avascular and have less contrast enhancement. However, unlike renal AML, 50% of hepatic AMLs lack considerable fat content. Because of this variable fat content, it is difficult to accurately distinguish AML from other hepatic tumours.

Prasad SR, et al. Fat-containing lesions of the liver: Radiologic-pathologic correlation. *Radiographics*. 2005;25:321–31.

45. D. Fat embolism appears in 6 hours and clears in 7–10 days.

Lung contusion turns out to be the most common manifestation of blunt trauma to the chest. Contusions become visible on chest radiographs within 6 hours post-trauma and resolve within 3–7 days. Massive contusion can lead to pulmonary oedema and diffuse alveolar damage (DAD). Aspiration appears within minutes and clears in 24–48 hours unless it triggers an infection with subsequent pneumonia. Pneumonia appears after 5–7 days and clears in 2–4 weeks. Lung infarction due to pulmonary embolism manifests after 3–5 days and clears in approximately 3 weeks. Fat embolism appears after 24–48 hours and clears in 7–10 days. ARDS with diffuse alveolar damage appears after 24–48 hours and clears in 4–6 weeks.

Stark P, Stark HE. Pulmonary manifestations of trauma. *Contemp Diagnos Radiol*. 2010;33(16):1–5.

46. A. High on DWI, low on ADC and corresponding low signal intensity on T2W MRI

T2-weighted images are the 'workhorse' images for prostate cancer. The glandular peripheral zone appears high in signal, whereas the central stroma has lower signal intensity on T2-weighted images. Tumours are lower in signal intensity than normal peripheral zone glandular tissue on T2-weighted images. Peripheral zone cancers are usually round or ill-defined. Various conditions, such as prostatitis, haemorrhage, atrophy, benign prostatic hyperplasia (BPH) and post-treatment changes can mimic cancer. Cancers in the central gland are even more challenging to detect than peripheral zone cancers, because the signal characteristics of the normal and hypertrophic central gland are usually similar to those of the tumour on T2-weighted images. Prostate cancers often include tightly packed glandular elements with increased cellular density and diminished extracellular spaces, which can be detected as high-signal-intensity foci on raw DW-MRI (restricted diffusion) but are low in signal on apparent diffusion coefficient (ADC) maps. ADC maps reflect the amount of diffusion present – the lower the diffusion, the darker the lesion.

Turkbey B, et al. Imaging techniques for prostate cancer: Implications for focal therapy. *Nat Rev Urol*. 2009;6(4): 191–203.

47. D. Soft-tissue calcifications

Acute arthritis may be the first manifestation of sarcoidosis. It is mainly oligoarticular but occasionally polyarticular, and rarely monoarticular. Ankles are the most commonly involved joints. Enthesitis, tendinosis and tenosynovitis are well recognised, especially around the ankle. The triad of acute arthritis, bilateral hilar adenopathy and erythema nodosum is known as *Lofgren syndrome*. Chronic arthritis tends to involve the shoulders, hands, wrists, ankles and knees. Dactylitis can be seen; it is very similar to that seen in patients with psoriatic arthritis.

Osseous involvement causes cystic, reticular or destructive lesions involving mainly the hands and feet (lace-like pattern) but can affect the skull, ribs, sternum, vertebrae, nasal bones, pelvis, tibia and femur as well. MRI shows multiple bony lesions with high T2-weighted and intermediate T1-weighted signal, although diffuse involvement is also recognised. Sarcoid myopathy can also be acute and mimic polymyositis.

Abril A, Cohen MD. Rheumatologic manifestations of sarcoidosis. *Curr Opin Rheumatol*. 2004;16(1):51–5. Manaster BJ, et al. *The Requisites: MSK Imaging*. 4th edn. Philadelphia, PA: Mosby, 2013:486–7.

48. C. Sturge–Weber syndrome

Sturge–Weber syndrome is a rare neurocutaneous disorder characterised by abnormal vascular malformation involving the skin (ophthalmic branch of the trigeminal nerve) and leptomeninges of the brain. The facial capillary port-wine stain is usually ipsilateral to the leptomeningeal venous angiomatosis. Tram-track cortical calcification (T2 hypointensity) and cortical atrophy is probably secondary to underlying ischaemia. Associated calvarial thickening, enlarging diploic space and increased pneumatisation of mastoid air cells (Dyke–Davidoff–Mason Syndrome) and ipsilateral enlargement of choroid plexus may also be seen. Angioma of the choroid of the eye is also a characteristic finding.

Moore KR, et al. *Diagnostic Imaging: Paediatric Neuroradiology*, 1st edn. Salt Lake City: Amirsys, 2007.

49. B. Hepatocellular adenoma

Hepatic adenomas were virtually unknown prior to 1960, the year in which oral contraceptives were introduced. Although the precise pathogenic mechanism of hepatic adenomas is still unknown, the use of oestrogen-containing or androgen-containing steroid medications clearly increases their prevalence, number and size within the affected population and often within individual patients. Moreover, this causal relationship is related to dose and duration, with the greatest risk encountered in patients taking large doses of oestrogen or androgen for prolonged periods of time. In women who have never used oral contraceptives, the annual incidence of hepatic adenoma is about 1 per million. This increases to 30–40 per million in long-term users of oral contraceptives. Another risk group for hepatocellular adenoma are patients with Type I glycogen storage disease. In these patients, the adenomas are also more likely to be multiple and to undergo malignant transformation, although the latter is still quite rare. Adenomas rarely undergo malignant transformation to HCC, even after years of maintaining a stable appearance.

Grazioli L, et al, Hepatic adenomas: Imaging and pathologic findings. *Radiographics*. 2001;21:877–94.

50. C. Metastatic angiosarcoma

Squamous cell carcinomas are regarded as the most common type of cavitating metastases, although adenocarcinomas are also implicated. Metastatic sarcomas can also cavitate, and a pneumothorax can be complicated.

Angiosarcoma represents the most common non-lymphoid malignant tumour of the spleen. Imaging reveals splenomegaly and an ill-defined heterogeneous mass.

Adam A, et al. *Grainger & Allison's Diagnostic Radiology: A Textbook of Medical Imaging*. 5th edn. New York: Churchill Livingstone, 2008:1764–5.

Seo JB, et al. Atypical pulmonary metastases: Spectrum of radiologic findings. *Radiographics*. 2001; 21(2): 403–17.

51. E. The higher the tumour grade, the greater the grade of enhancement

DCE-MRI evaluates the vascularity of tumours by providing quantitative kinetic parameters that reflect the flow of blood and the permeability of the vessels. DCE-MRI increases the specificity of prostate tumour detection. Tumours show early enhancement and early washout of the contrast agent – the higher the tumour grade, the higher would be the permeability parameters (K^{trans} – wash-in, K_{ep} – washout). A disadvantage of DCE-MRI is that small, low-grade tumours may not demonstrate abnormal enhancement. Furthermore, abnormal enhancement patterns can also be seen in patients with BPH, which can make assessment of the central gland difficult. However, in the glandular peripheral zone and anterior gland, DCE-MRI can be helpful in identifying lesions that are not suspected on T2-weighted images. The degree of enhancement on DCE-MRI correlates positively with tumour grade.

Turkbey B, et al. Imaging techniques for prostate cancer: Implications for focal therapy. *Nat Rev Urol.* 2009; 6(4):191–203.

52. A. Melorheostosis

Melorheostosis is a very rare non-hereditary disease of unknown aetiology. Patients can present with pain and restricted movements of the joint, but the disease is usually asymptomatic and is discovered incidentally. Some patients may have thickening and fibrosis of overlying skin, resembling scleroderma or joint contractures. Radiographic features include dense irregular bone running down the cortex of a tubular long bone, which can cross the joint. This has the appearance of flowing/molten wax and is usually limited to one side of cortex, although the internal or external cortex may be affected. The lower limbs are the most commonly affected. Other notable features are discrepant leg length on the affected side and the presence of adjacent ossified soft-tissue masses (27%).

Dähnert W. *Radiology Review Manual.* 7th edn. Philadelphia, PA: Lippincott Williams & Wilkins, 2011.
Sutton D. *Textbook of Radiology and Imaging.* 7th edn. Edinburgh: Churchill Livingstone, 2003.

53. B. Multiple sclerosis

The spinal cord is known to be frequently involved in MS or in combination with lesions in the brain; as many as 25% of cases have been found to involve only the spinal cord. Most spinal cord lesions occur in the cervical cord. Cervical spinal MRI is particularly useful when the patient is suspected to have MS and brain lesions are absent. On T2-weighted spinal imaging, most plaques are peripherally located (commonly dorsolateral) and less than two vertebral body segments in length. The lesions tend to be multifocal and present as well-circumscribed foci with an increased T2 signal intensity. With acute spinal cord lesions, enhancement is frequently seen. Spinal cord atrophy, which may reflect axonal loss, may also be observed and is believed to be an important element in disability. Though rarely seen in other diseases, asymptomatic lesions of the spinal cord can be present in MS and may help lead to the correct diagnosis.

Unlike its applicability to the brain, FLAIR imaging appears unreliable in the detection of MS lesions in the spinal cord. The short inversion time inversion-recovery (STIR) sequence has been found to be sensitive for lesion detection, particularly diffuse lesions.

Ge Y. Multiple sclerosis: The role of MR imaging. *AJNR Am J Neuroradiol.* 2006;27(6):1165–76.
Poonawalla AH, et al. Cervical spinal cord lesions in multiple sclerosis: T1-weighted inversion-recovery MR imaging with phase-sensitive reconstruction. *Radiology.* 2008;246(1):258–64.

54. D. Autoimmune haemolytic anaemia

Mature cystic teratoma can be associated with complications from rupture, malignant degeneration or (most commonly) torsion. Mature cystic teratomas affected by torsion are larger than average (mean diameter 11 cm vs. 6 cm); this enlargement could be the result of the torsion rather than the cause of it.

Most mature cystic teratomas can be diagnosed at US. However, the US diagnosis is complicated by the fact that these tumours may have a variety of appearances. Three manifestations occur most commonly. The most common manifestation is a cystic lesion with a densely echogenic tubercle (Rokitansky nodule) projecting into the cyst lumen. The second manifestation is a diffusely or partially echogenic mass with the echogenic area usually demonstrating sound attenuation owing to sebaceous material and hair within the cyst cavity.

Outwater EK, et al. Ovarian teratomas: Tumor types and imaging characteristics. *Radiographics.* 2001;21:475–90.

55. E. Elevated CA-125 levels are commonly seen in children with germ cell tumours.

Mature cystic teratoma, often called *dermoid cyst* when the ectodermal elements predominate, is the most common ovarian tumour in children and adolescents, accounting for approximately 50% of all paediatric ovarian neoplasms. CA-125 levels are more frequently elevated in patients with epithelial ovarian cancers than in those with germ cell tumours (GCTs). CA-125 levels should not be routinely obtained in children, particularly in premenarcheal girls, as epithelial ovarian tumours are extremely rare before menarche. The serum AFP level is elevated in patients with GCTs such as yolk sac tumours, immature teratomas, embryonal carcinomas and mixed GCTs with yolk sac elements.

Heo SH, et al. Review of ovarian tumors in children and adolescents: Radiologic-pathologic correlation. *Radiographics*. 2014;34:2039–55.

56. E.   Haemangioma

The classic haemangioma is an asymptomatic lesion that is discovered at routine examination or autopsy. At US, the typical appearance is a homogeneous, hyperechoic mass with well-defined margins and posterior acoustic enhancement. The CT findings consist of a hypoattenuating lesion on non-enhanced images. After intravenous administration of contrast material, arterial-phase CT shows early, peripheral, globular enhancement of the lesion. The attenuation of the peripheral nodules is equal to that of the adjacent aorta. Venous-phase CT shows centripetal enhancement that progresses to uniform filling .This enhancement persists on delayed-phase images.

At MR imaging, haemangiomas are characterised by well-defined margins and high signal intensity on T2-weighted images, which is identical to that of cerebrospinal fluid. Specificity is improved by using serial gadolinium-enhanced gradient-echo imaging. The gadolinium intake is similar to the intake of iodinated contrast material during enhanced CT. With T2-weighted spin-echo and dynamic gadolinium-enhanced T1-weighted gradient-echo sequences, the sensitivity and specificity of MR imaging are 98% and the accuracy is 99%. The imaging features of a haemangioma depend on its size; typical haemangiomas are mostly less than 3 cm in diameter.

Vilgrain V, et al. Imaging of atypical haemangiomas of the Liver with pathologic correlation. *Radiographics*. 2000;20:379–97.

57. A.   Surgery is preferred over embolisation

Treatment of pulmonary AVMs is with either surgery or embolotherapy, with the latter being the preferred option. Indications for treatment include intolerance to exercise, aneurysms greater than 2 cm in diameter or feeding arteries of 3 mm or larger, which are associated with increased risk of stroke and brain abscess.

Coils and Amplatzer plugs are used for large vessel permanent occlusion, like embolisation of pulmonary AVM.

Lubarsky M, et al. Embolization agents – Which one should be used when? Part 1: Large-vessel embolization. *Semin Intervent Radiol*. 2009;26(4):352–7.
Poole PS, Ferguson EC. Revisiting pulmonary arteriovenous malformations: Radiographic and CT imaging findings and corresponding treatment options. *Contemp Diagnos Radiol*. 2010; 33(8):1–5.

58. A.   Hyperintense on T1W imaging and hypointense on T2W imaging

T1-weighted images are important in prostate cancer staging, because they show the presence of haemorrhage secondary to a recent biopsy; haemorrhage is almost always hyperintense compared with normal parenchyma on T1-weighted MRI. Haemorrhage typically appears low in signal on T2-weighted MRI and mimics cancer.

Turkbey B, et al. Imaging techniques for prostate cancer: Implications for focal therapy. *Nat Rev Urol*. 2009;6(4):191–203.

59. D.   Paget disease (acute phase)

Paget disease is a multifocal skeletal condition whereby bone remodelling becomes abnormal and eventually exaggerated. It typically affects middle-aged to elderly people and has acute and chronic phases with differing radiographic appearances. The acute phase, also known as the active or osteolytic phase, is characterised by aggressive bone resorption secondary to disordered osteoclastic activity. This manifests as lucency within the medulla of the long bones, typically in a flame shape or 'blade of grass' configuration. Over time, osteoblastic activity overtakes the osteoclastic resorption, resulting in osteosclerosis, cortical thickening and increased trabeculation. Giant cell tumour is a benign neoplasm of the mature skeleton, seen almost exclusively in those under 30 years of age. Although osteomyelitis can result in bony lucency, it is typically patchy with a moth-eaten texture.

Dähnert W. *Radiology Review Manual.* 6th edn. Philadelphia, PA: Lippincott Williams & Wilkins, 2007:145.

60. D. Superior sagittal sinus thrombosis

In neonates, shock and dehydration is a common cause of venous sinus thrombosis. In older children it is often local infection; in adults, coagulopathies are more common than infection. In women, OCP use and pregnancy are strong risk factors.

Imaging findings of cerebral venous thrombosis can be categorised as direct, as when there is visualisation of cortical or dural sinus thrombus (delta sign on unenhanced CT and empty delta sign on post-contrast CT venogram), or indirect, as when there are ischaemic or vascular changes related to the venous outflow disturbance. Venous infarction manifests as a low-attenuation lesion with or without subcortical haemorrhage.

Brain lesions are related to a venous distribution. Bilateral parasagittal hemispheric lesions are suggestive of superior sagittal sinus thrombosis. Ipsilateral temporo-occipital and cerebellar lobe lesions can be found in transverse sinus thrombosis. In bilateral thalamic lesions, deep cerebral venous thrombosis should be suspected.

Rodallec MH, et al. Cerebral venous thrombosis and multidetector CT angiography: Tips and tricks. *Radiographics.* 2006;26 Suppl 1:S5–18; discussion S42–3.
Simons B, et al. Cerebral venous thrombosis. Radiology assistant. http://www.radiologyassistant.nl/en/p4befacb3e4691/cerebral-venous-thrombosis.html [accessed on 18 February 2017].

61. D. Hypointense to surrounding liver on the enhanced portal venous phase

Typically, FNH is iso- or hypointense on T1-weighted images, is slightly hyper- or isointense on T2-weighted images and has a hyperintense central scar on T2-weighted images. FNH shows intense homogeneous enhancement in the arterial phase and enhancement of the central scar in the later phases of gadolinium-enhanced imaging.

FNH does not have a tumour capsule, although the pseudocapsule surrounding some FNH lesions may be quite prominent. The pseudocapsule of FNH results from compression of the surrounding liver parenchyma by the FNH, perilesion vessels and inflammatory reaction. The pseudocapsule is usually a few millimetres thick and typically shows high signal intensity on T2-weighted images. The pseudocapsule may show enhancement on delayed contrast-enhanced images.

A central scar is present at imaging in most patients with FNH. The amount of scar tissue within FNH and the size of the central scar may vary. The central scar is typically high in signal intensity on T2-weighted images and low in signal intensity on T1-weighted images. It shows visible enhancement on delayed contrast-enhanced images. High signal intensity of the central scar may be caused by the inflammatory reaction around the ductular proliferation as well as the vessels within the septa and central scar. The central scar is not a specific finding of FNH and can be seen in a variety of other focal liver lesions, such as giant haemangiomas.

Hussain SM, et al. Focal nodular hyperplasia: Findings at state-of-the-art MR imaging, US, CT, and pathologic analysis. *Radiographics.* 2004;24:3–19.

62. C. Osler–Rendu–Weber syndrome

Osler–Rendu–Weber syndrome is an uncommon genetic disorder characterised by arteriovenous malformations in the skin, mucous membranes and visceral organs. The brain, gastrointestinal tract, skin, lung and nose are the primary sites affected.

Pulmonary AVM typically appears as a round or oval mass of uniform density, which can be lobulated but with well-circumscribed and sharply defined margins. The feeding arteries are seen radiating from the hilum of the lung, and the draining veins are seen coursing towards the left atrium.

Multiple ischaemic strokes in different arterial territories at different ages characterise the embolic mechanism in HHT. Brain abscess is the most serious neurologic complication in PAVM. Typically in HHT these abscesses are multiple and recurrent, affecting the superficial layers of the cerebral lobes (mostly the parietal lobe).

Carette MF, et al. Imaging of hereditary hemorrhagic telangiectasia. *Cardiovasc Intervent Radiol.* 2009;32(4): 745–57.
Poole PS, Ferguson EC. Revisiting pulmonary arteriovenous malformations: Radiographic and CT imaging findings and corresponding treatment options. *Contemp Diagnos Radiol.* 2010;33(8):1–5.

63. C. Low serum estradiol levels

Ovarian hyperstimulation syndrome is usually iatrogenic secondary to ovarian stimulant drug therapy for infertility but may occur as a spontaneous event in pregnancy and is associated with raised serum estradiol levels. The syndrome consists of ovarian enlargement with extravascular accumulation of exudates leading to weight gain, ascites, pleural effusions, intravascular volume depletion with hemoconcentration and oliguria in varying degrees, with increased risk of thrombosis and stroke. Pain, abdominal distention, nausea and vomiting are frequently seen. The imaging findings are similar at US, CT and MR imaging and reflect ovarian enlargement by distended corpora luteal cysts of varying sizes. Because the enlarged follicles are often peripheral in location, a spoked wheel appearance has been described. Ascites, pleural effusion and pericardial effusion are also described. Familiarity with ovarian hyperstimulation syndrome and the appropriate clinical setting should help avoid the incorrect diagnosis of an ovarian cystic neoplasm.

Bennett GL, et al. Gynecologic causes of acute pelvic pain: Spectrum of CT findings. *Radiographics.* 2002; 22(4):785–801.

64. A. A comparison radiograph of the contralateral knee

The appearance is likely to represent post-traumatic cortical desmoid. It is also known as *avulsive cortical irregularity* or *Bufkin lesion.* It results from chronic avulsive stress at the femoral region of the medial head of the gastrocnemius. It is usually an incidental finding. One-third of cases are bilateral and a comparison photograph of the contralateral knee is helpful to assess the other side.

If plain films are not helpful, an MRI can be useful to assess soft tissues. Post-traumatic cortical desmoid does not involve soft tissues.

Adam A, et al. *Grainger & Allison's Diagnostic Radiology: A Textbook of Medical Imaging.* 5th edn. New York: Churchill Livingstone, 2008:1783–4.

65. B. Tuberous sclerosis

Tuberous sclerosis is a neuroectodermal disorder, characterised by the classic triad of adenoma sebaceum, seizures and mental retardation. CNS findings include subependymal hamartomas, which can calcify (classic calcified subependymal nodules), giant cell astrocytoma (at the foramen of Monro, often replacing the third ventricle), cortical tubers and heterotopic islands of grey in white matter. Pulmonary involvement includes interstitial fibrosis at lung bases, LAM, multiple lung cysts and chylothorax. Cardiac involvement includes rhabdomyoma, aortic aneurysm and congenital cardiomyopathy. Renal involvement includes AML, cysts and RCCs. Ocular lesions include optic nerve glioma and hamartoma. Other visceral abnormalities include splenic tumour and pancreatic and hepatic adenomas.

Dähnert W. *Radiology Review Manual.* 7th edn. Philadelphia, PA: Lippincott Williams & Wilkins, 2011: 333–5.

66. C. Bronchial atresia

This is the classic description of a mucocoele. Congenital bronchial atresia is a congenital abnormality caused by focal interruption of a lobar, segmental or subsegmental bronchus with associated peripheral mucous impaction (bronchocoele/mucocoele) and associated hyperinflation of the obstructed lung segment. The apicoposterior segmental bronchus of the left upper lobe is most commonly affected. The condition is usually benign and asymptomatic and is often an incidental chest X-ray finding. Mean age at diagnosis is 17 years and symptoms, if present, include recurrent pulmonary infection, mild wheeze and dyspnoea.

The typical appearance of Swyer–James syndrome is that of a small, hyperlucent lung, with overexpansion of the contralateral lung. A diffuse pattern of scarring or irregular vessels may also be present. Cystic fibrosis is unlikely in a previously well individual. Kartagener syndrome appears as bilateral bronchiectasis. Allergic bronchopulmonary aspergillosis is a possibility, but the minor symptoms fit best with bronchial atresia.

Dähnert W. *Radiology Review Manual*. 7th ed. Philadelphia, PA: Lippincott Williams & Wilkins, 2011:481.

67. D. The most common malignant germ cell tumour is a dysgerminoma.

Germ cell tumours are the most common type of ovarian neoplasm, with one-third of these being malignant in children and adolescents. A dysgerminoma is the most common malignant germ cell tumour and is associated with gonadal dysgenesis.

The majority of germ cell tumours are mature cystic teratomas (also known as *dermoid cysts*), which account for 50% of all paediatric ovarian neoplasms. These are bilateral in 10% of cases.

Heo SH, et al. Review of ovarian tumors in children and adolescents: Radiologic-pathologic correlation. *Radiographics*. 2014;34:2039–55.

68. E. CT imaging best demonstrates the pericyst, matrix and daughter cysts.

Hydatid disease is a severe and common parasitic disease that is endemic to the Mediterranean basin and other sheep-raising areas. Humans become infected by ingesting the eggs of the tapeworm *Echinococcus granulosus*, either by eating contaminated food or from contact with dogs. The ingested embryos invade the intestinal mucosal wall and proceed to the liver via the portal venous system. Although the liver filters out most of these embryos, those that are not destroyed become hepatic hydatid cysts.

US findings are variable and range from purely cystic to solid-appearing pseudotumours. Wavy bands of delaminated endocyst (water lily sign) may be noted internally. Daughter cysts, sometimes surrounded by echogenic debris (matrix), are frequently seen. Calcifications, varying from tiny to massive, are often present peripherally.

At CT, a hydatid cyst usually appears as a well-defined, hypoattenuating lesion with a distinguishable wall. Coarse wall calcifications are present in 50% of cases, and daughter cysts are identified in approximately 75%. Because of its superb contrast resolution, MR imaging best demonstrates the pericyst, the matrix or hydatid sand (debris consisting of freed scolices) and the daughter cysts. The pericyst is seen as a hypointense rim on both T1-weighted and T2-weighted images because of its fibrous composition and the presence of calcifications. The hydatid matrix appears hypointense on T1-weighted images and markedly hyperintense on T2-weighted images; when present, daughter cysts are hypointense relative to the matrix on both T1-weighted and T2-weighted images.

Mortele KJ, et al. The infected liver: Radiologic-pathologic correlation. *Radiographics*. 2004;24:937–55.

69. E. Bronchial dehiscence

Immediate complications (<24 hours)
- Malpositioned monitoring tubes and lines
- Donor–recipient size mismatch
- Hyperacute rejection

Early complications (24 hours to 1 week)
- Ischaemia-reperfusion injury (reperfusion oedema)
- Acute pleural complications

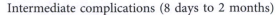

Intermediate complications (8 days to 2 months)
- Acute rejection
- Bronchial anastomotic complications like dehiscence
- Infections

Primary late complications (2–4 months)
- Bronchial stenosis and bronchomalacia
- Viral infection
- Pulmonary embolism and infarction
- Complications that affect the native lung

Secondary late complications (≥4 months)
- Mycobacterial infection
- Chronic rejection
- Cryptogenic organising pneumonia
- Posttransplantation lymphoproliferative disorder
- Upper-lobe fibrosis
- Recurrence of primary disease
- Bronchogenic carcinoma

Krishnam MS. Post-operative complications of lung transplantation: Radiologic findings along a time continuum. *Radiographics*. 2007;27(4):957–74.

70. C. MRI

Uterine dehiscence is characterised by incomplete rupture of the uterine wall, usually involving the endometrium and myometrium but with an intact overlying serosal layer. MR imaging may be better than CT in evaluating for uterine dehiscence because of its multiplanar capability and greater soft-tissue contrast and its ability to help identify an intact serosal layer.

Rodgers SK, et al. Imaging after cesarean delivery: Acute and chronic complications. *Radiographics*. 2012;32(6): 1693–712.

71. D. Posterior translation of tibia

An ACL injury results in anterior translation of the tibia. The 'kissing contusions' from a pivot shift mechanism of injury results in marrow oedema in the posterolateral region of the tibial plateau and the mid portion of the lateral femoral condyle. A deep lateral femoral sulcus, more than 1.5 mm, may be appreciated on plain film. Uncovering of the posterior horn of the lateral meniscus is associated with the anterior translation of the tibia. The PCL tends to buckle after an ACL injury resulting in a reduced PCL angle less than 105 degrees.

Ng WHA, et al. Imaging of the anterior cruciate ligament. *World J Orthop*. 2011;2(8):75–84.
Sanders TG, et al. Bone contusion patterns of the knee at MR imaging: Footprint of the mechanism of injury. *Radiographics*. 2000;20:S135–51.

72. C. Basal meningitis suggests neurosyphilis.

The finding of diffuse cerebral atrophy in HIV can be accompanied by diffuse, confluent, ill-defined areas of abnormally increased signal intensity on T2-weighted MR images of the periventricular white matter. No enhancement is noted. These findings were initially attributed to CMV infection, as autopsy studies have shown that a high percentage of AIDS patients had concomitant CMV infection of the CNS. It was subsequently recognised that HIV is neurotrophic and directly infects the CNS; these global abnormalities were then attributed to a subacute encephalitis caused by HIV. It now seems likely that both HIV and CMV can cause subacute encephalitis and encephalopathy; these conditions have an identical non-specific imaging appearance. CMV encephalopathy appears to manifest itself late in the illness, whereas

HIV rather than H1V dementia (although usually presenting late) can occasionally be the AIDS-defining illness.

In addition to subacute encephalitis, CMV infection can manifest as a more virulent ventriculoencephalitis. This is most often seen in concert with CMV infection elsewhere in the body (such as CMV retinitis) and is usually a late manifestation of AIDS. The infection appears to begin in the ependymal or subependymal region and spread into the adjacent brain. The ventricles are enlarged, and hypoattenuation on CT or increased signal intensity on T2-weighted MRI is noted in the periventricular white matter. Ill-defined periventricular enhancement can also be seen following injection of contrast medium. Meningitis – particularly basilar meningitis – and hydrocephalus occur often in the setting of neurotuberculosis. Meningitis manifests on CT scans and MR images as prominent enhancement and thickening of the meninges and it can be associated with infarcts secondary to vascular stenosis or occlusion. Neurosyphilis, which is being diagnosed with increased frequency among patients with AIDS, can cause infarcts secondary to arteritis.

Walot I, et al. Neuroimaging findings in patients with AIDS. *Clin Infect Dis.* 1996;22(6):906–19.

73. D.   Hilar lymph nodes are more common in MRSA

Radiological findings of MRSA pneumonia reported in the current literature are limited to descriptions of necrotising pneumonia. The frequencies of bronchial wall thickening and centrilobular nodules were significantly higher in patients with MSSA than MRSA pneumonia. Moreover, the frequency of centrilobular nodules with a tree-in-bud pattern was significantly higher in patients with MSSA than MRSA pneumonia. There were no significant differences in other CT findings including ground-glass opacity and consolidation between the two groups. Ground-glass change and bronchial wall thickening were the two most common CT findings in both groups. There were no significant differences in zonal distributions between the two groups. Both groups showed unilateral or bilateral opacities and predominantly upper zone changes.

The frequency of pleural effusion was significantly higher in patients with MRSA than in those with MSSA pneumonia. There was no difference in hilar or mediastinal lymphadenopathy.

Morikawa K, et al. Meticillin-resistant *Staphylococcus aureus* and meticillin-susceptible *S. aureus* pneumonia: Comparison of clinical and thin-section CT findings. *Br J Radiol.* 2012;85(1014):e168–75.

74. A.   Klippel–Trénaunay syndrome

Klippel–Trénaunay syndrome is a sporadic rare mesodermal abnormality that usually affects a single lower limb. It is characterised by a triad of a port-wine naevus (unilateral cutaneous capillary haemangioma, often in a dermatomal distribution on the affected limb), overgrowth of distal digits/entire extremity (involving soft tissue and bone) and varicose veins on the lateral aspect of the affected limb. Although the other options can produce limb hypertrophy, they would not be expected to show all the features of the triad described.

Auyeung KM, et al. Klippel–Trénaunay syndrome presenting in a child with vascular malformation. *J Hong Kong Coll Radiol.* 2002;5:227–9.
Dähnert W. *Radiology Review Manual.* 7th edn. Philadelphia, PA: Lippincott Williams & Wilkins, 2011.

75. C.   They are high signal intensity on T1W MR images.

Biliary hamartomas, also known as *biliary microhamartomas* or *von Meyenburg complex*, are composed of one or more dilated duct-like structures lined by biliary epithelium and accompanied by a variable amount of fibrous stroma. Biliary hamartomas are typically multiple round or irregular focal lesions of nearly uniform size (up to 15 mm) scattered throughout the liver. These lesions are often discovered incidentally, and if the patient has a primary neoplasm they can be mistaken for metastatic disease. The lesions are hypoattenuating at CT, hypointense at T1-weighted MR imaging and hyperintense at T2-weighted imaging. If the echo time is increased at T2-weighted imaging, the signal intensity of these lesions increases further and approaches that

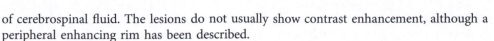

of cerebrospinal fluid. The lesions do not usually show contrast enhancement, although a peripheral enhancing rim has been described.

The differential diagnoses for biliary hamartomas include metastatic disease and simple hepatic cysts. Biliary hamartomas are relatively uniform in size, whereas metastatic lesions are usually more heterogeneous in size and in attenuation or signal intensity. Compared with biliary hamartomas, hepatic cysts are rarely as uniformly small or numerous, whereas the cysts in autosomal dominant polycystic disease are usually larger and more numerous.

Brancatelli G, et al. Fibropolycystic liver disease: CT and MR imaging findings. *Radiographics*. 2005;25:659–70.

76. B. HELLP syndrome

HELLP (haemolysis, elevated liver enzymes, low platelets) syndrome is one of the hypertensive disorders of pregnancy, occurring in 4%–12% of pre-eclamptic patients, from vascular endothelial injury, which results in intravascular deposition of fibrin with end organ damage and can occur prior to or after delivery. Disseminated intravascular coagulation (DIC) is seen in 20%–40% of patients. Other major complications include placental abruption, acute renal failure, pulmonary oedema, pleural and pericardial effusions, hepatic infarction, haematoma and rupture. Pelvic pain may occur in the setting of haemoperitoneum.

Spontaneous intrahepatic haemorrhage and rupture likely result from toxaemia-related vasculopathy with endothelial damage, leading to haemorrhage. Supportive therapy is usually offered initially, with capsular rupture necessitating surgery. Embolisation of the hepatic artery may be attempted. CT is important in initial diagnosis and for serial follow-up. Findings may include subcapsular or intrahepatic haemorrhage, capsular rupture and areas of confluent necrosis secondary to infarction. Intravenous contrast-enhanced CT allows identification of active arterial extravasation, which cannot be seen on US.

Fitz-Hugh–Curtis syndrome refers to the development of perihepatitis in association with pelvic inflammatory disease.

Bennett GL, et al. Gynecologic causes of acute pelvic pain: Spectrum of CT findings. *Radiographics*. 2002; 22(4):785–801.

77. C. SAPHO syndrome

The acronym SAPHO (synovitis, acne, palmoplantar pustulosis, hyperostosis and osteitis), which was coined in 1987, is applied to occurrences of a wide spectrum of aseptic neutrophilic dermatoses in association with aseptic osteoarticular lesions. The sternoclavicular joint (most frequently affected) is involved in 65%–90% of cases. Hyperostosis and osteosclerosis are characteristic findings at conventional radiography and CT. Other findings include joint erosion and ankylosis. In the presence of active lesions, MR imaging with T2-weighted or STIR sequence may depict bone marrow oedema, a feature that helps differentiate active lesions from chronic ones. The 'bull's head' sign (i.e., increased radiotracer uptake in the sternal manubrium and both sternoclavicular joints at delayed scintigraphy) is highly specific for the diagnosis of SAPHO and may obviate biopsy.

Acute septic arthritis of the sternoclavicular joint is an uncommon infectious condition that is usually monoarticular and insidious in onset. Changes that are visible at CT include destruction of the articular surface, widening of the joint space, gas and fluid collections in the chest wall and mediastinum, and mediastinal soft-tissue stranding. MR images in addition may depict bone marrow oedema.

The sternoclavicular joint can be affected by osteoarthrosis, RA, and seronegative and crystalline arthropathy, which depict their respective specific features on imaging; however, imaging is often non-specific.

Restrepo CS, et al. Imaging appearances of the sternum and sternoclavicular joints. *Radiographics*. 2009;29(3): 839–59.

78. D. HSV encephalitis

Herpes simplex virus (HSV) is notable for its typical imaging appearance and because it is readily treatable when diagnosed early but potentially devastating in cases of delayed diagnosis. The typical appearance of HSV encephalitis includes parenchymal oedema (hypoattenuating on CT; hyperintense on FLAIR) with variable patchy or gyriform enhancement and variable degrees of restricted diffusion; parenchymal haemorrhage and necrosis may occur in severe or untreated cases. MRI findings are seen earlier in the course of infection than CT findings, with DWI changes most sensitive among routine sequences. The classic distribution includes bilateral (though asymmetric) involvement of the limbic system (most notably the mesial temporal lobes, i.e., the hippocampus, amygdala and parahippocampal gyrus). Other cortical regions may also be involved, while the basal ganglia are typically spared.

Mitchell BC, Dehkharghani S. Imaging of intracranial infectious diseases in adults. *Appl Radiol*. 2014;43:6–15.

79. A. Long or short segments of marked stricture in the main pancreatic duct

IPMNs are a group of neoplasms in the biliary duct or pancreatic duct that cause cystic dilatation from excessive mucin production and accumulation. There are three main types of pancreatic IPMNs: main duct, branch duct and combined. A main duct IPMN commonly causes dilatation of the papilla, with bulging of the papilla into the duodenal lumen. Filling defects caused by mural nodules or mucin may be seen at MRCP or ERCP. At CT and MR imaging, filling defects caused by mural nodules enhance, while filling defects caused by mucin do not enhance.

Nikolaidis P, et al. Imaging features of Benign and malignant ampullary and periampullary lesions. *Radiographics*. 2014;34:624–41.

80. B. Gas locules in the fluid is most specific

Thoracic empyema is defined as purulent content in the pleural cavity.

Empyemas usually form an obtuse angle with the chest wall and are lenticular in shape (bi-convex) in comparison to the crescentic shape of pleural effusion. Empyema also shows enhancing thickened pleura, the split pleura sign (which differentiates it from peripheral lung abscesses), septations, associated consolidation or infected foci like subdiaphragmatic abscess, and so on. Gas can be present in both an empyema and pulmonary abscess.

Jannette C, Stern EJ. *Chest Radiology*. Philadelphia, PA: Lippincott Williams & Wilkins, 2008:146.

81. A. Uterine dehiscence

Uterine dehiscence is characterised by incomplete rupture of the uterine wall, usually involving the endometrium and myometrium but with an intact overlying serosal layer. Uterine dehiscence is a very difficult imaging diagnosis. The presence of a bladder flap haematoma greater than 5 cm and larger pelvic haematomas should be considered abnormal and highly suspicious for uterine dehiscence in the proper clinical setting. MR imaging may be better than CT in checking for uterine dehiscence because of its multiplanar capability and greater soft-tissue contrast, with its ability to help identify an intact serosal layer. Uterine rupture is the most severe potential complication of caesarean delivery and is defined as separation of all layers of the uterine wall, including the serosal layer, with abnormal communication between the uterine cavity and the peritoneal cavity. The presence of gas/blood within the uterine defect extending from the endometrial cavity to the extrauterine parametrium in association with haemoperitoneum increases the likelihood of rupture in the appropriate clinical setting.

Rodgers SK, et al. Imaging after cesarean delivery: Acute and chronic complications. *Radiographics*. 2012;32(6): 1693–712.

82. B. Primary osteomyelitis is more common than secondary osteomyelitis.

Primary osteomyelitis of the sternum is uncommon, with only a small number of cases reported in the literature. It may occur in patients with a history of intravenous drug abuse, AIDS, haemoglobinopathy or other immune deficiency states. *Staphylococcus aureus* infection is the most common cause of sternal osteomyelitis. Secondary osteomyelitis of the sternum is more common than the primary form, particularly after sternotomy. This is a potentially severe complication because of the risk of mediastinitis. Risk factors for secondary osteomyelitis include obesity, insulin-dependent diabetes and internal mammary artery grafts.

The presence of one or more sternal fractures implies high-energy trauma. The importance of sternal fractures lies in the high frequency of associated injuries. Spontaneous fractures of the sternum have occurred in the presence of a neoplasm (e.g., multiple myeloma, metastasis), strain from heavy lifting, labour and bone insufficiency (e.g., in osteoporosis).

Sternoclavicular dislocation is a rare occurrence; anterior (or presternal) displacement is more common, but posterior (or retrosternal) displacement is more frequently associated with life-threatening complications caused by the compression of vital structures such as the trachea, great vessels and nerves. CT provides a detailed depiction of the sternoclavicular joint and helps characterise dislocation.

Restrepo CS, et al. Imaging appearances of the sternum and sternoclavicular joints. *Radiographics*. 2009;29(3): 839–59.

83. D. Ultrasound neck with FNA

The National Institute for Health and Clinical Excellence (NICE) guidance on cancer services published in 2004, entitled Improving Outcomes in Head and Neck Cancers, recommended that specialist clinics should be set up for the assessment of patients with head and neck lumps, structured in a similar way to one-stop breast lump clinics with radiologist and cytopathologist present, and availability of US and fine-needle aspiration (FNA) for initial assessment.

US is well established as a primary investigation for patients presenting with a lump in the neck, and FNA cytology is also established as initial investigation for lesions in the head and neck. The cost-effectiveness and diagnostic accuracy of FNA can be increased by using US guidance and the presence of an on-site cytopathologist.

Ganguly A, et al. The benefits of on-site cytology with ultrasound-guided fine needle aspiration in a one-stop neck lump clinic. *Ann R Coll Surg Engl*. 2010;92(8):660–4.

84. A. Acute appendicitis

The plain film findings and clinical history are suggestive of acute appendicitis, which is the most common reason for abdominal surgery in children. It is one of the most common causes of intestinal obstruction in children. Other causes include adhesions, intussusception, incarcerated inguinal hernia, malrotation with volvulus and Meckel's diverticulum.

The primary imaging modality in suspected acute appendicitis remains controversial. Several authors advocate plain films, US and CT as primary diagnostic sets, with various arguments. On plain films, a faecolith or appendicolith with small bowel obstruction (seen in 10% of cases) and displacement of bowel gas from the right iliac fossa are all typical signs of acute appendicitis. However, an abdominal US examination is the preferred imaging modality of choice for investigation of acute appendicitis in children rather than abdominal radiograph.

Acute cholecystitis and renal colic are not common diagnoses in children. Intussusception most often occurs between 3 months and 1 year of age.

Donnelly LF. *Pediatric Imaging: The Fundamentals*. Philadelphia, PA: Saunders Elsevier, 2009:113–14.

85. D. VHL syndrome – renal and pancreatic cysts

The description of the posterior fossa tumour is typical of either a pilocytic astrocytoma or haemangioblastoma. The multiple flow voids suggest a haemangioblastoma. VHL syndrome is an autosomal dominant condition with haemangioblastomas, renal cysts, clear cell renal carcinoma, phaeochromocytoma, pancreatic cysts and islet cell tumours.

Neurofibromatosis Type 1 presents with cutaneous lesions, multiple T2 hyperintensities and plexiform neurofibromas. Neurofibromatosis Type 2 presents with bilateral acoustic schwannomas. Sturge–Weber syndrome is a combination of a facial port-wine stain and cortical calcification. It usually presents with seizures. Li–Fraumeni syndrome is a hereditary cancer syndrome with a susceptibility to breast cancer, sarcomas and brain tumours (astrocytoma and choroid plexus carcinoma). Renal and pancreatic cysts are not typical features of any of the others.

Herron J, et al. Intra-cranial manifestations of the neurocutaneous syndromes. *Clin Radiol.* 2000;55: 82–98.

86. D. Serous cystadenoma

In 70% of cases, Serous cystadenomas demonstrate a polycystic or microcystic pattern consisting of a collection of cysts (usually more than six) that range from a few millimetres up to 2 cm in size. Fine, external lobulations are a common feature, and enhancement of septa and the cyst wall may be seen. A fibrous central scar with or without a characteristic stellate pattern of calcification is seen in 30% of cases and, when demonstrated with CT or MR imaging, is highly specific and is considered to be virtually pathognomonic for serous cystadenoma. Pancreatic ductal dilatation is an uncommon finding in these patients. The macrocystic or oligocystic variant of these tumours is very uncommon and is seen in less than 10% of cases. Either of these variants can take the form of a single dominant macrocavity, in which case it will appear as a unilocular cyst or may contain fewer large (2 cm) cysts. The latter variant is classified as a macrocystic lesion and may be difficult to differentiate from a mucinous cystic tumour. Mucinous cystic neoplasms (mucinous cystadenomas) mainly involve the body and tail of the pancreas and do not communicate with the pancreatic duct. At CT/MR, they are multilocular macrocystic lesions occasionally containing debris or hemorrhage. The complex internal architecture of the cyst, including septa and an internal wall, is best appreciated at MR imaging and endoscopic US, allowing differentiation from serous cystadenomas. Although peripheral eggshell calcification is not frequently seen at CT, it is specific for a mucinous cystic neoplasm and is highly predictive of malignancy. Pseudopapillary tumour is a solid tumour with a cystic component. Others in this group are islet cell tumour, pancreatic adenocarcinoma, and metastasis.

Sahani DV, et al. Cystic pancreatic lesions: A simple imaging-based classification system for guiding management. *Radiographics.* 2005;25:1471–84.

87. C. Fissural and septal nodules

Frequently, the CT findings are far more extensive than expected from a review of the plain chest radiograph. The lung abnormalities show a characteristic peripheral or peribronchial distribution, and the lower lung lobes are more frequently involved. In some cases, the outermost subpleural area is spared. The lung opacities vary from ground glass to consolidation; in the latter, air bronchograms and mild cylindrical bronchial dilatation are a common finding. These opacities have a tendency to migrate, changing location and size, even without treatment. They are of variable size, ranging from a few centimetres to an entire lobe. Some patients present with nodular opacities on the chest radiograph. Lung volumes are preserved in most patients.

Mueller-Mang C, et al. What every radiologist should know about idiopathic interstitial pneumonias. *Radiographics.* 2007;27(3):595–615.

88. C. Leiomyosarcoma

The presence of fat in a retroperitoneal tumour limits the differential diagnosis. A mass that is homogeneous and well defined and consists almost entirely of fat represents lipoma.

When the mass is somewhat irregular and ill-defined but contains fat, a diagnosis of liposarcoma should be considered. Liposarcomas are the most common sarcomas of the retroperitoneum.

Extremely hypervascular tumours such as paragangliomas sometimes contain haemorrhagic necrosis and manifest with fluid–fluid levels. Necrotic portions within tumours have low attenuation without contrast enhancement at CT and are hyperintense at T2-weighted MR imaging. Necrosis is usually seen in tumours of high-grade malignancy such as leiomyosarcomas, which have central necrosis more commonly than other sarcomas. Lymphomas grow and extend into spaces between pre-existing structures and surrounding vessels without compressing their lumina, manifesting with the 'CT angiogram sign' or 'floating aorta sign'. Some tumours, like lymphangioma, are completely cystic in appearance. Solid tumours with a partially cystic portion include neurogenic tumours.

Nishino M, et al. Primary retroperitoneal neoplasms: CT and MR imaging findings with anatomic and pathologic diagnostic clues. *Radiographics*. 2003;23(1):45–57.

89. A. McCune–Albright syndrome

Fibrous dysplasia is a relatively common benign skeletal disorder typically seen in adolescents and young adults. It can be monostotic (affecting one bone) or polyostotic (affecting multiple bones). Polyostotic fibrous dysplasia is commonly associated with café au lait spots, with irregular edges ('coast of Maine'), in contrast to regular edges ('coast of California') observed in neurofibromatosis.

Multiple endocrine disorders are described in association with fibrous dysplasia. McCune–Albright syndrome refers to the triad of polyostotic fibrous dysplasia (usually unilateral), café au lait spots and precocious puberty. Fibrous dysplasia is also associated with hyperthyroidism, hyperparathyroidism, acromegaly, diabetes mellitus and Cushing syndrome.

Mazabraud syndrome refers to the association of polyostotic fibrous dysplasia with multiple soft-tissue myxomas, which are typically intramuscular. Cherubism is a special form of fibrous dysplasia with symmetric involvement of both the maxilla and mandible. It typically affects men and tends to regress after adolescence.

Kransdorf MJ, et al. Fibrous dysplasia. *Radiographics*. 1990;10(3):519–37.

90. A. Pleomorphic adenoma

Nearly 80% of benign parotid neoplasms are pleomorphic adenomas. The most common malignancy of the parotid gland is mucoepidermoid carcinoma and that of the submandibular gland is adenoid cystic carcinoma. On non-enhanced and enhanced T1-weighted series, no histologic discrimination is possible because almost all masses are low in intensity and enhance.

Benign cysts (mucous retention cyst, lympho-epithelial cyst, first branchial cleft cyst, ranula, etc.) appear hyperintense on T2-weighted images, and, depending on the presence of haemorrhage, infection or hyperproteinaceous fluid, the T1-weighted image may show intermediate (solid-appearing) intensity. For this reason, administration of contrast material is helpful because cysts usually enhance on their periphery, whereas pleomorphic adenomas enhance solidly.

Adenoid cystic carcinoma has a very high rate of perineural spread (50%–60%). Cystic degeneration of a benign-appearing neoplasm suggests a Warthin tumour or pleomorphic adenoma. Multiple parotid masses are usually due to lymphadenopathy or Warthin tumours, the latter appearing almost exclusively in the parotid gland, usually in the tail of the gland in older men.

Specific signs predictive of malignancy were T2 hypointensity of the parotid tumour, ill-defined margins, diffuse growth, infiltration of subcutaneous tissue and lymphadenopathy. The predilection of deep lobe involvement was only indicative but not significant for malignancy. However, involvement of both lobes was significant for malignant lesions. Clinically, involvement of the facial nerve is highly suspicious of a malignant mass.

For determination of benign disease, a strong signal intensity on T2-weighted images, well-defined borders and a location in the superficial lobe were significant MR imaging findings for benignity. The degree of tumour enhancement after contrast administration did not help to distinguish benign from malignant tumours, though there was a tendency towards strong enhancement of benign tumours

Christe A, et al. MR imaging of parotid tumors: Typical lesion characteristics in MR imaging improve discrimination between benign and malignant disease. *AJNR Am J Neuroradiol.* 2011;32(7): 1202–7.

Yousem DM, et al. Major salivary gland imaging. *Radiology.* 2000;216(1):19–29.

91. C. Communication with the pancreatic duct

In 70% of cases, these benign tumours Serous cystadenomas demonstrate a polycystic or microcystic pattern consisting of a collection of cysts (usually more than six) that range from a few millimetres up to 2 cm in size. Fine, external lobulations are a common feature, and enhancement of septa and the cyst wall may be seen. A fibrous central scar with or without a characteristic stellate pattern of calcification is seen in 30% of cases and, when demonstrated at CT or MR imaging, is highly specific and is considered to be virtually pathognomonic for serous cystadenoma. Pancreatic ductal dilatation is an uncommon finding in these patients. In 20% of cases, these tumours are composed of microcysts in a honeycomb pattern and appear as well-marginated, 'spongy' lesions with soft-tissue or mixed attenuation and a sharp interface with the vascular structures at CT. In patients with indeterminate CT findings, further characterisation with MR imaging or endoscopic US may be possible. At MR imaging, the microcysts may be seen as numerous discrete foci with bright signal intensity on T2-weighted images. Likewise, endoscopic US can help accurately depict these small microcysts as discrete small anechoic areas. Because of the benign nature of serous cystadenomas, some surgeons recommend imaging surveillance of microcystic tumours as being sufficient in asymptomatic patients.

Unlike IPMN, serous or mucinous cystadenomas do not communicate with the pancreatic duct.

Sahani DV, et al. Cystic pancreatic lesions: A simple imaging-based classification system for guiding management. *Radiographics.* 2005;25:1471–84.

92. D. Right middle lobe and lingular bronchiectasis

HRCT scanning is more sensitive than chest radiographs for detecting the abnormalities of Mycobacterium avium complex (MAC) lung disease. The presence of bronchiectasis and multiple small nodules are predictive of MAC lung disease with pleural thickening or adhesions, usually adjacent to the pulmonary parenchymal abnormalities in about 50% of cases. Other reported abnormalities include atelectasis, consolidation, tree-in-bud and ground-glass opacities. Bronchiectasis is more common in MAC lung disease than MTB. Some nodules will disappear with successful treatment.

It has been suggested that MAC-related cavities tend to be thinner with less surrounding parenchymal opacification. In the absence of underlying lung disease, they primarily involve the right middle lobe or lingular. Pleural effusions are not common in MAC.

Field SK, et al. *Mycobacterium avium* complex pulmonary disease in patients without HIV infection. *Chest.* 2004;126(2):566–81.

93. B. Pial angioma demonstrated by leptomeningeal enhancement

The clinical picture is very suggestive of Sturge–Weber syndrome. The major pathological abnormality in Sturge–Weber syndrome is a meningeal tangle of vessels, commonly referred to as an *angioma*, which is ordinarily confined to the pia mater. This pathological process consists of multiple capillaries and small venous channels that are matted together on the surface of

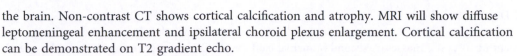

the brain. Non-contrast CT shows cortical calcification and atrophy. MRI will show diffuse leptomeningeal enhancement and ipsilateral choroid plexus enlargement. Cortical calcification can be demonstrated on T2 gradient echo.

The other options suggest different diagnoses respectively: posterior fossa haemangioblastoma – VHL; bilateral acoustic schwannomas – neurofibromatosis Type 2; multiple white matter T2 hyperintensities – unidentified bright spots in neurofibromatosis Type 1; multiple T1-weighted hyperintensities and cerebellar hypoplasia – neurocutaneous melanosis.

Herron J, et al. Intra-cranial manifestations of the neurocutaneous syndromes. *Clin Radiol.* 2000;55:82–98.

94. E. Soft-tissue rim sign

Before a tumour can be described as primarily retroperitoneal, the possibility that the tumour originates from a retroperitoneal organ must be excluded. When a mass deforms the edge of an adjacent organ into a 'beak' shape, it is likely that the mass arises from that organ (beak sign). When a large mass arises from a small organ, the organ sometimes becomes undetectable. This is known as the phantom organ sign. When a tumour compresses an adjacent plastic organ (e.g., gastrointestinal tract, inferior vena cava) that is not the organ of origin, the organ is deformed into a crescent shape (negative embedded organ sign). In contrast, when part of an organ appears to be embedded in the tumour (positive embedded organ sign), it is likely that the tumour originates from the involved organ. Hypervascular masses are often supplied by feeding arteries that are prominent enough to be visualised at CT or MR imaging, a finding that provides an important key to understanding the origin of the mass. Some tumours grow and extend into spaces between pre-existing structures and surrounding vessels without compressing their lumina. Lymphangiomas, ganglioneuromas and lymphomas are examples of such tumours manifesting with the CT angiogram sign' or 'floating aorta sign'.

The soft-tissue rim sign is described with distal ureteric calculus.

Nishino M, et al. Primary retroperitoneal neoplasms: CT and MR imaging findings with anatomic and pathologic diagnostic clues. *Radiographics.* 2003;23(1):45–57.

95. D. Osteophytes

Synovial hyperplasia and formation into pannus is the fundamental pathogenesis of RA. Hyperaemia is the first step in the inflammatory cascade that can be identified with imaging. Power Doppler, contrast-enhanced sonography and MR imaging (especially T1-weighted contrast-enhanced sequences with spectral fat saturation and water-weighted inversion-recovery images) are very helpful in identifying the pathologic condition. X-rays are often normal at this stage.

MR imaging is an excellent tool for assessing synovial swelling and volume. The use of a T1-weighted spin-echo sequence early after intravenous contrast material administration is highly recommended, as it helps differentiate effusion and synovium. Plain radiograph shows soft-tissue swelling, joint effusion and joint widening. Para-articular osteoporosis is cited as an early sign of joint involvement in RA. Up to 47% of patients may develop erosions within 1 year after onset of RA. MR imaging demonstrates erosions first. Sometimes, contrast enhancement helps distinguish erosions and pre-erosions from simple and degenerative bone cysts, which are less likely to enhance.

Joint subluxation, loose bodies (rice bodies) and ankylosis are other destructive/late features. Rotator cuff tear is often associated at the shoulder, and superior subluxation of the humeral head is often evident.

Osteophytosis are a feature of osteoarthrosis.

Sommer OJ, et al. Rheumatoid arthritis: A practical guide to state-of-the-art imaging, image interpretation, and clinical implications. *Radiographics.* 2005;25(2):381–98.

96. D. Branchial cyst

Second branchial cleft anomalies comprise 95% of all branchial cleft lesions, most commonly presenting as cystic masses. A second branchial cleft cyst (BCC) can occur anywhere in the lateral aspect of the neck but is classically seen as a well-marginated anechoic mass with a thin, well-defined wall at the anteromedial border of the sternocleidomastoid muscle at the junction of its upper and middle third. It may show thick walls or internal septations or echoes. On CT, it is seen as a well-circumscribed, non-enhancing mass of homogenous low attenuation. Wall thickening and enhancement may occur due to associated inflammation.

Metastatic nodes from head-and-neck malignancy, especially papillary carcinoma of the thyroid, are the most common types of nodal metastases presenting as cystic masses in the neck. Eighty percent of the cystic masses in patients over 40 years of age are due to necrotic lymph nodes.

On US, a central cystic area with thick irregular walls or an eccentric solid component may be seen. These solid areas usually demonstrate increased peripheral and intralesional vascularity on Doppler. The presence of punctate calcification within the solid component of the cystic node warrants careful search for primary papillary carcinoma in the thyroid gland. Occasionally necrosis within a metastatic lymph node may be very florid, mimicking a congenital cyst, such as a second BCC.

Mittal MK, et al. Cystic masses of neck: A pictorial review. *Indian J Radiol Imaging*. 2012;22(4):334–43.

97. B. Mounier–Kuhn syndrome

Mounier–Kuhn syndrome is characterised by distinct tracheobronchial dilation that is due to atrophy of the muscular and elastic tissues in the trachea and main bronchial wall. Diagnosis is often made by using CT, through which abnormally large air passages are detected. In adults, the diagnostic criteria are trachea >30 mm, right main bronchus >20 mm and the left main bronchus >18 mm. Upper zone emphysema, lower zone bronchiectasis and tracheal diverticulae are recognised.

Connective-tissue diseases, ataxia-telangiectasia, ankylosing spondylitis, Ehlers–Danlos syndrome, Marfan syndrome, Kenny–Caffey syndrome, Brachmann–de Lange syndrome and cutis laxa are also associated with secondary tracheobronchial enlargement. All of these conditions should be considered in the differential diagnosis.

Williams–Campbell syndrome is a rare form of congenital cystic bronchiectasis, in which distal bronchial cartilage is defective with preservation of central bronchi and trachea.

Celik B, et al. Mounier-Kuhn syndrome – A rare cause of bronchial dilation. *Tex Heart Inst J*. 2011;38(2):194–6.

98. E. Side-branch intraductal papillary mucinous neoplasm

IPMNs can be classified as main duct, branch duct (side-branch) or mixed IPMNs, depending on the site and extent of involvement. Main duct IPMN is a morphologically distinct entity and cannot be included in the discussion of pancreatic cysts. However, a side-branch IPMN or a mixed IPMN (in which a side-branch tumour extends to the main pancreatic duct) can have the morphologic features of a complex pancreatic cyst, making clear-cut distinction from a mucinous cystic neoplasm difficult. Identification of a septated cyst that communicates with the main pancreatic duct is highly suggestive of a side-branch or mixed IPMN. However, it is important to be aware that lack of communication with the main pancreatic duct at imaging does not exclude an IPMN. Currently, MR cholangiopancreatography is considered the modality of choice for demonstrating the morphologic features of the cyst (including septa and mural nodules), establishing the presence of communication between the cystic lesion and the pancreatic duct, and evaluating the extent of pancreatic ductal dilatation. Because these lesions are considered premalignant, surgical resection has typically been recommended. The occurrence of malignancy is significantly higher in main duct and mixed IPMNs than in side-branch IPMNs. Therefore, in cases of side-branch IPMN, the treatment decision should be based on the risk–benefit ratio,

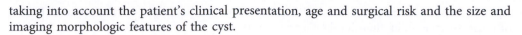

taking into account the patient's clinical presentation, age and surgical risk and the size and imaging morphologic features of the cyst.

Sahani DV, et al. Cystic pancreatic lesions: A simple imaging-based classification system for guiding management. *Radiographics*. 2005;25:1471–84.

99. B. T1W TSE

T1-weighted images are the most sensitive in children less than 1 year of age. T2-weighted images are the most sensitive in children between the ages of 1 and 2 years, demonstrating a gradual shift from hyperintense to hypointense relative to grey matter. The only area to remain hyperintense after the age of 2 years, and often for quite some time, is the peritrigonal region. FLAIR unsurprisingly follows the same pattern as T2 but lags behind somewhat. Both T1-weighted and T2-weighted images should be used to assess myelination. All children should achieve the adult appearance of white matter by 36–40 months.

Barkovich AJ. Concepts of myelin and myelination in neuroradiology. *Am J Neuroradiol*. 2000;21:1099–109.
Barkovich AJ, et al. Normal maturation of the neonatal and infant brain: MR imaging at 1.5 T. *Radiology*. 1988;166:173–80.

100. C. Haemorrhagic cyst

Haemorrhagic ovarian cysts are likely caused by bleeding into a corpus luteum. The majority have typical US features that allow a confident diagnosis to be made. A reticular pattern of internal echoes due to fibrin strands is a strong predictor of a haemorrhagic cyst. This pattern has also been referred to as having a fishnet, lacy, cobweb or spiderweb appearance. Although a clot may occasionally simulate a solid nodule, it is usually recognisable by its concave outer margin and/or absence of detectable flow at colour or power Doppler US. Bloodclot can sometimes be recognised on a grey-scale US scan by its jellylike movement when pressure is applied with the transducer. A fluid level occasionally occurs in a haemorrhagic cyst.

Brown DL, et al. Adnexal masses: US characterization and reporting. *Radiology*. 2010;254(2):342–54.

101. C. 2

The MRI sequences typically used are STIR, T1W, and T2W. The grading of such fractures is based on the MR findings and are as follows:

Grade 1 – Periosteal oedema on STIR, no marrow change
Grade 2 – Periosteal oedema on STIR + marrow change on T2-weighted only
Grade 3 – Periosteal oedema on STIR plus marrow changes on T2-weighted and T1-weighted
Grade 4 – Visible fracture line

Fredericson M, et al. Tibial stress reaction in runners: Correlation of clinical symptoms and scintigraphy with a new magnetic resonance imaging grading system. *Am J Sports Med*. 1995;23:472–81.

102. A. Cystic hygroma

A cystic hygroma is the most common form of lymphangioma and constitutes about 5% of all benign tumours of infancy and childhood. The overwhelming majority (about 80%–90%) are detected by the time the patient is 2 years old.

These lesions are characteristically infiltrative in nature and do not respect fascial planes; hence recurrence post-surgery is not uncommon.

On US scans, most cystic hygromas manifest as a multilocular predominantly cystic mass with septa of variable thickness. The echogenic portions of the lesion correlate with clusters of small, abnormal lymphatic channels. Fluid–fluid levels can be observed with a characteristic echogenic, haemorrhagic component layering in the dependent portion of the lesion. The most common pattern is that of a mass with low or intermediate signal intensity on T1-weighted images and hyperintensity on T2-weighted images. Infrequently, this lesion may be hyperintense on

T1-weighted images, a finding associated with clotted blood or high lipid (chyle) content. In the case of haemorrhage, fluid–fluid levels may be observed.

Koeller KK, et al. Congenital cystic masses of the neck: Radiologic-pathologic correlation. *Radiographics*. 1999; 19(1):121–46; quiz 152–3.

103. C. Lack of tapering of a bronchus

Bronchiectasis is defined as an 'irreversible localised or diffuse dilatation, usually resulting from chronic infection, proximal airway obstruction, or congenital bronchial abnormality'. On chest radiographs, bronchiectasis manifests as tram tracks, parallel line opacities, ring opacities and tubular structures. CT is substantially more sensitive than chest radiography for showing bronchiectasis, which is characterised by lack of bronchial tapering, bronchi visible in the peripheral 1 cm of the lungs, and an increased broncho-arterial ratio producing the so-called signet-ring sign. Mucoid impaction, segmental atelectasis and secondary bronchial wall thickening are all associated secondary signs.

Cantin L, et al. Bronchiectasis. *AJR Am J Roentgenol*. 2009;193:W158–71.

104. D. The submucosal gas in pneumatosis cystoides intestinalis can mimic colonic polyps on a barium enema when viewed *en face*.

Pneumatosis is the presence of gas bubbles within the wall of the involved segment of bowel. The patterns of pneumatosis vary from circular to linear to bubble and curvilinear gas collections. Such patterns can differentiate benign and clinically worrisome pneumatosis intestinalis. The circular form is usually benign and most often seen with pneumatosis cystoides intestinalis and affect the whole colon. Pseudopneumatosis is more common in the right colon because of the presence of liquid fecal matter.

Linear or bubble- like air can be due to both benign and life- threatening causes, and its radiographic appearance alone does not allow differentiation between them. In PI due to benign causes, the bowel wall is usually normal.

Additional CT findings such as soft-tissue thickening of the bowel wall, free fluid and peri-intestinal soft-tissue stranding are more frequently associated with clinically worrisome than benign pneumatosis intestinalis.

Portal venous gas is differentiated from biliary gas by its characteristic tubular branching lucencies that extend to the periphery of the liver, whereas biliary air is more central.

Ho LM, Paulson EK, Thompson WM. Pneumatosis intestinalis in the adult: benign to life-threatening causes. *AJR Am J Roentgenol*. 2007;188:1604–1613.

105. D. Visualisation of a heartbeat

Ninety-five percent of ectopic pregnancies are tubal; they occur mostly in the ampulla (70%). An adnexal mass that is separate from the ovary is the most common finding of a tubal pregnancy and is seen on US images. Although not common, an adnexal mass is more specific for an ectopic pregnancy when it contains a yolk sac or a living embryo. The tubal ring sign is the second most common sign of a tubal pregnancy. The tubal ring sign describes a hyperechoic ring surrounding an extrauterine gestational sac. A related finding is the 'ring of fire' sign, which is recognised by peripheral hypervascularity of the hyperechoic ring. The term *previously* described the high-velocity, low-impedance flow surrounding an ectopic adnexal pregnancy. Peripheral hypervascularity is a non-specific finding of the ring of fire sign and may also be seen surrounding a normal maturing follicle or a corpus luteal cyst. Location of the ring of fire in an ovary distinguishes a corpus luteal cyst from an ectopic pregnancy where the ring is extra-ovarian.

Intrauterine findings of an ectopic pregnancy include a 'normal endometrium', a pseudo–gestational sac, a trilaminar endometrium and a thin-walled decidual cyst. Extrauterine findings of ectopic pregnancy include pelvic free fluid, hematosalpinx and haemoperitoneum.

Lin EP, et al. Diagnostic clues to ectopic pregnancy. *Radiographics*. 2008;28(6):1661–71.

106. D. Peritrigonal region

Myelin development correlates with functional milestones.

By 2 years, the infant brain should resemble the adult brain with the exception of the peritrigonal area, which is the last area to myelinate. This area can remain unmyelinated long after the age of 2 years. This can be seen on MRI as persistent T2-weighted and FLAIR hyperintensity and should not be confused with a pathological process. The process of myelination is predictable and follows a few simple rules: central to peripheral, caudal to rostral, dorsal to ventral. At birth, the cerebellum, brainstem and posterior limb of the internal capsule should normally be myelinated. The anterior limb should myelinate by 2 months.

Barkovich AJ. Concepts of myelin and myelination in neuroradiology. *Am J Neuroradiol.* 2000;21:1099–109.

107. E. Pleural plaque secondary to asbestos exposure

There are many causes of HPOA, most of which are pulmonary in origin: intrathoracic malignant tumours, including metastasis, mesothelioma, bronchogenic carcinoma and lymphoma; benign tumours, including benign pleural fibroma, thymoma and pulmonary haemangiomas; chronic pulmonary infection (e.g., bronchiectasis and lung abscesses); and cyanotic congenital heart disease. Extrathoracic causes include ulcerative colitis, Crohn's disease, Whipple disease, liver disease (e.g., cirrhosis, liver abscesses and primary biliary cirrhosis) and gastric and pancreatic carcinomas. Although asbestosis (i.e., asbestos-induced pulmonary fibrosis) is a known cause of HPOA, pleural plaques are not. Radiological abnormalities most commonly affect the lower limb or forearm bones with cortical thickening and lamellar periosteal proliferation. Hypertrophic pulmonary osteoarthropathy is commonly present in conjunction with finger clubbing. If the underlying condition is treated, then this often quickly leads to remission of their symptoms and about a month later to resolution of the radiological findings.

Dähnert W. *Radiology Review Manual.* 7th edn. Philadelphia, PA: Lippincott Williams & Wilkins, 2011:110.

108. B. Dentigerous cyst

Odontogenic keratocysts are believed to arise from the dental lamina and other sources of odontogenic epithelium. At radiography, an odontogenic keratocyst usually appears as a unilocular, lucent lesion with smooth, corticated borders that is often associated with an impacted tooth. Such lesions are indistinguishable from dentigerous cysts at radiography. They are more likely to show aggressive growth than other odontogenic cysts and may have undulating borders and a multilocular appearance; these characteristics make odontogenic keratocysts indistinguishable from ameloblastomas.

The dentigerous (follicular) cyst is the most common type of non-inflammatory odontogenic cyst and the most common cause of a pericoronal area of lucency associated with an impacted tooth. At radiography, dentigerous cysts appear as well-defined, round or ovoid, corticated, lucent lesions around the crowns of unerupted teeth, usually third molars. The roots of the involved tooth are often outside the lesion and in mandibular bone.

Scholl RJ, et al. Cysts and cystic lesions of the mandible: Clinical and radiologic-histopathologic review. *Radiographics.* 1999;19(5):1107–24.

109. A. High-density mucus plugging

A 'finger-in-glove' pattern can be seen at chest radiography in ABPA that corresponds to mucoid bronchial impaction at chest CT. CT findings in ABPA include cystic or varicoid bronchiectasis, a tree-in-bud pattern of nodules, bronchial wall thickening and air trapping with a central or proximal upper-lobe predominance. High-attenuating (>70–100 HU) bronchial contents at CT represent fungal debris containing iron and manganese.

The classic diagnostic triad in patients with cystic fibrosis includes an abnormal sweat chloride test result and manifestations of pulmonary and pancreatic disease. Upper-lobe predominance is seen in many but not all cases; a diffuse distribution is also a common sign.

Normal to increased lung volumes are typical in CF and indicate air trapping and small airways disease. CT images show extensive cystic and cylindrical bronchiectasis and bronchial wall and peribronchial interstitial thickening. Findings are typically more extensive in patients with bronchiectasis due to cystic fibrosis than in patients with bronchiectasis due to other causes. Nodular opacities throughout the lungs correlate with areas of mucoid bronchial or bronchiolar impaction. Tree-in-bud nodules indicate the diffuse bronchiolitis that typically occurs in cystic fibrosis. In addition, a mosaic pattern of attenuation secondary to air trapping due to obstructed bronchi and bronchioles is commonly seen.

Milliron B, et al. Bronchiectasis: Mechanisms and imaging clues of associated common and uncommon diseases. *Radiographics*. 2015;35(4):1011–30.

110. D.   Surgical placement of a jejunostomy tube

Pneumatosis is the presence of gas bubbles within the wall of the involved segment of bowel. It is seen in a wide variety of conditions. It is widely divided into two groups: primary (idiopathic) and secondary. Conditions associated with secondary pneumatosis include obstruction; pulmonary disease such as COPD and asthma; vascular conditions such as ischaemia and infarction; inflammatory conditions such as Crohn's and UC; necrotising enterocolitis; drugs such as steroids and chemotherapy; and collagen vascular diseases such as scleroderma, SLE and dermatomyositis.

Feczko PJ, et al. Clinical significance of pneumatosis of the bowel wall. *Radiographics*. 1992;12:1069–78.

111. E.   Solid component with intense enhancement on Doppler

Endometriomas typically appear as complex cysts, either unilocular or multilocular, that have a ground-glass appearance due to diffuse, homogeneous, low- to medium-level internal echoes. Similar internal echoes may occur in haemorrhagic cysts, dermoids and some ovarian carcinomas. Thus, it is important to carefully evaluate for other features like a solid component that would suggest a different diagnosis. An endometrioma is very likely when there are diffuse internal echoes in a cystic mass lacking other US features. Additional features reported include echogenic foci in the wall and small solid areas along the wall, most likely representing solid endometrial tissue, which can mimic malignant cysts. Endometrial solid deposits are less likely to be vascular on Doppler compared to tumour, but the role of Doppler imaging is unclear. A small percentage (probably <15%) of endometriomas have less-typical US features such as anechoic fluid, a fluid–fluid level, heterogeneity or calcification. Endometriomas may occasionally simulate a solid mass, especially when they are chronic. Rarely, endometroid or clear cell carcinoma may develop within an endometrioma; this is more likely in women over 45 years of age and in endometriomas larger than 9 cm.

Brown DL, et al. Adnexal masses: US characterization and reporting. *Radiology*. 2010;254(2):342–54.

112. B.   Sclerotic bone lesions

The patient has tuberous sclerosis, an inherited autosomal dominant multisystem disorder with multifocal systemic hamartomas. Osseous manifestations include cyst-like lesions, hyperostosis of the inner table of the calvaria, osteoblastic changes, periosteal new bone formation and scoliosis. These osseous lesions can occur anywhere in bone, commonly in the calvaria, short tubular bones of the hand or foot, spine and pelvis. The cyst-like lesions are usually irregularly circumscribed and have a sclerotic appearance peripherally.

Dähnert W. *Radiology Review Manual*. 7th edn. Philadelphia, PA: Lippincott Williams & Wilkins, 2011.

113. B.   Retrosternal goitre

Most thyroid masses in the mediastinum represent downward retrosternal extension of multinodular colloid goitre. They usually have a well-defined outline, which may be spherical and lobulated. Round or irregular well-defined areas of calcification may be seen in benign areas, whereas amorphous cloud-like calcification is occasionally seen within carcinomas.

Almost all intrathoracic masses displace and narrow the trachea, which is well recognised in plain film. On US, the inability to see the inferior extent of a thyroid mass is suggestive of retrosternal extension. CT is the best modality for initial investigation because it confirms the finding, displays its anatomical location and provides information should the lesion not be a retrosternal goitre. Clinically within 30 seconds after raising both arms simultaneously (Pemberton's manoeuvre), marked facial plethora (Pemberton's sign) develops, indicating compression of the jugular veins by the enlarged multinodular goitre.

Adam A, et al. *Grainger & Allison's Diagnostic Radiology: A Textbook of Medical Imaging.* 5th edn. New York: Churchill Livingstone, 2008:244.
Basaria S, Salvatori R. Pemberton's sign. *N Engl J Med.* 2004;350:1338.
Umeoka S, et al. Pictorial review of tuberous sclerosis in various organs. *Radiographics.* 2008;28(7):e32.

114. E.   Central to peripheral, caudal to rostral, dorsal to ventral

Myelination begins at 16 weeks *in utero* and is far from complete at term birth. It continues during the first 2 years of life until it reaches the level of myelination seen in a normal adult brain. Learning development coincides with myelination. CT and MRI can be used to assess myelination. On CT, unmyelinated white matter will appear hypodense. Unmyelinated white matter will appear hypointense on T1-weighted and hyperintense on T2-weighted. This can be confusing as many other conditions of interest in the neonate can cause T2-weighted hyperintensity. Knowing the pattern of normal myelination is therefore essential when interpreting paediatric neuroimaging.

Barkovich AJ. Concepts of myelin and myelination in neuroradiology. *Am J Neuroradiol.* 2000;21:1099–109.

115. B.   Sarcoidosis

Bronchiectasis with Upper or Mid-Lung Predominance
- Cystic fibrosis
- ABPA
- Sarcoidosis
- TB

Bronchiectasis with Anterior Predominance
- Atypical mycobacterial infection
- ARDS

Bronchiectasis with Lower Lung Predominance
- Pulmonary fibrosis
- Chronic aspiration
- Kartagener's syndrome
- Common variable immunodeficiency
- α_1-Antitrypsin deficiency

Bronchiectasis with Central Predominance
- Mounier–Kuhn syndrome
- Williams–Campbell syndrome

Milliron B, et al. Bronchiectasis: Mechanisms and imaging clues of associated common and uncommon diseases. *Radiographics.* 2015;35(4):1011–30.

116. C.   Heterogeneous content is detected within the mass on CT.

This uncommon, typically benign tumour is found mainly in young, non-Caucasian women between the second and third decades of life. It seems to have a predilection for Asian and African American women, although rare cases have been reported in children and men.

Although most solid pseudopapillary tumours (SPTs) exhibit benign behaviour, malignant degeneration does occur. Patients with SPT of the pancreas are often clinically asymptomatic. They may present with a gradually enlarging abdominal mass or complain of vague abdominal pain or discomfort. The abdomen is usually non-tender on palpation, but obstructive symptoms may occur if the tumour grows large enough to compress adjacent viscera.

There are usually no abnormalities in clinical laboratory tests (e.g., serum amylase levels) or in pancreatic cancer markers (e.g., CA19–9, carcinoembryonic antigen, fetoprotein). The diagnosis is not uncommonly made incidentally at abdominal examination, US or CT performed for other reasons.

SPT of the pancreas has distinctive pathologic features. The mass may occur anywhere in the pancreas but is most frequently found in the head or tail. At gross examination, the mass is usually large (mean maximum dimension 9.3 cm) and well encapsulated and contains varying amounts of necrosis, haemorrhage and cystic change.

Coleman KM, Whitehouse RW. Solid-pseudopapillary tumour of the pancreas. *Radiographics*. 2003;23: 1644–8.

117. B. Hydrosalpinx

Hydrosalpinx should be suspected based on location and configuration. Characteristically, it is a tubular-shaped cystic structure that is separate from the ipsilateral ovary. Its configuration may reveal indentations on the opposite sides of the wall referred to as the 'waist sign'. The waist sign in combination with a tubular-shaped cystic mass has been found to be pathognomonic of a hydrosalpinx. Incomplete septa, due to the wall of the tube folding on itself, or small mural nodules, due to thickening of endosalpingeal folds (termed 'beads on a string'), are also typical and are more predictive of hydrosalpinx when the mass is tubular in shape. The distinction from tumour nodule is easier when one recognises that the mass is separate from the ovary. Additionally, the solid component of the rare fallopian tube carcinoma is usually larger and less numerous than the multiple small nodules due to thickened endosalpingeal folds.

Brown DL, et al. Adnexal masses: US characterization and reporting. *Radiology*. 2010;254(2):342–54.

118. B. Mid-shaft of the second metatarsal

Stress fractures of the metatarsals account for between 9% and 24.6% of stress fractures in athletes. Plain radiographic evaluation may reveal normal appearances. Two to three weeks after the injury, periosteal bone reaction may be visible on radiographs. MRI has high sensitivity in the diagnosis of these fractures, depicting oedema of the bone marrow and periosteum. A hypointense fracture line may also be visible on MRI. The most common site of metatarsal stress fractures are the distal shaft and neck of the second and third metatarsals, especially in long-distance runners. They are usually thinner than the first metatarsal and bear a large amount of weight during the 'push off' phase of running. Stress fractures of the fifth metatarsal base occurring approximately 1.5 cm distal to the tubercle, at the junction of the metaphysis and diaphysis (Jones' fracture), deserve special mention as high-performance athletes with this injury, because of their propensity to be delayed or non-union, and refracture, may benefit from early operative intervention.

Liong SY, Whitehouse RW. Lower extremity and pelvic stress fractures in athletes. *Br J Radiol*. 2012;85(1016): 1148–56.

119. D. US neck with FNA

Thyroid scanning using pertechnetate (99MTc) is traditionally used to screen thyroid nodules for malignancy. The finding of a hyperfunctioning or 'hot' nodule (uptake of tracer within the nodule with suppression of uptake in the surrounding normal thyroid tissue) excludes malignancy in almost all patients. A non-functioning or 'cold' nodule was thought to indicate increased risk of malignancy, with 5%–15% of these being malignant.

FNA should be the first-line investigation for assessment of all solitary nodules or a dominant nodule in a multinodular goitre. US is well established as a primary investigation for patients presenting with a lump in the neck; moreover, the cost-effectiveness and diagnostic accuracy of FNA can be increased by using US guidance and the presence of an on-site cytopathologist.

Ganguly A, et al. The benefits of on-site cytology with ultrasound-guided fine needle aspiration in a one-stop neck lump clinic. *Ann R Coll Surg Engl.* 2010;92(8):660–4.

Mackenzie EJ1, Mortimer RH. 6: Thyroid nodules and thyroid cancer. *Med J Aust.* 2004;180(5):242–7.

120. B.   Discharge with reassurance

This is a description of the normal appearances of the thymus for a child of this age. The wavy margins result from interdigitation of soft thymic tissue in the intercostal spaces. Sometimes a definite notch (unilateral or bilateral) can be seen at the junction of the inferior aspect of the gland and the cardiac silhouette. The thymus gradually involutes with age and may acutely shrink during periods of bodily stress. During the recovery period, it grows back to its original size or even larger, a phenomenon known as *thymic rebound hyperplasia*. The thymus becomes less evident between 2 and 8 years of age, after which it cannot be visualised on the frontal chest X-ray.

Nasseri F, Eftekhari F. Clinical and radiologic review of the normal and abnormal thymus: Pearls and pitfalls. *Radiographics.* 2010;30:413–28.

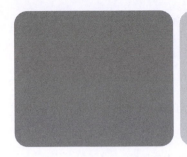

Time: 3 hours

1. An 18-year-old girl with chronic cough and recurrent chest infections shows symmetrical upper lobe predominant varicoid and cystic bronchiectasis on HRCT. Review of older abdominal plain films shows calcification across the central upper abdomen at the T12/L1 level. What is the likely diagnosis?
   A. Cystic fibrosis (CF)
   B. Sarcoidosis
   C. William–Campbell syndrome
   D. ABPA
   E. Kartagener's syndrome

2. A 53-year-old woman with upper abdominal discomfort was sent for an abdominal US, which showed a hypoechoic mass in the pancreas. A CT was performed, which reported a possible serous cystadenoma. Which one of the following statements regarding serous cystadenomas of the pancreas is true?
   A. They are rich in mucin.
   B. They are rich in glycogen.
   C. They have malignant potential.
   D. They appear only as a unilocular cyst on CT.
   E. They are more common in men than in women.

3. A 2-year-old boy with proptosis and cat's eye was investigated with CT for persistent headache. Axial images showed a densely calcified mass replacing the right eyeball. The optic nerve was also calcified and surrounded by tumour, which had replaced most of the periorbital fat. The optic canal was expanded with extension of the mass in the middle cranial fossa. What is the diagnosis?
   A. Malignant melanoma of the choroid
   B. Rhabdomyosarcoma
   C. Coats' disease
   D. Neuroblastoma metastasis
   E. Retinoblastoma

4. A 29-year-old woman with three previous miscarriages, not explained by any hormonal, biochemical or metabolic abnormality, was being investigated for a structural cause to explain the recurrent miscarriage. A pelvic MRI was scheduled, as it was the most definitive investigation for congenital structural anomalies and/or uterine masses. Which one of the following descriptions would suggest the diagnosis of uterus didelphys?
   A. Two separate uterine cavities with two cervices and two proximal vagina
   B. Two separate uterine cavities with two cervices

C. Two separate uterine horns with common uterine cavity, with one cervix

D. External indentation of the uterine fundus with one uterine cavity

E. Single uterine horn connected to a single fallopian tube

5. With regard to stress fractures affecting the lower limb in athletes, all of the following statements are correct, except

A. Anterior tibial stress fractures have a higher propensity of non-union.

B. Fibular stress fractures affect the proximal end.

C. Femoral stress fractures can affect the neck or shaft.

D. 'Female athlete triad' is associated with femoral and sacral fractures.

E. Tibial stress fracture can be transverse or longitudinal.

6. A 3-year-old girl is referred to an endocrine clinic with unilateral jaw swelling noted at the dentist. Her general practitioner has also reported that she has signs of precocious puberty. An X-ray of the facial bones demonstrates expansion of the frontal bone and right side of the mandible. She is likely to have which other associated condition?

A. Neurofibromatosis

B. Madelung deformity

C. Lisch nodule

D. Hyperthyroidism

E. Hypothyroidism

7. A 35-year-old man known to the ENT for sinonasal disease presents to the chest clinic with productive cough. The house officer examining the patient struggled to hear the heart sounds properly. HRCT, among other findings, shows left lower lobe bronchiectasis without any central endobronchial mass to explain the focal bronchiectasis. What is the likely diagnosis?

A. Cystic fibrosis (CF)

B. Sarcoidosis

C. William–Campbell syndrome

D. Allergic bronchopulmonary aspergillosis (ABPA)

E. Kartagener's syndrome

8. A 56-year-old man with gallstone pancreatitis is referred for a CT of the abdomen. The CT shows multiple cysts around the tail of the pancreas with further cysts in the lesser sac and left paracolic gutter. These are reported as pseudocysts. Which one of the following statements regarding pancreatic pseudocysts is false?

A. They usually take 4–6 weeks to mature.

B. They can be multiple.

C. They have an epithelial lining.

D. They may communicate with the pancreatic ductal system.

E. They may be extrapancreatic in location.

9. A woman who was 20 weeks pregnant was referred to the US department by her midwife for a routine anomaly scan. The scan was reported as showing features consistent with congenital diaphragmatic hernia. All of the following are prenatal US findings suggestive of a diaphragmatic hernia, except

A. Failure to visualise the stomach in the left upper quadrant

B. Cardiac dextroposition

C. Echogenic mass in the left hemithorax

D. Compressed left lung

E. Increased abdominal circumference

10. A 52-year-old woman presents to the orthopaedic outpatient clinic with a painful forefoot. On examination, there was a painful response elicited by Mulder's manoeuvre. Which one of the following statements concerning Morton neuromas in the forefoot is false?
    A. They are often seen in young and middle-aged women.
    B. The inter space between the third and fourth toes is the most commonly affected site.
    C. The characteristic MR finding is a nodule with low signal intensity on T1W images.
    D. Ultrasound is a sensitive modality in identifying the lesion.
    E. Gradient echo MR sequences elicit blooming artefact in the lesion.

11. A 54-year-old man with suspicious findings on US was recommended for an MRI of the orbits for further evaluation. Sagittal MR images of the globe showed a focal area of thickening in the posterior aspect of the globe with hyperintense signal on T1W sequence and strongly hypointense signal on T2W sequence. What is the diagnosis?
    A. Malignant melanoma of the choroid
    B. Rhabdomyosarcoma
    C. Coats' disease
    D. Neuroblastoma metastasis
    E. Retinoblastoma

12. A previously healthy 9-month-old is admitted with tachypnoea and fever. His white cell count and neutrophils are elevated. His temperature is 39.2°C. An AP CXR demonstrates a well-defined 5 cm rounded lung opacity with well-formed borders. What is the most likely diagnosis?
    A. Bronchogenic cyst
    B. Pulmonary metastases
    C. Neuroblastoma
    D. Congenital cystic adenomatoid malformation
    E. Round pneumonia

13. A 77-year-old man with chronic inflammatory disease and renal failure is known to have secondary amyloidosis. All of the following are features of amyloid involvement of the respiratory system, except
    A. Interstitial septal thickening
    B. Cavitating nodules
    C. Focal amyloidoma
    D. Calcification of central airways
    E. Calcification in peripheral consolidation

14. An US of the abdomen in a 43-year-old woman with a known underlying chronic condition demonstrates small cysts in the pancreas. She is sent for a dual-phase CT for further characterisation. The scan shows multiple true cysts with no obvious suspicious features. Which one of the following conditions is associated with true pancreatic cysts?
    A. Tuberous sclerosis
    B. Von Hippel–Lindau disease
    C. Neurofibromatosis Type 1
    D. Autosomal recessive polycystic kidney disease
    E. Multiple neuroendocrine neoplasia

15. A woman who is 22 weeks pregnant is referred for routine anomaly scan to the US department. US shows that the ventricular atrium measure 14 mm at the level of the posterior margin of the glomus of the choroids plexus on an axial plain through the level of the thalami. What is the next appropriate step?
    A. Repeat US in 4 weeks.
    B. Amniocentesis.

C. Foetal MRI.

D. Check maternal oestradiol levels.

E. It is a normal finding.

16. Which of the following is not a recognised radiographic finding in a patient with haemochromatosis?

   A. Chondrocalcinosis

   B. Arthropathy with iron deposition in the synovium

   C. Generalised increased bone density

   D. Joint space narrowing

   E. Osteophyte formation

17. A 9-year-old girl with a long history of cough, wheeze, sinusitis, headache and weight loss presented to the GP with an acute history of increasing breathlessness. Sweat test analysis shows 80 mmol/L of sodium chloride in forearm sweat (normal <40 mmol/L). All of the following are typical features on a chest X-ray, except

   A. Hyperinflation

   B. Bronchial dilatation

   C. Cystic areas in the lung

   D. Linear interstitial opacities

   E. Dextrocardia

18. A 55-year-old woman with asymmetrical bilateral proptosis is referred for an orbital MRI to exclude retro-orbital mass lesions. MRI reveals diffuse swelling of all extraocular muscles, with the swelling primarily involving the belly of the muscle without involvement of the tendinous insertions. The muscles are isointense to normal in signal on T1W images and hypointense on T2W images. What is the diagnosis?

   A. Orbital pseudotumour

   B. Thyroid opthalmopathy

   C. Lymphoma orbit

   D. Steroid therapy

   E. Obesity

19. A 62-year-old man with progressive cough and shortness of breath has bilateral patchy ground-glass change with areas of dependent and non-dependent septal thickening in the basal lung zones on HRCT. Which of the following is incorrect about drug-induced lung disease?

   A. Diffuse alveolar damage occurs with Gold.

   B. Chronic nitrofurantoin toxicity results in high-density consolidation.

   C. High-density liver is seen in amiodarone toxicity.

   D. There is no correlation between dose of methotrexate and toxicity.

   E. NSIP is generally the most common change on HRCT.

20. A 50-year-old man is sent for an urgent contrast CT of the abdomen following a history of abdominal pain. The CT is unremarkable apart from inflammatory stranding in the omentum. All of the following are clinical features of omental infarction, except

   A. Occurrence in patients of all ages

   B. Massive rectal bleeding

   C. Slightly higher incidence in men

   D. Acute right-sided abdominal pain

   E. Rarely, a palpable mass at the site of abdominal pain

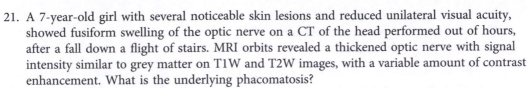

21. A 7-year-old girl with several noticeable skin lesions and reduced unilateral visual acuity, showed fusiform swelling of the optic nerve on a CT of the head performed out of hours, after a fall down a flight of stairs. MRI orbits revealed a thickened optic nerve with signal intensity similar to grey matter on T1W and T2W images, with a variable amount of contrast enhancement. What is the underlying phacomatosis?
    A. Neurofibromatosis type 2
    B. Neurofibromatosis type 1
    C. Von Hippel-Lindau disease
    D. Tuberous sclerosis
    E. Down's syndrome

22. Foetal MRI usually is performed in a scanner with a magnet strength of
    A. 0.5 Tesla
    B. 1.5 Tesla
    C. 1 Tesla
    D. 3 Tesla
    E. 0.1 Tesla

23. A patient arrives in the A&E department having been involved in a road traffic collision. He is haemodynamically stable. The Glasgow Coma Scale (GCS) at the scene was 14. On arrival in A&E, he is found to have a bruised left forehead. He suddenly becomes unresponsive, with a GCS of 4, and is intubated. As the on-call radiologist you are called to perform a head CT. Which of the following would make an epidural haemorrhage least likely?
    A. Biconvex hyperdensity
    B. Overlying skull fracture
    C. Crossing of suture line
    D. Homogenous fluid of 50 HU
    E. Homogenous fluid of 80 HU

24. A 12-month-old presents with loss of appetite, fever and shortness of breath. Chest X-ray demonstrates a well-circumscribed paraspinal mass with a sharp pleuro-pulmonary surface. There is some calcification within the mass and the intercostal space at that level is widened. What is the most likely diagnosis?
    A. Bronchogenic cyst
    B. Neuroblastoma
    C. Ganglioneuroma
    D. Left lower lobe pneumonia
    E. Teratoma

25. Foetal MRI is most commonly organised to evaluate inconclusive but potentially significant findings detected on ultrasound or to characterise definite abnormality detected on anomaly scan. Which one of the following MR imaging sequences is the most popular for foetal imaging?
    A. Fast spin echo T1W images
    B. STIR
    C. Fat-suppressed T1W images
    D. Single-shot, fast spin echo (SS FSE) T2W images
    E. FLAIR

26. A 45-year-old man with proptosis of the right eye is referred for an MRI for further evaluation. MRI reveals uniform swelling involving all the extraocular muscles and a markedly dilated superior ophthalmic vein. What is the likely diagnosis?
    A. AVM of the optic nerve
    B. Carotid-cavernous fistula

C. Haemangioma

D. Lymphatic malformation of the orbit

E. Thyroid opthalmopathy

27. A 4-day-old infant presents with poor feeding and lethargy. She was born at term following premature rupture of membranes. Chest X-ray demonstrates bilateral patchy infiltrates with small effusions. What is the most likely diagnosis?

A. Hyaline membrane disease

B. Meconium aspiration

C. Transient tachypnoea of the newborn

D. Group B streptococcal pneumonia

E. Congenital listeriosis

28. All the following statements regarding HRCT changes in cytotoxic drug-induced lung disease are true, except

A. Bleomycin toxicity has a poor prognosis.

B. Paclitaxel is associated with pulmonary injury.

C. There is no correlation between carmustine dose and toxicity.

D. Diffuse alveolar damage (DAD) is the most common manifestation.

E. Bleomycin toxicity can be increased by concomitant oxygen therapy.

29. A 66-year-old person is sent for an urgent CT of the abdomen post-contrast. The CT is unremarkable apart from inflammatory stranding in the omentum. No peritoneal nodules or ascites are detected on the CT and the report states possible omental infraction. All of the following are expected to be seen on the CT, except

A. Cake-like or whorled structure of mixed attenuation

B. Small amount of free peritoneal fluid

C. The fat-ring sign

D. Minimal reactive lymphadenopathy

E. Haziness of the fat anterior to the colon

30. A skeletal survey is performed on a 2-year-old boy with short stature. The lateral film of the spine reveals abnormal vertebral bodies with a central anterior 'beak' and generalised flattening. Radiographs of the hands shows a pointed proximal fifth metacarpal base with a notch at the ulnar aspect. Which of the following is the most likely diagnosis?

A. Hunter syndrome

B. Hurler syndrome

C. Morquio syndrome

D. Achondroplasia

E. Nail-patella syndrome

31. Which one of the following statements regarding rheumatoid arthritis-associated thoracic manifestation is true?

A. Thoracic involvement occurs early in the disease.

B. Pleural effusions is usually bilateral.

C. COP is a recognised pattern on HRCT in rheumatoid lungs.

D. Fibrosis mostly affects the upper lobes.

E. Cavitation in nodules suggests some other disease.

32. A 39-year-old hypotensive man involved in an RTA was sent for an urgent CT of the abdomen and pelvis to evaluate for solid organ or bowel injury. Which one of the following statements concerning imaging in blunt trauma to the liver is false?

A. Non-surgical treatment has become the standard of care in haemodynamically stable patients with blunt liver trauma.

    B. Hepatic lacerations demonstrate jagged edges.

    C. CT is the diagnostic modality of choice for the evaluation of blunt liver trauma in haemodynamically stable patients.

    D. CT features of blunt liver trauma include lacerations, subcapsular or parenchymal hematomas, active haemorrhage, juxtahepatic venous injuries, periportal low attenuation and a flat inferior vena cava.

    E. Follow-up MRI is required in patients with high-grade liver injuries to identify potential complications that require early intervention.

33. A 45-year-old man with proptosis of the right eye is referred for an MRI for further evaluation. MRI reveals a moderately large, well-defined intraconal retrobulbar mass, which is isointense to muscle on T1W images and markedly hyperintense to fat on T2W images. What is the most likely diagnosis?

    A. Retinoblastoma

    B. Rhabdomyoma

    C. Haemangioma

    D. Orbital pseudotumour

    E. Metastatic lymphoma

34. A 32-year-old woman is referred by her family doctor to the gynaecology clinic with history of congestive dysmenorrhoea, dyspareunia, fever and vaginal discharge. She had used a coil regularly in the past, which was later discontinued due to recurrent bouts of pelvic inflammation. Which one of the following statements concerning pelvic inflammatory disease is false?

    A. Pyosalpinx can have a high T1 signal.

    B. A tubular, fluid-filled structure with enhancing walls suggests pyosalpinx.

    C. Delay in treatment can lead to tubo-ovarian abscess.

    D. Intense enhancement of inflamed areas on contrast-enhanced T1W MRI.

    E. High signal in inflammatory stranding in peritubal fat on T1 fat-suppressed images.

35. A 40-year-old woman with short stature presents with early-onset hearing loss. Diagnostic workup reveals micromelic dwarfism, diffuse demineralisation and thinning of cortical bone, mild scoliosis and old fractures of the vertebral bodies and long bones. There was evidence of poor dentition. Which of the following is the most likely diagnosis?

    A. Hypophosphatasia

    B. Osteogenesis imperfecta

    C. Paget disease

    D. Osteoporosis

    E. Achondroplasia

36. A macrosomic neonate (secondary to maternal diabetes) is noted to be in mild respiratory distress following delivery by caesarean section (CS). A chest X-ray demonstrates mild cardiomegaly mild hyperexpansion and small pleural effusions of the lungs. No focal lung abnormality is seen. What is the most likely diagnosis?

    A. Respiratory distress syndrome

    B. Meconium aspiration

    C. Staphylococcal pneumonia

    D. Group B streptococcal pneumonia

    E. Transient tachypnea of the newborn

37. A 6-year-old child is admitted to the emergency department presenting with diffuse abdominal pain, arthralgia and bilateral lower limb palpable purpura. Which of the following findings on an abdominal US examination is least expected?

    A. Ileocaecal intussusception

    B. Bowel wall thickening

C. Multifocal hepatic lesions

D. Bilaterally enlarged, echogenic renal cortices

E. Ascites

38. All of the following are musculoskeletal manifestations of rheumatoid arthritis that can be seen on chest radiographs, except

A. Subacromial abutment of humeral head

B. Superior rib notching

C. Global loss of shoulder joint space

D. Erosion of medial aspect of clavicle

E. Erosion superolaterally in the humeral head

39. A 46-year-old man with syncopal episodes is found to be profoundly hypoglycaemic on each of the episodes. He is not on any antidiabetic medication. What imaging investigation would you suggest for further evaluation?

A. CT of the chest and liver

B. CT of the brain

C. MRA of the circle of Willis

D. Dual-phase CT of the pancreas

E. US of the abdomen

40. A 33-year-old woman with progressive congestive dysmenorrhoea, deep dyspareunia and infertility is being evaluated for possible endometriosis. All of the following are typical MR findings of endometriosis, except:

A. Hypointense cysts on T1W images

B. Hyperintense cysts on T2W images

C. Multilocular cysts

D. Thick-walled cysts

E. Hypointense wall thickening on T1W and T2W images

41. A 6-year-old boy presents with increasing pain within his upper back, which came on insidiously over a few weeks. The child is otherwise well. A radiograph of his thoracic spine reveals collapse of the T9 vertebral body. The disc spaces are preserved; there is no kyphosis, and no involvement of the posterior elements. Which of the following is the most likely diagnosis?

A. Ewing's sarcoma

B. Metastasis

C. Tuberculosis

D. Fracture

E. Eosinophilic granuloma

42. A 6-year-old boy presents with progressive proptosis of the right eye. CT shows a homogenous hypodense mass in the upper outer corner of the right orbit associated with thinning of the roof. No infiltration of the surrounding fat is evident. On MRI, the mass returns a similar signal to that of orbital fat and showed thin ring enhancement. What is the diagnosis?

A. Lymphoma

B. Pleomorphic adenoma of lacrimal gland

C. Epidermoid cyst

D. Dermoid cyst

E. Sebaceous cyst

43. A 42-year-old man presented with right-sided proptosis with mass in the inner canthus of the eye. An axial CT scan showed soft-tissue density and expansion of the right anterior

ethmoid air cells bulging into the orbit. The extraocular muscles were displaced but not involved. What is the diagnosis?

A. Encephalocele
B. Anterior ethmoid mucocoele
C. Destructive midline granuloma
D. Wagner's disease
E. Esthesioneuroblastoma

44. A 62-year-old man, who has undergone solid organ transplant, is found to be profoundly neutropaenic and presents with progressive fever, cough and shortness of breath. He is acutely unwell. Chest X-ray shows bilateral patchy air space opacities and bronchoalveolar lavage showed *Aspergillus* organisms. HRCT is organised to confirm pulmonary invasive aspergillosis. All the following are typical imaging features, except:

A. Nodules with surrounding ground-glass change
B. Pulmonary sequestra
C. Peripheral wedge-shaped consolidation
D. Air crescent sign
E. Central bronchiectasis

45. A 2-year-old child presents with fever, erythema of the oral mucosa with chest and abdominal pain. Echocardiography reveals the presence of a coronary arterial aneurysms. An underlying vasculitis is suspected. Which of the following statements is least accurate in this clinical setting?

A. Aneurysms are typically seen in the proximal segments of the coronary arteries.
B. Aneurysms less than 5 mm in diameter are considered small.
C. Smaller aneurysms have a higher likelihood of thrombosis.
D. Multiple coronary artery aneurysms are more common than isolated aneurysms.
E. The most common site for a coronary aneurysm is in the left anterior descending artery.

46. A 61-year-old man with difficulty in swallowing was sent by his family doctor for a barium swallow. The examination showed a smooth filling defect in the mid-lower oesophagus with minor hold-up of contrast and proximal oesophageal dilatation. CT performed for further evaluation did not show any extra oesophageal organ involvement or lymphadenopathy. The most common mesenchymal tumour of the oesophagus is

A. Lipoma
B. Gastrointestinal stromal tumour
C. Haemangioma
D. Leiomyosarcoma
E. Leiomyoma

47. A 22-year-old woman who had undergone a caesarean section presents with cyclic voiding symptoms but no haematuria. Cystoscopy shows a filling defect and MRI is performed. Axial T2W MRI shows hypointense irregular focal wall thickening on the left posterolateral aspect of the bladder, without any fat stranding or associated lymph nodes, suggesting intrinsic bladder endometriosis. Which of the following statements is false, regarding deep pelvic endometriosis?

A. Subperitoneal invasion of endometriotic tissue must exceed 5 mm.
B. Endometriotic nodules can have high T2W signal.
C. Low-signal nodular thickening of uterosacral ligament on T2W images.
D. Ureteric endometriosis is mostly intrinsic.
E. Obliteration of pouch of Douglas is recognised in advanced disease.

48. A 7-year-old boy fell off a bike onto his outstretched left hand. X-ray showed a fracture of the left distal radius involving the epiphyseal plate that extends into the metaphysis. The epiphysis was split into two fragments. What is the Salter–Harris classification?
    A. 1
    B. 2
    C. 3
    D. 4
    E. 5

49. An 81-year-old man with bilateral calcified and uncalcified pleural plaques, basal predominant fibrotic lungs and unilateral pleural effusion is sent for a CT scan with high suspicion of primary pleural mesothelioma. CT and pleural fluid aspirate confirmed mesothelioma. Which of these is not a feature of unresectability?
    A. Extension into peritoneal cavity
    B. Involvement of endothoracic fascia
    C. Pericardial involvement
    D. Multiple sites of extension into the chest wall
    E. Direct extension into the ribs and spine

50. A 70-year-old man with a history of weight loss and iron deficiency anaemia is referred for a CT colonography study. There is no malignancy on the scan but a 5 cm cystic structure is seen next to the distal ileum, in keeping with a duplication cyst. The most common site of a duplication cyst of the gastrointestinal tract is the
    A. Oesophagus
    B. Stomach
    C. Duodenum
    D. Jejunum
    E. Ileum

51. A 33-year-old woman is referred by her family doctor to the infertility clinic for further investigations to identify any potentially treatable cause of infertility. Which one of the following statements regarding intracavitary uterine abnormalities as a cause of infertility is false?
    A. Uterine synechiae is a complication of D&C.
    B. Synechiae appear as linear filling defects on HSG.
    C. Submucosal leiomyomas distort endometrial cavity.
    D. Submucosal leiomyomas can obstruct fallopian tubes.
    E. Cervical factor infertility is the most common cause of infertility.

52. A 45-year-old man with ulceration of the nasal septum was investigated further with CT sinuses. CT showed bone destruction involving the nasal cavity, turbinates and paranasal sinuses without associated soft-tissue masses. Chest radiograph of the same person done to exclude infection showed multiple nodules of varying sizes.
    A. Churg–Strauss disease
    B. Ethmoid carcinoma
    C. Polyarteritis nodosa
    D. Granulomatosis with polyangitis
    E. Leprosy

53. A 30-year-old sustains a knee injury while skiing. MRI shows that there is a high signal in the lateral femoral condyle and the posterolateral part of the lateral tibial plateau. What is the most likely injury?
    A. ACL
    B. PCL

C. MCL

D. LCL

E. MPFL (Medial patellofemoral ligament)

54. A 14-year-old girl with chronic constitutional symptoms and sinonasal disease presents to the outpatient department. A CT of the paranasal sinuses reveals diffuse sinusitis and thickening of the paranasal sinus walls. On a plain chest radiograph, a cavitating pulmonary lesion is identified.

Which of the following vasculitides would be the most likely diagnosis?

A. Kawasaki's disease

B. Cogan's syndrome

C. Takayasu's arteritis

D. Granulomatosis with polyangiitis

E. Polyarteritis nodosa

55. A 77-year-old man with a high-risk occupational history and progressive limitation of exercise tolerance was sent for a staging CT of the chest to investigate a persistent right-sided pleural effusion. All of the following pulmonary CT features are suggestive of asbestos exposure, except:

A. Basal fibrosis

B. Calcified pleural plaques

C. Diffuse pleural thickening

D. Round atelectasis

E. High-density consolidation

56. A 65 year old known diabetic woman is acutely unwell and presents with increasing epigastric tenderness. She is referred by the surgeons for an urgent contrast enhanced CT of the abdomen. The CT shows features consistent with emphysematous gastritis. All of the following are expected CT findings, except:

A. Air in the stomach wall

B. Pneumoperitoneum

C. Pneumobilia

D. Portal venous gas

E. Irregular gastric mucosal fold thickening

57. A 31-year-old woman was referred for a hysterosalpingogram for assessment of tubal anatomy and patency. The left fallopian tube was normal but no pelvic spillage was observed on the right, subject to proximal obstruction of the tube on the right. Which of the following conditions is not a cause of obstruction in the fallopian tube?

A. Granulomatous salpingitis

B. Intraluminal endometriosis

C. Congenital atresia

D. Peritubal adhesions

E. Tubal spasm

58. A 29-year-old man with history of discharge from the right ear underwent a CT of the temporal bones for further evaluation. Coronal CT images showed enlargement of the epitympanic recess and erosion of the walls and scutum with an associated soft-tissue mass. Only fragments of the ossicular chain could be identified. What is the diagnosis?

A. Cholesterol granuloma

B. Acquired attic cholesteatoma

C. Congenital cholesteatoma

D. Carcinoma of the middle ear

E. Malignant otitis externa

59. An 8-year-old boy presents with a 5-week history of left hip pain and limp. Several previous pelvic X-rays were normal. A bone scan shows reduced uptake in the left femoral epiphysis. A line drawn from the lateral aspect of the femoral neck intersects the femoral head. What is the most likely diagnosis?
    A. SUFE
    B. Transient synovitis
    C. Perthes disease
    D. Developmental dysplasia of the hip
    E. Sickle cell disease

60. A 6-year-old boy with abdominal pain and jaundice was sent for a specialist review because the GP identified abnormal LFTs (raised bilirubin, raised AST and ALT). Viral serology for hepatitis B and C were negative. Twenty-four-hour urinary copper excretion was >100 microgram (normal <40 microgram). An abnormal ring was noted in the eye on slit lamp examination. All of the following can be seen on US of the abdomen, except:
    A. Mild hepatomegaly
    B. Small echogenic liver
    C. Abnormally large kidneys
    D. Ascites
    E. Abnormally large spleen

61. A 3-year-old patient with Beckwith–Wiedemann syndrome presents for an abdominal US study. The clinical indication states 'routine screening for malignancy'. Which tumour is not commonly associated with the underlying syndrome?
    A. Rhabdomyosarcoma
    B. Wilms tumour
    C. Neuroblastoma
    D. Renal rhabdoid tumour
    E. Hepatoblastoma

62. A 37-year-old woman with known history of inflammatory bowel disease presented to the gastroenterologist with worsening abdominal and systemic symptoms. All of the following extra-intestinal manifestations of inflammatory bowel disease parallel the activity of the disease, except:
    A. Erythema nodosum
    B. Enteropathic spondylitis
    C. Uveitis
    D. Monoarticular peripheral arthritis
    E. Pulmonary embolism

63. Which one of the following statements regarding penetrating aortic atherosclerotic ulcers is true?
    A. They can progress to pseodoaneurysm.
    B. They are contrast-filled outpouchings surrounded by an intramural hematoma.
    C. They occur early in atherosclerotic disease.
    D. They can progress to aortic rupture.
    E. Intramural haematoma signifies its aggressive nature.

64. A 26-year-old woman was referred by her family doctor to the infertility clinic for further investigations. She was scheduled to have a transvaginal US evaluation in the radiology department. All of the following are presumptive findings of ovulation on transvaginal ultrasound, except:
    A. Reduction in size of the dominant follicle
    B. Continued increase in size of the follicle

C. Loss of clearly defined follicular margin

D. Appearance of internal echoes in the follicle

E. Increased fluid in the pouch of Douglas

65. A 26-year-old man with facial pain shows a large, well-demarcated expansile cystic lesion in the petrous apex with erosion of the internal auditory meatus. No associated erosion of the scutum is identified, and the tympanic membrane is intact. MRI reveals a corresponding high-signal lesion on both T1W and T2W sequences. What is the diagnosis?

A. Cholesterol granuloma

B. Acquired cholesteatoma

C. Congenital cholesteatoma

D. Carcinoma of petrous temporal bone

E. Arachnoid cyst

66. A 6-year-old girl complains of pain in her left shoulder. X-ray shows a lucent lesion in the proximal humeral epiphysis. The lesion has sclerotic borders with specks of calcification within the lesion. What is the most likely diagnosis?

A. Simple bone cyst

B. Aneurysmal bone cyst (ABC)

C. Non-ossifying fibroma

D. Fibrous cortical defect

E. Chondroblastoma

67. Which one of the following extra-intestinal manifestations of inflammatory bowel disease is more likely to occur in patients with Crohn's disease than in those with ulcerative colitis?

A. Sclerosing cholangitis

B. Pyoderma gangrenosum

C. Gallstones

D. Erythema nodosum

E. Pulmonary embolism

68. A 33-year-old man presents with conductive hearing loss, pulsatile tinnitus and hoarseness of voice. CT showed erosion of the jugular fossa with upward extension of soft-tissue mass into the middle ear cavity. MRI shows an intermediate signal mass on T1W images with high signal on T2W sequence interspersed with signal voids. Intense enhancement was seen on post gadolinium images. What is the diagnosis?

A. Carotid body tumour

B. Non-specified skull base tumour

C. Neurofibroma of the XII nerve

D. Glomus jugulare

E. Osteoblastoma of transverse process of C2

69. A 66-year-old man with acute onset of chest pain radiating to the back is sent for an urgent post-contrast CT of the chest to exclude aortic dissection. There is no evidence of a dissection or a penetrating aortic ulcer, but the scan is reported as showing an acute intramural haematoma in the descending thoracic aorta. All of the following are characteristic CT findings, except:

A. It is subintimal in location.

B. It appears as a crescent of high density.

C. MRI can help differentiate it from slow flow in false lumen of dissection.

D. The aortic wall appears thinned out.

E. They can progress to aortic rupture.

70. A 27-year-old woman is being investigated for infertility. No anatomical abnormality of the uterus was identified on US examination of the pelvis, and she was referred for further investigations to assess tubal patency. Patency of the fallopian tubes is best imaged by:
    A. MRI
    B. Transvaginal US
    C. Hysterosalpingography
    D. Sonohysterography
    E. Transabdominal US

71. A 10-year-old girl complains of severe pain in her left hip. Plain X-ray shows there is a 5 mm lucent lesion in the medial femoral neck. On MRI, there is a 2 mm central focus, which is isointense on T1W and high on T2W images. There is surrounding high signal on T2W image. Dynamic imaging reveals peak enhancement on arterial phase with early partial washout of the lesion. There is slower progressive enhancement of the adjacent bone marrow. What is the likely diagnosis?
    A. Osteoid osteoma
    B. Osteoblastoma
    C. Stress fracture
    D. Cortical desmoid
    E. Osteochondroma

72. On a routine neonatal clinical examination, the paediatric registrar notes a simple sacral dimple at the natal cleft. It is blind-ended without any associated tuft of hair at the site of the dimple. What is the most reasonable subsequent management plan?
    A. No further management is required.
    B. Ultrasonography of the spine.
    C. Ultrasonography of the spine and cranial contents.
    D. MRI of the spine.
    E. MRI of the brain and spine.

73. A 4-year-old child falls onto an outstretched arm while on the playground. A radiograph of the elbow demonstrates the presence of a posterior fat pad adjacent to the distal humerus. There is no cortical defect or obvious fracture on the radiograph. What is the most likely underlying pathology?
    A. Osteomyelitis
    B. Supracondylar fracture
    C. Head of radius fracture
    D. Clinoid fracture of the ulna
    E. Septic elbow joint effusion

74. All of the following structures are present in the centre of the secondary pulmonary lobule, except:
    A. Respiratory bronchiole
    B. Pulmonary artery
    C. Pulmonary vein
    D. Lymphatics
    E. Bronchovascular interstitium

75. A 34-year-old woman with primary sclerosing cholangitis presents with worsening LFTs. All of the following are potential complications of primary sclerosing cholangitis in patients with inflammatory bowel disease, except:
    A. Cholangiocarcinoma
    B. Cholangitis

C. Choledocholithiasis

D. Liver cirrhosis

E. Hepatic haemangioma

76. A woman who was 32 weeks pregnant presented to the labour ward with acute onset of sudden severe abdominal pain developing over a period of 24 hours. Clinically there was tenderness in the right lower quadrant with features of guarding and exacerbation with movement. Which one of the following statements regarding the use of MRI for evaluation of an acute abdomen during pregnancy is *false*?

A. It has no known carcinogenic effects.

B. It has no known teratogenic effects.

C. It can be used when an initial US examination is equivocal.

D. The result of the study potentially affects the immediate care of the mother or foetus.

E. MR contrast agent is routinely used in pregnancy.

77. Which technique reduces artefact from hip prosthesis during MRI?

A. Use of a magnet with a higher field strength

B. Use of FSE imaging rather than GE imaging

C. Alignment of prosthesis perpendicular to the magnetic field

D. Using a narrower bandwidth

E. Use of the magic angle

78. A 19-year-old man shows a large mass in the nasopharynx on CT sinuses. Post-contrast images confirmed an intensely vascular mass extending into the pterygopalatine fossa and infratemporal fossa with forward displacement of the posterior wall of the maxillary sinus. Coronal images showed erosion of the base of the pterygoid plate. What is the diagnosis?

A. Inverted papilloma

B. Nasopharyngeal carcinoma

C. Juvenile angiofibroma

D. Lymphoma

E. Midline granuloma

79. A 41-year-old woman was referred for a pelvic US by her family doctor after she complained of pelvic heaviness. US revealed a complex primarily solid-looking mass in the adnexa, which was thought to be ovarian in origin. A pelvic MRI was scheduled for further evaluation and characterisation. All of the following adnexal masses usually present on both T1W and T2W MR imaging with low signal intensity, except:

A. Mucinous cystadenoma

B. Brenner tumour

C. Ovarian fibroma

D. Fibrothecoma

E. Exophytic leiomyoma

80. A neonate on the intensive care unit is referred for a chest and abdominal radiograph. There are several support lines and tubes *in situ*. Which of the following is inappropriately located?

A. The umbilical venous catheter (UVC) tip within the inferior vena cava, just below/at the level of the right atrium

B. The umbilical arterial catheter (UAC) tip at the L1 vertebral level

C. The endotracheal tube (ETT) tip at the T2 vertebral level

D. The nasogastric tube (NGT) tip located below the diaphragm within a gastric air shadow

E. The central venous catheter tip located at the cavo-atrial junction

81. A 66-year-old man presented to the A&E department with progressive chest tightness and shortness of breath. ECG was normal and inflammatory markers were normal. Chest X-ray was abnormal and an HRCT was requested. HRCT showed a diffuse interstitial pattern of small nodular opacities. All of the following may be associated with this finding, except:
    A. Sarcoidosis
    B. Talcosis
    C. Scleroderma
    D. Hypersensitivity pneumonitis
    E. Small nodular metastasis

82. A 37-year-old woman with known history of inflammatory bowel disease presented to the gastroenterologist with worsening abdominal and systemic symptoms. All of the following are extra-intestinal musculoskeletal manifestations of inflammatory bowel disease, except:
    A. Neuropathic osteoarthropathy
    B. Enteropathic spondylitis
    C. Hypertrophic osteoarthropathy
    D. Sacroiliitis
    E. Monoarticular peripheral arthritis

83. On your routine MR reporting session, a lumbar spine shows normal alignment and multilevel low signal on both T1 and T2 in the intervertebral discs centrally, with disc space narrowing. What is the most likely diagnosis?
    A. CPPD
    B. Ochronosis
    C. Amyloidosis
    D. Renal osteodystrophy
    E. Gout

84. A 64-year-old man with nasal obstruction and bloody nasal discharge showed a large heterogeneous mass in the nasopharynx on CT sinuses. There was loss of normal parapharyngeal fat planes with non-enhancement of the ipsilateral jugular vein. What is the diagnosis?
    A. Inverted papilloma
    B. Nasopharyngeal carcinoma
    C. Juvenile angiofibroma
    D. Lymphoma
    E. Midline granuloma

85. A 77-year-old man with progressive worsening of breathing and chest pain presented to his family doctor, who sent him for a chest X-ray to exclude infection. The chest X-ray showed multiple ring shadows and he was sent for an HRCT. The HRCT confirmed the presence of multiple small cystic spaces in both lungs. All of the following disorders of the lung can be associated with this HRCT pattern, except:
    A. Tuberous sclerosis
    B. Langerhans cell histiocytosis
    C. Lymphocytic interstitial pneumonia
    D. End-stage interstitial fibrosis
    E. Coal worker's pneumoconiosis

86. A 67-year-old man with worsening abdominal pain and LFTs shows a peripheral mass in the right lobe of the liver. Contrast-enhanced dynamic MRI done for further characterisation confirmed the lesion seen on US, with evidence of liver capsular retraction consistent with

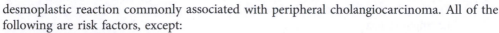

desmoplastic reaction commonly associated with peripheral cholangiocarcinoma. All of the following are risk factors, except:
A. Radium exposure
B. Chronic hepatitis
C. Primary sclerosing cholangitis
D. Thorotrast exposure
E. Clonorchis sinensis infection

87. A 59-year-old woman with an apparent lump in the lower abdomen, weight loss and new onset tremor was sent for an MRI of the pelvis to investigate. Sagittal T2W MRI showed a multiloculated, heterogeneous left ovarian lesion with very low signal intensity. Corresponding axial in-phase and out-of-phase images revealed a hypointense mass with chemical shift artefact in its ventral aspect. Axial post-contrast T1W MRI showed significant enhancement of the ovarian lesion. What is the diagnosis?
A. Brenner tumour
B. Struma ovarii
C. Ovarian thecofibroma
D. Mucinous cystadenoma
E. Endometrioma

88. Posteromedial corner (PMC) of the knee involves the following structures:
A. Semimembranosus tendon and posterior oblique ligament
B. Popliteus muscle and arcuate ligament
C. Iliotibial band and biceps femoris
D. Gastrocnemius and PCL
E. Medial retinaculum and medial collateral ligament

89. A 53-year-old man with lump in the right side of the neck was investigated with US. US showed a solid lesion closely related to the carotid artery. Axial CT showed a large, well-defined mass bulging into the nasopharynx. Multiplanar reconstructed images revealed characteristic splaying of the carotid bifurcation. What is the diagnosis?
A. Glomus jugulare
B. Glomus tympanicum
C. Thymic cyst
D. Carotid body tumour
E. Glomus vagale

90. While reporting a plain radiograph of the knee in a 5-year-old child, you notice premature closure of the distal femoral growth plate. Which of the following features in the clinical history would not explain this?
A. Localised radiotherapy to the leg
B. Hypervitaminosis A
C. Osteomyelitis
D. Previous trauma to the knee
E. Hyperparathyroidism

91. A 45-year-old trumpet player presented with a lump in the right side of the neck, which appeared to grow in size when the man was playing the trumpet and become less prominent when he was relaxed. CT showed clearly defined, round, radio lucency in the soft tissue of the right side of the neck lateral to the larynx. A normal barium swallow report was available in the system for suspected swallowing difficulty performed at a different hospital. What is the likely diagnosis?
A. Internal laryngocele
B. External laryngocele

C. External laryngocele with infection
D. Laryngomalacia
E. Tracheomalacia

92. A 67-year-old man with a progressive restrictive pattern of pulmonary function test and increasing chest tightness was sent for an HRCT for characterisation. HRCT showed nodular septal thickening with further bronchovascular nodules and thickening. Which one of the following disorders is most likely to be the cause?
A. Pneumoconiosis
B. Lymphangitis
C. Lymphocytic interstitial pneumonia
D. Hypersensitivity pneumonitis
E. Churg–Strauss syndrome

93. A 48-year-old man with a history of alcohol excess is admitted with a variceal bleed. Regarding upper gastrointestinal varices, which of the following statements is correct?
A. They are the result of hepatopetal blood flow from the left gastric vein and splenic vein to the superior mesenteric vein.
B. Oesophageal varices tend to bleed more severely than gastric varices.
C. Splenic portography is the first-line investigation for assessment.
D. Barium studies can detect gastric varices in approximately 75% of cases evidenced by lobulated folds and polypoidal fundal masses.
E. Gastric varices bleed more frequently than oesophageal varices.

94. A 67-year-old woman with bilateral lower limb swelling and increasing abdominal girth was scheduled to have an ultrasound as first-line investigation. Ultrasound revealed a complex primarily cystic mass in the adnexa with some solid components. A pelvic MRI was organised for further characterisation. All of the following are MR imaging features of ovarian mucinous cystadenomas that help differentiate them from ovarian serous cystadenomas, except:
A. Large size
B. Solid component suggesting malignancy
C. More commonly multilocular than unilocular
D. Higher signal intensity on T1W MRI
E. Lower signal intensity on T2W MRI

95. Which of the following anatomical variants and its associated clinical symptom is incorrect?
A. Os acromiale – impingement
B. Conjoint spinal nerve roots – muscle weakness
C. Positive ulnar variance – TFC tear
D. Discoid meniscus – locking
E. Os naviculare – pain behind the heel

96. A child is referred with a presumed diagnosis of a mucopolysaccharidosis. A skeletal survey demonstrates multiple features in keeping with dysostosis multiplex. Which one of the following radiographic features is not part of this syndrome?
A. J-shaped sella
B. Tilting of the radius and ulna away from each other
C. Arrowhead terminal phalanx
D. Calvarial thickening
E. Proximal pointed metacarpals

97. A patient with cancer has developed bone marrow suppression as a result of chemotherapy and complains of fever and dyspnoea. A chest HRCT scan shows

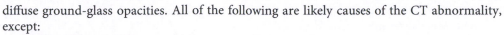

diffuse ground-glass opacities. All of the following are likely causes of the CT abnormality, except:

A. Pneumocystis carinii pneumonia
B. Pulmonary oedema
C. Chemotherapy drug toxicity
D. Desquamative interstitial pneumonia
E. Respiratory syncytial virus infection

98. A 65-year-old man is admitted with intractable retching and sudden onset epigastric pain. A nasogastric tube could not be passed into the stomach. Regarding gastric volvulus, which one of the following statements is correct?

A. Aetiology is related to unusually short gastrohepatic and gastrocolic mesenteries.
B. Sliding/para-oesophageal hernia does not predispose to gastric volvulus.
C. Organo-axial volvulus is more common than mesentero-axial volvulus and creates a 'mirror-image' stomach.
D. Mesentero-axial volvulus rotates around a line from cardia to pylorus.
E. Organo-axial volvulus is associated with 'upside down stomach' appearance.

99. A 31-year-old woman with a complex cystic adnexal mass on the left identified on pelvic ultrasound was referred for a pelvic MRI with a view towards further characterisation of the mass lesion. Which of the following statements regarding ovarian tumour is incorrect?

A. Granulosa cell tumour is associated with endometrial hyperplasia.
B. The presence of fat is specific for teratoma.
C. Immature teratoma is mainly cystic.
D. Dysgerminoma is associated with raised HCG level.
E. Brenner tumour is associated with calcification.

100. A 48-year-old woman with mid and lower back pain and shortness of breath presented to the the A&E department. Plain radiographs showed diffusely osteopaenic bones and an old superior end plate depression fracture of L1. CTPA showed acute pulmonary emboli. Plain X-ray of her hand done a year ago at a different hospital showed a metacarpal index of 9.8. What is your diagnosis?

A. Marfan's syndrome
B. Homocystinuria
C. Systemic lupus erythematosus
D. Acromegaly
E. Soto's syndrome

101. A 22-year-old man with a rapidly enlarging painful right maxilla showed an opacified right maxillary antrum on plain radiograph with destruction of the lateral wall. Axial CT showed extensive new bone formation on both sides of the anterolateral wall of the maxillary antrum with sun ray spiculations anteriorly. What is the diagnosis?

A. Ewing's sarcoma
B. Synovial sarcoma
C. Antral carcinoma
D. Myeloma
E. Osteogenic sarcoma

102. A chest radiograph of a 3-year-old child demonstrates marked right lower zone consolidation with a large pneumatocoele. A diagnosis of necrotising pneumonia is made. What is the most likely causative organism?

A. *Staphylococcus aureus*
B. *Streptococcus pyogenes*

C. *Bordatella pertussis*

D. *Mycobacterium tuberculosis*

E. *Aspergillus*

103. A 3-month-old full-term infant with normal antenatal history presents with multiple seizures. On clinical examination, there is no facial asymmetry, dysmorphology or opthalmoplegia. There is marked hypotonia of the limbs. An MRI of the brain revealed a reduction in the number of cortical sulci and shallow Sylvian fissures. What is the most likely diagnosis?
    A. Holoprosencephaly
    B. Lissencephaly
    C. Band heterotopia
    D. Hemimegalancephaly
    E. Schizencephaly

104. A 35-year-old woman who is a heavy smoker now complains of slowly progressive dyspnoea. A chest HRCT scan shows patches of ground-glass opacity interspersed with low-density centrilobular nodules. She does not have any pets at home. The most likely cause of this CT abnormality is:
    A. Cytomegalovirus pneumonia
    B. Respiratory bronchiolitis interstitial lung disease
    C. Hypersensitivity pneumonitis
    D. Pulmonary alveolar proteinosis
    E. Non-specific interstitial pneumonia

105. A 38-year-old patient presents with right-sided abdominal pain. She underwent renal transplantation 2 years previously for autosomal dominant polycystic kidney disease. A CT scan of the abdomen revealed oedematous terminal ileum, caecum and ascending colon. Which of the following is the most likely diagnosis in this patient?
    A. Appendicitis
    B. Tuberculosis
    C. Crohn's disease
    D. Typhlitis
    E. Ischaemic bowel

106. All of the following are recognised indications for foetal MRI, except
    A. Congenital anomalies of the brain and spine
    B. Masses in the face or neck
    C. Thoracic masses including CCAM, CDH
    D. Assessment of polyhydramnios
    E. Foetal surgical assessment of meningomyelocele

107. Which one of the following is not a feature of benign osteochondroma?
    A. Presence of variably mineralised/ossified cartilage cap
    B. Bursae formation
    C. Cartilage cap thickness of less than 8 mm
    D. Cartilage cap thickness of more than 2.5 cm
    E. Invagination of cartilaginous cap into the medullary component of the lesion

108. A moderately large, elongated lesion is seen posteriorly in the thoracic spinal canal on the MRI of a 36-year-old apyrexial, systemically healthy man with lower limb weakness. The signal from the fluid is noted to be identical to CSF elsewhere. No history of trauma was present. What is the diagnosis?
    A. Extradural arachnoid cyst
    B. Extradural abscess

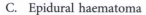

C. Epidural haematoma

D. Syrinx

E. Cystic meningioma

109. A 45-year-old smoker was sent for an HRCT for disease characterisation. HRCT showed patchy ground-glass density bilaterally. Some regions of the peripheral lung were normal while other areas showed a fine reticular pattern representing thickened interlobular and intralobular septa associated with the abnormal ground-glass opacity. No honeycombing was seen. All of the following can produce this appearance except:

A. Lipoid pneumonia

B. RBILD

C. Good pasture syndrome

D. Alveolar proteinosis

E. ARDS

110. A staging CT is performed on a patient with biopsy-proven gastric cancer. The tumour involves serosa, and enlarged nodes are present 3.5 cm from the primary tumour. No distant lesion is identified. Which one of the following is the correct TNM stage?

A. T1 N0 M0

B. T1 N1 M1

C. T2 N1 M0

D. T2 N2 M0

E. T3 N2 M0

111. An 11-year-old girl with tiredness and delayed menarche was sent by her GP to the paediatric clinic for further evaluation. Elevated urinary adrenocorticosteroid metabolites were noted. US abdomen showed large echogenic adrenal masses bilaterally. MRI showed bilateral adrenal myelolipoma. What is the diagnosis?

A. Hyperparathyroidism

B. Grave's disease

C. Cystic fibrosis

D. Congenital adrenal hyperplasia

E. Congenital hypothyroidism

112. A 27-year-old woman was referred for a pelvic ultrasound by her family doctor to investigate irregular periods. Pelvic ultrasound revealed enlarged ovaries bilaterally with multiple peripheral cysts of similar size arranged like a garland around centrally increased ovarian stroma. All of the following are associated clinical features commonly observed in this clinical scenario, except:

A. Hypertension

B. Obesity

C. Insulin resistance

D. Menorrhagia

E. Hirsutism

113. An elderly woman with progressive worsening of back pain is initially investigated with plain films of the spine. Plain radiographs show Grade III collapse of L3 with Grade II collapse of at least two other mid-thoracic vertebrae. MRI suggested osteoporotic collapse as the most likely cause. Which one of the following is the expected progression of osteoporotic vertebral compression fractures as seen on MR imaging?

A. A partial return to normal fatty marrow.

B. No change.

C. The progression is unpredictable.

D. An increase in oedema and fibrovascular tissue.

E. A decrease in normal fatty marrow.

114. A 53-year-old man with acute left leg pain in the distribution of the left L5 nerve was referred for an MRI of the lumbar spine. MRI revealed a well-defined lesion with low signal on T1W images and high signal on T2W images in the lateral aspect of the spinal canal, in close relation to the L4/5 facet joint. What is the diagnosis?

A. Ganglion

B. Synovial cyst

C. Neurofibroma

D. Arachnoid cyst

E. Tarlov cyst

115. A 45-year-old man presents to the A&E department with acute onset of dyspnoea. Serum biochemistry reveal an elevated creatinine consistent with established renal failure, and a chest HRCT scan shows isolated, diffuse ground-glass opacity. The most likely cause of the CT abnormality is:

A. Pulmonary alveolar proteinosis

B. Pneumocystis carinii pneumonia

C. Acute interstitial pneumonia

D. Respiratory bronchiolitis interstitial lung disease

E. Diffuse alveolar haemorrhage

116. A 58-year-old inpatient, admitted 10 days before for an acute exacerbation of chronic obstructive pulmonary disease, develops profuse watery diarrhoea and severe cramp-like abdominal pain. Abdominal X-ray is unremarkable, but CT demonstrates circumferential wall thickening of the rectum extending to the mid-transverse colon, an 'accordion sign' in the sigmoid colon, pericolonic fat stranding and ascites. What is the most likely diagnosis?

A. Radiation enteritis

B. Ischaemic colitis

C. Diverticulitis

D. Amoebiasis

E. Clostridium difficile colitis

117. A 29-year-old woman with a pelvic mass on US is sent for MRI. Axial TSE MRI shows a well-defined, ovoid solid mass with low signal on T1W images and intermediate signal with multiple round internal cysts on T2W images. Gadolinium-enhanced TSE T1 FS image shows the mass as having a moderately enhancing solid portion. All the following ovarian tumours typically show solid enhancing elements, except

A. Sclerosing stromal tumour

B. Sertoli–Leydig cell tumour

C. Struma ovarii

D. Serous cystadenoma

E. Cystadenofibroma

118. Which of the following is a joint that is not characteristically involved in primary osteoarthritis (OA)?

A. Distal interphalangeal joint (DIPJ)

B. First metatarsophalangeal joint (MTPJ)

C. Metacarpophalangeal joint (MCPJ)

D. Knee

E. Lumbar spine

119. Cervical spine MRI of a 37-year-old woman with neck pain, tingling and numbness in the left C5–C7 distribution showed a well-defined intradural mass with signal characteristic similar to spinal cord in both T1W and T2W sequences. The cord was displaced posteriorly without any intrinsic signal change. Intense enhancement was noted on the post-contrast images with a dural tail. What is the diagnosis?

    A. Neurofibroma
    B. Schwannoma
    C. Epidural abscess
    D. Intraspinal aneurysm
    E. Meningioma

120. A 3-day-old neonate presents with bilious vomiting and clinical suspicion for malrotation. Which of the following imaging features would best fit with this diagnosis?

    A. A duodeno-jejunal (DJ) flexure located left of the midline, above the gastric pylorus
    B. A double bubble sign on supine abdominal radiograph
    C. Retroperitoneal location of the third part of the duodenum
    D. Superior mesenteric artery located to the right of the superior mesenteric vein
    E. Distended bowel loops throughout the whole abdomen on plain radiography

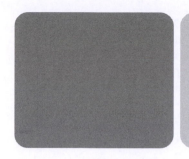

CHAPTER 10
TEST PAPER 5

Answers

1. A. Cystic fibrosis (CF)

The classic diagnostic triad in patients with cystic fibrosis includes an abnormal sweat chloride test result and manifestations of pulmonary and pancreatic disease. Upper lobe predominance is seen in many but not all cases; a diffuse distribution is also common. Normal to increased lung volumes are typical in CF and indicate air trapping and small airways disease. CT images show extensive cystic and cylindrical bronchiectasis and bronchial wall and peribronchial interstitial thickening. Findings are typically more extensive in patients with bronchiectasis due to cystic fibrosis than in patients with bronchiectasis due to other causes. Nodular opacities throughout the lungs correlate with areas of mucoid bronchial or bronchiolar impaction. Tree-in-bud nodules indicate the diffuse bronchiolitis that typically occurs in cystic fibrosis. In addition, a mosaic pattern of attenuation secondary to air trapping due to obstructed bronchi and bronchioles is commonly seen.

Milliron B, et al. Bronchiectasis: Mechanisms and imaging clues of associated common and uncommon diseases. *Radiographics*. 2015;35(4):1011–30.

2. B. They are rich in glycogen.

Serous cystadenomas are benign cystic neoplasms of the pancreas that occur frequently in older women (median age 65 years). Serous cystadenomas are composed of numerous small cysts that are conjoined in a honeycomb-like formation. The size of these cysts ranges from 0.1 to 2.0 cm but typically is less than 1 cm. The cysts are lined by glycogen-rich epithelium and separated by fibrous septa that radiate from a central scar, which may be calcified. This formation has led to the use of the more descriptive term *microcystic pancreatic lesion*. Serous cystadenomas are usually discovered incidentally at imaging; however, those that are large may cause symptoms such as abdominal pain or, more rarely, jaundice. Progressive enlargement of serous cystadenomas – especially those with a size of 4 cm or more at initial manifestation may be seen at serial follow-up imaging examinations performed over a period of months or years. Multiple serous cystadenomas may occur in von Hippel–Lindau disease.

At MR imaging, a serous cystadenoma appears as a cluster of small cysts within the pancreas, with no visible communication between the cysts and the pancreatic duct. The cysts show signal intensity of simple fluid on T2-weighted images, and the thin fibrous septa between them enhance on delayed contrast-enhanced MR images.

Kalb B, et al. MR imaging of cystic lesions of the pancreas. *Radiographics*. 2009;29:1749–65.

3. E. Retinoblastoma

Retinoblastoma is the most common tumour of the globe in children. It is seen in children less than 3 years, presenting with leukocoria; 75% are unilateral and unifocal, 25% are bilateral or unilateral multifocal. When seen bilaterally in conjunction with pineoblastoma, it is called *trilateral retinoblastoma*.

CT is preferred and shows clumped or punctate calcification (95%) in the posterior aspect of the eye, extending into the vitreous humor with minimal enhancement. Absence of calcification makes retinoblastoma unlikely. On MRI, retinoblastomas are hyperintense on T1-weighted and hypointense on T2-weighted images, possibly due to calcification or paramagnetic tumour protein. MRI is better at depicting tumour extension along optic nerves and intracranially. CT is better at showing bone destruction including expansion of the optic canal.

Adam A, et al. *Grainger & Allison's Diagnostic Radiology: A Textbook of Medical Imaging*, 5th edn. New York: Churchill Livingstone, 2008:1396–7.

4. A. Two separate uterine cavities with two cervices and two proximal vagina

Uterus didelphys results from complete failure of Müllerian duct fusion. Each duct develops fully with duplication of the uterine horns, cervix and proximal vagina. A fundal cleft greater than 1 cm has been reported to be 100% sensitive and specific in differentiation of fusion anomalies (didelphys and bicornuate) from reabsorption anomalies (septate and arcuate). Bicornuate uterus involves duplication of uterus with possible duplication of cervix (bicornuate unicollis or bicornuate bicollis).

Behr SC, et al. Imaging of Müllerian duct anomalies. *Radiographics*. 2012;32(6):E233–50.

5. B. Fibular stress fractures affect the proximal end.

The tibia is the most commonly involved bone, accounting for up to almost half of stress fractures reported in some series. Two types of tibial stress fractures have been described – transverse and longitudinal. Transverse fractures are more common and can occur on the compression side (posterior) or tension side (anterior). Posterior transverse fractures of the tibial shaft are most commonly seen in long-distance runners. Tension stress transverse fractures of the anterior tibial shaft occur more commonly in jumpers and have a higher propensity for non-union and progression to an acute complete fracture.

The most common site of fibular stress fracture in runners is the lower fibula, just proximal to the tibiotalar syndesmosis.

Femoral neck stress fractures are associated with the classic 'female athlete triad' of amenorrhoea, osteoporosis and eating disorders. Femoral neck stress fractures are often classified as tension side (superolateral or transverse) or compression side (inferolateral), with the contention that tension side fractures are associated with poorer prognosis and are potentially unstable. The femoral shaft is particularly susceptible to repetitive stresses on the medial compression side of the femur at the junction of the proximal and middle thirds.

Fractures of the sacrum have predominantly been described in long-distance runners, particularly women, but have also been reported in hockey players. Sacral stress fractures are also associated with the female athlete triad.

Liong SY, Whitehouse RW. Lower extremity and pelvic stress fractures in athletes. *Br J Radiol*. 2012;85 (1016):1148–56.

6. D. Hyperthyroidism

The child has McCune–Albright syndrome (MAS), which is defined as the association of polyostotic fibrous dysplasia (PFD), precocious puberty, café au lait spots and other endocrinopathies caused by the hyperactivity of various endocrine glands. Among the endocrine syndromes described in association with MAS are (1) hyperthyroidism, (2) acromegaly, (3) gonadotrophinomas, (4) hyperprolactinaemia, (5) Cushing syndrome, (6) hyperparathyroidism, (7) gynaecomastia and (8) hypophosphataemic rickets.

Lisch nodules are associated with neurofibromatosis. Fibrous dysplasia in MAS can involve any bone but most commonly affects the long bones, ribs, skull and facial bones. There is no association between Madelung deformity and MAS.

Dähnert W. *Radiology Review Manual*, 7th edn. Philadelphia, PA: Lippincott Williams & Wilkins, 2011:82.

7. E. Kartagener's syndrome

Kartagener's syndrome refers to the clinical combination of situs inversus, chronic sinusitis and bronchiectasis in a subset of patients with ciliary dyskinesia.

Patients with primary ciliary dyskinesia typically have varicoid bronchiectasis preferentially affecting the lower lungs, particularly the right middle lobe and lingula, with chronic volume loss and consolidation. Tree-in-bud nodules related to infection and mucous plugging secondary to impaired clearance are also frequently seen. The associated finding of dextrocardia can be seen at chest radiography in cases of Kartagener's syndrome.

Milliron B, et al. Bronchiectasis: Mechanisms and imaging clues of associated common and uncommon diseases. *Radiographics*. 2015;35(4):1011–30.

8. C. They have an epithelial lining.

Overall, pseudocysts are the most common cystic lesions of the pancreas. These lesions occur in the setting of pancreatitis, resulting from haemorrhagic fat necrosis and encapsulation of pancreatic secretions by granulation tissue and a fibrous capsule. The MR imaging appearance of pseudocysts may evolve over time; they are often irregularly marginated early in their formation but become well circumscribed, with a thickened enhancing wall, over a period of several weeks. Blood products and necrotic or proteinaceous debris are commonly present and produce intrinsically increased T1 signal intensity. The thickened and enhancing cyst wall seen on images corresponds to a thick rim of granulation tissue and fibrosis that is uniformly seen at histologic analysis. Other changes of acute or chronic pancreatitis are frequently seen in association with pseudocysts, and MR imaging may be the imaging modality of choice for depicting the features of parenchymal pancreatic disease.

MR imaging has proved superior to CT for demonstrating internal complexity in pseudocysts. Furthermore, the signal intensity increase in tissues surrounding a complicated pseudocyst on T2-weighted fat-suppressed images correlates with the degree of inflammation present. However, in patients with a pseudocyst, the cause of inflammation is more likely to be chemical irritation than infection, and it may be impossible to differentiate between an infectious process and other possible causes on the basis of imaging features alone. Clinical manifestations may be similarly unhelpful, since the symptoms of chemical irritation may be identical to those of sepsis. Moreover, pancreatic pseudocysts may dissect along abdominopelvic fascial planes to sites remote from the pancreas (e.g., liver, pleura or mediastinum).

Fistulation may occur between a pseudocyst and one or more vascular structures.

Kalb B, et al. MR imaging of cystic lesions of the pancreas. *Radiographics*. 2009;29:1749–65.

9. E. Increased abdominal circumference

The hallmarks of the diagnosis, in the first trimester as well as later in pregnancy, are the presence of the stomach, bowel or liver in the chest, shift of the mediastinum and displacement of the heart to the contralateral side. Increase in abdominal circumference is not a feature; the contrary can however be observed and can be a clue. In 50% of affected foetuses, there are associated chromosomal abnormalities or other malformation. The hernia results from abnormal formation or fusion of the pleuroperitoneal membranes with the septum transversum, and it is surgically correctable. Neonatal death results from pulmonary hypoplasia and pulmonary hypertension.

Daskalakis G, et al. First trimester ultrasound diagnosis of congenital diaphragmatic hernia. *J Obstet Gynaecol Res*. 2007;33(6):870–2.

10. E. Gradient echo MR sequences elicit blooming artefact in the lesion.

Morton neuromas are masses composed of interdigital perineural fibrosis and nerve degeneration. Morton neuroma occurs between the metatarsal heads, most commonly between the third and fourth toes. Morton neuroma is more common in women, and high-heeled shoes have been implicated as a causative factor. Pain at the metatarsal head, often radiating to the toes, is characteristic.

The MRI appearance is that of a tear-drop-shaped soft-tissue mass between the metatarsal heads, projecting inferiorly into the plantar subcutaneous fat and located plantar to the intermetatarsal ligament. The mass is typically intermediate in signal intensity on T1-weighted images. It is iso- or hypointense relative to fat on T2-weighted images, resulting in poor lesion conspicuity. The use of gadopentetate dimeglumine is helpful because intense enhancement typically occurs on fat-suppressed T1-weighted images, increasing the conspicuity of the lesion.

Ashman CJ, et al. Forefoot pain involving the metatarsal region: Differential diagnosis with MR imaging. *Radiographics.* 2001;21(6):1425–40.
Stadnick ME. Morton Neuroma. MRI Web Clinic – January 2006.

11. A. Malignant melanoma of the choroid

Primary orbital melanoma is the most common primary intraocular malignancy in adults. MR imaging is superior to CT in the evaluation of choroidal melanomas, as melanin has intrinsic T1 and T2 shortening effects, thereby manifesting with increased T1 signal intensity and decreased T2 signal intensity. CT is non-specific, often demonstrating a hyperattenuating choroidal mass.

MR imaging is also valuable for identifying other features, such as large tumour size, extraocular extension and ciliary body infiltration, all of which also portend a poorer prognosis. In addition, MR imaging is superior to CT for identifying retinal detachment and extrascleral spread.

Notably, approximately 20% of melanomas are amelanotic, thereby lacking characteristic T1 and T2 shortening effects on MR images. In addition, MR signal characteristics may not always allow melanoma to be reliably distinguished from ocular metastases.

Tailor TD, et al. Orbital neoplasms in adults: Clinical, radiologic, and pathologic review. *Radiographics.* 2013;33(6):1739–58.

12. E. Round pneumonia

Round pneumonia usually occurs in children under the age of 8 years. It is most commonly seen with bacterial pneumonia (pneumococcus). The mass has an alarming appearance on CXR; however, further investigation is only warranted if there is concern regarding the diagnosis. A CXR as soon as 48 hours later often shows dissipation of the mass into more typical consolidation, or complete resolution following antibiotic treatment. It is most common in the superior segment of the lower lobes. It is important to make the diagnosis to avoid unnecessary CT.

Bronchogenic cyst is often an incidental finding and often has a compressive effect unlike round pneumonia. Thoracic neuroblastoma may be an incidental finding, but the clinical history given is more in keeping with an infective process. Congenital cystic adenomatoid malformation (CCAM) is usually diagnosed antenatally or in the neonatal period. Indeed, in the newborn, 80% of cases of CCAM present with some degree of respiratory distress secondary to mass effect and pulmonary compression or hypoplasia.

Dähnert W. *Radiology Review Manual*, 7th edn. Philadelphia, PA: Lippincott Williams & Wilkins, 2011:420.

13. B. Cavitating nodules

Amyloidosis refers to a group of disorders characterised by the deposition of abnormal protein material in extracellular tissue.

Tracheobronchial amyloidosis generally presents with symptoms of airway obstruction. Classic radiological signs include nodular and irregular narrowing of the tracheal lumen, airway wall thickening and calcified amyloid deposits. Lobar or segmental collapse may be seen.

Pulmonary involvement by amyloid may be localised or diffuse. Radiologically, the diffuse parenchymal and alveolar septal forms of amyloid deposits appear as non-specific diffuse interstitial or alveolar opacities. HRCT reveals interlobular septal thickening with a predominant basilar and peripheral distribution, small well-defined nodules (2–4 mm) and confluent consolidations located predominantly in the subpleural regions. Some nodules may show calcifications.

Nodular amyloid deposits appear in multiple sites; focal deposits are less common. Amyloid nodules are generally in the lower lobes and peripheral and subpleural areas. They are sharply defined with lobulated contours, contain calcification (in about 50%), are of multiple shapes and sizes and grow slowly with no regression. Cavitation is very rare.

Vieira IG, et al. Pulmonary amyloidosis with calcified nodules and masses – A six-year computed tomography follow-up: A case report. *Cases J.* 2009;2:6540.

14. B.   Von Hippel–Lindau disease

Pancreatic involvement in VHL disease includes simple pancreatic cysts (50%–91%), serous microcystic adenomas (12%) and rarely adenocarcinomas. Pancreatic neuroendocrine tumours (5%–17%) also occur. Combined lesions occur, but neuroendocrine tumours and cystic lesions only rarely exist together. The reported prevalence of pancreatic involvement in VHL disease varies from 0% in some family groups to 77% in others.

Pancreatic cysts are extremely rare in the general population; therefore, the presence of a single cyst in an individual undergoing VHL disease screening because of a family history makes it highly likely that the person has VHL disease. In general, cystic pancreatic lesions in VHL disease are asymptomatic or associated with only mild symptoms. As a result, they are typically detected during screening examinations and may therefore facilitate the identification of gene carriers. In addition, pancreatic lesions may be the only abdominal manifestation and may precede any other manifestation by several years; thus, recognition permits earlier diagnosis of VHL disease.

Leung RS, et al. Imaging features of von Hippel–Lindau disease. *Radiographics.* 2008;28:65–79.

15. C.   Foetal MRI

Ultrasound imaging is the screening modality of choice for initial evaluation of the foetal central nervous system. However, using MRI additional abnormalities were identified in 50% of the foetuses. Measurement of the hydrocephalus should be in the true axial plane at the atria of the lateral ventricle and glomus of the choroid plexus. The ventricle is measured from the inner margin of the medial ventricular wall to the inner margin of the lateral wall. Ventriculomegaly can be divided into three subgroups, borderline (10–12 mm), mild (>12–15 mm) and severe (>15 mm).

Morris JE, et al. The value of in-utero magnetic resonance imaging in ultrasound diagnosed foetal isolated cerebral ventriculomegaly. *Clin Radiol.* 2007;62(2):140–4.

16. C.   Generalised increased bone density

Haemochromatosis may either be primary or secondary. It is most commonly primary and congenital with an autosomal recessive (AR) inheritance. It is relatively common in Caucasian populations with an incidence of 1 in 300 to 1 in 400. Men are affected about 10 times more commonly than women, and at an earlier age.

It is often characterised radiographically by beak-like osteophytes projecting from the second and third metacarpal heads.

The other hallmark radiographic findings of haemochromatosis include the following: generalised osteoporosis (not increased bone density), arthropathy with iron deposition in the synovium (50%), joint space narrowing and enlargement of metacarpal heads. Chondrocalcinosis is also relatively common in this condition, most often affecting the knees and triangular fibrocartilage.

Dähnert W. *Radiology Review Manual*, 7th edn. Philadelphia, PA: Lippincott Williams & Wilkins, 2011:105.

17. E.   Dextrocardia

Cystic fibrosis is an AR disorder leading to a defect in the CF transmembrane receptor (CFTR) protein resulting in defective ion transport in exocrine glands.

In CF, abnormal function of sweat glands result in higher concentrations of sodium chloride in the sweat; >40 mmol/L is suspicious and >60 mmol/L is diagnostic of CF.

Spirometry shows an obstructive pattern with reduced FVC and increased lung volumes. Chest X-ray shows hyperinflation, bronchial dilatation, bronchiectasis and its associated signs, cystic spaces, increases interstitial and linear/reticular opacities, and increased AP dimension on lateral chest X-ray. CF is not routinely associated with dextrocardia.

Dextrocardia is a component of Kartagener's syndrome (immotile cilia syndrome), which is associated with bronchiectasis and sinusitis but not with an abnormal sweat test.

Tasker RC, et al. *Oxford Handbook of Paediatrics*. Oxford: Oxford University Press, 2008:282.

18. B. Thyroid opthalmopathy

Graves ophthalmopathy is the most common cause of exophthalmos in adults. In Graves ophthalmopathy, classically spindle-shaped enlargement of the extraocular muscles is observed, with sparing of the tendinous insertion. The inferior, medial, superior and lateral rectus muscles (listed in order of decreasing frequency of involvement) may be involved. These findings are usually bilateral and symmetric; however, they may also be unilateral.

Idiopathic orbital inflammatory syndrome, also known as *orbital pseudotumour*, is the second most common cause of exophthalmos. It is a non-granulomatous orbital inflammatory process with no known local or systemic cause. In idiopathic orbital inflammatory syndrome, unlike Graves ophthalmopathy, there is tendinous involvement of the extraocular muscles.

LeBedis CA, Sakai O. Nontraumatic orbital conditions: Diagnosis with CT and MR imaging in the emergent setting. *Radiographics*. 2008;28(6):1741–53.

19. B. Chronic nitrofurantoin toxicity results in high-density consolidation.

Nitrofurantoin is used to treat urinary tract infections. Acute pulmonary toxicity manifests radiologically with diffuse bilateral, predominantly basal heterogeneous opacities. Non-specific interstitial pneumonia (NSIP) is the most common histopathologic manifestation of chronic toxicity.

Methotrexate-induced pulmonary drug toxicity occurs in 5%–10% of patients. There is no correlation between the development of drug toxicity and the duration of therapy or total cumulative dose. NSIP is the most common manifestation; hypersensitivity pneumonitis and cryptogenic organising pneumonia (COP) are less common.

Diffuse alveolar damage and NSIP are the most common manifestations of gold-induced lung disease, with COP being less common.

NSIP is the most common manifestation of amiodarone-induced lung disease. Pleural effusion is recognised. COP is less common and occurs in association with NSIP. A distinctive feature of amiodarone toxicity is focal, homogeneous, peripheral, high-attenuation pulmonary opacities due to incorporation of amiodarone into Type II pneumocytes. The combination of high-attenuation abnormalities within the lung, liver or spleen is characteristic of amiodarone toxicity.

Rossi SE, et al. Pulmonary drug toxicity: Radiologic and pathologic manifestations. *Radiographics*. 2000;20(5):1245–59.

20. B. Massive rectal bleeding

Primary omental infarction is often a haemorrhagic infarction resulting from vascular compromise related to the tenuous blood supply to the right edge of the omentum or to kinking of veins, usually those on the right side, deep within the anterior pelvis in the inferior extent of the omentum. Some omental infarcts are related to a combination of the reduced arterial and venous blood flow that occurs in hypercoagulable states, congestive heart failure and vasculitis. Secondary omental infarction may occur after a traumatic injury as a result of surgical trauma or inflammation of the omentum. Often, the site of secondary infarction is near the surgical site rather than in the right lower quadrant, the typical location of primary omental infarction.

Patients with omental infarction usually present with subacute onset of pain in the right lower quadrant, often with a slightly elevated white blood cell count. Other gastrointestinal symptoms such as vomiting, nausea and fever are absent. Establishing a preoperative diagnosis of omental infarction is difficult because it often mimics acute appendicitis or cholecystitis. In most cases, the radiologist makes the diagnosis after cross-sectional imaging has been performed.

Omental infarction demonstrates a variety of imaging appearances at CT. Classically; it appears as a fatty, large (>5 cm) encapsulated mass, with soft-tissue stranding adjacent to the ascending colon. Early or mild infarction may manifest as mild haziness in the fat anterior to the colon.

Kamaya A, et al. Imaging manifestations of abdominal fat necrosis and its mimics. *Radiographics.* 2011;31:2021–34.

21. B. Neurofibromatosis type 1

The imaging appearance of optic nerve gliomas is characteristic, such that biopsy is rarely performed. MR imaging is the modality of choice, particularly for assessing involvement of the orbital apex, optic chiasm, hypothalamus and other intracranial structures. The lesions are typically isointense on T1-weighted images and isointense to hyperintense on T2-weighted images. Enhancement is variable, and cystic spaces may be seen. Calcifications are rare. A rim of T2 hyperintensity is often observed at the tumour periphery, a finding that may mimic an expanded subarachnoid space. However, this finding corresponds histopathologically to leptomeningeal infiltration and proliferation (so-called arachnoidal gliomatosis).

The appearance of optic nerve gliomas is different in patients with and without NF1. In patients with NF1, the optic nerve often appears tortuous, kinked or buckled and diffusely enlarged. In patients without NF1, gliomas tend to be fusiform. Isolated chiasmal gliomas are more likely in the absence of neurofibromatosis, and chiasmal involvement is also more common in patients who do not have neurofibromatosis.

Tailor TD, et al. Orbital neoplasms in adults: Clinical, radiologic, and pathologic review. *Radiographics.* 2013;33(6):1739–58.

22. B. 1.5 Tesla

Foetal MR imaging is routinely performed on 1.5T MR scanners.

Glen OA, Barkovich AJ. Magnetic resonance imaging of the fetal brain and spine: An increasingly important tool in prenatal diagnosis, Part 1. *AJNR Am J Neuroradiol.* 2006;27:1604–11.

23. C. Crossing of suture line

Epidural (extradural) haematomas do not generally cross suture lines, unless associated with a diastatic fracture of the suture. Extradural haematomas are biconvex, extra-axial fluid collections associated with skull vault fracture. Fresh blood is 30–50 HU; coagulated blood is 50–80 HU.

Dähnert W. *Radiology Review Manual*, 6th edn. Philadelphia, PA: Lippincott Williams & Wilkins, 2007:286.

24. B. Neuroblastoma

About 34% of mediastinal masses are posterior and 88% of these are neurogenic in origin (most of which arise from the ganglion cells in the paravertebral sympathetic chain). The remaining 12% of posterior mediastinal masses are foregut cysts, malignant lymphoma, Hodgkin disease or non-Hodgkin lymphoma. Neuroblastoma is most common in the under 5-year-olds and ganglioneuroma is most common in those older than 10 years.

Radiographic appearances are as described in the question. Cross-sectional imaging is useful to delineate the extent of the mass and any spinal involvement. Left lower lobe pneumonia can be confused with tumour, and this is a known diagnostic pitfall. Bronchogenic cyst is typically middle mediastinal.

Merten DF. Diagnostic imaging of mediastinal masses in children. *AJR Am J Roentgenol.* 1992;158:825–32.

25. D. Single-shot, fast spin-echo (SS-FSE) T2W images

Because foetal MR imaging is performed without maternal or foetal sedation, image acquisition is susceptible to foetal motion; therefore, foetal MR imaging is performed primarily using ultrafast MR imaging techniques known as single-shot, fast spin-echo (SS-FSE) or half-Fourier acquired single-shot, turbo spin-echo (HASTE). Using these rapid pulse sequences, a single T2-weighted image can be acquired in less than 1 second, reducing the likelihood of foetal motion during image acquisition. Because each image is acquired separately, foetal motion typically affects only the particular image that was acquired while the foetus moved.

Glen OA, Barkovich AJ. Magnetic resonance imaging of the fetal brain and spine: An increasingly important tool in prenatal diagnosis, Part 1. *AJNR Am J Neuroradiol.* 2006;27:1604–11.

26. B. Carotid-cavernous fistula

Caroticocavernous fistulas are abnormal communications between the carotid artery and the cavernous sinus, either directly or via intradural branches of the internal or external carotid arteries.

The pattern of venous drainage, either anterior into the ophthalmic veins or posterior into the petrosal sinuses, often dictates the clinical findings and radiographic appearance. Anterior drainage typically leads to the most dramatic ocular findings and enlargement of the superior orbital vein, the latter often detectable with CT or MRI. However, superior orbital vein enlargement is not specific to CCF. Additional radiographic findings with variable prevalence include lateral bulging of the cavernous sinus wall and enlargement of extraocular muscles on CT or MRI, and abnormal cavernous sinus flow voids on MRI. Direct visualisation of flow-related hyperintensity on the source images of three-dimensional time-of-flight MRA can be extremely helpful in CCF detection, with 83% sensitivity and 100% specificity, far superior to standard MRI.

Rucker JC, et al. Magnetic resonance angiography source images in carotid cavernous fistulas. *Br J Ophthalmol.* 2004;88(2):311.

27. D. Group B streptococcal pneumonia

Group B streptococcal pneumonia is associated with premature rupture of the membranes during labour. The disease may have an early onset with septicaemia and fulminant progression to severe respiratory distress, shock and respiratory failure within 24 hours or a late onset 1–12 weeks after birth, which is frequently associated with meningitis. Neonatal pneumonia can closely mimic hyaline membrane disease clinically and is the most frequent cause of septicaemia in the neonate. Infection may resemble hyaline membrane disease very closely, especially in smaller infants. However, extensive granular confluent infiltrates whose distribution is often less uniform than those of hyaline membrane disease are more commonly seen. There is also less atelectasis than in hyaline membrane disease. Pleural effusions are not uncommon and the lung volume is normal.

The differential diagnosis includes hyaline membrane disease, which usually has a uniform distribution of pulmonary opacities, never has pleural effusions and has a decreased lung volume; meconium aspiration, which usually has nodular non-homogeneous densities, may have pleural effusions and usually has an increased lung volume; and finally, transient tachypnoea of the newborn, which usually has non-homogeneous densities and may have pleural fluid.

Arthur R. The neonatal chest X-ray. *Paediatr Respir Rev.* 2001;2:311–23.

28. C. There is no correlation between carmustine dose and toxicity.

Cyclophosphamide and busulfan are the most common drugs that cause lung injury. Diffuse alveolar damage (DAD) is the most common manifestation of cyclophosphamide-induced lung disease, with NSIP and COP being less common. There is no relationship between development of lung injury and dose and duration of therapy.

Carmustine is one of the few drugs for which there is a clear relationship between cumulative dose and lung injury. Lung injury can occur at low doses if the patient has undergone thoracic radiation therapy. DAD is the most common manifestation, with NSIP being less common.

DAD is the most common manifestation of bleomycin-induced lung disease, with NSIP and COP being less common. The risk of developing lung injury is increased in the elderly, in patients on oxygen therapy, with a history of prior thoracic irradiation, or in whom therapy is restarted in 6 months of discontinuation. The prognosis is poor, with most patients dying of respiratory failure within 3 months.

Paclitaxel may commonly cause pulmonary toxicity.

Rossi SE, et al. Pulmonary drug toxicity: Radiologic and pathologic manifestations. *Radiographics*. 2000;20(5):1245–59.

29. C.   The fat-ring sign

Omental infarction demonstrates a variety of imaging appearances on CT. Classically; it appears as a fatty, large (>5 cm) encapsulated mass, with soft-tissue stranding adjacent to the ascending colon. Early or mild infarction may manifest as mild haziness in the fat anterior to the colon.

Omental torsion is a rare cause of omental infarction and occurs when a portion of the omentum twists upon itself, leading to vascular compromise. In omental torsion, swirling of the vessels is often visible within the omentum. Although most cases of omental infarction are on the right side, left-sided infarction also may spontaneously occur.

Unusual locations of infarction are more commonly seen in the setting of surgical trauma or post-operative changes that result in altered omental vascular supply and subsequent infarction. Similar to epiploic appendagitis, the adjacent colon is usually spared, although rarely the colonic wall may be thickened, a result of direct extension of omental inflammation. The fat-ring sign is seen in epiploic appendagitis, not omental infarction.

Kamaya A, et al. Imaging manifestations of abdominal fat necrosis and its mimics. *Radiographics*. 2011;31:2021–34.

30. C.   Morquio syndrome

The mucopolysaccharidoses are a group of inherited diseases characterised by abnormal storage and excretion in the urine of various mucopolysaccharides. These patients have short stature and characteristic plain film findings. A characteristic finding in the hands is a pointed proximal fifth metacarpal base that has a notched appearance to the ulnar aspect. There is generalised flattening of the vertebral bodies (platyspondyly) (cf. not a feature of Hurler syndrome). Hunter and Hurler syndromes demonstrate an anterior vertebral beak that is inferiorly positioned, whereas Morquio syndrome demonstrates an anterior vertebral beak that is centrally positioned. Although achondroplasia can cause rounded anterior beaking in the vertebra of the upper lumbar spine, the findings described within the hands are more typical of the mucopolysaccharidoses.

Brant WE, Helms CA. *Fundamentals of Diagnostic Radiology*, 3rd edn. Philadelphia, PA: Lippincott Williams & Wilkins, 2006.
Dähnert W. *Radiology Review Manual*, 7th edn. Philadelphia, PA: Lippincott Williams & Wilkins, 2011.

31. C.   COP is a recognised pattern on HRCT in rheumatoid lungs.

Thoracic involvement develops in patients with disease progression. Pleural disease is the most common thoracic manifestation and pleural thickening is the most common finding, more than pleural effusion. Pleural effusions are usually unilateral and may be loculated. They usually occur late in the disease and are commonly associated with pericarditis and subcutaneous nodules. HRCT shows basal and peripheral predominant fibrosis. Rarely upper lobe fibrosis, mimicking tuberculosis (TB), can occur. There is increased prevalence of lung cancer in fibrotic rheumatoid lung disease. Nodules are multiple and well circumscribed, often forming thick-walled cavities. Obliterative bronchiolitis results in air trapping and mosaic pattern. COP is also seen on HRCT.

Mayberry JP, et al. Thoracic manifestations of systemic autoimmune diseases: Radiographic and high-resolution CT findings. *Radiographics*. 2000;20(6):1623–35.

32. E. Follow-up MRI is required in patients with high-grade liver injuries to identify potential complications that require early intervention.

Non-surgical treatment has become the standard of care in haemodynamically stable patients with blunt liver trauma. The use of helical CT in the diagnosis and management of blunt liver trauma is mainly responsible for the notable shift during the past decade from routine surgical to non-surgical management of blunt liver injuries. CT is the diagnostic modality of choice for the evaluation of blunt liver trauma in haemodynamically stable patients and can accurately help identify hepatic parenchymal injuries, help quantify the degree of haemoperitoneum and reveal associated injuries in other abdominal organs, retroperitoneal structures and the gastrointestinal tract. The CT features of blunt liver trauma include lacerations, subcapsular or parenchymal hematomas, active haemorrhage, juxtahepatic venous injuries, periportal low attenuation and a flat inferior vena cava. It is important that radiologists be familiar with the liver injury grading system based on these CT features that was established by the American Association for the Surgery of Trauma. CT is also useful in the assessment of delayed complications in blunt liver trauma, including delayed haemorrhage, hepatic or perihepatic abscess, post-traumatic pseudoaneurysm and haemophilia, and biliary complications such as biloma and bile peritonitis. Follow-up CT is needed in patients with high-grade liver injuries to identify potential complications that require early intervention.

Yoon W, et al. CT in blunt liver trauma. *RadioGraphics*. 2005;25:87–104.

33. C. Haemangioma

Although not true neoplasms, cavernous malformations are the most common benign orbital mass in adults. Although these masses are commonly referred to as *cavernous haemangiomas*, many pathologists prefer the term *cavernous malformation*.

On CT images, cavernous malformations are typically well circumscribed, homogeneous and ovoid. The majority occur at the lateral aspect of the intraconal space. Conal and extraconal cavernous malformations are rare. Phleboliths are virtually never seen. Cavernous malformations tend to displace and surround adjacent structures, such as extraconal muscles and the optic nerve, rather than cause direct invasion. Osseous remodelling may be present, although bone erosion is rare. At MRI performed with T1-weighted sequences, cavernous malformations are isointense relative to muscle; the lesions appear uniformly hyperintense on T2-weighted images, with no flow voids. Internal septations may be identified on T2-weighted images. At multiphase CT, enhancement of cavernous malformations is poor on early arterial phase images, owing to the scant arterial supply. Delayed venous phase images demonstrate progressive filling of the mass from periphery to centre, with complete filling within 30 minutes. This enhancement pattern may permit differentiation of cavernous malformations from other vascular lesions with rich arterial supply, such as capillary haemangioma (a paediatric diagnosis), haemangiopericytoma and arteriovenous malformations.

Rhabdomyosarcoma is the most common soft-tissue malignancy of childhood and most common primary orbital malignancy. CT shows moderately well-defined to ill-defined margins, irregular shape and mild–moderate contrast enhancement. Adjacent bony destruction occurs in 40%. Globe distortion and extension to the paranasal sinuses may also be seen. Calcification is rare unless post-treatment. MR typically shows bright T2 signal, distinguishing rhabdomyosarcoma from other tumours such as chloroma (granulocytic sarcoma), lymphoma and metastatic neuroblastoma.

Khan SN, Sepahdari AR. Orbital masses: CT and MRI of common vascular lesions, benign tumors, and malignancies. *Saudi J Ophthalmol*. 2012;26(4):373–83.

Tailor TD, et al. Orbital neoplasms in adults: Clinical, radiologic, and pathologic review. *Radiographics*. 2013;33(6):1739–58.

34. E. High signal in inflammatory stranding in peritubal fat on T1 fat-suppressed images

Pelvic inflammatory disease (PID) affects women of reproductive age and can lead to infertility, ectopic pregnancy and chronic pelvic pain. In acute cases when dilated fallopian tubes are detected, it is extremely important to be able to differentiate tubal torsion from a pyosalpinx. A tubal torsion and a hematosalpinx may have a similar appearance to that of a fluid-filled tube on T2-weighted and STIR images; on T1-weighted images, however, a fluid-filled tube has low signal intensity. Layering is common with haemorrhagic lesions, and tubal torsion may have a comma-shaped appearance. A pyosalpinx may have a similar appearance to that of a hydrosalpinx, but a hydrosalpinx usually has thinner walls. An abscess usually has low T1-weighted and high T2-weighted signal, but there can be a large variation in the signal intensity on T1-weighted and heterogeneity on T2-weighted images. Thick, irregular walls are typical of abscesses.

The T1 signal of pyosalpinx/TO abscess varies according to haemorrhagic/proteinaceous content. On post-contrast T1-weighted images, pyosalpinx shows wall enhancement. Enhancement of the surrounding inflamed fat can also be evident. Inflammatory fat stranding is also seen on fat-suppressed T2-weighted sequences.

Febronio EM, et al. Acute pelvic inflammatory disease: Pictorial essay focused on computed tomography and magnetic resonance imaging findings. *Radiol Bras.* 2012;45(6):345–50.

Tukeva TA, et al. MR imaging in pelvic inflammatory disease: Comparison with laparoscopy and US. *Radiology.* 1999;210(1):209–16.

35. B. Osteogenesis imperfecta

Osteogenesis imperfecta is an inherited disorder that results from mutations in either the *COL1A1* or *COL1A2* gene of Type I collagen. The disease is usually apparent at birth or in childhood, but more mild forms of the disease may not be apparent until adulthood. The disease is classified into Types I–IV, with Type I, the mildest form, being described in the question. The presenile hearing loss is caused by otosclerosis. The differential diagnosis can be resolved by the extraskeletal manifestations (blue sclerae and dentinogenesis imperfecta). The other types are Type II, lethal perinatal; Type III, severe progressive; and Type IV, moderately severe.

Adam A, et al. *Grainger & Allison's Diagnostic Radiology: A Textbook of Medical Imaging*, 5th edn. New York: Churchill Livingstone, 2008:1092–3.

36. E. Transient tachypnoea of the newborn

Although RDS is seen in association with maternal diabetes and caesarean section, hyperexpansion is not a feature of RDS. Transient tachypnoea of the newborn appears soon after birth (<4 hours) and has been identified as occurring with caesarean birth and infant sedation. Longer labour intervals, macrosomia of the foetus, and maternal asthma have also been associated. It may be accompanied by chest retractions, by expiratory grunting, or by cyanosis (which can be relieved with minimal oxygen). Recovery is usually complete within 3 days.

The lungs are usually affected diffusely and symmetrically, and the condition is commonly accompanied by small pleural effusions. The clinical course of transient tachypnoea is relatively benign when compared with the severity suggested by chest films. Radiographic resolution by the second or third day characterises this entity and differentiates it from other possible disorders; if radiographic resolution is not complete by the third day or if respiratory symptoms persist longer than 5 days, an alternative diagnosis should be sought.

Findings of transient tachypnoea of the newborn on chest radiographs may include mild, symmetrical lung overaeration, prominent perihilar interstitial markings and small pleural effusions. The radiographic appearance at times can mimic the diffuse, granular appearance of hyaline membrane disease but without pulmonary underaeration. Neonates with transient tachypnoea are usually delivered at term. Radiographic lung changes may also resemble the coarse, interstitial pattern seen with other causes of pulmonary oedema or the irregular pattern of lung opacification seen in meconium aspiration syndrome.

Arthur R. The neonatal chest X-ray. *Paediatr Respir Rev.* 2001;2:311–23.

37. C. Multifocal hepatic lesions

Henoch–Schonlein purpura is the most common vasculitis of childhood affecting small blood vessels. Clinical manifestations may include non-thrombocytopenic purpura, arthritis, abdominal pain, gastrointestinal haemorrhage and glomerulonephritis. Imaging is useful to depict end-organ damage.

Ultrasound findings may include bowel wall oedema, submucosal and intramural haemorrhage, intussusception, hypoperistalsis, bowel dilatation, ascites, normal or enlarged echogenic kidneys, and also possible intramural haematomas within the urinary bladder and ureters. Non-specific findings on scrotal ultrasound may be identified such as hydroceles, scrotal wall thickening and inflammation of the spermatic cord and epididymis.

Khanna G, et al. Pediatric vasculitis: Recognizing multisystemic manifestations at body imaging. *Radiographics.* 2015;35:849–65.

38. D. Erosion of the medial aspect of the clavicle

Bone changes of rheumatoid arthritis seen on chest X-ray include resorption of the lateral end of the clavicles, erosive arthritis of the shoulders (most commonly superolateral aspect of humeral head), global loss of shoulder joint space, superior rib notching, atrophy and rotator cuff tear.

Sommer OJ, et al. Rheumatoid arthritis: A practical guide to state-of-the-art imaging, image interpretation, and clinical implications. *Radiographics.* 2005;25(2):381–98.

39. D. Dual-phase CT pancreas

Insulinomas are the most common functioning pancreatic endocrine tumours (PET), accounting for just over 40% of all functioning PETs. They have an incidence of two to four per million people each year. They tend to manifest earlier and have a smaller size than other functioning and non-functioning endocrine tumours,

Insulinomas usually are sporadic, but they account for 10%–30% of functioning PETs in patients with Multiple endocrine neoplasia (MEN1) and they have been reported in patients with neurofibromatosis Type 1.

In 1935, Whipple and Frantz described the classic clinical triad of insulinomas: symptoms of hypoglycaemia, low blood glucose and relief of symptoms with administration of glucose. Hypoglycaemia typically manifests during fasting or after exercise, and patients often self-medicate by eating frequent small meals. On CT and MR imaging, insulinomas are typically homogeneous and hyperenhancing. The use of coronal images may help differentiate these small hyperenhancing lesions from nearby.

Lewis RB, et al. Pancreatic endocrine tumors: Radiologic-clinicopathologic correlation. *RadioGraphics.* 2010;30:1445–64.

40. A. Hypointense cysts on T1W images

Findings of an adnexal mass with high T1-weighted signal and high T2-weighted signal (although slightly lower T2 signal than simple or functional cyst) is highly specific for an endometrioma. The main differential for high T1-weighted cysts are haemorrhagic functional cysts and mature cystic teratoma. Cystic teratoma is differentiated by means of T1-weighted fat-suppressed images. Endometriomas tend to have higher T1 and lower T2 signal than haemorrhagic cysts, due to higher protein content and viscosity (described as T2 shading). Multifocal lesions and bilateral lesions also favour endometriosis. Hemosiderin-laden macrophages combined with the fibrous nature of the cyst wall give it a low-signal-intensity appearance on both T1- and T2-weighted images. Wall thickening, septae and nodularity are also recognised.

Woodward PJ, et al. Endometriosis: Radiologic-pathologic correlation. *Radiographics.* 2001;21(1):193–216.

41. E. Eosinophilic granuloma

The vast majority of 'vertebra plana' lesions in relatively healthy children are caused by an eosinophilic granuloma. The other available options are all possible, but less common, differential diagnoses. There is usually preservation of the disc space and no kyphosis. The posterior elements are rarely involved.

Dähnert W. *Radiology Review Manual*, 7th edn. Philadelphia, PA: Lippincott Williams & Wilkins, 2011.
Sutton D. *Textbook of Radiology and Imaging*, 7th edn. Edinburgh: Churchill Livingstone, 2003.

42. D. Dermoid cyst

Dermoid cysts represent the most common congenital lesion of the orbit and account for one-third of all childhood orbital tumours.

CT shows an ovoid, well-demarcated cystic lesion; there may be fat (50%) or calcification (15%) present. Bone remodelling and thin rim enhancement is described. The majority occur in the extraconal location, occupying the superolateral aspect of the anterior orbit (related to the frontozygomatic suture). MRI shows high signal on T1-weighted images, if containing fat or proteinaceous material with low to isointense signal on T2-weighted images. Thin rim enhancement is seen on T1 FS images post-administration of gadolinium, unless the lesion has ruptured.

Grant LA, Griffin N. *Grainger & Allison's Diagnostic Radiology Essentials*. Orbital tumours. New York, NY: Churchill Livingstone Elsevier Limited, 2013:826.
Jung WS, et al. The radiological spectrum of orbital pathologies that involve the lacrimal gland and the lacrimal fossa. *Korean J Radiol: Off J Korean Radiol Soc*. 2007;8(4):336–42.

43. B. Anterior ethmoid mucocoele

Paranasal sinus mucocoeles are benign, expansile cystic masses covered by respiratory epithelium, resulting from accumulation and retention of mucus secretion in cases where the sinus drainage is obstructed. They primarily occur in the frontal sinuses (60%–65%) but may also be found in ethmoid sinuses (20%–25%).

Usually, mucocoeles are seen as an isodense or mildly hyperdense sinus opacity in relation to the cerebral tissue, but in cases of acute infection it may appear as a more dense and peripherally enhanced image. The neighbouring bone structure is remodelled with areas of thickening, expansion and erosion. Additionally, in the areas of greater fragility, one may observe herniation into adjacent structures, displacing structures rather than invading them. Invasion would suggest malignancy.

The radiological appearance at MRI varies with the time of evolution of the disease. Initially, the contents will be predominantly aqueous, so the corresponding image will be hypointense on T1-weighted sequences and hyperintense on T2-weighted sequences. Over time, the protein contents may increase, resulting in hyperintense images both on T1-weighted and T2-weighted sequences.

Carvalho BV, et al. Typical and atypical presentations of paranasal sinus mucocele at computed tomography. *Radiol Bras*. 2013;46(6):372–5.

44. E. Central bronchiectasis

Angioinvasive pulmonary aspergillosis occurs almost exclusively in immunocompromised patients with severe neutropenia. Characteristic CT findings include nodules surrounded by a halo of ground-glass attenuation (halo sign) or pleura-based, wedge-shaped areas of consolidation. In neutropenia patients, the halo sign is highly suggestive of angioinvasive aspergillosis. However, a similar appearance has been described in infection by Mucorales, *Candida*, herpes simplex virus (HSV), cytomegalovirus (CMV), Wegener's granulomatosis, Kaposi's sarcoma and haemorrhagic metastases. Separation of fragments of necrotic lung (pulmonary sequestra) from adjacent parenchyma results in air crescents similar to those seen in mycetomas. The air crescent sign is usually seen after initiation of treatment and with resolution of the neutropenia. Airway invasive aspergillosis shows multiple centrilobular nodules and the tree-in-bud pattern.

Franquet T, et al. Spectrum of pulmonary aspergillosis: Histologic, clinical, and radiologic findings. *Radiographics*. 2001;21(4):825–37.

45. C. Smaller aneurysms have a higher likelihood of thrombosis

Kawasaki's disease is a common paediatric vasculitis of medium-sized vessels, with coronary vasculitis being the hallmark manifestation. It is the leading cause of acquired heart disease in children in developed countries.

Coronary arterial aneurysms typically occur within the subacute phase of the disease and may be associated with sudden cardiac death. The aneurysms typically develop in the proximal segments of major coronary arteries and affect the left anterior descending artery followed by the proximal right coronary arteries in frequency of location. Smaller aneurysms, (<5 mm in diameter) are more likely to regress than larger aneurysms (>8 mm in diameter), which have a higher likelihood of thrombosis and infarction.

Khanna G, et al. Pediatric vasculitis: Recognizing multisystemic manifestations at body imaging. *Radiographics*. 2015;35:849–65.

46. E. Leiomyoma

Leiomyomas are neoplasms of mature smooth muscle cells and are the most common benign oesophageal neoplasm, although they are about 50 times less common than oesophageal carcinoma. They are also the most common mesenchymal tumours of the oesophagus, unlike in the remainder of the gastrointestinal tract, where GISTs predominate.

Oesophageal leiomyomas are nearly twice as common in men as in women and have been reported in patients between 4 and 81 years of age, although they rarely occur in the paediatric population. Most patients are asymptomatic, but dysphagia and pain may develop, depending on the size of the lesion and amount of encroachment on the oesophageal lumen, in contrast to patients with malignant oesophageal tumours.

Affected individuals usually have long-standing symptoms, with a duration of more than 2 years in most cases. Treatment options include endoscopic resection, surgical enucleation and observation. Oesophageal leiomyomas have a benign clinical course and typically do not recur after surgery.

Lewis RB, et al. Oesophageal neoplasms: Radiologic-pathologic correlation. *Radiographics*. 2013;33:1083–110.

47. D. Ureteric endometriosis is mostly intrinsic.

Deep pelvic endometriosis is defined as subperitoneal invasion by endometriotic lesions that exceeds 5 mm in depth. Involvement of anatomic structures such as the uterosacral ligaments or the vaginal or rectal wall should be suspected when these structures have a hypointense thickened or nodular appearance on T2-weighted images. Intermingled high T2 signal would be secondary to ectopic endometrial glands. On T1-weighted or fat-suppressed T1-weighted MR images, these foci may have either high or low signal intensity, depending on the presence or absence of bloody content. Some endometriomas may show restricted diffusion on DWI, probably due to intracystic blood clots. Enhancement may or may not occur post-contrast, depending on the proportions of inflammatory reaction, glandular tissue and fibrosis. Bladder endometriosis should be considered in anyone who presents with urinary tract symptoms after having undergone hysterectomy or other gynaecologic surgical procedure. Because vesical endometriosis seldom invades the mucosa, MR imaging may show abnormalities although cystoscopy is normal. As with bladder involvement, extrinsic endometriosis is the most common form of ureteral involvement. On MR imaging, ureteral endometriosis usually appears as irregular hypointense nodules on T2-weighted images. Deep retroperitoneal endometriotic lesions of the posterior compartment involve the rectovaginal pouch, retrocervical area, uterosacral ligaments, posterior vaginal fornix, rectovaginal septum and rectum. Obliteration of the pouch of Douglas occurs when retrocervical lesions extend to the anterior rectal wall.

Coutinho A Jr, et al. MR imaging in deep pelvic endometriosis: A pictorial essay. *Radiographics*. 2011;31(2):549–67.

48. D. 4

Physeal Salter–Harris fractures are divided into two categories on the basis of the involved physeal regions: (1) horizontal fractures without involvement of the germinal or proliferative zone of the physis and (2) longitudinal fractures that extend through all zones of the physis into the epiphysis.

Horizontal fractures (Salter–Harris Types I and II) result in bridge formation in 25% of cases, whereas longitudinal fractures (Salter–Harris Types III and IV) result in bridge formation in 75% of cases.

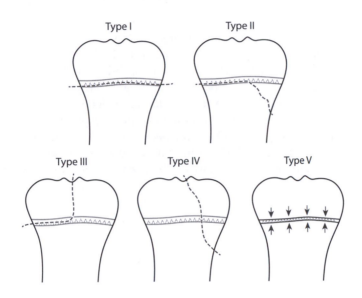

Jaimes C, et al. MR imaging of normal epiphyseal development and common epiphyseal disorders. *Radiographics*. 2014;34(2):449–71.

49. B. Involvement of endothoracic fascia

Malignant mesothelioma occurs mainly in the pleura and peritoneum but can arise in the pericardium or tunica vaginalis testis. It is the most common primary neoplasm of the pleura and has a strong association with asbestos exposure, particularly crocidolite. Mesothelioma is not known to arise from plaques.

There is a new TNM staging system for diffuse malignant pleural mesothelioma that emphasises the criteria for determinate local tumour extension and regional lymph node status, to identify patients with potentially curable early disease (T1a and b); potentially resectable but not necessarily curable (T2 and T3); and unresectable local tumour spread (T4). Signs of unresectability include multifocal extension into chest wall with or without rib or spine destruction, extension through diaphragm into peritoneum, extension into contralateral pleura, extension into mediastinal organs, extension through pericardium and direct extension into heart. Localised tumour extension into the endothoracic fascia (T3) is potentially resectable.

Roach HD, et al. Asbestos: When the dust settles an imaging review of asbestos-related disease. *Radiographics*. 2002;22:S167–84.

50. E. Ileum

Enteric duplication cysts are an uncommon congenital abnormality. They can occur anywhere along the digestive tract on the mesenteric side. The small intestine is most commonly involved, with the order from most to least common being the ileum, jejunum and duodenum. Most duplication cysts manifest during the first year of life, although some occasionally manifest in older patients. Children can present with a variety of symptoms including abdominal distention, vomiting, bleeding, a palpable abdominal mass and rarely urinary frequency and hesitancy. Complications include perforation, intussusception, bowel obstruction from adjacent pressure or mass effect, volvulus and associated malignancy. Malignant lesions arising from duplication cysts are rare, particularly in children.

Tong SC, et al. Ileocaecal enteric duplication cyst: Radiologic-pathologic correlation. *Radiographics.* 2002;22:1217–22.

51. E. Cervical factor infertility is the most common cause of infertility.

Intrauterine filling defects seen at HSG may be caused by air bubbles in the contrast material injection, intrauterine adhesions, submucosal leiomyomas, endometrial polyps or blood clots. Intrauterine adhesions, or synechiae, may be the result of previous pregnancy, dilation and curettage, surgery or infection. They appear as irregular linear filling defects at HSG; the endometrial cavity may appear distorted or may not expand as expected with contrast. Even subcentimetric endometrial polyps and submucosal leiomyomas may interfere with embryo transfer and implantation. Submucosal leiomyomas distort the normal-appearing endometrium. Uterine contour irregularities observed at HSG can be due to adenomyosis, uterine leiomyomas and Müllerian duct anomalies. Submucosal leiomyoma located near the uterine cornua may obstruct the ipsilateral fallopian tube. Cervical abnormalities include *cervical factor infertility*, an inadequate quality or volume of cervical mucus, a condition that accounts for approximately 10% of cases of female infertility, and cervical stenosis.

Steinkeler JA, et al. Female infertility: A systematic approach to radiologic imaging and diagnosis. *Radiographics.* 2009;29(5):1353–70.

52. D. Granulomatosis with polyangitis

CT scanning is likely to reveal a common mucosal thickening similar to that encountered in chronic sinusitis. However, the presence of bony erosions of the sinonasal wall is very suspect of the diagnosis of a granulomatous disease. Bone erosion commonly affects the lamina papyracea (orbital wall), inter sino-nasal wall and nasal septum. Bone destruction usually involves the nasal septum and then extends to the sinonasal wall, destroying the turbinates. Differential diagnoses including traumatic lesions (accidental, iatrogenic) or toxic lesions (cocaine abuse, chromium salts) should be considered. Isolated septal perforation should suggest the diagnosis of GP. There are no specific imaging findings to distinguish GP from 'lethal midline granuloma', but the destructive lesions seem to be more extensive in lethal midline granuloma.

Pulmonary nodules and masses are the most common radiologic findings of Wegener's granulomatosis.

Benoudiba F, et al. Sinonasal Wegener's granulomatosis: CT characteristics. *Neuroradiology.* 2003;45:95–9.
Martinez F, et al. Common and uncommon manifestations of Wegener granulomatosis at chest CT: Radiologic-pathologic correlation. *Radiographics.* 2012;32:51–69.

53. A. ACL

The pivot shift injury is a non-contact injury commonly seen in skiers or US football players. The resulting bone contusion (pivot shift oedema) pattern involves the posterior aspect of the lateral tibial plateau and the midportion of the lateral femoral condyle. The exact location of the lateral femoral condyle injury depends on the degree of flexion of the knee at injury. Another recently described bone contusion pattern associated with the pivot shift injury is oedema within the posterior lip of the medial tibial plateau. Pivot shift oedema is typically associated with ACL tear, most commonly mid-substance.

Dashboard oedema is seen at the anterior aspect of the tibia and, occasionally, at the posterior surface of the patella. The associated soft-tissue injuries include disruption of the PCL (most commonly mid-substance) posterior joint capsule.

Hyperextension of the knee can result in kissing contusion involving the anterior aspect of the tibial plateau and the anterior aspect of the femoral condyle. ACL, PCL and meniscal injury can be associated depending on the force.

The classic bone contusion pattern seen after lateral patellar dislocation includes involvement of the anterolateral aspect of the lateral femoral condyle and the inferomedial aspect of the patella. This is associated with tear of MPFL.

With clip injury (pure valgus stress), bone marrow oedema is usually most prominent in the lateral femoral condyle secondary to the direct blow, whereas a second smaller area of oedema may be present in the medial femoral condyle secondary to avulsive stress to the MCL (mostly at the femoral attachment).

Sanders TG, et al. Bone contusion patterns of the knee at MR imaging: Footprint of the mechanism of injury. *Radiographics.* 2000;20:S135–51.

54. D. Granulomatosis with polyangiitis

Granulomatosis with polyangiitis (GPA), previously known as *Wegener's granulomatosis*, affects small to medium-sized vessels and most commonly involves the upper and lower respiratory tracts and kidneys. In comparison to adults, children are more likely to have multi-organ involvement with renal disease, subglottic stenosis, nasal deformity and pulmonary findings. Differential diagnosis of GPA may include those that present with pulmonary-renal features such as mixed connective tissue diseases, Goodpasture syndrome or systemic lupus erythematosus.

Takayasu arteritis is a large-vessel vasculitis with characteristic abnormalities of the aorta and its main branches. Kawasaki's disease and polyarteritis nodosa (PAN) are medium vessel vasculitides. The hallmark imaging feature in Kawasaki's disease includes coronary artery aneurysms. In PAN, angiographic findings of aneurysms, stenoses or occlusions of medium-sized vessels is a key diagnostic criterion. This is predominantly seen in renal and mesenteric arteries, although not pathognomonic.

Cogan's syndrome is an autoimmune disorder characterised by interstitial keratitis and bilateral audiovestibular deficits. It may be associated with a systemic vasculitis and typically presents in young adulthood.

Khanna G, et al. Pediatric vasculitis: Recognizing multisystemic manifestations at body imaging. *Radiographics.* 2015;35:849–65.

55. E. High-density consolidation

Pleural disease is the most commonly encountered manifestation of asbestos-related disease. Benign pleural effusions are thought to be the earliest pleural-based phenomenon. The most common manifestation of asbestos exposure is pleural plaques that usually arise from the parietal pleura but may arise from visceral pleura. Calcification is reported in 10%–15%. The classic distribution of plaques is the posterolateral chest wall, lateral chest wall, the dome of the diaphragm (virtually pathognomonic) and the mediastinal pleura. The apices and costophrenic angles are typically spared. Diffuse pleural thickening is less specific for asbestos exposure. Asbestos-related round atelectasis is also known as asbestos pseudotumour and is related to fibrosis in the superficial layers of the pleura. *Asbestosis* is the term given to lung fibrosis caused by asbestos. The changes are more pronounced in the lower lobes and subpleurally but often extend to involve the middle lobe and lingula. Malignant mesothelioma and bronchogenic carcinoma are known associations. High-density consolidation is typical of amiodarone lung changes.

Roach HD, et al. Asbestos: When the dust settles an imaging review of asbestos-related disease. *Radiographics.* 2002;22:S167–84.

56. C. Pneumobilia

Of all the hollow viscera, the stomach is the least commonly affected by gas-forming infections. Of the 30 reported cases in the literature, caustic ingestion (37%) and alcohol abuse (22%) were found to be the most common causes. Other predisposing conditions include recent gastroduodenal surgery, trauma and gastric infarction. Caustic ingestion of acid is thought to promote coagulative necrosis of the gastric lumen, whereas ingestion of an alkaline substance leads to liquefactive necrosis; in either case, the end result is mucosal damage and super infection with gas-forming bacteria. There are no predilections with regard to age, sex or diabetic status. Clinical manifestation may be dramatic, ranging from acute sepsis to gastric haemorrhage and, rarely, vomiting of the necrotic stomach cast.

CT is considered the modality of choice for detection of intramural gas and evaluation for the presence of pneumoperitoneum or portal venous gas. CT may also demonstrate irregular mucosal fold thickening and may be used to monitor response to treatment or disease progression. An important differential diagnosis to consider is benign gastric emphysema. Gas collections form within the gastric wall without associated infection by gas-forming organisms. Gas may enter the wall from the lumen, peritoneal surface or oesophageal or duodenal connection and is usually associated with violent coughing, vomiting or severe obstructive pulmonary disease. Gastric fold inflammation and thickening are not present, and the patient is usually asymptomatic with spontaneous resolution expected.

Grayson DE, et al. Emphysematous infections of the abdomen and pelvis: A pictorial review. *Radiographics.* 2002;22:543–61.

57. D. Peritubal adhesions

The differential diagnosis of tubal occlusion typically includes tubal spasm, infection and prior surgery. Rare causes include granulomatous salpingitis due to tuberculosis, intraluminal endometriosis, parasitic infection and congenital atresia of the fallopian tubes. When tubal occlusion in the proximal or interstitial portion of the fallopian tube is seen at hysterosalpingography, a tubal spasm should be considered as the possible cause. Delayed radiography may be performed to help differentiate tubal spasm from true tubal occlusion. A spasmolytic agent such as glucagon also may be administered to relax the uterine muscle and relieve a tubal spasm.

Peritubal adhesions show peritubal pooling of contrast material rather than occlusion of fallopian tubes.

Steinkeler JA, et al. Female infertility: A systematic approach to radiologic imaging and diagnosis. *Radiographics.* 2009;29(5):1353–70.

58. B. Acquired attic cholesteatoma

Cholesteatomas are composed of densely packed desquamated keratinising squamous cells, arising from a peripheral shell of inward-facing epithelium. The role of CT is to assess the extent of disease and exclude complications. Key findings on HRCT include soft-tissue opacification in the attic, aditus (non-dependent location) and/or mastoid air cells, erosion of the scutum, disruption of ossicular chain (long process of incus erosion is common), presence of disease in sinus tympani and erosions of the tegmen tympani, semicircular canal, facial nerve canal and inner ear. In cases of clinical suspicion of intracranial extension, perform contrast CT/MRI to rule out intracranial complications.

Congenital cholesteatoma is difficult to differentiate from acquired type, but clinical features help; it is commonly seen in children with intact tympanic membrane and absence of previous otologic disease.

Anbarasu A, et al. Soft tissue attenuation in middle ear on HRCT: Pictorial review. *Indian J Radiol Imaging.* 2012;22:298–304

59. B. Transient synovitis

Acute transient synovitis is the most common non-traumatic cause of hip pain in young children. It tends to affect children between 2 and 9 years of age and boys are affected two to four times more often. Where history is typical no imaging may be required; ultrasound can be used to identify the effusion. Initial bone scan uptake can be reduced, mimicking SUFE, but can increase later on.

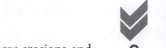

Juvenile arthritis affects children above 4–5 years of age. Radiographs may show erosions and loss of joint space. MRI and ultrasound are more sensitive for soft-tissue changes, allowing demonstration of synovitis, distinguishing pannus from simple effusion and identifying cartilage destruction and cortical erosions.

Septic arthritis is an emergency. The majority of patients are less than 2 years old and are usually unwell with pain on passive movement of the hip.

Avascular necrosis (AVN) of the femoral head is a condition induced by compromised blood supply, resulting in progressive destruction of bone. It is most commonly idiopathic (Perthes) but may be seen following trauma, infection, steroid treatment and in association with haematological diseases, such as sickle cell anaemia. Perthes disease usually affects children between 4 and 10 years of age and is more common in boys. Plain radiography is insensitive at early changes. The epiphysis may appear small, sclerotic or flattened with subchondral lucency or more marked fragmentation. Where symmetrical changes are seen, hypothyroidism or epiphyseal dysplasia should be considered. Meyer's dysplasia mimics Perthes disease unilaterally by appearance but is asymptomatic.

Jain N, et al. Radiological approach to a child with hip pain. *Clin Radiol.* 2013;68(11):1167–78.

60. C. Abnormally large kidneys

There are several causes of chronic liver failure in children: chronic hepatitis (hepatitis B and C), biliary atresia, drug induced (e.g., paracetamol), alpha-1-antitrypsin deficiency, Wilson's disease, cystic fibrosis, IBD (inflammatory bowel disease), Budd–Chiari syndrome, TPN (total parenteral nutrition) induced and so on.

Abnormal sweat test (>60 mmol/L of sodium chloride) suggests CF, while reduced serum copper and caeruloplasmin and raised 24-hour urinary copper suggests Wilson's disease. US shows hepatomegaly, echogenic liver, splenomegaly, ascites and varices.

Kayser–Fleischer rings from copper deposition in the eye are pathognomonic but may require slit lamp examination to visualise. Adolescent patients can present with neurological symptoms.

Enlarged kidneys are not a feature of Wilson's disease and may be seen in the acute phase of glomerulonephritis, ATN, renal vein thrombosis, amyloidosis, lymphoma, diabetes, glycogen storage disease, polycystic kidney disease and so on.

Dähnert W. *Radiology Review Manual*, 7th edn. Philadelphia, PA: Lippincott Williams & Wilkins, 2011.
Tasker RC, et al. *Oxford Handbook of Paediatrics*. Oxford: Oxford University Press, 2008.

61. D. Renal rhabdoid tumour

Rhabdoid tumour is a rare, highly aggressive malignancy of early childhood. It is not related to Wilms tumour or rhabdomyosarcoma and was recently recognised as a distinct pathologic entity. Its name is derived from its histologic appearance, which resembles that of a tumour of skeletal muscle origin, although a myogenic origin has not been proved.

Rhabdoid tumour occurs exclusively in children, comprising 2% of paediatric renal malignancies. Approximately 80% occur in patients less than 2 years of age and 60% in patients less than 1 year of age, with the majority (25%) diagnosed between 6 and 12 months of age. The median age at diagnosis is 11 months, with the lesion reported at up to 9 years of age.

Lowe LH, et al. Pediatric renal masses: Wilms tumor and beyond. *RadioGraphics.* 2000;20:1585–603.

62. E. Pulmonary embolism

Extra-intestinal manifestations of inflammatory bowel disease:

Musculoskeletal System
Arthritis
Colitic type, ankylosing spondylitis, isolated joint involvement, hypertrophic osteoarthropathy: clubbing, periostitis

Miscellaneous Manifestations
Osteoporosis, aseptic necrosis, polymyositis

Dermatologic and Oral Systems
Reactive Lesions
Erythema nodosum, pyoderma gangrenosum, aphthous ulcers, necrotising vasculitis
Specific Lesions
Fissures, fistulas, oral Crohn's disease, drug rashes
Nutritional Deficiencies
Acrodermatitis enteropathica, purpura, glossitis, hair loss, brittle nails
Associated Diseases
Vitiligo, psoriasis, amyloidosis

Hepatopancreatobiliary System
Primary sclerosing cholangitis, bile-duct carcinoma
Associated Inflammation
Autoimmune chronic active hepatitis, pericholangitis, portal fibrosis, cirrhosis, granulomatous disease
Metabolic manifestations
Fatty liver, gallstones associated with ileal Crohn's disease

Ocular System
Uveitis/iritis, episcleritis, scleromalacia, corneal ulcers, retinal vascular disease

Metabolic System
Growth retardation in children and adolescents, delayed sexual maturation

Renal System
Calcium oxalate stones

Levine JS, Burakoff R. Extra intestinal manifestations of inflammatory bowel disease. *Gastroenterol Hepatol (N Y)*. 2011;7(4):235–41.

63. C. They occur early in atherosclerotic disease.
In a penetrating aortic ulcer (PAU), an atheromatous plaque ulcerates and burrows through the intima into the aortic media. This leads to haemorrhage into the wall (intramural hematoma). The mural haematoma may break through into the adventitia to form a pseudoaneurysm, or it may rupture. Ulceration of an aortic atheroma occurs in patients with advanced atherosclerosis. On imaging, a penetrating aortic ulcer can be distinguished from an atheromatous plaque by presence of a focal, contrast-filled outpouching surrounded by an intramural hematoma, which confirms the aggressive behaviour of the lesion. The atheromatous plaque with ulceration but without penetration through the intima shows irregular margins, but no contrast material extends beyond the level of intima, which is frequently calcified, and no intramural hematoma is present. PAU can present with chest or back pain.

Macura KJ, et al. Pathogenesis in acute aortic syndromes: Aortic dissection, intramural hematoma, and penetrating atherosclerotic aortic ulcer. *AJR Am J Roentgenol*. 2003;181:309–16.

64. B. Continued increase in size of follicle
Ovulation is sonographically determined by the follicle suddenly disappearing or regressing in size, irregular margins, intrafollicular echoes, follicles becoming more echogenic, free fluid in the pouch of Douglas and increased perifollicular blood flow velocities on Doppler.

Bakos O, et al. Ultrasonographical and hormonal description of the normal ovulatory menstrual cycle. *Acta Obstet Gynecol Scand*. 1994;73(10):790–6.

65. A. Cholesterol granuloma

Cholesterol granulomas of the temporal bone can occur in the mastoid segment, the middle ear and the petrous apex. They are the most common primary petrous apex lesions.

Temporal bone CT reveals an expansile, sharply defined and often rounded mass of the petrous apex with cortical thinning and trabecular breakdown. The general appearance is that of a slowly progressive benign process. There is central soft-tissue density without an internal matrix, a calcification or residual septations. If the lesion is sufficiently enlarged, frank bony dehiscence is observed.

On MRI, cholesterol granulomas are typically hyperintense on both T1 and T2-weighted sequences because of the accumulation of blood breakdown products and proteinaceous debris. Small lesions may be relatively homogeneous, whereas large lesions show more heterogeneity. Often cholesterol granulomas have a distinct hypointense peripheral rim on T2-weighted images due to hemosiderin deposition. After contrast administration, there may be subtle peripheral enhancement secondary to inflammatory response but no central enhancement that would indicate solid tissue.

Chapman PR, et al. Petrous apex lesions: Pictorial review. *AJR Am J Roentgenol*. 2011;196(3 Suppl):WS26–37.

66. E. Chondroblastoma

Chondroblastomas are rare, benign, cartilaginous tumours that affect the epiphysis of children. On MR images, chondroblastomas are seen as epiphyseal lesions with high T2 signal intensity surrounded by a halo of oedema in the adjacent marrow and soft tissues. A characteristic thin (<1 mm) low-signal-intensity ring that corresponds to peripheral sclerosis is seen in more than 90%. Fluid–fluid levels similar to Aneurysmal bone cyst (ABCs) are seen in 20%–30% of cases. Differential considerations include epiphyseal osteomyelitis and osteoid osteoma.

Neuroblastoma metastasis and Langerhans cell hystiocytosis can also affect the epiphyses.

Simple bone cyst (SBC), fibrous cortical defects and ABC affect the metaphysis.

Jaimes C, et al. MR imaging of normal epiphyseal development and common epiphyseal disorders. *Radiographics*. 2014;34(2):449–71.

67. D. Erythema nodosum

Pyoderma gangrenosum (PG) has been reported in 1%–10% of ulcerative colitis (UC) patients and 0.5%–20% of Crohn's disease (CD) patients. There is no significant difference between genders. There have been conflicting data regarding the distribution of PG among CD and UC; however there is no statistically significant difference between the two groups.

Erythema nodosum is more common in CD than in UC. The occurrence of lesions parallels intestinal disease activity, and lesions frequently resolve when bowel disease subsides; thus, treatment is usually aimed at the underlying bowel disease. At times, erythema nodosum can precede bowel exacerbations and can require treatment with oral steroids. Based on these findings, patients with idiopathic EN should be evaluated for IBD.

Levine JS, Burakoff R. Extra intestinal manifestations of inflammatory bowel disease. *Gastroenterol Hepatol (N Y)*. 2011;7(4):235–41.

68. D. Glomus jugulare

About 80% of all paragangliomas are either carotid body tumours or glomus jugulare tumours. The typical CT appearance of a carotid body tumour is a well-defined soft-tissue mass within the carotid space of the infrahyoid neck. The underlying hypervascularity of the tumour results in homogeneous and intense enhancement following intravenous administration of contrast material. Splaying of the common carotid bifurcation is very suggestive of a carotid body tumour.

On high-resolution CT scans of the temporal bones, expansion and erosion of the jugular foramen characterise the glomus jugulare tumour. The tumour spreads along the paths of least resistance and is initially directed superiorly owing to the intrinsic weakness of this part of the jugular fossa. Subsequently, the hypotympanum, mesotympanum and the sinus tympani are invaded. Ossicular chain destruction is common. Inferior spread of the tumour produces infiltration of the IJV (internal jugular vein) and infratemporal fossa.

Paragangliomas typically exhibit a low signal intensity on T1-weighted images and high signal intensity on T2-weighted sequences. As with CT, homogeneous and intense enhancement is noted following the intravenous administration of contrast material. Multiple serpentine and punctate areas of signal void characterise the typical paraganglioma with all MR sequences; these areas are variably distributed throughout the mass and are believed to represent flow voids in the larger intratumoural vessels (salt-and-pepper appearance).

Rao AB, et al. Paragangliomas of the head and neck: Radiologic-pathologic correlation. *Radiographics*. 1999;19:1605–32.

69. D. The aortic wall appears thinned out.

Aortic intramural hematoma may occur as a primary event in hypertensive patients from spontaneous bleeding from the vasa vasorum into the media or may be caused by a penetrating atherosclerotic ulcer. Intramural hematoma can also develop in blunt chest trauma with aortic wall injury. The hematoma propagates along the media layer of the aorta. Consequently, intramural hematoma weakens the aorta and may progress either to outward rupture of the aortic wall or to inward disruption of the intima, the latter leading to communicating aortic dissection. Intramural hematoma can be distinguished from mural thrombus by identification of the intima: mural thrombus lies on top of the intima, which is frequently calcified, whereas intramural hematoma is subintimal. On unenhanced CT, intramural hematoma is hyperdense. MR imaging aids in the distinction of slow flow in the false lumen of a dissection from no flow in an intramural hematoma. Dynamic post-contrast MR imaging is more sensitive for excluding slow flow in the thickened aortic wall, which would indicate aortic dissection rather than intramural hematoma.

Macura KJ, et al. Pathogenesis in acute aortic syndromes: Aortic dissection, intramural hematoma, and penetrating atherosclerotic aortic ulcer. *AJR Am J Roentgenol*. 2003;181:309–16.

70. C. Hysterosalpingography

Hysterosalpingography provides optimal depiction of the fallopian tubes, allowing detection of tubal patency, tubal occlusion, tubal irregularity and peritubal disease. An imaging evaluation for female infertility typically begins with an assessment of tubal patency at hysterosalpingography, which may be followed by pelvic US, pelvic MRI or both to further characterise any additional findings.

Steinkeler JA, et al. Female infertility: A systematic approach to radiologic imaging and diagnosis. *Radiographics*. 2009;29(5):1353–70.

71. A. Osteoid osteoma

Osteoid osteoma is a benign bone tumour that occurs most frequently in men and boys between 7 and 25 years old. Most patients experience pain that worsens at night and is promptly relieved by the administration of salicylates. Typical radiographic findings of osteoid osteoma include an intracortical nidus, which may display a variable amount of mineralisation, accompanied by cortical thickening and reactive sclerosis in a long bone shaft. The nidus is round or oval and usually smaller than 2 cm. At CT, the nidus is well defined and round or oval with low attenuation. The nidus has low to intermediate signal intensity on T1-weighted images and variable signal intensity on T2-weighted images, depending on the amount of mineralisation present in the centre of the nidus. Oedema in adjacent bone marrow and soft tissue and joint effusion may also be seen. Enhancement of a hypervascular nidus may be seen at dynamic CT.

Chai JW, et al. Radiologic diagnosis of osteoid osteoma: From simple to challenging findings. *Radiographics*. 2010;30(3):737–49.

72. A. No further management is required.

Typical indications for spinal US in newborns and infants are skin-covered masses and midline cutaneous malformations of the back (e.g., dimple, haemangiomatous or hairy lesion), which are suggestive of associated dysraphic anomalies of the spinal cord. Spinal dysraphism is often associated with tethering of the spinal cord. The US appearance of tethering is a low-lying or blunt-ended conus medullaris due to abnormal fixation of the spinal cord. Moreover, movement of the spinal cord and cauda equina can be evaluated with real-time US with M-mode scanning. Typically, the tethered cord is positioned eccentrically and demonstrates reduced or absent movement. Dorsal dermal sinus manifests as a small dimple or pinpoint ostium, which is often associated with an area of hyperpigmented, angiomatous skin or hypertrichosis and occurs in a midline location or rarely in a paramedian location. Soft-tissue asymmetry and bone anomalies are common findings. Typical complications are infections such as recurrent meningitis, epidural or subdural abscess, and intramedullary spinal cord abscess. In particular, dorsal dermal sinus occurring in a paramedian location is often associated with an intraspinal dermoid or epidermoid cyst, which causes compression of neural structures with neurologic symptoms. For these reasons, dorsal dermal sinus has to be differentiated from simple sacral dimple or pilonidal sinus. The latter two anomalies do not extend to neural structures.

Unsinn KM. US of the spinal cord in newborns: Spectrum of normal findings, variants, congenital anomalies, and acquired diseases. *RadioGraphics*. 2000;20:923–38.

73. B. Supracondylar fracture

The value of the fat pad sign is greatest as a predictor of an intra-articular disease process at the elbow in the absence of any radiographically visible bone abnormality. Fat pad displacement is independent of fracture displacement and comminution. This applies in particular to elbow examination in children, who often have very slight structural changes at presentation. Supracondylar fractures account for 60% of all elbow fractures in children, followed by fracture of the lateral epicondyle (15%) and separation of the medial epicondylar ossification centre (10%). In adults, fracture of the radial head or neck accounts for just under 50% of all fractures at the elbow, followed by fracture of the olecranon (20%) and dislocations and fracture dislocations.

Goswami GK. The fat pad sign. *Radiology*. 2002;222:419–20.

74. C. Pulmonary vein

The secondary pulmonary lobule, as defined by Miller, refers to the smallest unit of lung structure marginated by connective tissue septa. Secondary pulmonary lobules are irregularly polyhedral in shape and vary in size, measuring from 1 to 2.5 cm in diameter.

Airways, pulmonary arteries and veins, lymphatics and the various components of the pulmonary interstitium are all represented at the level of the secondary lobule. Each secondary lobule is supplied by a small bronchiole, pulmonary artery and lymphatic branches centrally and is marginated by connective tissue, the interlobular septa, that contain pulmonary veins and lymphatics.

Webb WR. Thin-section CT of the secondary pulmonary lobule: Anatomy and the image – The 2004 Fleischner lecture. *Radiology*. 2006;239(2):322–38.

75. E. Hepatic haemangioma

There is no association between PSC and hepatic haemangiomas.

PSC is an idiopathic, chronic, fibrosing inflammatory disease of the bile ducts that eventually leads to bile-duct obliteration, cholestasis and biliary cirrhosis. A strong association with inflammatory bowel disease, especially ulcerative colitis, is noted (70% of cases). Although the cause of PSC is unknown, most experts believe it to be an autoimmune process because PSC may be associated with other autoimmune diseases such as retroperitoneal fibrosis, mediastinal fibrosis and Sjögren syndrome. The rate of progression is unpredictable, with up to 49% of symptomatic patients eventually developing biliary cirrhosis and liver failure. Treatment is usually palliative and includes medical therapy with orally administered agents such as ursodiol (ursodeoxycholic acid) or endoscopic or percutaneous mechanical dilation of dominant strictures. Currently, orthotropic liver transplantation is the only curative therapy for PSC.

Vitellas KM, et al. Radiologic manifestations of sclerosing cholangitis with emphasis on MR cholangiopancreatography. *RadioGraphics*. 2000;20:959–75.

76. E. MR contrast agent is routinely used in pregnancy.

The present data have not conclusively documented any deleterious effects of MR imaging exposure on the developing foetus. Therefore no special consideration is recommended for the first, versus any other, trimester in pregnancy. Nevertheless, as with all interventions during pregnancy, it is prudent to screen women of reproductive age for pregnancy before permitting them access to MR imaging environments. If pregnancy is established, consideration should be given to reassessing the potential risks versus benefits of the pending study in determining whether the requested MR examination could safely wait to the end of the pregnancy before being performed. Pregnant patients can be accepted to undergo MR scans at any stage of pregnancy if the information requested from the MR study cannot be acquired by means of non-ionising means (e.g., ultrasonography), the data are needed to potentially affect the care of the patient or foetus during the pregnancy, or the referring physician believes that it is not prudent to wait until the patient is no longer pregnant to obtain these data.

MR contrast agents should not be routinely provided to pregnant patients. The decision to administer a gadolinium-based MR contrast agent to pregnant patients should be accompanied by a well-documented risk–benefit analysis. There should be overwhelming potential benefit to the patient or foetus outweighing the theoretical but potentially real risks of long-term exposure of the foetus to free gadolinium ions. Studies have demonstrated that at least some of the gadolinium-based MR contrast agents readily pass through the placental barrier and enter the foetal circulation. From here, they are filtered in the foetal kidneys and then excreted into the amniotic fluid. In this location, the gadolinium-chelate molecules are in a relatively protected space and may remain for an indeterminate amount of time before finally being reabsorbed and eliminated. The longer the chelated molecule remains in the amniotic cavity, the greater the potential for dissociation of the potentially toxic gadolinium ion from its ligand. It is unclear what impact such free gadolinium ions might have if they were to be released in any quantity in the amniotic fluid. Certainly, deposition into the developing foetus would raise concerns of possible secondary adverse effects. The risk to the foetus of gadolinium-based MR contrast agent administration remains unknown; it may be harmful.

Kanal E, et al. ACR Guidance document on MR safe practices: 2013. *J Magn Reson Imag.* 2013;37(3):501–30.

77. B. Use FSE imaging rather than GE imaging

Several strategies help in reduction of susceptibility artefact from hip prosthesis. Some of these are as follows:

- Reduced magnetic field strength
- Increasing bandwidth during slice selection and readout
- Increasing matrix size: 512 pixels
- Maintain good SNR (signal to noise ratio) by increasing number of excitations NEX (number of excitation)
- Use spin echo (FSE) instead of gradient echo (GRE) where possible
- STIR for fat suppression (spectral frequency selective fat suppression performs better in a homogeneous field)
- Use of shorter echo spacing
- Use smaller water–fat shift
- Use thinner slices

- Align prosthesis parallel to the magnetic field
- Use view-angle tilting (VAT)

Hargreaves BA, et al. Metal-induced artifacts in MRI. *AJR Am J Roentgenol.* 2011;197(3):547–55.

78. C. Juvenile angiofibroma

Juvenile angiofibroma presents characteristic imaging signs. The diagnosis by CT is based upon the site of origin of the lesion in the pterygopalatine fossa. There are two constant features: (1) a mass in the posterior nasal cavity and pterygopalatine fossa; (2) erosion of bone behind the sphenopalatine foramen with extension to the upper medial pterygoid plate.

The characteristic features on MRI are due to the high vascularity of the tumour, causing signal voids and strong post-contrast enhancement.

Lloyd G, et al. Imaging for juvenile angiofibroma. *J Laryngol Otol.* 2000;114:727–30.

79. A. Mucinous cystadenoma

The solid fibrous component of fibroma, fibrothecoma and cystadenofibroma characteristically demonstrates very low T2 signal intensity. With T1-weighted sequences, fibrothecomas demonstrate non-specific hypo- to isointensity with mild enhancement following the intravenous administration of a gadolinium chelate. Brenner tumour is an uncommon epithelial-stromal tumour. The fibrous components, as well as calcifications (when present), are markedly hypointense on T2-weighted MR images. Exophytic subserosal leiomyoma have low T2 signal with low to intermediate T1 signal on MRI. The 'bridging vessel' sign represents tortuous vascular structures passing between the uterus and the lesion and may be seen at US; however, this sign is most clearly depicted at gadolinium-based contrast material–enhanced T1-weighted imaging or T2-weighted imaging, which nicely demonstrate vascular flow voids.

The bridging vessel sign confirms that the lesion originates from the uterus and excludes an ovarian origin.

Mucinous cystadenomas show a complex cystic structure with high signal on T2-weighted images.

Khashper A, et al. T2-hypointense adnexal lesions: An imaging algorithm. *Radiographics.* 2012;32(4):1047–64.

80. B. The umbilical arterial catheter (UAC) tip at the L1 vertebral level

The umbilical venous catheter (UVC) tip should lie within the inferior vena cava, just below or at the level of the right atrium.

The tip of a UAC should be optimally positioned between the T6 and T9 levels so that it does not interfere with major upper abdominal arterial branches.

The endotracheal tube (ETT) tip should lie at the T2 vertebral level.

The nasogastric tube (NGT) tip should be located below the diaphragm within a gastric air shadow.

The central venous catheter tip should be located at the cavo-atrial junction.

Jain SN. A pictorial essay: Radiology of lines and tubes in the intensive care unit. *Indian J Radiol Imaging.* 2011;21(3):182–90.

81. C. Scleroderma

There are three possible HRCT distributions of nodules: perilymphatic, random and centrilobular.

The causes of perilymphatic nodules include sarcoidosis, lymphangitis carcinomatosa, silicosis, amyloidosis (rare) and lymphoid interstitial pneumonia (rare). The causes of random nodules include miliary TB, miliary spread of fungal infection, metastasis and sarcoidosis (rare). The causes of centrilobular nodules include endobronchial infection, endobronchial tumour, aspiration, respiratory bronchiolitis interstitial lung disease (RB-ILD), hypersensitivity pneumonitis (HP), histiocytosis, vascular causes (oedema and haemorrhage) and talcosis.

Elicker B, et al. High-resolution computed tomography patterns of diffuse interstitial lung disease with clinical and pathological correlation. *J Bras Pneumol.* 2008;34(9):715–44.

82. A. Neuropathic osteoarthropathy

Extra intestinal manifestations of inflammatory bowel disease:

Musculoskeletal System

Arthritis

Colitic type, ankylosing spondylitis, isolated joint involvement, hypertrophic osteoarthropathy: clubbing, periostitis

Miscellaneous Manifestations

Osteoporosis, aseptic necrosis, polymyositis

Dermatologic and Oral Systems

Reactive Lesions

Erythema nodosum, pyoderma gangrenosum, aphthous ulcers, necrotising vasculitis

Specific Lesions

Fissures, fistulas, oral Crohn's disease, drug rashes

Nutritional Deficiencies

Acrodermatitis enteropathica, purpura, glossitis, hair loss, brittle nails

Associated Diseases

Vitiligo, psoriasis, amyloidosis

Hepatopancreatobiliary System

Primary sclerosing cholangitis, bile-duct carcinoma

Associated Inflammation

Autoimmune chronic active hepatitis, pericholangitis, portal fibrosis, cirrhosis, granulomatous disease

Metabolic Manifestations

Fatty liver, gallstones associated with ileal Crohn's disease

Ocular System

Uveitis/iritis, episcleritis, scleromalacia, corneal ulcers, retinal vascular disease

Metabolic System

Growth retardation in children and adolescents, delayed sexual maturation

Renal System

Calcium oxalate stones

Levine JS, Burakoff R. Extra intestinal manifestations of inflammatory bowel disease. *Gastroenterol Hepatol (N Y)*. 2011;7(4):235–41.

83. B. Ochronosis

Causes of intervertebral disc calcification include the following:

- Degenerative disc disease is a relative common cause for disc calcification.
- Alkaptonuria, or ochronosis, results in dense central calcification affecting the nucleus pulposus and is associated with generalised osteopaenia. Changes often start at the lumbar spine.
- Ankylosing spondylitis is a recognised cause; associated findings helping in narrowing the diagnosis.
- Calcium pyrophosphate dehydrate deposition disease (CPPD), haemochromatosis and hypervitaminosis D can result in calcification of the annulus fibrosus.
- Transient intervertebral disc calcification is seen in children, typically in the cervical spine and spontaneously regresses.
- Other recognised causes of disc calcification include juvenile chronic arthritis, amyloidosis, poliomyelitis, acromegaly, hyperparathyroidism, trauma and post-operative discs.

Burgener FA, et al. *Differential Diagnosis in Conventional Radiology*. New York: Thieme, 2008.

Eisenberg RL. *Clinical Imaging: An Atlas of Differential Diagnosis*. Philadelphia, PA: Lippincott Williams & Wilkins, 2003.

84. B. Nasopharyngeal carcinoma

Imaging is crucial in delineating the extent of local tumour extension, as well as detecting nodal metastases, which are present in the vast majority of patients at the time of diagnosis (75%–90%). Nasopharyngeal carcinoma (NPC) usually presents with intermediate signal intensity, higher than the muscle signal, on T2-weighted images, low signal intensity on T1-weighted images and enhance to a lesser degree than does normal mucosa. Eighty-two percent of NPCs arise in the posterolateral recess of the pharyngeal wall (Rosenmüller fossa).

Larger/more aggressive tumours may extend into any direction, eroding the base of skull and passing via the Eustachian tube, foramen lacerum, foramen ovale or directly through bone into the clivus, cavernous sinus and temporal bone. Invasion of the parapharyngeal space is associated with an increased risk of distant metastases and tumour recurrence. Following administration of contrast, the tumour mass and nodal metastases usually demonstrate heterogeneous enhancement. Careful assessment of cervical lymph nodes is essential due to the high rate of nodal involvement at the time of diagnosis. Cranial nerve involvement and venous occlusion is best demonstrated on post-contrast MRI.

Razek AAKA, King A. MRI and CT of nasopharyngeal carcinoma. *AJR Am J Roentgenol.* 2012;198(1):11–18.

85. E. Coal worker's pneumoconiosis

Many diffuse lung diseases may manifest cysts as the primary abnormality, although lymphangioleiomyomatosis and Langerhans cell histiocytosis (LCH) are the most common to present with diffuse lung cysts. Others include lymphocytic interstitial pneumonia, follicular bronchiolitis, amyloidosis, light-chain deposition disease, Birt–Hogg–Dube syndrome, end-stage fibrosis (honeycombing) and cystic metastasis (leiomyosarcoma, synovial cell sarcoma, epithelioid cell sarcoma and endometrial stromal sarcoma).

Seaman DM, et al. Diffuse cystic lung disease at high-resolution CT. *AJR Am J Roentgenol.* 2011;196:1305–11.

86. B. Chronic hepatitis

There are a number of recognised risk factors for cholangiocarcinoma that all share the common feature of chronic biliary inflammation. Among these risk factors, infection with liver flukes (e.g., *Opisthorchis viverrini* and *Clonorchis sinensis*) and hepatolithiasis are common causes of cholangiocarcinoma in endemic areas. Dietary or endogenous nitrosamine compounds associated with parasitic infections also play an important role as cofactors in carcinogenesis, probably due to the carcinogenic effect of nitrosamine compounds on the proliferation of epithelial cells of the bile duct. Cholangiocarcinoma arising from a cirrhotic liver may be surrounded by a fibrotic pseudocapsule, which is an unusual finding in cholangiocarcinoma arising from a non-cirrhotic liver. In such cases, capsular retraction is noted along the tumour surface. This capsular retraction may be seen in some hepatocellular carcinomas (HCCs) with cirrhotic stroma but is more suggestive of cholangiocarcinoma. Cholangiocarcinoma can develop in a congenital choledochal cyst, with a lifetime risk of 10%–15%. In addition, a European study showed that a history of alcohol-related liver disease, cirrhosis, various bile-duct diseases, chronic inflammatory bowel disease or diabetes may increase the risk of development of cholangiocarcinoma.

Chung YE, et al. Varying appearances of cholangiocarcinoma: Radiologic-pathologic correlation. *Radiographics.* 2009;29:683–700.

87. B. Struma ovarii

Struma ovarii is a rare ovarian lesion that accounts for 2% of ovarian teratomas. Struma ovarii is a highly specialised form of ovarian teratoma and is composed entirely or predominantly of thyroid tissue. About 5% of patients develop clinical evidence of hyperthyroidism. At US, struma ovarii has a non-specific solid, cystic appearance. MRI demonstrates a loculated cystic mass with variable signal characteristics. Cystic spaces may show marked T2 hypointensity and intermediate T1 signal intensity due to the thick, gelatinous colloid of the struma. Some locules may contain microscopic fat, as indicated by signal drop-off and chemical shift artefact on opposed-phase T1-weighted MRI. Struma ovarii typically demonstrates strong enhancement of the solid components on post-contrast T1-weighted MRI. Struma ovarii are benign in 95% of cases and usually occur in premenopausal women; therefore, preoperative diagnosis is essential to avoid unnecessary radical surgery.

Khashper A, et al. T2-hypointense adnexal lesions: An imaging algorithm. *Radiographics*. 2012;32(4):1047–64.

88. A. Semimembranosus tendon and posterior oblique ligament

The PMC contains the structures lying between the posterior margin of the longitudinal fibres of the superficial medial collateral ligament and the medial border of the posterior cruciate ligament. The PMC has five major components: the semimembranosus tendon and its expansions, the oblique popliteal ligament (OPL), the posterior oblique ligament (POL), the posteromedial joint capsule (or simply the posteromedial capsule) and the posterior horn of the medial meniscus.

Lundquist RB, et al. Posteromedial corner of the knee: The neglected corner. *Radiographics*. 2015;35(4):1123–37.

89. D. Carotid body tumour

A carotid body paraganglioma arises within the carotid body and characteristically splays the bifurcation of the CCA. As the tumour enlarges, it encases but does not narrow the calibre of the ECA and ICA. With disease progression, the lesion may involve the lower cranial nerves and adjacent pharynx. Superior extension to the skull base and invasion into the intracranial cavity has also been reported.

The typical CT appearance of a carotid body tumour is a well-defined soft-tissue mass within the carotid space of the infrahyoid neck. The underlying hypervascularity of the tumour results in homogeneous and intense enhancement following intravenous administration of contrast material. Splaying of the common carotid bifurcation is very suggestive of a carotid body tumour.

The characteristic CT appearance is that of a uniloculated or multiloculated, hypoattenuated cystic mass adjacent to the carotid space. The mass may extend into the mediastinum. The signal intensity of thymic cysts on MR images is low on T1-weighted and high on T2-weighted images.

The glomus tympanicum tumour manifests as a small discrete mass arising from the cochlear promontory and confined to the tympanic cavity. Ossicular destruction is not typical, although encasement is frequent in larger lesions. The vagal paraganglioma appears similar to the carotid body tumour with some exceptions. These masses displace both the ECA and ICA anteromedially, separating these vessels from the IJV. In addition, extension into the suprahyoid carotid space is seen in approximately two-thirds of vagal paragangliomas, whereas it is uncommon with carotid body tumours (up to 8%).

Koeller KK, et al. Congenital cystic masses of the neck: radiologic-pathologic correlation. *Radiographics*. 1999;19(1):121–46.
Rao AB, et al. Paragangliomas of the head and neck: Radiologic-pathologic correlation. *Radiographics*. 1999;19:1605–32.

90. E. Hyperparathyroidism

Physeal fracture is the most common cause of bone bridging across the growth plate, but growth arrest may also be due to other insults: infection, therapeutic irradiation, metabolic or haematologic abnormality, tumour, burn, frostbite, electrical injury, sensory neuropathy, microvascular ischaemia or insertion of metal. Premature fusion of the growth plate has also been reported in patients with hypervitaminosis A.

Craig JG, et al. Premature partial closure and other deformities of the growth plate: MR imaging and three-dimensional modelling. *Radiology*. 1999;210(3):835–43.

91. B.   External laryngocele

Simply stated, a laryngocele is a dilated laryngeal saccule, and there are three types: internal, external and mixed. Approximately 40% of laryngoceles are internal; these laryngoceles are confined to the larynx and do not pierce the thyrohyoid membrane. External laryngoceles (26% of cases) extend through the thyrohyoid membrane at the point of insertion of the superior laryngeal nerve and vessels (neurovascular bundle). The component superficial to the thyrohyoid membrane is dilated, and the saccular portion inside the membrane is normal in size. Finally, mixed laryngoceles (44% of cases) have abnormal dilatation of the saccule on both sides of the thyrohyoid membrane. The association of laryngocele with laryngeal carcinoma is well documented: Investigators worldwide have reported an increased frequency of laryngoceles in patients with laryngeal carcinoma.

On CT scans, a laryngocele appears as a well-defined, smooth mass in the lateral aspect of the superior paralaryngeal space. Internal laryngoceles will be limited by the thyrohyoid membrane. External and mixed laryngoceles lie superficial to the thyrohyoid membrane at the point of insertion of the superior laryngeal nerve and vessels (neurovascular bundle). The attenuation of these lesions may vary, depending on the amount of secretions, air and soft tissue from an associated laryngeal neoplasm.

Koeller KK, et al. Congenital cystic masses of the neck: Radiologic-pathologic correlation. *Radiographics.* 1999;19(1):121–46.

92. B.   Lymphangitis

The most common malignancy associated with lymphangitis carcinomatosa is bronchogenic carcinoma, most commonly adenocarcinoma, followed by breast, GI malignancies (stomach and colon) and prostate cancer.

Chest CT is more specific and sensitive than CXR for the diagnosis of lymphatic metastasis. On HRCT, there is variable, smooth, irregular or nodular thickening of the interlobular septae and bronchovascular bundles, which often have a beaded appearance. Another characteristic feature is either smooth or nodular thickening of the peribronchovascular interstitium. Similar changes can be seen along the fissures. In many patients, the abnormality is unilateral or patchy. Pleural effusion and hilar adenopathy are associated.

Prakash P, et al. FDG PET/CT in assessment of pulmonary lymphangitic carcinomatosis. *AJR Am J Roentgenol.* 2010;194:231–6.

93. D.   Barium studies can detect gastric varices in approximately 75% of cases evidenced by lobulated folds and polypoidal fundal masses

Gastrointestinal varices occur as a result of hepatofugal flow from the left gastric vein and splenic vein to the superior mesenteric vein. This usually occurs secondary to liver cirrhosis but isolated splenic vein occlusion (with pancreatic disease) can also be the cause. Gastric varices bleed less frequently but more severely than oesophageal varices.

Dähnert W. *Radiology Review Manual*, 7th ed. Philadelphia, PA: Lippincott Williams & Wilkins, 2011:852.

94. B.   Solid component suggesting malignancy

Serous tumours are more common in both the benign and malignant categories. They are usually unilocular, whereas malignancies may demonstrate solid components and multilocularity. The signal is usually low to intermediate on T1 and high on T2-weighted images. At CT, diffuse psammomatous calcifications may cause these tumours or their implants to have very high attenuation.

Mucinous ovarian tumours are less common. Mucinous ovarian tumours are generally cystic but unlike serous tumours may be very large and tend to be multiloculated. They often have variable signal intensity in the loculi owing to proteinaceous or mucinous contents and haemorrhage. The signal intensity of mucin on T1-weighted images varies depending on the degree of mucin concentration (watery mucin has a lower T1 signal than thicker mucin). On T2-weighted images, corresponding signal intensities are flipped, so watery mucin has a higher signal and thicker mucin appears hypointense.

Jeong YY, et al. Imaging evaluation of ovarian masses. *Radiographics*. 2000;20(5):1445–70.

95. E. Os naviculare – pain behind the heel

The os acromiale has been implicated as a risk factor for the development of impingement syndrome. Hypertrophic osteophytes may arise at the synchondrosis of an os acromiale, and the os acromiale is thought to increase the incidence of osteoarthritis at the AC joint.

Medial side foot pain (os naviculare syndrome) is the most common presenting feature of accessory navicular bone; the pain is aggravated by walking, running and weight-bearing activities.

Positive ulnar variance is associated with ulnar impaction syndrome or ulnocarpal abutment with TFC degeneration and ulnar-sided wrist pain.

Discoid meniscus is an uncommon anatomical variant, more commonly affecting the lateral meniscus. Although frequently asymptomatic, it is prone to cystic degeneration with subsequent tears. Clinical presentation may be with pain, locking or clicking.

All kinds of neurological deficits and clinical symptoms may occur with conjoined nerve roots. Besides the different phenotypes of low back or sciatic pain, the most common complaints are numbness and muscular weakness.

Bancroft LW, Bridges MD. *MRI Normal Variants and Pitfalls*. Philadelphia, PA: Lippincott Williams & Wilkins, 2008.
Böttcher J, et al. Conjoined lumbosacral nerve roots: current aspects of diagnosis. *Eur Spine J*. 2004;13(2):147–51.
Cerezal L, et al. Imaging findings in ulnar-sided wrist impaction syndromes. *Radiographics*. 2002;22(1):105–21.
Davlin CD, Fluker C. Bilateral os acromiale in a Division I basketball player. *J Sports Sci Med*. 2003;2:175–9.
Manaster BJ, et al. *Musculoskeletal Imaging*. Philadelphia, PA: Mosby Inc, 2007.

96. C. Arrowhead terminal phalanx

Mucopolysaccharidoses (MPS) represent a heterogeneous group of inheritable lysosomal storage diseases in which the accumulation of undegraded glycosaminoglycans (GAGs) leads to progressive damage of affected tissues. The typical symptoms include organomegaly, dysostosis multiplex, mental retardation and developmental delay.

Dysostosis multiplex is represented by several bone malformations found in the skull, hands, legs, arms and column. Some of the other common skeletal manifestations include macrocephaly with dolichocephaly, facial anomalies, obtuse angle of mandible with prognathism, paddle- or oar-shaped ribs, atlanto-axial instability, malformed vertebral bodies, hip dysplasia, coxa valga, proximal humeral notching, inferior tapering of ileum, rounded iliac wings, bullet-shaped phalanges and hypoplastic and irregular carpal and tarsal bones. The abnormal storage of GAGs leads to liver and spleen enlargement; it also damages cartilage layers and synovial recesses in the joints.

Palmucci S, et al. Imaging findings of mucopolysaccharidoses: a pictorial review. *Insights Imaging*. 2013;4(4):443–59.

97. D. Desquamative interstitial pneumonia

Opportunistic Infections
- Pneumocystis pneumonia (PCP)
- CMV pneumonia
- HSV pneumonia
- Respiratory syncytial virus bronchiolitis

Chronic Interstitial Diseases
- HP
- Desquamative interstitial pneumonia (DIP)
- RB-ILD
- NSIP
- Acute interstitial pneumonia (AIP)
- Lymphocytic interstitial pneumonia (LIP)
- Sarcoidosis

Acute Alveolar Disease
- Pulmonary oedema
- ARDS
- Diffuse alveolar haemorrhage

Others
- Drug toxicity
- Pulmonary alveolar proteinosis
- COP
- Bronchoalveolar carcinoma

DIP is associated with smoking but not in immunocompromised host.

Miller WT. Isolated diffuse ground-glass opacity in thoracic CT: Causes and clinical presentations. *AJR Am J Roentgenol.* 2005;184:613–22.

98. C. Organo-axial volvulus is more common than mesentero-axial volvulus and creates a 'mirror-image' stomach

The aetiology of gastric volvulus is related to unusually long gastrohepatic and gastrocolic mesenteries. Organo-axial volvulus rotates around a line from the cardia to the pylorus, whereas the axis of rotation in mesentero-axial volvulus runs from the lesser to the greater curve of stomach. Mesentero-axial volvulus is associated with 'upside-down' stomach appearance, whereas organo-axial volvulus is associated with a 'mirror-image' stomach.

Dähnert W. *Radiology Review Manual*, 7th edn. Philadelphia, PA: Lippincott Williams & Wilkins, 2011:852.

99. C. Immature teratoma is mainly cystic.

Ovarian tumours associated with endometrial hyperplasia or carcinoma includes endometrioid carcinoma, granulosa cell tumour and, occasionally, thecoma or fibrothecoma. Although rare, endometrioid carcinoma is the most common malignant neoplasm that arises from endometriosis. The presence of fat opacity or fat signal intensity in an ovarian lesion is highly specific for a teratoma. Mature cystic teratomas are predominantly cystic with dense calcifications, whereas immature teratomas are predominantly solid with small foci of lipid material and scattered calcifications. Ovarian tumours that are frequently associated with calcifications include serous epithelial tumour, fibrothecoma, mature or immature teratoma and Brenner tumour. Malignant germ cell tumours include dysgerminoma (raised HCG level) and endodermal sinus tumours (α-fetoprotein level) and are found in younger patients.

Jung SE, et al. CT and MR imaging of ovarian tumors with emphasis on differential diagnosis. *Radiographics.* 2002;22(6):1305–25.

100. B. Homocystinuria

Homocystinuria is an AR disorder secondary to deficiency of cystathionine synthase. Arachnodactyly (metacarpal index >8.4 or >9.4; depending reference standard used) is seen in one in three patients (cf. 100% in Marfan syndrome). Lens dislocation is downwards and inwards (cf. upwards and outwards in Marfan syndrome). Homocystinuria is also associated with osteoporosis, bowing/fractures, pectus deformities and biconcave vertebra. There is increased propensity of thromboembolic phenomena due to increased stickiness of platelets. Death is often from occlusive vascular disease.

Sotos syndrome is an autosomal dominant syndrome considered a form of cerebral gigantism.

Dähnert W. *Radiology Review Manual*, 7th edn. Philadelphia, PA: Lippincott Williams & Wilkins, 2011:107–8.

101. E. Osteogenic sarcoma
Fewer than 10% of osteosarcomas arise in the craniofacial bones, with most such tumours developing in the mandible and maxilla. The most common sites of involvement are the body of the mandible and the alveolar ridge or the antral area of the maxilla. It may be secondary to radiation, fibrous dysplasia, Paget disease, trauma, osteomyelitis, ossifying fibroma and giant cell tumour.

On CT, the tumour displays a spectrum of bone changes from well-demarcated borders, notably the low-grade osteosarcoma (uncommon), to lytic bone destruction with indefinite margin and variable cortical bone erosion, to the osteoblastic form, where the bone is sclerotic. The majority of osteosarcomas have matrix mineralisation, calcifications of the osteoid or osteoid-like substance within the tumour and some tumours show a sunburst effect caused by radiating mineralised tumour spiculae.

Ewing's sarcoma can also occur in this area, although the expected age would be younger. On CT, it often shows the characteristic onion-skin appearance of periosteal reaction and less often a sunburst type of periosteal reaction.

Razek AAKA. Imaging appearance of bone tumors of the maxillofacial region. *World J Radiol.* 2011;3(5): 125–34. doi:10.4329/wjr.v3.i5.125.

102. A. *Staphylococcus aureus*
Pneumatocoeles are thin-walled, air-filled intraparenchymal cysts that develop secondary to localised bronchiolar and alveolar necrosis, which allow one-way passage of air into the interstitial space. They commonly occur in immunocompetent patients and are most commonly associated with *S. aureus*, followed by *Staphylococcus pneumoniae* infections. Although there is no clear correlation between the development of pneumatocoeles and mechanical ventilation, patients receiving mechanical ventilation have an increased risk for developing complications related to pneumatocoeles, including an increase in their size. Other than in hyperimmunoglobulin E syndrome, there is no known genetic or familial tendency for pneumatocoeles.

The majority of pneumatocoeles (more than 85%) resolve spontaneously, partially or completely over weeks to months without clinical or radiographic sequelae.

Al-Saleh S, et al. Necrotizing pneumonia complicated by early and late pneumatoceles. *Can Respir J.* 2008;15(3):129–132.
Dähnert W. *Radiology Review Manual*, 7th edn. Philadelphia, PA: Lippincott Williams & Wilkins, 2011.

103. B. Lissencephaly
Lissencephaly (smooth brain) is a severe malformation of the cerebral cortex that results from impaired neuronal migration during the third and fourth months of gestation. The affected brain shows either an absence or a paucity of gyri (agyria or pachygyria, respectively).

The most common clinical manifestations include severe psychomotor retardation, developmental delay, seizures and failure to thrive. The prognosis depends on the degree of failure of cortical development. In severe cases, death occurs in infancy or early childhood. Prenatal diagnosis of an affected foetus allows appropriate counselling and optimisation of obstetric management. Abnormal cortical development is the main manifestation of lissencephaly, although other associated cranial and extracranial abnormalities may be present.

Ghai S, et al. Prenatal US and MR imaging findings of lissencephaly: Review of fetal cerebral sulcal development. *Radiographics.* 2006;26:389–4.

104. B. Respiratory bronchiolitis interstitial lung disease

RB-ILD is a smoking-related interstitial lung disease. The distribution at HRCT is mostly diffuse. The key HRCT features of RB-ILD are centrilobular nodules in combination with ground-glass opacities and bronchial wall thickening. Coexisting moderate centrilobular emphysema is common, given that most patients have a smoking history.

Mueller-Mang C, et al. What every radiologist should know about idiopathic interstitial pneumonias. *Radiographics.* 2007;27(3):595–615.

105. D. Typhlitis

Typhlitis, also known as *neutropenic colitis*, is a recognised acute colitis affecting the caecum ± the terminal ileum and ascending colon with a predisposition for children with leukaemia, lymphoma and patients on immunosuppressive treatment (i.e., neutropenia). The CT findings include circumferential wall thickening of the caecum, which may extend to the terminal ileum and ascending colon, pericaecal fluid and localised fat stranding. Intestinal TB may be primary or secondary to haematogenous spread from pulmonary TB, and predominantly affects the colon and ileum. Appendicitis may also produce caecal wall thickening, but it is usually asymmetric in nature and rarely extends into the terminal ileum. Backwash ileitis is a chronic complication of ulcerative colitis in which the terminal ileum is affected with a patulous ileocaecal valve, absent peristalsis and granularity of the mucosa. Pseudomembranous colitis usually has a predisposition for the distal colon but may affect the colon in its entirety.

Dähnert W. *Radiology Review Manual*, 7th edn. Philadelphia, PA: Lippincott Williams & Wilkins, 2011:889–90.

106. D. Assessment of polyhydramnios

The most common indications for foetal MRI are neurological. MRI is commonly used to investigate underlying aetiologies of ventriculomegaly and morphologic brain abnormalities that are not as readily depicted with US such as dysgenesis of corpus callosum, malformations of cortical development and posterior fossa anomalies. Foetal MRI may detect subtle neural tube defects not shown by US and determine the level of the defect in myelomeningocele for potential foetal surgery. The next common indication for foetal MRI is evaluation of suspicious thoracic masses. MRI has the advantage over US in differentiating the liver and bowel loops from lung tissue or masses; this aids in differentiating a congenital diaphragmatic hernia from a pulmonary mass. MRI could be helpful in providing tissue characterisation of foetal abdominal masses when US study is non-specific. MRI is particularly useful in the assessment of pregnancies complicated by oligohydramnios, which can limit the diagnostic sensitivity of US.

Saleem SN. Fetal MRI: An approach to practice: A review. *J Adv Res.* 2014;5(5):507–23.

107. D. Cartilage cap thickness of more than 2.5 cm

Pain and increase in the size of osteochondroma raises suspicion of peripheral chondrosarcomatous transformation. MRI, in particular T2-weighted images, evaluate thickness of cartilage cap. A cap thickness of more than 2.5 cm is suspicious and warrants tissue diagnosis.

Osteochondromas can be solitary or multiple. Multiple osteochondromas are known as diaphyseal aclasis. Multiplicity is not necessarily a feature/predictor of malignancy.

Osteochondromas can sometimes turn malignant and become peripheral chondrosarcomas. Sudden pain and increase in size of an osteochondroma raises suspicion of peripheral chondrosarcoma.

Neurovascular compromise can be secondary to compression by osteochondroma and does not indicate malignancy. Fracture and bursae formation are related to symptomatic osteochondromas and may be present in benign osteochondromas.

Bernard et al. Improved differentiation of benign osteochondromas from secondary chondrosarcomas with standardized measurement of cartilage cap at CT and MR imaging. *Radiology.* 2010;255(3):857–65.

108. A. Extradural arachnoid cyst

Spinal extradural arachnoid cyst (SEAC) is a rare disease and uncommon cause of compressive myelopathy. SEACs can be found in any location, although they are mostly reported to be located at the mid-thoracic to the thoraco-lumbar junction, commonly in a posterior position. The underlying cause is thought to be a dural defect. The cause of dural defect can be congenital or acquired. Trauma, arachnoiditis or iatrogenic cause can result in a small dural tear and subsequent CSF accumulation to develop SEACs.

MRI shows an elongated cystic mass, low on T1-weighted and high on T2-weighted images. CT myelography shows communication between the subarachnoid space and the cyst, confirming a dural tear.

Choi SW, et al. Spinal extradural arachnoid cyst. *J Korean Neurosurg Soc.* 2013;54(4):355–8. doi:10.3340/jkns.2013.54.4.355.

109. B. RB-ILD

The 'crazy-paving' pattern at thin-section CT of the lungs is characterised by scattered or diffuse ground-glass attenuation with superimposed interlobular septal thickening and intralobular lines.

Although originally described in cases of alveolar proteinosis, this pattern has subsequently been reported in a variety of conditions including *Pneumocystis carinii* pneumonia, bronchioloalveolar carcinoma, sarcoidosis, NSIP, COP, lipoid pneumonia, ARDS and pulmonary haemorrhage syndromes including idiopathic pulmonary haemosiderosis, Wegener granulomatosis, Churg–Strauss syndrome, Goodpasture syndrome, collagen-vascular diseases, drug-induced coagulopathy and haemorrhage associated with malignancy.

Rossi S, et al. 'Crazy-paving' pattern at thin-section CT of the lungs: Radiologic-pathologic overview. *Radiographics.* 2003;23(6):1509–19.

110. D. T2 N2 M0

Staging

T1 = Limited to mucosa or submucosa
T2 = Tumour involves muscle/serosa
T3 = Tumour penetrates through serosa
T4a = Tumour involves adjacent contagious tissues
T4b = Invasion of adjacent structures, diaphragm, abdominal wall and so on
N1 = Involvement of perigastric nodes within 3 cm of primary along greater or lesser curvature
N2 = Involvement of regional nodes >3 cm from primary along branches of coeliac axis
N3 = Para-aortic, hepatoduodenal, retropancreatic, mesenteric nodes
M1 = Distant metastases

Dähnert W. *Radiology Review Manual*, 7th edn. Philadelphia, PA: Lippincott Williams & Wilkins, 2011:492.

111. D. Congenital adrenal hyperplasia

Classic congenital adrenal hyperplasia (CAH) is due to deficiency of enzymes in the steroidogenesis pathway and can present as a severe salt-wasting form that usually appears with acute adrenal insufficiency in early infancy (men in 7–10 days of birth) and a simple virilising form in which patients demonstrate masculinisation of external genitalia (women) or signs of virilisation in early life in men. Non-classic (late onset) CAH presents in pubertal girls with symptoms of mild androgen excess.

Most lesions are asymptomatic and may be discovered incidentally. Larger lesions (typically over 4 cm in size) can present with retroperitoneal haemorrhage or related symptoms. They are associated with Cushing syndrome, congenital adrenal hyperplasia (21-hydroxylase deficiency) and Conn syndrome (primary hyperaldosteronism).

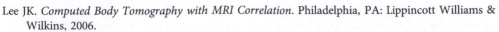

Lee JK. *Computed Body Tomography with MRI Correlation.* Philadelphia, PA: Lippincott Williams & Wilkins, 2006.

Tasker RC, McClure RJ, Acerini CL (eds.) *Oxford Handbook of Paediatrics.* Oxford: Oxford University Press, 2008.

112. D. Menorrhagia

Polycystic ovarian syndrome (PCOS) is the most common endocrine abnormality in women of reproductive age and carries with it significant health risks, including infertility, endometrial hyperplasia, diabetes (insulin resistance), obesity and cardiovascular disease (hypertension, hyperlipidaemia, coronary artery and cerebrovascular events). Patients with PCOS have hyperandrogenism, hirsutism and ovarian dysfunction (oligo- or anovulation) and present with oligo-amenorrhea.

Lee TT, Rausch ME. Polycystic ovarian syndrome: Role of imaging in diagnosis. *Radiographics.* 2012;32(6):1643–57.

113. A. A partial return to normal fatty marrow.

The signal intensity of the fractured vertebral body would appear low on T1-weighted images in the acute phase and would gradually be restored to normal intensity from the periphery to the centre of the body, as healing progresses. On T2-weighted images, the signal intensity of the fractured vertebral body would appear high, with or without some strongly lowered area in it, in the acute phase, and would be gradually restored to normal intensity with time.

Acute fracture and metastatic compression fracture can both show enhancement post-contrast injection. However, contrast enhancement decreases with time in benign vertebral fractures as normal marrow signal is restored.

Cho T, et al. MRI findings on healing process of vertebral fracture in osteoporosis. *J Orthop Sci.* 1(1):16–33.

114. B. Synovial cyst

Intraspinal synovial cysts are extradural lesions that arise from the synovial lining of the facet joints. Most cysts are found at the L4–L5 facet joint, as this is the level where the most biomechanical spinal motion occurs.

The differential diagnosis for synovial cysts includes arachnoid cysts, perineural (Tarlov) cysts, schwannomas and migrated herniated disk fragments. The MR imaging characteristics and the neuroanatomic location of the cyst help distinguish synovial cysts from these other lesions.

Extradural arachnoid cysts are cerebrospinal fluid-filled outpouchings of the arachnoid membranes that extend through a defect in the dura mater. Two-thirds of these lesions occur in the thoracic spine; this helps to differentiate these masses from synovial cysts, which occur most frequently in the lumbar spine. Perineural cysts can be distinguished from synovial cysts because perineural cysts are separate from the facet and are intimately associated with the nerve root. Likewise, schwannomas can be distinguished from synovial cysts on MR images by their intimate association with the nerve root. Furthermore, the propensity for schwannomas to enhance homogeneously after administration of a gadolinium-containing contrast agent helps one distinguish this entity from synovial cysts, which typically demonstrate only rim enhancement. Migrated disk fragments are sometimes found dorsal to the thecal sac, which complicates their differentiation from synovial cysts. They can, however, be distinguished reliably by their relationship to the ligamentum flavum, their signal intensity characteristics and their lack of degenerative changes in the facet joint. Migrated disk fragments are typically located anterior to the ligamentum flavum, whereas synovial cysts are located dorsal to or inseparable from the ligamentum flavum. Furthermore, migrated disk fragments are usually lobulated and have lower signal intensity on T2-weighted MR images than do the spherically shaped synovial cysts.

Marichal DA, et al. Case 101: Lumbar facet synovial cyst. *Radiology.* 2006;241(2):618–21.

115. E. Diffuse alveolar haemorrhage

Anti-glomerular basement membrane antibody disease (Goodpasture syndrome) is defined by a triad of diffuse pulmonary haemorrhage, glomerulonephritis and circulating anti-glomerular basement membrane antibodies. Findings at chest radiography may occasionally be normal despite the presence of diffuse pulmonary haemorrhage. Diffuse pulmonary haemorrhage can also occur in patients with systemic lupus erythematosus, typically in the context of established disease associated with extrapulmonary manifestations such as glomerulonephritis.

Mayberry JP, et al. Thoracic manifestations of systemic autoimmune diseases: Radiographic and high-resolution CT findings. *Radiographics*. 2000;20(6):1623–35.

116. E. Clostridium difficile colitis

Given the clinical history of recent antibiotic therapy and the introduction to a nosocomial environment, one must always consider *Clostridium difficile* colitis in the presence of multiple episodes of watery diarrhoea. CT, the most sensitive examination for *C. difficile* colitis, may demonstrate circumferential colon wall thickening with a predisposition for the rectum (but may affect the entire colon), a 'target' sign (due to submucosal oedema and mucosal hyperaemia), pericolonic fat stranding and ascites. The accordion sign is typical in severe cases of *C. difficile* colitis and appears as intraluminal contrast media trapped between multiple thickened oedematous folds of bowel wall – the appearance mimics an accordion. There is no history to suggest radiation enteritis and the involvement of the rectum and distal colon excludes amoebiasis as a likely cause. Ischaemic colitis may have a similar appearance but is usually segmental in nature, dependent on the arterial distribution.

Dähnert W. *Radiology Review Manual*, 7th edn. Philadelphia, PA: Lippincott Williams & Wilkins, 2011:882.

117. D. Serous cystadenoma

Ovarian tumours with highly enhancing solid portions, although uncommon, include sclerosing stromal tumour, Sertoli–Leydig cell tumour, struma ovarii and cystadenofibroma.

Jung SE, et al. CT and MR imaging of ovarian tumors with emphasis on differential diagnosis. *Radiographics*. 2002;22(6):1305–25.

118. C. Metacarpophalangeal joint (MCPJ)

Primary OA describes degenerative joint disease with no local aetiological factor. It is age related and caused by high mechanical forces of a repetitive nature on a normal joint.

Secondary OA describes degenerative changes within a joint with an underlying aetiological factor. These may include trauma, CPPD, inflammatory arthritis, haemochromatosis, developmental dysplasia of the hip (DDH), AVN or loose bodies.

The joints most commonly involved in primary OA are distal interphalangeal, proximal interphalangeal, first carpometacarpal joint, hips, knees, spine and first metatarsophalangeal. The joints commonly spared include metacarpophalangeal, wrist, elbow, shoulder and ankles.

Weissleder R, et al. *Primer of Diagnostic Imaging*, 4th edn. Philadelphia, PA: Mosby Elsevier, 2007:450–2.

119. E. Meningioma

Meningiomas are well circumscribed and show avid enhancement on contrast-enhanced imaging. On CT, they are iso/hyperattenuating. The hyperattenuation reflects the cellular nature of these lesions, but the presence of calcification also contributes. Hyperostosis may be seen but is not as common as in the intracranial forms. This is due, in part, to the more prominent epidural fat within the spine. They are most commonly isointense on both T1-weighted and T2-weighted imaging. Some may be hyperintense on T2-weighted imaging, and flow voids may be seen. If they are densely calcified, they will show low signal on both T1-weighted and T2-weighted imaging. Meningiomas prominently enhance on contrast-enhanced imaging, and a dural tail may be observed.

On MRI, paragangliomas are well circumscribed and hyperintense on T2-weighted imaging and avidly enhance on contrast-enhanced imaging. The classic salt and pepper appearance associated with head and neck paragangliomas may be seen. The entire spine should be imaged because of the possibility of intradural metastasis. Because of the highly vascular nature, prominent flow voids in and around the tumour commonly occur. A low-signal hemosiderin rim may be seen on T2-weighted images.

Neurofibromas and schwannomas can be difficult to differentiate by imaging. Both tumours may widen the neuroforamina, erode bone and cause vertebral body scalloping on CT. On MRI, both neoplasms are isointense on T1-weighted imaging and hyperintense on T2-weighted imaging; however, schwannomas may have mixed signal intensity on T2-weighted imaging because of the mixture of cells. A central area of lower T2 signal may be seen in neurofibromas and is referred to as the 'target sign'.

Karl A. Soderlund, et al. Radiologic-pathologic correlation of pediatric and adolescent spinal neoplasms: Part 2, intradural extramedullary spinal neoplasms. *AJR Am J Roentgenol.* 2012;198(1):44–51.

120. D. Superior mesenteric artery located to the right of the superior mesenteric vein

The upper GI series remains the imaging reference standard for the diagnosis of malrotation with or without volvulus. The normal position of the DJ junction is to the left of the left-sided pedicles of the vertebral body at the level of the duodenal bulb on frontal views and posterior (retroperitoneal) on lateral views. In children with acute duodenal obstruction, the upper GI series may depict a Z-shaped configuration of the duodenum in the presence of obstructing peritoneal bands or a corkscrew-shaped duodenum in the presence of volvulus. In children who have bowel malrotation without volvulus, the upper GI series shows an abnormal position of the DJ junction.

The detection of the double bubble sign suggests duodenal obstruction. In infants in whom the radiograph demonstrates a double bubble, one should consider both intrinsic and extrinsic causes of obstruction. The intrinsic causes are duodenal atresia, duodenal stenosis and duodenal webs; the extrinsic causes include annular pancreas, malrotation of the gut with obstruction produced by mid-gut volvulus or by Ladd bands and preduodenal position of the portal vein. The proximal left-sided bubble is the air- and fluid-filled stomach. The duodenum represents the second bubble to the right of the midline.

The third part of the duodenum is a retroperitoneal structure. Normally SMV is to the right of the SMA. Distended bowel loops throughout the abdomen would exclude any significant mid-gut obstruction.

Applegate KE, et al. Intestinal malrotation in children: a problem-solving approach to the upper gastrointestinal series. *Radiographics.* 2006;26(5):1485–500.

Traubici J. The double bubble sign. *Radiology.* 2001;220(2):463–4.

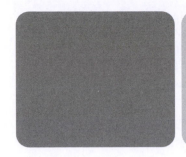

CHAPTER 11
TEST PAPER 6

Questions

Time: 3 hours

1. A Computed tomography (CT) chest is done in a 6-month-old girl with a history of premature birth, chronic lung disease and MRSA pneumonia. It shows a large gas-containing, thin-walled cavity in the right lung, consistent with a pneumatocoele. All the following are true regarding a pneumatocoele, except:
   A. They are gas-filled, thin-walled spaces surrounded by lung.
   B. They can be associated with lung contusion.
   C. Most pneumatocoeles resolve spontaneously.
   D. Pneumatocoeles do not cause mediastinal shift.
   E. They can have fluid levels.

2. A 58-year-old patient is reported to have a carcinoid tumour of the gastrointestinal (GI) tract on an abdominal computed tomography scan. What is the most common primary site of GI carcinoids?
   A. Stomach
   B. Colon
   C. Rectum
   D. Small bowel
   E. Appendix

3. A 53-year-old man with history of haematuria which shows a gel-like polypoid filling defect on cystoscopy is sent for an MRI. The MRI shows a low T1 signal, heterogeneous T2 signal (central high and peripheral low) lesion. On post-contrast T1W FS images, the peripheral portion enhances more than the central potion, resembling a ring-like pattern. What is the diagnosis?
   A. Endometriosis
   B. Inflammatory pseudotumour
   C. Malakoplakia
   D. Cystitis glandularis
   E. Eosinophilic cystitis

4. A 33-year-old man presented with fever and sudden-onset back pain. Inflammatory markers were slightly raised. MRI spine showed high signal in the L3/4 disc space on T2W and STIR images, with enhancement of the disc extending to the adjacent end plates on post-contrast sequences. What is the diagnosis?
   A. Metastasis
   B. Prolapsed intervertebral disc
   C. Sequestrated disc
   D. Discitis
   E. Epidural abscess

5. A 65-year-old woman with progressive increase in knee pain and limited mobility is referred by her GP to have a plain X-ray of the knee. Plain films show bilateral chondrocalcinosis along with some other arthritic features. Which one of the following conditions is the most common cause of chondrocalcinosis?
   A. Calcium pyrophosphate dihydrate crystal deposition disease
   B. Hydroxyapatite crystal deposition disease
   C. Primary synovial osteochondromatosis
   D. Intraarticular synovial cell sarcoma
   E. Chronic renal failure

6. A 14-year-old boy with family history of pulmonary chondroma in his elder brother is investigated with a CT of the chest and abdomen. The CT shows a 3 × 3 cm calcified perihilar lung mass and a large mixed density mass in the left upper quadrant, anterior to the spleen inseparable from the stomach. What other finding(s) would you expect on the CT?
   A. Bilateral renal carcinoma
   B. Hepatoblastoma
   C. Multiple cysts in the lung, kidney and pancreas
   D. Wilms tumour on the right
   E. Multiple extra-adrenal neuroblastomas

7. Transverse US image of a foetal thorax with a four-chamber view of the heart demonstrates homogeneous intermediate echogenicity of the right lung. The heart is mildly rotated to the right and there are cystic areas in the left side of the thorax suggesting a diaphragmatic hernia. All of the following are true regarding investigation of congenital lung anomalies, except:
   A. Meconium shows high T1 and low T2 signal on MRI.
   B. Normal lung reduces in T2 intensity as it matures.
   C. Secondary pulmonary hypoplasia is more common than primary.
   D. Interventricular septum determines the cardiac axis.
   E. Echogenicity of lung advances as gestation advances.

8. A 42-year-old man who sustained a comminuted acetabular fracture underwent a CT of his pelvis for further characterisation and treatment planning. The CT report described it as an anterior column acetabular fracture. Which one of the following anatomic structures must be disrupted on the CT?
   A. Ilioischial line
   B. Iliopectineal line
   C. Sacroiliac joint
   D. Anterior wall
   E. Posterior wall

9. A 29-year-old woman has come to the A&E department with 3 months' history of shortness of breath after her second miscarriage. She had an episode of pulmonary embolism during her first pregnancy and epilepsy in her teens. Chest radiograph done in the A&E department shows progressive enlargement of cardiac silhouette and left-sided pleural effusion. What is the likely diagnosis?
   A. Systemic lupus erythematosus (SLE)
   B. Rheumatoid arthritis
   C. Wegner's disease
   D. Polyarteritis nodosa (PAN)
   E. Homocystinuria

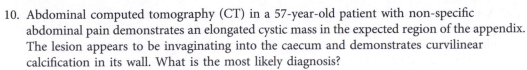

10. Abdominal computed tomography (CT) in a 57-year-old patient with non-specific abdominal pain demonstrates an elongated cystic mass in the expected region of the appendix. The lesion appears to be invaginating into the caecum and demonstrates curvilinear calcification in its wall. What is the most likely diagnosis?
    A. Lipomatosis of ileocaecal valve
    B. Carcinoid tumour of the appendix
    C. Mucocoele of the appendix
    D. Epiploic appendagitis
    E. Myxoglobulosis

11. Tuberculous spondylitis is diagnosed in a 44-year-old woman with progressive neurological deficit with severe discovertebral destruction and compression of the spinal cord at the T11–12 level on sagittal T2W & STIR MR images. Post-contrast images show a rim-enhancing anterior abscess that does not encase the intercostal arteries. All of the following features are more likely to represent tuberculosis spondylitis compared to pyogenic spondylitis, except:
    A. Subligamentous spread
    B. Three or more vertebral level involvement
    C. Skip lesions
    D. Homogenous enhancement of the disc
    E. Paraspinal calcification

12. A CT cystogram is being performed on a 40-year-old man brought to the A&E department, after a fall from a roof. Blood is seen at the external urethral meatus on examination. The CT scan shows focal thickening of the urinary bladder wall, with no extravasation outside the bladder. Which of the following is the most likely injury sustained?
    A. Bladder contusion
    B. Intraperitoneal bladder rupture
    C. Extraperitoneal bladder rupture
    D. Combined intraperitoneal and extraperitoneal bladder rupture
    E. Subserosal bladder rupture

13. A 28-year-old man with sudden-onset of heart murmur and a normal chest radiograph is admitted for progressive shortness of breath on exertion over the recent months. There is a positive family history for heart murmurs and sudden death of a sibling at the age of 30 years. While in the hospital he developed an acute, severe bout of central chest pain, which prompted an urgent CT of the chest. The CT of the chest shows dissection of an enlarged ascending aorta. What is the diagnosis?
    A. Homocystinuria
    B. Marfan syndrome
    C. Ehlers–Danlos syndrome
    D. Pseudoxanthoma elasticum
    E. Mucopolysaccharidosis

14. A 59-year-old patient is admitted with general lethargy, weight loss and gradual abdominal distension. Diagnostic work-up included an abdominal CT scan, which demonstrated thickening of the peritoneal surfaces and a large, multiloculated dense ascites, causing secondary scalloping of the liver edge. What is the most likely location of the primary tumour?
    A. Stomach
    B. Appendix
    C. Pancreas
    D. Liver
    E. Rectum

15. A 44-year-old woman with recurrent urinary tract infections is referred for a renal tract ultrasound. This demonstrates normal kidneys and multiple fluid-filled cysts within the bladder wall. Which of the following is the most likely cause?
    A. Transitional cell carcinoma
    B. Cystitis cystica
    C. Emphysematous cystitis
    D. Eosinophilic cystitis
    E. Interstitial cystitis

16. A 22-year-old man presents to the A&E department with a painful swollen ankle following a twisting injury. Plain X-rays showed no fracture, although diffuse soft-tissue swelling was evident. The ankle mortise was intact. Incidental note was made of a benign lesion in the mid-shaft of the fibula, which the reporting radiologist described as a *fibrous cortical defect*. Which one of the following statements regarding this entity is false?
    A. They are smaller than non-ossifying fibromas.
    B. Pathological fractures tend to end in non-union.
    C. Both show dense sclerotic border on CT.
    D. They commonly affect the metaphysis of long bones.
    E. They are uncommon in the upper extremity.

17. A 43-year-old man presents to the A&E department with severe headache and is sent for an urgent CT brain, which is normal. MRI shows loss of normal flow void in the basal cisterns with intense enhancement along the cisterns on post-contrast images. What is the likely diagnosis?
    A. Subarachnoid haemorrhage
    B. Lymphoma
    C. TB meningitis
    D. Ruptured dermoid cyst
    E. Creutzfeldt-Jakob disease (CJD)

18. A 6-year-old child is admitted to the emergency department with a head injury. The emergency department consultant demands an urgent CT of the head. Which of the following risk factors would warrant a CT of the head within 1 hour of the injury?
    A. Two episodes of vomiting after the head injury
    B. Amnesia of events 10 minutes preceding the head injury
    C. Fall from a playground-climbing frame of 3 metres in height
    D. GCS of 13 on initial clinical assessment
    E. Abnormal drowsiness

19. An 8-year-old boy attends the emergency department after his bicycle collides with an oncoming car. The ambulance crew have immobilised his cervical spine and report that the patient was complaining of severe neck ache. All of the following risk factors warrant a CT of the cervical spine without obtaining a plain radiograph, except
    A. The patient is already attending the department for a CT of the head.
    B. Fall from a height of more than 1 metre.
    C. Loss of sensation in the upper arms.
    D. GCS of 13 on initial assessment.
    E. The child needs to be intubated.

20. A 34-year-old man with history of measles infection showed marked cerebral atrophy on MRI with high signal in the deep white matter bilaterally on T2 and FLAIR images. What is the most likely diagnosis?
    A. Adrenoleukodystrophy
    B. Alexander's disease

C. CJD

D. Progressive multifocal leukoencephalopathy (PML)

E. Subacute sclerosing panencephalitis

21. A 25-year-old man presents with left hip/groin pain after exercise that worsens on internal rotation of the hip. A plain AP radiograph of the pelvis shows an osseous protrusion at the femoral head–neck junction, and the measured alpha angle is greater than 55 degrees. Which of the following is the most likely diagnosis?

A. Pincer type femoro-acetabular impingement

B. Cam-type femoro-acetabular impingement

C. Missed congenital hip dislocation

D. Focal acetabular over-coverage

E. Protrusio acetabuli

22. Chest radiograph of a currently asymptomatic 84-year-old man shows a large well-defined soft-tissue density mass in the left apex with a sharp inferior margin. There is underlying rib abnormality, suggesting previous surgery and sheet-like pleural calcification in the left mid and lower zone. What is the diagnosis?

A. Aspergilloma

B. Plombage

C. Pancoast tumour

D. Bronchogenic cyst

E. Lymphoma

23. An adult patient was admitted to hospital with abdominal pain, jaundice and a palpable epigastric mass. Ultrasound demonstrated isolated dilatation of the common bile duct with otherwise normal appearance of the proximal biliary tree. What is the most likely diagnosis based on the sonographic findings?

A. Choledochal cyst

B. Caroli disease

C. Choledochocoele

D. Common bile duct diverticulum

E. Impacted common bile duct calculus

24. A 40-year-old patient emigrating from an African country is investigated for stone disease because of left-sided renal angle pain. CT of the kidneys, ureters and bladder (KUB) confirms a left renal calculus but also shows thin curvilinear calcification outlining a normal-sized bladder with involvement of the distal ureters only. Which of the following is the most likely cause?

A. Tuberculosis

B. *Escherichia coli* infection

C. Transitional cell carcinoma

D. Malakoplakia

E. Schistosomiasis

25. An asymptomatic military recruit showed a well-defined 2 × 2 cm solitary pulmonary nodule in the right lower zone on a plain chest radiograph. On close inspection, the nodule showed faint calcification. CT performed for further characterisation showed areas of fat density on pixelometry. What is the diagnosis?

A. Tuberculoma

B. Aspergilloma

C. Hamartoma

D. Carcinoid

E. Haemangioma

26. You are performing an abdominal ultrasound scan on a woman who has been complaining of chronic abdominal pain. There is a large 20 cm multiloculated, ovoid anechoic mass in the right lobe of liver. The internal septations are well visualised and hyperechoic. Further investigation with CT demonstrates enhancement of its thick wall and internal septations. What is the most likely diagnosis?

A. Simple hepatic cyst

B. Choledochal cyst

C. Echinococcal cyst

D. Caroli disease

E. Biliary cystadenoma

27. An intravenous urogram is performed on a 70-year-old diabetic for recurrent *E. coli* urinary tract infections. This demonstrates multiple small, smooth, plaque-like mural defects of the bladder and distal ureteric walls. Which of the following is the most likely cause?

A. Emphysematous cystitis

B. Malakoplakia

C. Leukoplakia

D. Haemorrhagic cystitis

E. Bladder outflow obstruction

28. A 45-year-old woman presents with right hip pain. An AP radiograph of the hip shows a large lucent lesion with stippled calcification and a wide destructive-appearing zone of transition. Which of the following is the most likely diagnosis?

A. Osteomyelitis

B. Osteosarcoma

C. Chondrosarcoma

D. Fibrous dysplasia

E. Chondromyxoid fibroma

29. A 37-year-old woman with progressive worsening of headache had a facial series done following an injury to the face when she fell while skating. PA view of the skull and OM view did not show any fractures. Incidental note was made of enlarged optic canals. All of the following are associated with this, except

A. NF1

B. Optic glioma

C. Sarcoidosis

D. Sphenoid mucocoele

E. Ophthalmic artery aneurysm

30. A 1-year-old child is admitted with seizures and found to have bilateral subdural haematomas. There is concern regarding non-accidental injury and a full skeletal survey is requested. According to the Royal College of Radiologists guidelines, which radiograph(s) would not be routinely included in a full skeletal survey?

A. PA radiograph of the right hand

B. AP radiograph of the left tibia and fibula

C. AP radiograph of the cervical spine

D. Lateral radiograph of the lumbar spine

E. Right oblique radiograph of the chest

31. A term neonate is found in respiratory distress with shortness of breath and tachypnoea on Day 1 of life. An urgent chest radiograph demonstrates a right-sided pneumothorax.

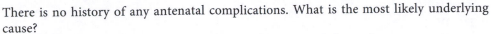

There is no history of any antenatal complications. What is the most likely underlying cause?

A. Respiratory distress syndrome (pulmonary surfactant deficiency)
B. Group B streptococcus infection
C. Congenital pulmonary airway malformation (CPAM)
D. Meconium aspiration
E. Congenital diaphragmatic hernia (CDH)

32. A 58-year-old man who worked in the mines for several years presented with progressive shortness of breath on exertion. Extensive interstitial thickening and small nodules bilaterally with large masses of consolidation in the upper lobes were noted on the most recent chest radiograph. Comparison with previous films suggested central migration of the consolidation like upper lobar masses. What is the diagnosis?

A. Pneumoconiosis with progressive massive fibrosis
B. End-stage sarcoidosis
C. End-stage Langerhans Cell Histiocytosis (LCH)
D. Cryptogenic fibrosing alveolitis
E. Old TB

33. A patient is admitted to hospital with progressively worsening jaundice and raised bilirubin levels. Ultrasound of the abdomen, demonstrates a large hyperechoic focus casting a shadow within the neck of the gallbladder, causing secondary dilation of the common hepatic and intrahepatic bile ducts proximally. The distal common bile duct (CBD) was normal.
What is the most likely diagnosis?

A. Caroli disease
B. Choledochocoele
C. Caroli syndrome
D. Mirizzi syndrome
E. Cholangiocarcinoma

34. A 30-year-old man is admitted with lower abdominal pain following a road traffic accident in which he was an unrestrained passenger. Blood is seen in his urine and a bladder injury is suspected. Regarding extraperitoneal bladder rupture, which of the following is incorrect?

A. It is more common than intraperitoneal rupture.
B. A flame-shaped extravasation of contrast can often be seen.
C. It is usually caused by puncture from a pelvic fracture.
D. Contrast most commonly extravasates into the retropubic space of Retzius.
E. The bladder dome is the most common site of injury.

35. A 4-year-old child presents with short stature and failure to grow. Plain radiographs reveal multiple abnormalities, including generalised increased density of long bones with thickened cortices, widened cranial sutures, Wormian bones, a hypoplastic mandible and shortened pointed distal phalanges. Which of the following is the most likely diagnosis?

A. Pyknodysostosis
B. Osteopetrosis
C. Cleidocranial dysostosis
D. Osteosclerosis
E. Kinky hair syndrome

36. A man with nasopharyngeal squamous cell carcinoma undergoes MRI staging. A pathological node is seen lateral to the IJV. It lies below the hyoid bone but above the vocal cords. At which level is this likely to be located?

A. I
B. II

C. III
D. IV
E. V

37. CT of the chest in a 68-year-old man who worked for 20 years in a coal mine, showed an ill-defined 3-cm spiculated nodule in the apical segment of the lower lobe of the left lung. The lesion was avid on PET and showed high signal on axial T2W MRI thorax. All of the following are true regarding lung cancer and progressive massive fibrosis except:
A. T2W is useful in differentiating lung cancer from PMF.
B. PET CT is useful in differentiating lung cancer from PMF.
C. PMF shows low signal compared to muscle on T1W MRI.
D. PMF commonly shows peripheral enhancement on contrast MRI.
E. Histopathologic analysis should still be performed for diagnosis.

38. A patient is admitted to hospital with jaundice and recent weight loss. Abdominal ultrasound demonstrates marked dilation of the intrahepatic ducts, extending to the liver surface. Note is also made of an isoechoic mass at the porta hepatis. Which of the following is the most likely diagnosis?
A. Primary sclerosing cholangitis
B. Klatskin tumour
C. Mirizzi syndrome
D. Choledochal cyst
E. Caroli disease

39. A 17-year-old girl is admitted following a road traffic accident where she was a restrained passenger. She has low-volume haematuria following catheterisation. Pre- and post-intravenous (IV) contrast CT is performed after administering contrast via her urinary catheter. The pre-contrast CT shows contrast within the peritoneal cavity around loops of bowel and there is irregularity of the bladder wall at the dome of the bladder. No contrast blushes are seen on the arterial-phase CT. Which of the following is the most likely injury?
A. Extraperitoneal bladder rupture
B. Intraperitoneal bladder rupture
C. Subserosal bladder rupture
D. Iliac artery injury with haemorrhage
E. Pelvic haematuria from occult fracture

40. A 65-year-old man presents with severe upper thoracic back pain, of insidious onset, with little relief from analgesia. Lateral radiographs of his thoracic spine reveals uniformly increased density within the T7 and T9 vertebral bodies, with retention of the vertebral body size and contour. Which of the following is the most likely cause for this finding?
A. Bone metastasis
B. Osteoid osteoma
C. Tuberous sclerosis
D. Osteopetrosis
E. Fluorosis

41. A 40-year-old man was punched in the face during an altercation. Clinical examination showed left facial swelling with left-sided ophthalmoplegia and diplopia. X-rays showed a left maxillary fracture. What is the likely cause of the patient's symptoms?
A. Superior orbital fissure syndrome
B. Cavernous sinus thrombosis

C. Carotico-cavernous fistula

D. Post-traumatic ophthalmoplegia

E. Cerebral venous sinus thrombosis

42. While reporting a plain radiograph of a 10-year-old girl patient's left hand, you notice that her bone age is delayed. There is no indication of the patient's underlying condition on the request form. The bones of the hand are otherwise unremarkable.

Which of the following conditions may offer a possible explanation?

A. Hypothyroidism

B. Achondroplasia

C. Haemophilia

D. Cushing syndrome

E. Precocious puberty

43. A 42-year-old man with cough and haemoptysis, swelling of ankles and hand, raised urea, and creatinine on recent blood biochemical profile, presented to the A&E department with bloody nasal discharge. A Chest radiograph was performed. What do you expect the chest radiograph to show given the clinical scenario?

A. Miliary nodules

B. Few varying sized nodules, some with cavitation

C. Perihilar infiltrates in a batwing pattern

D. Bilateral upper lobe fibrosis

E. Tramline and gloved finger opacities

44. An 87-year-old female patient from a nursing home presents with a history of severe abdominal pain and diarrhoea. She has a past medical history of transient ischaemic attacks and two non-ST elevation myocardial infarctions. Blood results show an elevated lactate level and raised white cell count. CT report states that the most likely cause is ischaemic colitis. What is the most likely CT finding?

A. Thick-walled caecum with distended appendix

B. Dilated loop of bowel in the left iliac fossa with spiralling vessels

C. Thick-walled oedematous loops of bowel with branching lucencies peripherally in liver

D. Thick-walled oedematous colon with ascites

E. Dilated small bowel loops with branching linear lucency at the porta hepatis

45. A 60-year-old male smoker attends for a CT scan following an ultrasound scan that showed unilateral hydronephrosis. The scan shows a lobulated irregular bladder wall mass that enhances in the portal venous phase, to a greater extent than the bladder wall. Which of the following is the likely diagnosis?

A. Squamous cell carcinoma

B. Adenocarcinoma

C. Transitional cell carcinoma

D. Leiomyoma

E. Blood clot

46. A 40-year-old man had a cardiac CT and MRI to evaluate suspected cardiomyopathy. This revealed a well-defined incidental lesion within the T10 vertebral body, with coarse vertical trabeculae on CT, and high signal on both T1 and T2 sequences on MRI. The lesion enhanced with contrast on both modalities. What is the most likely diagnosis?

A. Plasmacytoma

B. Osteosarcoma

C. Osteopathia striata

D. Enostosis

E. Haemangioma

47. A 30-year-old woman presents with a painless neck mass. MRI confirms that this is a thin-walled cyst lying just anterior to the sternocleidomastoid. There is a tract from the bifurcation of the common carotid artery. What is the diagnosis?

A. Lymphangioma

B. Thyroglossal duct cyst

C. First branchial cleft cyst

D. Carotid body tumour

E. Second branchial cleft cyst

48. A neonate presents with an imperforate anus and a presacral mass. MRI of the abdomen demonstrates an enhancing lesion with fatty components and T2* susceptibility artefacts. What other imaging finding would you expect?

A. Syrinx within the spinal canal

B. Anterior beaking of the vertebral bodies

C. Sacrococcygeal bony defect

D. Developmental dysplasia of the hips

E. Multiple renal cysts

49. A 17-year-old boy presents with an enlarging swelling in the midline at the level of the hyoid bone. The GP suspects a thyroglossal cyst and sends him for an ultrasound. Which of the following appearances is consistent with a thyroglossal cyst?

A. Hyperechoic mass in the midline

B. Hyperechoic mass to the left of the midline

C. Anechoic mass in the midline

D. Hyperechoic mass with coarse internal echoes

E. Hypoechoic mass to the left of midline

50. A 69-year-old woman presented to her GP with one month's history of headache and progressive swelling of both hands and face and an 8 months' history of progressive weight loss. Chest radiograph showed widening of the mediastinum and a large mass in the right upper lobe with a midline trachea. What do you expect the CT chest to show?

A. Cavitating lung primary in RUL without mediastinal nodes

B. Right Pancoast tumour with rib destruction

C. RUL large and multiple small nodules of Wegener's granulomatosis

D. RUL lung primary with retrosternal goitre

E. RUL lung primary and SVC obstruction

51. A 63-year-old man presents to his general practitioner having noticed recent lower gastrointestinal bleeding. While waiting for his outpatient appointment he experiences massive lower gastrointestinal blood loss. The patient is unable to have a colonoscopy and is sent for an urgent angiogram. This demonstrates patency of the major mesenteric and coeliac vessels. An abnormal tuft of vessels with early filling of the accompanying mesenteric vein is noted at the caecum. No associated mass was seen. What is the most likely diagnosis?

A. Ischaemic colitis

B. Angiodysplasia

C. Haemorrhoids

D. Colon carcinoma

E. Diverticulitis

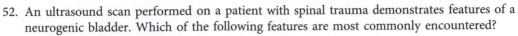

52. An ultrasound scan performed on a patient with spinal trauma demonstrates features of a neurogenic bladder. Which of the following features are most commonly encountered?
    A. Thin-walled bladder with decreased capacity
    B. Entirely normal bladder
    C. Thin-walled bladder with increased opacity
    D. Trabeculated bladder with increased opacity
    E. Trabeculated bladder with decreased capacity

53. A 40-year-old golfer presents with sudden-onset right medial palmar wrist pain during a golf swing. On examination, he has paraesthesia in the right fourth and fifth digits. Plain AP and oblique radiographs are normal. Which of the following is the most appropriate next investigation?
    A. Nerve conduction studies
    B. CT scan of the wrist with 1-mm slices
    C. Hook of hamate radiographic views
    D. MRI of the wrist
    E. Ultrasound scan of the wrist

54. All of the following statements regarding presacral mass lesions in children are true, except:
    A. Anterior sacral meningocoele is associated with Marfan syndrome.
    B. Rectal duplication cysts are high signal on T1W images.
    C. Tailgut cysts have high mucin content.
    D. Dermoid cysts have areas of high T1W signal, suggesting fat.
    E. Rectal duplication cysts may mimic lymphatic malformation.

55. A 5-year-old girl with history of seizures and learning difficulty is referred for an abdominal ultrasound due to non-specific abdominal pain. On imaging, you notice bilateral renal cysts and multiple hyperechoic lesions in the kidneys and spleen. The patient also has small red skin lesions on her face. What is the most likely unifying diagnosis?
    A. Sturge–Weber Syndrome
    B. Von Hippel–Lindau
    C. Autosomal dominant polycystic kidney disease
    D. Tuberous sclerosis
    E. PHACE syndrome

56. A patient with HIV is admitted to the medical ward with shortness of breath. Admission chest X-ray shows diffuse symmetrical air space change. There is no pleural effusion or mediastinal adenopathy. At what CD4 count would you expect *Pneumocystis jiroveci* to present as a potentially life-threatening complication?
    A. CD4 <0
    B. CD4 <50
    C. CD4 <100
    D. CD4 <200
    E. CD4 <400

57. A 64-year-old man presents with left lower quadrant pain. He is very tender on clinical examination and an urgent CT scan with contrast is performed. The radiologist suggests that the findings are in keeping with epiploic appendagitis. Which of the following best describes the CT findings in epiploic appendagitis?
    A. Accordion sign
    B. Pericolic fat stranding
    C. Ascites

D. Mucosal wall thickening with air-filled outpouchings

E. Pericolic focal hyperattenuation with a central area of fat density

58. A 16-year-old boy presents with recurrent urinary tract infections and an MRI Urogram is performed. This confirms ureteric duplication. Which of the following is correct regarding ureteric duplication?

A. The lower pole moiety inserts inferior to the upper pole moiety.

B. The lower pole moiety is more likely to obstruct than the upper pole moiety.

C. The upper pole moiety is often associated with an ectopic ureterocoele.

D. The upper pole moiety inserts horizontally and is associated with reflux.

E. Calyceal dilatation is usually seen in the lower pole.

59. A 25-year-old woman had radiographs of her pelvis and both her lower limbs following a road traffic accident. Although no fracture was identified, multiple incidental findings were observed, including bilateral posterior iliac horns, protuberant anterior iliac spines and rudimentary patellae. Which of the following is the most likely diagnosis?

A. Osgood–Schlatter

B. Bipartite patella

C. Diastrophic dysplasia

D. Protrusio acetabuli

E. Nail–patella syndrome

60. A 60-year-old woman with breast carcinoma presents with headaches. CT shows erosion of the right foramen ovale on bone windows. An MRI of the head and neck region is performed. Which of these options is a likely finding?

A. Fatty infiltration of the left side tongue muscles

B. Fatty atrophy of the right masticator muscles

C. Vocal cord deviation

D. Swelling of the right side of the face

E. Sensory loss of the right lower eyelid and cheek

61. A 5-month-old infant presents with one episode of urinary tract infection. The patient responds well to treatment and urinalysis reveals *E. coli* as the causative organism. There is no family history of ureteric reflux or renal disease. According to NICE guidelines, what imaging test(s) should be recommended?

A. Urgent urinary tract ultrasound

B. Routine urinary tract ultrasound within 6 weeks

C. Routine urinary tract ultrasound with DMSA within 4–6 months

D. Routine urinary tract ultrasound, DMSA and micturating cystourethrogram

E. Magnetic resonance cystourethrogram

62. A 55-year-old woman is found to have an incidental, pleurally based 7 cm ovoid mass with smooth tapered margins, on an otherwise unremarkable CT urography examination. MR imaging is performed for further assessment. Which of the following imaging characteristics is most suggestive of a diagnosis of benign mesothelioma?

A. T1 MR hypointense; T2 MR hyperintense; contrast enhancement on CT avid

B. T1 MR hypointense; T2 MR hyperintense; contrast enhancement on CT minor

C. T1 MR hyperintense; T2 MR hyperintense; contrast enhancement on CT avid

D. T1 MR hypointense; T2 MR hypointense; contrast enhancement on CT avid

E. T1 MR hyperintense; T2 MR hyperintense; contrast enhancement on CT minor

63. A patient with known ulcerative colitis is admitted as an emergency following an episode of acute abdominal pain. The clinicians are worried about toxic megacolon and request an

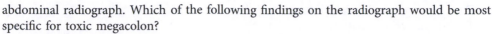

abdominal radiograph. Which of the following findings on the radiograph would be most specific for toxic megacolon?

A. Preservation of haustra
B. Thumbprinting of the mucosal wall
C. Descending colon diameter of 4.5 cm
D. Dilated transverse colon with mucosal islands
E. Pseudodiverticulae in the ascending colon

64. A 12-year-old boy undergoes ultrasound of his renal tract to investigate recurrent urinary tract infections. The kidneys initially appear to lie more inferiorly and anteriorly than would normally be expected. On closer examination, a bridge of renal tissue connects the lower poles of both kidneys and a diagnosis of horseshoe kidney is made. What structure has limited the ascent of the horseshoe kidney, causing its abnormal location?

A. Umbilical ligament
B. Coeliac axis
C. Inferior mesenteric artery
D. Superior mesenteric artery
E. Attachment to the dome of the bladder

65. A plain film of the knee of a 33-year-old man involved in an RTA shows an pure depression fracture involving the lateral tibial plateau. What would be the Schatzker classification?

A. Type I
B. Type II
C. Type III
D. Type IV
E. Type V

66. A 55-year-old postmenopausal woman is being treated with tamoxifen for breast cancer. Which of the following might occur as a side effect of this medication?

A. Increased size of her uterine fibroids
B. Reduction in size of her uterine fibroids
C. Formation of multiple ovarian cysts
D. Cervical stenosis
E. Thin atrophic endometrium

67. A 33-year-old man with chronic sinus disease is being considered for a functional endoscopic sinus surgery (FESS) operation. The ENT surgeon refers him for CT sinuses prior to surgery. Regarding the ethmoidal sinuses, the ethmoidal air cells occasionally pneumatise laterally and posteriorly around the frontal recess. What is the name of this anatomical variation?

A. Concha bullosa
B. Agger nasi cell
C. Haller cell
D. Onodi cell
E. Paradox middle turbinate

68. A 40-year-old man presents with dyspnoea and peripheral oedema and is found to have elevated jugular venous pressure. Echocardiography shows reduced mobility of the pericardium. Contrast-enhanced CT is performed. Which of the following features is least suggestive of a diagnosis of constrictive pericarditis?

A. Pleural effusion
B. Contrast reflux into the coronary sinus
C. Curvature of the interventricular septum to the right

D. Linear pericardial calcifications

E. Azygos vein dilatation

69. A 65-year-old woman with known history of gallstones is referred for an out-of-hours ultrasound scan to investigate fever, rigors and deranged liver function tests. Ultrasound demonstrates a common bile duct measuring 11 mm diameter and mild intrahepatic biliary dilatation, and a gallbladder containing multiple calculi associated with wall thickening, pericholecystic free fluid and a positive Murphy's sign. What diagnosis should be fed back to the referring clinicians?

A. Ascending cholangitis

B. Biliary colic

C. Acute cholecystitis

D. Primary sclerosing cholangitis

E. Impacted calculus in common bile duct

70. A 65-year-old woman presents to the orthopaedic clinic with left hip pain 3 years following a total hip joint replacement (THR). The plain radiograph shows focal radiolucencies around the prosthesis with smooth endosteal scalloping. The patient is systemically well with normal inflammatory markers. Presentation and radiographic appearances are characteristic of which of the following?

A. Mechanical loosening

B. Infection

C. Histiocytic response

D. Stress shielding

E. Heterotopic ossification

71. An X-ray of the mandible demonstrates a well-defined, unilocular cyst with corticated margins at the ramus. The patient is known to have a history of multiple skin lesions. What is the most likely diagnosis?

A. Radicular cyst

B. Residual cyst

C. Cementoma

D. Odontogenic keratocyst

E. Ameloblastoma

72. A tibia and fibula radiograph is performed on a 2-month-old baby for leg swelling. The radiologist notices fine periosteal reaction along the diaphysis of the tibia. Which one of the following statements is false regarding neonatal periosteal reaction?

A. Physiological periosteal reaction may be a normal finding in children up to the age of 6 months.

B. Commonly encountered sites of physiological periosteal reaction may include the humerus, tibia and femur.

C. If physiological periosteal reaction is present, it is typically asymmetric.

D. The initial presentation of non-accidental injury may include periosteal reaction of a long bone.

E. The presence of marked periosteal reaction may suggest an underlying congenital cardiac disease.

73. A 16-year-old boy presents with shin pain. A tibia and fibula radiograph demonstrates a well-defined, cortically based osteolytic lesion within the diaphysis measuring 4 cm cranio-caudally without periosteal reaction.

On MRI, the lesion is solitary, intermediate signal on T1 sequences (same as muscle) and high signal on T2. There is homogenous and avid enhancement post-contrast administration. There is no soft-tissue mass associated with the bony lesions.

Which one of the following differential diagnoses is the most likely?
A. Simple bone cyst
B. Non-ossifying fibroma
C. Fibrous cortical defect
D. Chondroid myxoid fibroma
E. Adamantinoma

74. A 73-year-old man is found to have a pulmonary nodule on routine chest radiograph. Pre- and post-contrast-enhanced CT of the chest is performed. Which one of the following features is least suggestive of benignity of the nodule?
A. Nodule enhancement of 10 Hounsfield units
B. A peripheral rim of enhancement
C. A flattened configuration of the nodule
D. Central calcification
E. Ground glass and solid components to the nodule

75. A 24-year-old man is investigated for weight loss and chronic abdominal pain. Small bowel MRI demonstrates thickened loops of small bowel. Small bowel follow-through confirms the presence of non-stenotic ulcers of the distal small bowel. Apart from Crohn's disease, which one of the following is the most common diagnosis?
A. Yersinia
B. Tuberculosis
C. Reiter syndrome
D. Lymphoma
E. Steroids

76. A 30-year-old woman with dysmenorrhoea and menorrhagia has had uterine artery embolisation of her fibroid uterus. She presents with lower abdominal pain and a malodorous vaginal discharge. Ultrasound demonstrates a distended debris- and fluid-filled uterine cavity with a separate hypoechoic large mass noted at the internal cervical os, causing cervical obstruction. Which of the following is the most likely explanation for these findings?
A. Embolisation and subsequent swelling surrounding a cervical fibroid
B. Detachment of a large subserosal pedunculated fibroid following embolisation
C. Detachment of a large submucosal fibroid following embolisation
D. Incidental large endometrial polyp close to the internal cervical os
E. Cervical carcinoma

77. A 20-year-old man was seen in the A&E department after an injury to his foot during a football game. On examination, there was tenderness on palpation in the forefoot. A plain film performed showed a step in the alignment of the medial aspect of the second metatarsal bone and middle cuneiform bone. The second to fourth metatarsal had moved laterally. Normal alignment was noted at the articulation between the first metatarsal and medial cuneiform bone. Which type of fracture is demonstrated on the plain film?
A. March fracture
B. Jones fracture
C. Lover's fracture
D. Homolateral Lisfranc fracture dislocation
E. Divergent Lisfranc fracture dislocation

78. A 20-year-old patient presents with long-standing halitosis and foul taste in the mouth. MRI showed a 1.5 cm smoothly marginated midline cystic mass in the posterior roof of the nasopharynx, which does not enhance with contrast. What is the likely diagnosis?
A. Fossa of Rosenmuller tumour
B. Rathke's pouch

C. Thornwaldt's cyst

D. Mucous retention cyst

E. Chronic sinus disease

79. 'Floating tooth' sign is not associated with which one of the following conditions?

A. Leukaemia

B. Multiple myeloma

C. Multifocal histiocytosis

D. Burkitt lymphoma

E. Mastocytosis

80. A 40-year-old man is diagnosed on the basis of a screening chest radiograph and a subsequent high-resolution thoracic CT scan with alveolar microlithiasis. Which one of the following is not an expected finding in this condition?

A. Raised serum calcium levels

B. Diffuse involvement of both lungs

C. Intense uptake on bone scintigraphy

D. Submillimetre micronodulations

E. Marked discrepancy between radiograph and clinical symptoms

81. A 42-year-old patient who has a long history of ileocolic Crohn's disease presents with weight loss and vomiting. On CT, there is a heterogeneous soft-tissue polypoidal mass halfway along the second part of the duodenum. No significant lymphadenopathy is noted. Which of the following is the most likely diagnosis?

A. Adenocarcinoma of the small bowel

B. Hamartomatous polyp

C. Lymphoma

D. Gastrointestinal stromal tumour (GIST)

E. Pancreatic carcinoma

82. Routine mammograms of a woman show a 1 cm retro-areolar lesion. Ultrasound demonstrates an 8 mm retro-areolar lesion with a dilated duct. Which of the following is the most likely diagnosis?

A. Papillomatosis

B. Ductal cancer

C. Ductal ectasia

D. Plasma cell mastitis

E. Papilloma

83. A 57-year-old woman presents with a dry mouth and dry eyes. Ultrasound of the parotids demonstrates multiple small hypoechoic areas. MRI demonstrates a speckled honeycomb appearance on T2W images. What is the most likely diagnosis?

A. Sarcoid

B. Pleomorphic adenoma

C. Sjogren's syndrome

D. Warthin's tumour

E. Mucoepidermoid carcinoma

84. Anteroposterior radiograph of the knee of a 14 year old boy shows proximal tibial physeal widening and irregularity. Because of continued knee pain worsening with activity, MR imaging is performed to exclude a meniscal tear. MRI shows substantial widening and irregularity of the proximal tibial physis. Physeal stress injury is diagnosed. All of the following are expected findings, except

A. Cartilage injury

B. Tongue of high signal extending into metaphysis

C. Bone bridging

D. Physeal irregularity

E. Diffuse low T1W signal to the bone adjacent to the physis

85. A 50-year-old man with chronic middle ear problems has a CT scan of the temporal bones, which shows a cholesteatoma. Regarding cholesteatoma, which of the following statements is false?

A. Cholesteatomas can be classified as either congenital or acquired.

B. Congenital cholesteatomas can be located everywhere in the temporal bone.

C. Primary acquired cholesteatomas develop behind an apparently intact tympanic membrane.

D. Pars flaccida (attic) cholesteatomas are located at the lower one-third portion of the tympanic membrane.

E. Pars tensa (sinus) cholesteatomas develop most often through a defect of the lower two-thirds portion of the tympanic membrane.

86. A 45-year-old woman is diagnosed with a biopsy-proven cancer. A lymph node is also demonstrated in the upper outer quadrant of the breast. Which of the following features is most suggestive of malignancy in the node?

A. Hyperechoic centre

B. Round and hypoechoic node

C. Posterior acoustic shadowing

D. A 1.5 cm node in the upper outer quadrant

E. Homogeneous enhancement on MRI

87. A 56-year-old man presents with dyspnoea. Chest radiography shows increased interstitial markings with a predominantly lower zone distribution bilaterally. A diagnosis of interstitial fibrosis is made on high-resolution CT. Which of the following conditions is least likely to show interstitial fibrosis with this distribution?

A. Systemic lupus erythematosus

B. Rheumatoid arthritis

C. Ankylosing spondylitis

D. Methotrexate-induced fibrosis

E. Scleroderma

88. A 60-year-old man with neurofibromatosis Type 1 presents with vague abdominal pain and bloating. A CT scan reveals a well-defined hyperenhancing rounded exophytic mass within the left upper quadrant, which has a broad base with the body of the stomach with no fat plane between the two. The spleen, transverse colon and left kidney are displaced by this mass. It measures 18 cm. There is no lymphadenopathy. Which of the following is the most likely diagnosis?

A. Ectopic pancreas

B. Gastric lipoma

C. Gastric adenocarcinoma

D. Malignant GIST (gastrointestinal stromal tumour)

E. Benign GIST (gastrointestinal stromal tumour)

89. With regard to ossification centres of the elbow in a child, which of the following statements is correct?

A. The absence of the internal epicondyle ossification centre suggests an avulsion injury, if the radial ossification centre is visible.

B. The absence of the lateral epicondyle ossification centre could be normal in a 12-year-old.

C. The trochlear ossification centre occurs before the capitellum ossification centre.

D. Lateral epicondyle avulsion injuries are more common that medial epicondyle avulsion injuries.

E. Medial epicondyle avulsion injuries are associated with excess forces from the common extensor tendon.

90. With regard to physeal stress injury in children, all of the following statements are true, except:
    A. Little Leaguer's shoulder refers to injury of the proximal humerus.
    B. Physeal injuries are more easily identified on MRI.
    C. Gymnast's wrist refers to injury to the distal radius.
    D. Gymnast's wrist results in negative ulnar variance.
    E. Little Leaguer's elbow refers to injury to the medial epicondyle of the humerus.

91. A 34-year-old man is undergoing preoperative assessment of his mitral valve using CT angiography. Which of the following combinations represents the optimal view and timing for visualising the mitral valve on CT?
    A. Two-chamber view in mid-systole
    B. Two-chamber view in mid-diastole
    C. Three-chamber view in mid-systole
    D. Three-chamber view in mid-diastole
    E. Four-chamber view in mid-diastole

92. A 43-year-old diabetic man underwent non-contrast CT of his abdomen and pelvis, which demonstrated a dense liver. He described erectile dysfunction and arthropathy mainly affecting his second and third metacarpophalangeal joints bilaterally but also affecting his hips. Which of the following is the most likely diagnosis?
    A. Amyloidosis
    B. Glycogen storage disease
    C. Wilson disease
    D. Haemophilia
    E. Haemochromatosis

93. A 50-year-old woman presents with refractory hypertension and palpitations. Urinary vanillylmandelic acid (VMA) levels are raised. A CT scan demonstrates normal adrenals. Which of the following should be the next line of investigation?
    A. Ultrasound (US) scan of adrenal glands.
    B. In-phase and out-of-phase MRI sequences to assess fatty content.
    C. Radionuclide imaging using an analogue of guanethidine such as metaiodobenzylguanidine (MIBG).
    D. Adrenal biopsy.
    E. Radionuclide imaging using radiolabelled analogues of cholesterol such as ^{131}I-6B-iodomethyl-19-norcholesterol (NP-59).

94. A 65-year-old male patient presents with back pain and loss of sensation in his left leg. An MRI scan of his lumbar spine reveals multiple lesions within the vertebral bodies of his lower spine, of varying sizes. These were of low signal on both T1 and T2 sequences. Which of the following is the most likely diagnosis?
    A. Myeloma
    B. Paget disease
    C. Prostate cancer metastases
    D. Renal cancer metastases
    E. Haemangiomas

95. A 40-year-old woman with long-standing history of epistaxis has been diagnosed with Wegener's granulomatosis. The following statements are true about Wegener's granulomatosis affecting the head and neck except:
    A. It may lead to destruction of the hard palate.
    B. Premaxillary and retroantral fat are rarely involved.
    C. Sarcoidosis may have a similar appearance.

D. Chronic disease may result in thickening of the paranasal sinuses.

E. The nasal septum may disappear in chronic disease.

96. A large posterior fossa mass arising from the roof of the fourth ventricle is identified on an MRI brain in an 8-year-old child. The lesion is poorly defined and does not contain any internal calcification or extension into the basal cisterns.

Which imaging feature of this lesion would be considered atypical?

A. Marked associated hydrocephalus

B. Avid contrast enhancement

C. Hyperdense appearance on CT

D. Absence of drop metastases on MRI spine imaging

E. Restricted diffusion on diffusion-weighted imaging (DWI)

97. A preterm neonate born at 24 weeks is referred for a cranial ultrasound study. A focus of increased echogenicity is present in the right caudothalamic groove extending into the lateral ventricle, without ventricular dilatation.

Which grade germinal matrix haemorrhage would this feature most represent?

A. Grade 1

B. Grade 2

C. Grade 3

D. Grade 4

E. Grade 5

98. A 50-year-old teacher with a neck lump is referred for an ultrasound, which revealed a thyroid nodule. Which of the following is an indication for FNA of a thyroid nodule?

A. Entirely cystic lesion

B. Presence of microcalcification

C. Presence of multiple cystic nodules

D. Every nodule above 2 cm

E. Every nodule that is hypervascular

99. A 62-year-old man is found to have a right-sided pleural effusion on imaging. Which of the following pathologies is more likely to result in a pleural effusion on the right side than on the left side?

A. Transection of the proximal thoracic duct

B. Traumatic rupture of the thoracic aorta (distal to left subclavian artery)

C. Spontaneous oesophageal rupture

D. Gastric carcinoma

E. Pancreatitis

100. A 26-year-old diabetic man who is known to binge drink is referred to you with deranged liver function tests following antibiotics for a chest infection. On ultrasound, you see a hyperechoic area anteriorly within the left lobe of liver within Segment 4. Which of the MRI sequences from the list below will be the most helpful in determining the nature of this lesion (although all would be required for a definitive diagnosis)?

A. In-phase and out-of-phase T1-weighted images

B. T1 and T2W images

C. Diffusion-weighted images and apparent diffusion coefficient

D. Dynamic contrast-enhanced phase images

E. T2 with TE of 80 ms and T2 with TE of 160 ms

101. When investigating adrenal disease, which of the following statements is incorrect?

A. Biochemical evaluation is usually the first line of investigation.

B. Delayed radiolabelled analogues of cholesterol, such as 1-6B-iodomethyl-19-nocholesterol (NP-59), are used to identify and localise masses that result in adrenal cortical dysfunction.

C. MIBG, an analogue of guanethidine, is used to image adrenal cortical disorders.

D. ^{131}I and ^{123}I-MIBG can be used to screen the whole body for sympathomedullary tissue.

E. ^{18}F fluorodeoxyglucose (FDG) can sometimes differentiate between benign adenomas and metastases.

102. A 20-year-old male patient presents to the A&E department following a skateboard injury. He has pain in his right clavicle and plain films are subsequently performed, which reveal elevation of the clavicle above the superior border of the acromion. What statement is true in regard to this injury?

A. The acromioclavicular (AC) ligament is ruptured but the coracoclavicular (CC) ligament is intact.

B. The joint capsule is ruptured but the CC ligament is intact.

C. The CC ligament is ruptured but the AC ligament is intact.

D. The AC ligament, CC ligament and joint capsule are ruptured but the deltoid attachment is intact.

E. The AC ligament and CC ligament are ruptured with detachment of the deltoid muscle.

103. You are reporting a CT pulmonary angiogram of 39-year-old man who presented with shortness of breath. You have excluded pulmonary embolism but are concerned about the appearances of the trachea, which has diffuse narrowing of the lumen with marked wall thickening. You decided to contact the A&E clinician to clarify patient symptoms. After further questioning, the patient admits to episodes of wheeze and stridor for over past few months. All of the following cause diffuse thickening of the wall with decreased diameter of the tracheal lumen, except:

A. Relapsing polychondritis

B. Tracheopathia osteoplastica

C. Tracheal Wegener's granulomatosis

D. Mounier–Kuhn disease

E. Tracheal sarcoidosis

104. A patient presents with deranged liver function tests, right upper quadrant pain, nausea, flushing and recurrent bouts of diarrhoea. The surgeon thinks the patient may have gallstone disease and requests a MRCP. A single 3 mm gallstone is noted within the gallbladder, but the bile ducts are within normal limits. A markedly hyperintense lesion on T2 is noted within the mesentery and a few of the small bowel loops in this region appear tethered. The lesion enhances avidly following administration of gadolinium. There are further hyperintense lesions noted throughout the liver, which also avidly enhance in the arterial phase. Which one of the following is the most likely diagnosis?

A. Metastatic melanoma

B. Cholangiocarcinoma with liver and mesenteric metastasis

C. Retractile mesenteritis

D. Carcinoid syndrome

E. Cholecystitis with mesenteric and liver abscesses

105. An adult patient undergoes ultrasound examination of the abdomen. He is known to have end-stage renal failure and has been on renal dialysis for 5 years. Incidentally, several round and well-defined anechoic lesions are demonstrated in both kidneys. These demonstrate posterior acoustic enhancement. There is no previous relevant family history and a previous ultrasound 5 years ago was normal. Which of the following is the most likely diagnosis?

A. Adult polycystic kidney disease

B. Multicystic dysplastic kidney

C. Multiple simple renal cysts

D. Cystic renal cell cancer

E. Uraemic cystic disease

106. An 80-year-old patient with history of rheumatoid arthritis, has been involved in a 40 mph head-on car crash. Air bags were deployed. You are asked to review a cervical spine trauma series. No fracture is identified. The patient has mid-cervical spine tenderness. The patient wants to go home. Which of the following is the best option?

A. Let the patient be discharged since trauma series is normal.

B. Repeat lateral and AP views.

C. Request a flexion and extension lateral cervical spine.

D. Cervical spine CT.

E. Bone scintigraphy.

107. All of the following statements are true with regard to stress fractures in young athletic children, except

A. Children with limb misalignment are at greater risk.

B. Stress fracture of the femoral neck involves the superior surface.

C. Shin splints show linear oedema limited to the medial tibia.

D. Distal femoral metaphysis are recognised sites for stress fracture.

E. Pars interarticularis fractures are due to repetitive extension and torsion.

108. A 7-year-old boy presents to his emergency department complaining of a limp and pain in his left hip. He is febrile and blood test results reveal raised inflammatory markers. The emergency department staff are concerned regarding an underlying diagnosis of septic arthritis.

Which one of the following statements regarding imaging in septic arthritis is false?

A. An ultrasonography can be performed to guide needle aspiration of an underlying hip effusion.

B. Destruction of underlying bone is normally seen at presentation on plain radiography.

C. The suggestion of underlying hip effusion may be identified on plain radiography of the pelvis.

D. An effusion normally collects in the anterior recess of the hip joint on ultrasound early in the process.

E. Septic arthritis is usually a mono-articular process.

109. A 42-year-old female patient with shortness of breath undergoes CT pulmonary angiogram for suspected pulmonary embolism (PE). In addition to the presence of subsegmental PE, the scan reveals two well-defined, rounded intraluminal polypoid masses on the posterior wall of the trachea and multiple small nodules in both lungs. Disseminated malignancy is suspected. Which primary malignancy is most likely to metastasize to the trachea?

A. Malignant melanoma

B. Ovarian carcinoma

C. Sarcoma

D. Transitional cell carcinoma of the urinary bladder

E. Pancreatic carcinoma

110. A middle-aged woman presents with a painful anterior neck lump, associated with a rash. Ultrasound of the thyroid demonstrates an enlarged hypoechoic and hypervascular gland. Follow-up imaging 4 months later shows resolution of the previous changes. What is the diagnosis?

A. Hashimoto's thyroiditis

B. De Quervain's thyroiditis

C. Multinodular goitre

D.   Papillary thyroid carcinoma

E.   Anaplastic carcinoma

111. A 72-year-old woman with B12 deficiency and achlorhydria has a barium meal. The stomach is featureless with no demonstrable rugal folds, and there is narrowing of the body of the stomach. Which of the following is the most likely diagnosis?
A.   Infectious gastritis
B.   Ménétrier disease
C.   Eosinophilic gastritis
D.   Atrophic gastritis
E.   Linitis plastica

112. A 26-year-old obese and unwell woman attends the A&E department with right-sided abdominal pain. She has a positive pregnancy test. The A&E doctor requests an abdominal and pelvic ultrasound, which demonstrates some fluid within Morrison's pouch. The pelvic area is not well demonstrated on transabdominal ultrasound due to the patient's obesity, but no intrauterine pregnancy is noted. Which of the following should happen next?
A.   Laparotomy
B.   CT of the abdomen and pelvis
C.   Transvaginal ultrasound
D.   MRI of the pelvis
E.   Laparoscopy

113. Which one of the following is not a radiographic hallmark of degenerative arthritis?
A.   Asymmetrical joint space narrowing
B.   Subchondral sclerosis
C.   Periarticular osteoporosis
D.   Subchondral cysts
E.   Osteophytes

114. A 30-year-old teacher presents with thyroid swelling and proptosis. Which of the following is true regarding Grave's ophthalmopathy?
A.   It commonly involves the medial rectus first.
B.   It commonly involves the tendons of the eye muscles.
C.   There is associated dilatation of the superior ophthalmic vein.
D.   There is decreased density of the orbital fat.
E.   It is an autoimmune disease unrelated to thyroid function.

115. A 78-year-old man presents with weight loss and frank haematuria. He had a stricture of his urethra dilated many years ago. He has no other relevant past history. Initial ultrasound and IVU show a normal upper urinary tract and bladder. As part of the standard work-up, he proceeds to flexible cystoscopy, but the urologist is unable to pass the cystoscope beyond the proximal penile urethra. He is therefore referred for an ascending urethrogram, which demonstrates an irregular filling defect in the bulbar urethra. Which of the following is the likeliest diagnosis?
A.   Prostatic carcinoma
B.   Transitional cell carcinoma of the urethra
C.   Squamous cell carcinoma of the urethra
D.   Adenocarcinoma of the urethra
E.   Recurrent benign stricture

116. A 34-year-old patient with a recent history of a prolonged stay in an intensive care unit following road traffic accident is referred to the respiratory clinic with symptoms of dyspnoea, expiratory wheeze and recurrent chest infections. A CT scan of the chest is performed.

Which one of the following is the most likely tracheal complication of the previous prolonged intubation in this patient?

A. Carrot-shaped trachea
B. Sabre-sheath trachea
C. Tracheomalacia
D. Tracheopathia osteoplastica
E. Tracheal diverticulum

117. You are performing a small bowel follow-through on a 42-year-old female patient because of abdominal pain, weight loss and anaemia. The patient has had a normal endoscopy and colonoscopy. There is separation of the ileal loops within the right side of the abdomen. Some of the ileal loops in this region appear compressed on one side and one of the loops appears aneurysmal. You also note the presence of a fistula between the distal ileum and colon. Except for these ileal loops, the remainder of the small bowel appears normal. Which one of the following is the most likely diagnosis?

A. Crohn's disease
B. Tuberculosis
C. Small bowel lymphoma
D. Metastatic serosal deposits
E. Coeliac disease

118. A 65-year-old man presents with pain, swelling and paraesthesia in his left thigh. Clinical examination revealed a large 10 × 6 cm soft-tissue mass within the left thigh. The mass is of soft-tissue density on CT and demonstrates avid contrast enhancement. There is no involvement of the adjacent bone. On MRI, the mass returns a predominantly low signal on T1W sequences and high signal on T2W sequences. Which of the following is the most likely diagnosis?

A. Lipoma
B. Liposarcoma
C. Osteosarcoma
D. Soft-tissue fibroma
E. Lipoblastoma

119. On a routine neonatal birth check, the paediatric registrar suspects an infant of having developmental dysplasia of the hip (DDH), and refers the him for a hip ultrasound. Which one of the following statements regarding hip ultrasound according to the Graf classification is correct?

A. A normal alpha angle is less than or equal to 60 degrees.
B. A normal beta angle is greater than 20 degrees.
C. The alpha angle is measured from the triangular labral fibrocartilage to the vertical cortex of the ilium.
D. The beta angle can help to determine the dysplasia subtype.
E. The acetabular angle is measured from the acetabular roof to the vertical cortex of the ilium.

120. CT of the head of a young man for chronic headache showed erosion of the left frontal sinus. Post-contrast showed focal meningeal enhancement with mucosal enhancement of the right frontal sinus. What is the most likely diagnosis?

A. Mucocoele
B. Inverted papilloma
C. Pott's puffy tumour
D. Antrochoanal polyp
E. HIV

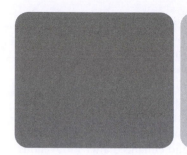

CHAPTER 12
TEST PAPER 6

Answers

1. D. Pneumatocoeles do not cause mediastinal shift.

Pneumatocoeles typically are post-infectious or post-traumatic, discrete, thin-walled, gas-containing collections within the lung parenchyma. They also may result from positive pressure ventilation–related barotrauma and ingestion of caustic material (e.g. hydrocarbons). Post-infectious pneumatocoeles most frequently complicate staphylococcal pneumonia and occur in infants. They typically appear within 1 week of onset of infection and most spontaneously disappear within weeks to months after the infection has resolved. Rarely, persistent pneumatocoeles may require percutaneous catheter drainage or surgical management. Post-traumatic pneumatocoeles result from blunt trauma. Such pneumatocoeles are typically observed within hours of the trauma and spontaneously resolve within 3 weeks. They generally spare the lung apices.

At CT, pneumatocoeles appear as well-defined parenchymal cystic structures, with a thin wall. They may be entirely filled with gas, or an air–fluid level may be seen. Contralateral mediastinal shift may be seen with large pneumatocoeles. They are associated with contusion in blunt trauma and can rupture to cause pneumothorax.

Dillman JR, et al. Expanding upon the unilateral hyperlucent hemithorax in children. *Radiographics*. 2011;31:723–41.

2. E. Appendix

Carcinoid tumours are the most common primary tumour of the small bowel and appendix. Gastrointestinal carcinoids account for about 85% of all carcinoid tumours, with the remaining 15% occurring in the lungs and bronchi. These tumours arise from the enterochromaffin cells of Kultchitsky; these express serotonin and other histamine-like substances. The appendix is the most common site of carcinoids, accounting for 30%–45%, the small bowel for 25%–35%, the rectum 10%–15%, the colon 5% and the stomach <3%. Most tumours are clinically silent but may cause pain, obstruction, weight loss and, rarely, bowel perforation. In rare cases (7% of small bowel carcinoids), the hormonal load from the tumour may overwhelm the liver's capacity to metabolise serotonin, causing a carcinoid syndrome–recurrent diarrhoea, right-sided endocardial fibroelastosis, wheezing/bronchospasm and flushing of the face and neck.

Dähnert W. *Radiology Review Manual*, 7th edn. Philadelphia, PA: Lippincott Williams & Wilkins, 2011: 826–28.

3. B. Inflammatory pseudotumour

Inflammatory pseudotumour is an interesting entity that has been reported in every organ of the body. At imaging, it usually appears as a solitary exophytic or polypoid bladder mass, which may be ulcerated. On T2-weighted MRI, it is heterogeneous, with a central hyperintense component surrounded by a low-signal-intensity periphery; on post-contrast images the periphery enhances, whereas the central region enhances poorly. The central region consists of necrotic tissue, and the periphery comprises fascicles of spindle cells in oedematous stroma with myxoid components, vessels and inflammatory cells (hence the name *pseudosarcomatous fibromyxoid tumour*). This structure may produce the pattern of ring-like enhancement observed on CT and MR images suggestive of the diagnosis, but histologic confirmation is essential. In young adults, the presence of luminal clot surrounding an enhancing bladder mass may also suggest this diagnosis.

MRI shows single or multiple masses. On T2-weighted images, cystitis glandularis shows low signal intensity with a central branching high-signal pattern. The hyperintense area shows the most contrast enhancement and corresponds to the vascular stalk. Eosinophilic cystitis nodules are hyperintense to muscle on T1, isointense on T2-weighted images, and enhanced after intravenous contrast administration.

Wong-You-Cheong JJ, et al. From the archives of the AFIP: Inflammatory and nonneoplastic bladder masses: Radiologic-pathologic correlation. *Radiographics*. 2006;26(6):1847–68.

4. D. Discitis

Pyogenic spondylitis most commonly involves the lumbar spine and one spinal segment, which consists of two vertebral bodies and the intervening disk. It typically displays low signal intensity on T1-weighted images, with a loss of definition of the vertebral end plate and of the adjacent vertebral bodies and high signal intensity on T2-weighted images. In the involved disk space, fluid-like signal intensity is seen on both T1 and T2 images. Following the intravenous administration of gadolinium-based contrast material, disk enhancement patterns from homogeneous to patchy non-confluent to peripheral enhancement may be seen. Infected bone marrow also enhances diffusely after contrast material is administered; contrast-enhanced fat-suppressed MR images are especially useful in demonstrating this marrow abnormality. MR imaging provides better definition of epidural extension of the inflammatory process and compression of the spinal cord and dural sac than other imaging modalities do. Paravertebral and epidural extension may appear in the form of either a phlegmon or an abscess with mixed signal intensity on both T1-weighted and T2-weighted images.

Hong SH, et al. MR imaging assessment of the spine: Infection or an imitation? *Radiographics*. 2009; 29(2):599–612.

5. A. Calcium pyrophosphate dihydrate crystal deposition disease

Pseudogout [calcium pyrophosphate dihydrate (CPPD) deposition disease] is a syndrome caused by the deposition of CPPD crystals in and about the joints of middle-aged or older adults. Three discrete manifestations of this deposition of CPPD crystals are recognised: (1) chondrocalcinosis, (2) typical arthropathy and (3) the clinical presentation of pain. Any combination of these features may suffice to suggest the diagnosis of pseudogout.

Other causes of chondrocalcinosis include the following:

Hyperparathyroidism
Gout
Wilson disease
Haemochromatosis
Ochronosis
Trauma
Osteoarthritis
Hypothyroidism
Hypomagnesaemia
Acromegaly
Oxalosis and hydroxyapatite deposition disease (HADD)

Dähnert W. *Radiology Review Manual*, 7th edn. Philadelphia, PA: Lippincott Williams & Wilkins, 2011:14.
Helms CA, et al. CPPD crystal deposition disease or pseudogout. *Radiographics*. 1982:2(1):40–52.

6. E. Multiple extra-adrenal neuroblastomas

The question describes the Carney triad: pulmonary chondroma, gastric GIST and multiple extra-adrenal neuroblastoma.

Cancer predisposition syndrome (CPS) is the term that is generally reserved to describe familial cancers in which a clear mode of inheritance can be established. Individuals may present with one or more key physical features or congenital anomalies (e.g. hemihypertrophy). Patients may have specific tumours that are known to be highly associated with a CPS (e.g. haemangioblastomas in VHL (Von Hippel-Lindau syndrome) disease).

Some physical features suggesting CPS are café-au-lait spots (NF1, NF2, Bloom's), angiofibromas (tuberous sclerosis, TS), pits in palms and soles (Gorlin), macrocephaly (Sotos, Cowden, Gorlin), macroglosia [BWS ((Beckwith–Wiedemann syndrome)], hyperpigmentation (NF1, Fanconi anaemia, Blooms), spotty skin pigmentation (Carney complex), hemihypertrophy (NF1, BWS, Klippel–Trénaunay syndrome), thumb malformation (Fanconi anaemia), aniridia [WAGR (Wilms tumor- anirida syndrome with genitourinary anomalies)] and so on.

Tumours associated with CPS include Wilms tumour (WAGR, BWS and several others), haemangioblastoma (VHL), clear cell renal carcinoma (VHL, TS), pheochromocytoma (VHL, MEN 2B, NF1), hepatoblastoma (BWS, Familial adenomatous polyposis, FAP), adrenocortical and breast carcinoma (Li–Fraumeni syndrome, LFS), optic glioma and neurofibrosarcoma (NF1), retinoblastoma (familial retinoblastoma), gastric cancer and GIST (FAP, NF1, Carney triad, HNPCC [hereditary non-polyposis colorectal cancer] or lynch syndrome, LFS, MEN1), neuroblastoma (NF1, BWS), rhabdomyosarcoma (LFS, NF1, BWS, hereditary retinoblastoma) and so on.

Screening tests and pathways have been established for several of these CPSs. These include US abdomen for BWS, LFS, FAP and VHL; prophylactic thyroidectomy for MEN 2; and so on.

Monsalve J, et al. Imaging of cancer predisposition syndromes in children. *Radiographics*. 2011;31(1):263–80.

7. B. Normal lung reduces T2 intensity as it matures.

At US, the foetal lungs normally appear homogeneous and are slightly more echogenic than the liver. The echogenicity of the lung increases as gestation advances. The presence of cysts or focal increased echogenicity of the lung parenchyma indicates a mass. The axis of the heart is determined relative to the interventricular septum.

At MR imaging, the trachea, bronchi and lungs demonstrate high T2 signal intensity relative to the chest wall muscles, because they contain a significant amount of fluid. As the lungs mature, there is increasing production of alveolar fluid, thereby increasing the T2 signal intensity of lung relative to the liver.

Pulmonary hypoplasia can be primary or secondary. Primary pulmonary hypoplasia is less common. The most common intrathoracic cause of secondary pulmonary hypoplasia is congenital diaphragmatic hernia. The herniated liver can be confused with a mass originating in the lung. Colour Doppler imaging may be helpful in identifying the portal and hepatic veins.

Meconium-filled large bowel is hyperintense on T1-weighted images and hypointense on T2-weighted images; therefore, intrathoracic herniation of the large bowel can easily be detected at MR imaging.

The most common extrathoracic cause of pulmonary hypoplasia is severe oligohydramnios, secondary to either foetal urogenital anomaly or premature rupture of membranes.

Biyyam DR, et al. Congenital lung abnormalities: Embryologic features, prenatal diagnosis, and postnatal radiologic-pathologic correlation. *Radiographics*. 2010;30(6):1721–38.

8. B. Iliopectineal line

On radiographs, the iliopectineal (or iliopubic) line represents the border of the anterior column, and the ilioischial line represents the posterior column.

Fracture involvement of the anterior and posterior columns is characterised by disruption of the iliopectineal line and ilioischial line, respectively. However, disruption of these lines may also be seen with other fracture patterns, such as a transverse fracture. Obturator ring and iliac wing involvement must also be present for classification as a both-column acetabular fracture.

Durkee NJ, et al. Classification of common acetabular fractures: Radiographic and CT appearances. *AJR Am J Roentgenol.* 2006;187(4):915–25.

9. A. Systemic lupus erythematosus (SLE)

Systemic Lupus Erythematosus (SLE) patients with antiphospholipid antibody (aPL-ab) syndrome present with arterial and veno-occlusive disease, thrombocytopenia and recurrent vascular thromboses and miscarriages. Patients with aPL-ab syndrome can present with recurrent strokes, Budd–Chiari syndrome, dural venous sinus thrombosis, ischaemic bowel and recurrent pulmonary embolism. Exudative pericardial effusions and pericarditis are common. Pleural effusions are the most common manifestation of SLE in the respiratory system and are bilateral in approximately 50% of patients.

Epileptic seizures are seen in 11% patients with SLE, with association of aPL-ab syndrome and stroke.

Lalani TA, et al. Imaging findings in systemic lupus erythematosus. *Radiographics.* 2004;24(4):1069–86.

10. C. Mucocoele of the appendix

Mucocoele of the appendix is an umbrella term used for the appearance of a cystic mass within the appendix that has varying pathological cause. Mucocoeles may be secondary to mucosal hyperplasia (25%), mucinous cystadenoma (63%) and mucinous cystadenocarcinoma (12%). The HU (Hounsfield Unit) value of the cystic lesion is variable from water density to soft-tissue density depending on the volume of mucin present within it. A CT scan is good at demonstrating the curvilinear or punctate rim-like calcification that is present in approximately 50% of cases. Ultrasound may demonstrate a right lower quadrant lesion with either cystic or mixed internal echogenicity depending on the amount of mucin. Rupture of mucocoeles may lead to pseudomyxoma peritonei with characteristic findings of multiple thin-walled cystic masses of varying sizes in the abdomen, scalloping of the liver and splenic margins and a gelatinous ascites. Myxoglobulosis is a rare variant of mucocoele with characteristic small, rounded calcific spherules.

Dähnert W. *Radiology Review Manual*, 7th edn. Philadelphia, PA: Lippincott Williams & Wilkins, 2011:877.

11. D. Homogenous enhancement of the disc

Spinal tuberculosis most commonly involves the thoracic spine and less often the lumbar spine. It is often difficult to differentiate between tuberculous and pyogenic spondylitis, both clinically and on images. MR imaging is very helpful for differentiating between tuberculous spondylitis and pyogenic spondylitis. A well-defined paraspinal mass with abnormal signal intensity; a thin, smooth abscess wall; subligamentous spread to three or more vertebral levels; and multiple vertebral or entire-body involvement are findings more suggestive of tuberculous spondylitis than of pyogenic spondylitis. The presence of skip lesions and of a large paraspinal cold abscess is also suggestive of tuberculous spondylitis. However, because they barely penetrate the anterior longitudinal ligament, neither an anterior paraspinal phlegmon or an abscess encasing the intercostal arteries, is seen in spinal tuberculosis. MR imaging is less sensitive than radiography or CT for identifying paraspinal calcifications, which are a distinctive imaging feature of spinal tuberculosis. Pyogenic spondylitis most commonly involves the lumbar spine and one spinal segment.

Hong SH, et al. MR imaging assessment of the spine: Infection or an imitation? *Radiographics.* 2009;29(2): 599–612.

12. A. Bladder contusion

Bladder contusion is the most common bladder injury following trauma. Unlike the other choices there is no contrast extravasation. The CT scans can show an intramural haematoma (seen as a focal ellipse-shaped thickening of the bladder wall). This may appear as a crescent-shaped filling defect on cystography. Subserosal bladder rupture is seen as an elliptical contrast extravasation adjacent to the bladder on CT. Both intraperitoneal and extraperitoneal bladder rupture can be seen as extravasation outside the bladder.

Brant WE, Helms CA. *Fundamentals of Diagnostic Radiology*, 3rd edn. Philadelphia, PA: Lippincott Williams & Wilkins, 2006:904–5.

Dähnert W. *Radiology Review Manual*, 7th edn. Philadelphia, PA: Lippincott Williams & Wilkins, 2011:999.

13. B. Marfan syndrome

Annulo-aortic ectasia, a condition characterised by dilated sinuses of Valsalva with effacement of the sinotubular junction, with normal calibre arch, is most commonly associated with Marfan syndrome. Other causes include homocystinuria, Ehlers–Danlos syndrome and osteogenesis imperfecta; however, annulo-aortic ectasia can be idiopathic, although onset and progression is more rapid in Marfan syndrome. Common cardiovascular manifestations, include annulo-aortic ectasia with or without aortic valve insufficiency, aortic dissection, aortic aneurysm, pulmonary artery dilatation and mitral valve prolapse, most of which are substantial contributors to mortality.

Homocystinuria presents with thromboembolic episodes like stroke. Murmurs related to AR or MR are not commonly associated with the other conditions.

Agarwal PP, et al. Multidetector CT of thoracic aortic aneurysms. *Radiographics*. 2009;29(2):537–52.

14. B. Appendix

The clinical picture and CT findings are characteristic for pseudomyxoma peritonei, a process of gradual accumulation of large amounts of gelatinous/mucinous material within the peritoneum. This accumulation of mucin is secondary to a ruptured mucocoele of the appendix. Characteristic CT findings include omental caking, thickening of the peritoneum and mesentery, large gelatinous ascites and scalloped contour of the liver and/or splenic borders. The ascites may vary from water density to a very thick soft-tissue density, which is dependent on the volume of mucin within the fluid. It is important to always scrutinise the appendix to identify the mucocoele once the secondary features are identified.

Dähnert W. *Radiology Review Manual*, 7th edn. Philadelphia, PA: Lippincott Williams & Wilkins, 2011:883.

15. B. Cystitis cystica

Cystitis cystica and cystitis glandularis are inflammatory processes of the bladder wall with multiple small, round, cyst-like elevations in the submucosa. They are often associated with irritants such as chronic infection, calculi or bladder outlet obstruction. The hallmark of emphysematous cystitis is gas within the bladder wall. The main risk factors are diabetes mellitus and bladder outflow obstruction. Eosinophilic cystitis can present with a nodular bladder wall, but the nodules would be echogenic on ultrasound in comparison with the fluid-filled cysts of cystitis cystica. In any event, all focal bladder abnormalities seen at imaging should be evaluated cystoscopically. In interstitial cystitis, the bladder wall becomes thick and trabeculated.

Brant WE, Helms CA. *Fundamentals of Diagnostic Radiology*, 3rd edn. Philadelphia, PA: Lippincott Williams & Wilkins, 2006:900.

16. B. Pathological fractures tend to end in non-union.

Benign bone tumours in the fibrous group include benign fibrous cortical defect (FCD), non-ossifying fibroma (NOF), osteo-fibrous dysplasia (OFD), fibrous dysplasia (FD) and fibroma. Benign fibrous cortical defects and non-ossifying fibromas are the most common tumours in the benign fibrous group. Benign cortical defects and non-ossifying fibromas are eccentric, cortical bone lesions, usually located in the metaphyses of long bones. Non-ossifying fibromas are usually larger than fibrous cortical defects. The most common locations for fibrous cortical defects are the distal femur, proximal tibia and distal tibia. They occur less commonly in the fibula and are relatively uncommon in the upper extremity.

On CT, both benign fibrous cortical defects and non-ossifying fibromas have a dense sclerotic border, and on MRI both are of low signal intensity on T1-weighted and T2-weighted images.

Pathologic fractures are more common with the larger non-ossifying fibroma variant. They tend to heal spontaneously.

Davé A, et al. Benign bone tumors part I: Benign fibrous bone tumors. *Contemp Diagn Radiol.* 2007;30(24):6.

17. C. TB meningitis

Tuberculous meningitis (TBM) is the most common manifestation of CNS tuberculosis across all age groups. The typical radiographic finding is abnormal meningeal enhancement, usually most pronounced in the basal cisterns. These findings are better seen at gadolinium-enhanced MR imaging than at CT. Appearances usually resolve relatively quickly with adequate treatment; however, radiographic resolution is delayed if there are thickened exudates. This appearance is non-specific and has a wide differential diagnosis that includes meningitis from other infective agents; inflammatory diseases such as rheumatoid arthritis and sarcoidosis; and neoplastic causes, both primary and secondary. The presence of high density within the basal cisterns on non-contrast CT scans is a very specific sign for TBM in children.

The most common complication of tuberculous meningitis is communicating hydrocephalus. Ischaemic infarcts are also common, being seen in 20%–40% of patients at CT, mostly within the basal ganglia or internal capsule resulting from vascular compression and occlusion of small perforating vessels. Cranial nerve (2, 3, 4 and 7) involvement is reported.

Andronikou S, et al. Definitive neuroradiological diagnostic features of tuberculous meningitis in children. *Pediatr Radiol.* 2004;34(11):876–85.
Burrill J, et al. Tuberculosis: A radiologic review. *Radiographics.* 2007;27(5):1255–73.

18. D. GCS of 13 on initial clinical assessment

According to the latest NICE guidelines, for children who have sustained a head injury and have any of the following risk factors, perform a CT head scan within 1 hour of the risk factor being identified:

- Suspicion of non-accidental injury
- Post-traumatic seizure but no history of epilepsy
- On initial emergency department assessment, GCS less than 14 or, for children under 1 year, GCS (paediatric) less than 15
- At 2 hours after the injury, GCS less than 15
- Suspected open or depressed skull fracture or tense fontanelle
- Any sign of basal skull fracture (haemotympanum, 'panda' eyes, cerebrospinal fluid leakage from the ear or nose, or Battle's sign)
- Focal neurological deficit
- For children under 1 year, presence of bruise, swelling or laceration of more than 5 cm on the head

For children who have sustained a head injury and have more than one of the following risk factors (and none of those mentioned above), perform a CT head scan within 1 hour of the risk factors being identified:

- Loss of consciousness lasting more than 5 minutes (witnessed)
- Abnormal drowsiness
- Three or more discrete episodes of vomiting

- Dangerous mechanism of injury (high-speed road traffic accident either as pedestrian, cyclist or vehicle occupant; fall from a height of greater than 3 metres; high-speed injury from a projectile or other object)
- Amnesia (antegrade or retrograde) lasting more than 5 minutes

Head injury: Assessment and early management. Clinical guideline [CG176]. Published date: January 2014. https://www.nice.org.uk/guidance/cg176 [accessed on 22 February 2017].

19. B. Fall from a height of more than 1 metre

According to the latest NICE guideline for spinal injury:

Perform MRI for children (under 16s) if there is a strong suspicion of

- Cervical spinal cord injury as indicated by the Canadian C-spine rule and by clinical assessment or
- Cervical spinal column injury as indicated by clinical assessment or abnormal neurological signs or symptoms, or both.

Consider plain X-rays in children (under 16s) who do not fulfil the criteria for MRI in recommendation but clinical suspicion remains after clinical assessment.

For imaging in children (under 16s) with head injury and suspected cervical spine injury, follow the recommendations in the NICE guideline on head injury.

For children with a head injury, perform a CT cervical spine scan if

- GCS is less than 13 on initial assessment.
- The patient has been intubated.
- Focal peripheral neurological signs.
- Paraesthesia in the upper or lower limbs.
- A definitive diagnosis is needed urgently (e.g. before surgery).
- The patient is having CT for head injury or multiregion trauma.
- There is strong clinical suspicion of injury despite normal X-rays.
- Plain X-rays are technically difficult or inadequate.
- Plain X-rays identify a significant bony injury.

CT is to be performed within 1 hour of the risk factor being identified.

Head injury: assessment and early management. Clinical guideline [CG176] Published date: January 2014. https://www.nice.org.uk/guidance/cg176 [accessed on 22 February 2017].
Spinal injury: assessment and initial management. NICE guideline [NG41] Published date: February 2016. https://www.nice.org.uk/guidance/ng41 [accessed on 22 February 2017].

20. E. Subacute sclerosing pan encephalitis

Creutzfeldt–Jakob disease (CJD) shows high signal intensities in the basal ganglia (putamen and caudate nucleus) and in the cortex on DW images. The high signal intensities in the basal ganglia are also prevalent on T2-weighted and FLAIR images. The cortical hyperintensities are usually not visualised on T2-weighted and FLAIR images (advantage of DW imaging).

Progressive multifocal leukoencephalopathy (PML) is a demyelinating disease of immunocompromised patients caused by human papovaviruses. Subacute sclerosing panencephalitis (SSPE) occurs several years after measles infection. SSPE typically starts with mental and behavioural abnormalities, myoclonia, tremor and seizures. Multifocal, hyperintense foci in white matter and the basal ganglia have been reported in PML and SSPE on T2-weighted images. On T2-weighted and FLAIR images, PML and SSPE are associated with white matter lesions, whereas CJD is not. The high-signal-intensity cortical lesions on DW images may be also a hallmark of CJD.

Stadnik TW, et al. Imaging tutorial: Differential diagnosis of bright lesions on diffusion-weighted MR images. *Radiographics.* 2003;23(1):e7.

21. B. Cam-type femoro-acetabular impingement

Femoro-acetabular impingement (FAI) is a major cause of premature osteoarthritis of the hip. It is split radiographically into two main types. Pincer-type impingement is the acetabular cause of FAI and is secondary to either focal or generalised over-coverage of the femoral head by the acetabulum. Cam-type impingement is the femoral cause and is secondary to an asphericity of the femoral head and offset of the femoral head–neck junction. Cam impingement is more common in young men and leads to a increased alpha angle (diagnostic > 55 degrees). The osseous bump at the head–neck junction may be located laterally, resulting in the 'pistol grip' deformity seen on AP pelvis.

Protrusio acetabuli occurs when the femoral head is overlapping the ilioischial line medially and may be idiopathic or secondary to causes such as rheumatoid arthritis, Paget disease Marfans syndrome and osteomalacia.

Tannast M, et al. Femoroacetabular impingement. Radiographic diagnosis – What the radiologist should know. *AJR Am J Roentgenol.* 2007;188:1540–52.

22. B. Plombage

In the pre-chemotherapy era, surgical management of pulmonary TB included thoracoplasty or plombage, in which an extrapleural space was created between parietal pleura and the chest wall, which was filled with materials such as fat, oil, wax packs, bone or methyl-methacrylate (Lucite) balls.

Appearance on chest radiograph depend on the material used, with associated chest wall deformity, resected ribs or stigma of pulmonary TB-like calcified granulomas, lymph nodes or sheets of pleural calcification.

Pancoast tumour when large would often be associated with destroyed ribs, and the description does not fit with an aspergilloma (visible air crescent) or bronchogenic cysts, which are homogenous and mostly located around the carina.

Garetier M, Rousset J. Clinical images: Thoracic balls. *CMAJ.* 2011;183:E1091.

23. A. Choledochal cyst

The Todani classification system is used to differentiate the cystic processes of the biliary tree into five groups. Type 1 cysts, known as *choledochal cysts*, are responsible for 90% of cystic biliary disease. These cysts are further subclassified into IA (dilation of the entire extrahepatic bile duct), IB (focal segmental dilation of the extrahepatic duct) and IC (dilation only affecting the common duct). Patients may present with the triad of vague abdominal pain, jaundice and a palpable epigastric mass, although this is only reported in 10%–20% of patients. Type 2 'cysts' are true diverticulae of the bile duct. Type 3, known as a *choledochocoele*, is a focal protrusion of CBD into the duodenum. Type 4, consists of multiple communicating intra and extra-hepatic duct cysts. Type 5, known as Caroli's disease, represents cystic dilatation of intra-hepatic ducts.

Dähnert W. *Radiology Review Manual*, 7th edn. Philadelphia, PA: Lippincott Williams & Wilkins, 2011:715.

24. E. Schistosomiasis

This is a classical description of schistosomiasis infection of the bladder, with curvilinear calcification spreading proximally from the bladder into the distal ureters. The bladder wall can otherwise appear normal but is often thick-walled or nodular. In tuberculosis, the calcification starts in the kidney and can then extend more distally. When involved, the bladder is usually contracted, rather than normal size. *Escherichia coli* infection is associated with emphysematous cystitis; bacterial infection can be associated with bladder calculi but not mural calcification. Calcification of transitional cell carcinoma can be linear, curvilinear or stippled; however, a mass or wall thickening would be expected and 97% of cases occur in over 45-year-olds. Malakoplakia is a rare condition and calcification in affected patients is uncommon.

Brant WE, Helms CA. *Fundamentals of Diagnostic Radiology*, 3rd edn. Philadelphia, PA: Lippincott Williams & Wilkins, 2006:900–1.

Davies SG, et al. *Aids to Radiological Differential Diagnosis*, 5th edn. Philadelphia, PA: Saunders Elsevier, 2009:227.

25. C. Hamartoma

Hamartoma is a benign neoplasm composed of mesenchymal tissues such as cartilage, fat, connective tissue, smooth muscle and calcification. Hamartoma are common benign tumours. Typical CT findings consist of a well-defined, smooth, round or lobulated nodule or mass with fat density in nearly two-thirds of cases, and popcorn-like calcification or central calcification in a quarter.

Furaya K, et al. Lung CT: Part 1, mimickers of lung cancer – Spectrum of CT findings with pathologic correlation. *AJR Am J Roentgenol*. 2012;199:4.

26. E. Biliary cystadenoma

Biliary cystadenomas are benign neoplasms originating in bile ducts, most commonly seen within the right lobe of liver. They rarely affect the extrahepatic biliary system. Women are affected more than men and typically present with chronic, vague abdominal pain. Biliary cystadenomas can reach up to 35 cm in size and are usually demonstrated as large multiloculated anechoic masses on ultrasound. A CT scan typically demonstrates a water density mass that shows enhancement of its walls and septations following administration of contrast, differentiating these from simple cysts. An echinococcal cyst (hydatid cyst) is a parasitic infection causing cystic transformation in the liver.

Dähnert W. *Radiology Review Manual*, 7th edn. Philadelphia, PA: Lippincott Williams & Wilkins, 2011:705.

27. B. Malakoplakia

Malakoplakia is a rare chronic inflammatory disease primarily affecting the bladder, with decreasing incidence with increasing proximity to the kidney. Small smooth papules, nodules or plaque-like mural defects of the affected urinary tract are characteristic. Malakoplakia can be associated with immunosuppression, diabetes mellitus, renal transplants or long-term corticosteroid use. Leukoplakia is characterised by soft-tissue flakes that can be passed in the urine during micturition. Haemorrhagic cystitis and emphysematous cystitis can occur with *E. coli* infections but are associated with intraluminal blood clots and gas deposits, respectively. Bladder outflow obstruction results in a thick-walled bladder with trabeculations.

Brant WE, Helms CA. *Fundamentals of Diagnostic Radiology*, 3rd edn. Philadelphia, PA: Lippincott Williams & Wilkins, 2006:900–1.
Dähnert W. *Radiology Review Manual*, 7th edn. Philadelphia, PA: Lippincott Williams & Wilkins, 2011:952.

28. C. Chondrosarcoma

The radiographic description is aggressive and the stippled calcification is suggestive of a chondroid matrix. The most likely diagnosis is therefore a chondrosarcoma. These may be primary or develop from an enchondroma or osteochondroma.

Although chondromyxoid fibroma would be a possibility in this age group, it is an exceedingly rare benign chondral lesion that would normally have well-defined, thickened sclerotic margins.

Chondrosarcomas are quite common tumours that may have relatively benign radiographic appearances. They are normally metaphyseal, located centrally within the skeleton and may exhibit endosteal scalloping. The diagnosis should also be considered in patients with increased pain or growth in centrally located enchondromas or osteochondromas. Surgical resection is the treatment of choice and the 5-year survival rate is approximately 75%.

Manaster BJ, et al. *The Requisites: MSK Imaging*, 3rd edn. Philadelphia, PA: Mosby, 2007:456–9.

29. C. Sarcoidosis

Causes of optic canal enlargement (more than 6.5 mm in diameter)
Common causes:
- Glioma of the optic nerve
- Meningioma of the optic nerve sheath
- Metastasis
- Neurofibromatosis with or without optic neurofibroma or glioma

Uncommon causes:

- Aneurysm of the ophthalmic artery or cavernous portion of internal carotid artery
- Arteriovenous malformation with ophthalmic artery involvement
- Carcinoma of ethmoid or sphenoid sinus
- Granuloma (e.g. tuberculosis, sarcoidosis)
- Increased intracranial pressure
- Mucocoele of sphenoid sinus
- Mucopolysaccharidoses (especially Hurler syndrome)
- Pituitary adenoma or craniopharyngioma extending anteriorly
- Pseudotumour of orbit
- Retinoblastoma with intracranial extension

Reeder MM. Gamut B-13; optic canal enlargement. In: *Reeder and Felson's Gamuts in Radiology.* Head and Neck, Reeder MM (ed.), New York: Springer Verlag, 2003:109–10.

30. C. AP radiograph of the cervical spine

The standard child protection skeletal survey for suspected non-accidental injury includes the following:

Skull
- AP, lateral and Townes view (the latter if clinically indicated).
- Skull X-rays should be taken even if a CT scan has been or will be performed.

Chest
- AP including the clavicles.
- Two oblique views to show ribs ('left and right oblique').

Abdomen
- AP including the pelvis and hips.

Spine
- Lateral: may require separate exposures of the cervical, thoracic and thoraco-lumbar regions.
- AP views of the cervical spine are rarely diagnostic at this age and should only be performed at the discretion of the radiologist.

Limbs
- AP of both upper arms
- AP of both forearms
- AP of both femurs
- AP of both lower legs
- PA of hands
- DP of feet

Where an abnormality is suspected, these views should be supplemented by the following:
- Lateral views of any suspected shaft fracture
- AP and lateral coned views when a fracture is suspected

Standards for Radiological Investigations of Suspected Non-accidental Injury, The Royal College of Radiologists, March 2008. ref: BFCR(08)1, available at https://www.rcr.ac.uk/system/files/publication/ field_publication_files/RCPCH_RCR_final_0.pdf.

31. D. Meconium aspiration

Meconium aspiration is the most common cause of neonatal respiratory distress in full-term or post-mature infants (hyaline membrane disease is the most common cause in premature infants).

Chest X-ray shows the following:

- Bilateral diffuse grossly patchy opacities (atelectasis + consolidation). Unlike hyaline membrane disease, air bronchogram is not a typical feature.
- Hyperinflation with areas of emphysema (air trapping).
- Spontaneous pneumothorax + pneumomediastinum (25%) requiring no therapy.
- Small pleural effusions (20%).
- Rapid clearing, usually within 48 hours.

Dähnert W. *Radiology Review Manual*, 7th edn. Philadelphia, PA: Lippincott Williams & Wilkins, 2011.

32. A. Pneumoconiosis with progressive massive fibrosis

On chest radiographs, large opacities (progressive massive fibrosis) may be seen in complicated coal worker pneumoconiosis, as in complicated silicosis.

The large opacities result from nodule coalescence and are observed commonly in the middle lung zone or peripheral one-third of the lung on axial chest images and in the upper lung zone on longitudinal images. The large opacities gradually migrate towards the hilum, leaving emphysematous lung tissue between the fibrotic tissue and the pleural surface.

Chong S, et al. Pneumoconiosis: Comparison of imaging and pathologic findings. *Radiographics*. 2006;26(1): 59–77.

33. D. Mirizzi syndrome

The sonographic findings of an impacted gallstone within the neck of bladder causing proximal biliary dilatation are diagnostic for Mirizzi syndrome. Mirizzi syndrome is caused by impaction of a large gallstone in the cystic duct, cystic duct remnant or gallbladder neck. The impacted stone causes external compression of the CBD, resulting in proximal dilation of the biliary tree. A choledochocoele is cystic dilatation of the CBD within the lumen of the duodenum. Caroli disease is a congenital disorder characterised by saccular dilatations of intrahepatic ducts. Caroli disease, in association with congenital hepatic fibrosis, polycystic kidney disease and others, is known as *Caroli syndrome.*

Dähnert W. *Radiology Review Manual*, 7th edn. Philadelphia, PA: Lippincott Williams & Wilkins, 2011:747.

34. E. The bladder dome is the most common site of injury.

Extraperitoneal bladder rupture accounts for 80% of bladder ruptures. A flame-shaped extravasation of contrast is a classic finding and can be seen to extend into the perivesical fat and into the retropubic space of Retzius, anterior abdominal wall, upper thigh or scrotum. The most common site of injury is close to the anterolateral aspect of the bladder base. It is usually caused by puncture from pelvic fractures.

Brant WE, Helms CA. *Fundamentals of Diagnostic Radiology*, 3rd edn. Philadelphia, PA: Lippincott Williams & Wilkins, 2006:904.

Dähnert W. *Radiology Review Manual*, 7th edn. Philadelphia, PA: Lippincott Williams & Wilkins, 2011:999.

35. A. Pyknodysostosis

Pyknodysostosis is a congenital abnormality that should be considered in the differential diagnosis of osteosclerosis. The patients are typically short, have hypoplastic mandibles, widened cranial sutures, Wormian bones, brachycephaly, clavicular dysplasia, thick skull base and hypoplasia or non-pneumatisation of the paranasal sinuses. The distinguishing feature is acro-osteolysis with sclerosis. The distal phalanges appear as if they have been put in a pencil sharpener – they are pointed and dense.

Brant WE, Helms CA. *Fundamentals of Diagnostic Radiology*, 3rd edn. Philadelphia, PA: Lippincott Williams & Wilkins, 2006.

Dähnert W. *Radiology Review Manual*, 7th edn. Philadelphia, PA: Lippincott Williams & Wilkins, 2011.

36. C. III

Clinical classification of neck nodes

Level I: Above hyoid bone

Level Ia: Previously called submental nodes

Level Ib: Previously called submandibular nodes

Level II: from skull base to level of lower body of hyoid bone

Posterior to back of submandibular gland

Anterior to back of sternocleidomastoid muscle

Level IIA: anterior, lateral, medial or posterior to internal jugular vein

Inseparable from internal jugular vein (if posterior to vein)

Previously classified as upper internal jugular nodes

Level IIB: Posterior to internal jugular vein with fat plane separating nodes and vein previously classified as upper spinal accessory nodes

Level III: From level of lower body of hyoid bone to level of lower cricoid cartilage arch, anterior to back of sternocleidomastoid muscle, previously known as *mid-jugular nodes.*

Level IV: From level of lower cricoid cartilage arch to level of clavicle

Level V: Posterior to back of sternocleidomastoid muscle from skull base to level of lower cricoid arch

Level VI: Between carotid arteries from level of lower body of hyoid bone to level superior to top of manubrium

Level VII: Between carotid arteries below level of top of manubrium

Silverman PM. Lymph node imaging: multidetector CT (MDCT). *Cancer Imaging.* 2005;5:S57–67.

37. B. PET CT is useful in differentiating lung cancer from PMF.

It is clinically and radiologically important to differentiate progressive massive fibrosis from lung cancer. MRI is a preferable option because lung cancer appears as high-signal lesion on T2-weighted images, whereas progressive massive fibrosis appears as a low-signal abnormality when compared with the signal of muscle on both T1-weighted and T2-weighted images. On post-contrast MR, progressive massive fibrosis appears peripherally enhanced more frequently than not. Histopathologic analysis should still be performed for diagnosis.

PET may show intensive uptake of FDG in the fibrotic mass in progressive massive fibrosis; hence differentiation from cancer may be difficult.

Chong S, et al. Pneumoconiosis: Comparison of imaging and pathologic findings. *Radiographics.* 2006; 26(1):59–77.

38. B. Klatskin tumour

Klatskin tumours are cholangiocarcinomas that involve the confluence of hepatic ducts and account for up to 70% of cholangiocarcinomas. Dilation of the intrahepatic ducts is the most frequent abnormal finding on ultrasound. Lobar atrophy may be very subtle on ultrasound but may be identified by secondary findings such as extension of dilated ducts to the liver surface and lobar ductal crowding. The tumour itself may be very difficult to identify on ultrasound but may present as an isoechoic or hyperechoic mass. Primary sclerosing cholangitis is a fibrotic process that affects the biliary tree causing multifocal strictures and may lead to biliary cirrhosis. Mirizzi syndrome is dilation of the proximal common bile duct and intrahepatic ducts secondary to external compression of a large gallstone impacted in the cystic duct/gallbladder neck.

Sainani NI, et al. Cholangiocarcinoma: Current and novel imaging techniques. *Radiographics.* 2008; 28:1263–87.

39. B. Intraperitoneal bladder rupture

Intraperitoneal bladder rupture occurs in around 20% of bladder ruptures. It can be caused by a sudden increase in intravesical pressure owing to blunt trauma and usually causes rupture to the bladder dome. Contrast can be seen in the peritoneal cavity, often outlining loops of bowel and extending up the paracolic gutters. Extraperitoneal bladder rupture is more common and is usually caused by puncture from pelvic fractures. Contrast can be seen in the retroperitoneal space, anterior abdominal wall, upper thighs or even the scrotum. It is important to distinguish between intraperitoneal and extraperitoneal rupture: intraperitoneal rupture requires surgical repair, whereas extraperitoneal rupture is managed conservatively. Contrast outside the bladder would not be seen on the pre IV contrast CT in cases of arterial damage or pelvic haematoma.

Brant WE, Helms CA. *Fundamentals of Diagnostic Radiology*, 3rd edn. Philadelphia, PA: Lippincott Williams & Wilkins, 2006:904.

40. A. Bone metastasis

The 'ivory vertebra' sign, as described in this case, refers to a diffuse and homogeneous increase in the density of a vertebral body, which retains its size and contours. It can occur in both adults and children but is more common in the former. In adults, ivory vertebra has been associated most commonly with fractures (compression or healing), haemangiomas, lymphoma, myelosclerosis, with metastatic disease (especially prostate, breast and carcinoid), chronic sclerosing osteomyelitis, Paget disease and renal osteodystrophy. An ivory vertebra at one or more vertebral levels in an elderly man is most compatible with a diagnosis of metastatic disease, commonly as the result of prostate carcinoma. The other options are all much less common causes of ivory vertebrae.

Graham TS. The ivory vertebra sign. *Radiology*. 2005;235:614–15.
Reeder MM (ed.), et al. *Reeder and Felson's Gamuts in Radiology: Comprehensive Lists of Roentgen Differential Diagnosis*, 4th edn. New York: Springer Verlag, 2003.

41. A. Superior orbital fissure syndrome

Because the upper transverse maxillary buttress forms the orbital floor, fractures of this buttress may cause various orbital complications, including inferior rectus muscle tears, globe rupture or impingement, optic nerve injury and orbital hematoma.

Superior orbital fissure syndrome is caused by extension of the fracture through the superior orbital fissure, with resultant injury to cranial nerves III, IV, V1 (the ophthalmic branch of the trigeminal nerve) and VI as they traverse the fissure into the orbit, thus causing ophthalmoplegia or diplopia (extra-ocular muscle paralysis) and ptosis (paralysis of the levator palpebrae superioris, which is supplied by cranial nerve III). Additional injury to the optic nerve (cranial nerve II) at the orbital apex results in orbital apex syndrome, with unilocular visual loss added to the list of signs and symptoms. Orbital apex syndrome is a surgical emergency because prompt intervention is necessary to prevent permanent blindness.

Winegar BA, et al. Spectrum of critical imaging findings in complex facial skeletal trauma. *RadioGraphics*. 2013;33:3–19.

42. A. Hypothyroidism

Causes of delayed bone age include the following:

- Constitutional: Familial and IUGR
- Metabolic: Hypothyroidism, hypopituitarism, hypogonadism (Turner syndrome), Cushing disease/steroid therapy, diabetes mellitus, rickets and malnutrition
- Systemic disease: Congenital heart disease, renal disease, coeliac disease, Crohn's disease, ulcerative colitis and anaemia
- Syndromes: Trisomies, Noonan disease, Cornelia de Lange, cleidocranial dysplasia, Lesch–Nyhan disease metatrophic dwarfism

Of these, in the absence of any other history or radiological abnormality, hypothyroidism is more likely until proven otherwise. Precocious puberty results in advanced bone age.

Dähnert W. *Radiology Review Manual*, 7th edn. Philadelphia, PA: Lippincott Williams & Wilkins, 2011.

43. B. Few varying sized nodules, some with cavitation

Wegener's granulomatosis, currently called *granulomatosis with polyangitis*, is a probable autoimmune disease characterised by systemic necrotising granulomatous destructive angitis, with a classic triad of respiratory tract inflammation, systemic small vessel vasculitis and necrotising glomerulonephritis.

Sinus disease classically includes destructive sinusitis, nasal septal ulceration, septal perforation and saddle nose deformity.

Chest radiograph shows interstitial fibrosis at the bases, which is usually asymptomatic. Multiple pulmonary nodules with cavitation are the most common and characteristic manifestation. Pleural effusions and mediastinal nodal enlargement are seen.

There are multiple causes of miliary nodules, described as innumerable small 1–4 mm lung nodules, described in miliary tuberculosis, fungal infection, metastasis (thyroid, renal, breast, melanoma, pancreas, trophoblastic tumour), sarcoidosis, pneumoconiosis, pulmonary haemosiderosis, varicella infection, hypersensitive pneumonitis, histiocytosis etc. Bilateral upper lobe fibrosis are classically described in TB, ankylosing spondylitis, sarcoidosis, silicosis, radiation and histiocytosis.

Dähnert W. *Radiology Review Manual*, 7th edn. Philadelphia, PA: Lippincott Williams & Wilkins, 2011:551–2.

44. C. Thick-walled oedematous loops of bowel with branching lucencies peripherally in the liver

The patient in this scenario has a history of atherosclerosis with end organ damage. This would make them at risk of developing ischaemic colitis. The area of bowel affected in this question is a watershed area and is most susceptible to ischaemic colitis. The other plain film findings described in this question include intramural gas and portal venous gas. These are very worrying signs and usually imply a poor outcome. Sigmoid volvulus would cause a coffee bean sign on plain film. The findings are also not suggestive of caecal volvulus or small bowel obstruction. Necrotising enterocoltis would cause intramural and portal venous gas; however, this is a condition of neonates. Dilated small bowel with gas at the porta hepatis, is classic description of gall stone ileus, with gas being in the biliary tree.

Pear BL. Pneumatosis intestinalis: A review. *Radiology*. 1998;207:13–19.

45. C. Transitional cell carcinoma

Transitional cell carcinoma of the bladder is the most common urinary tract malignancy in the UK and appears as a lobulated, irregular bladder wall thickening that enhances more greatly than the normal bladder wall. If hydronephrosis is present, this suggests muscle invasive disease. Squamous cell carcinoma can look like this but accounts for only 4% of all bladder malignancies and is therefore less likely unless there are specific risk factors such as schistosomiasis infection, chronic cystitis, bladder calculi or long-term catheterisation. Adenocarcinoma is rare and associated with urachal remnants or bladder extrophy. Leiomyomas appears as smooth bladder wall masses. Blood clots do not enhance and are often seen to change in size and position on sequential scans.

Brant WE, Helms CA. *Fundamentals of Diagnostic Radiology*, 3rd edn. Philadelphia, PA: Lippincott Williams & Wilkins, 2006:900–3.

46. E. Haemangioma

Vertebral hemangiomas are present in 5%–11% of all autopsies and are multiple in one-third of these cases. Lesions commonly occur in the vertebral bodies of the lower thoracic and lumbar spine, and radiographic appearances are those of coarse vertical trabeculations, giving a 'corduroy' or 'honeycomb' appearance. A CT scan may also demonstrate small punctuate areas of sclerosis, giving a 'polka-dot' appearance. On MRI, the lesions are of a mottled pattern with a characteristic low to high signal on T1-weighted sequences and high signal on T2-weighted sequences in proportion to the amount of adipose tissue. The lesions enhance strongly on both CT and MRI because of hypervascularity.

Dähnert W. *Radiology Review Manual*, 7th edn. Philadelphia, PA: Lippincott Williams & Wilkins, 2011.

47. E. Second branchial cleft cyst

The vast majority (95%) of branchial cleft anomalies arise from the second cleft. At least three-fourths of these anomalies are cysts, which typically occur between 10 and 40 years of age, in contrast to fistulas or sinuses, which manifest most commonly during the first decade of life. No gender predilection has been reported.

These cysts usually appear as painless, fluctuant masses in the lateral portion of the neck adjacent to the anteromedial border of the sternocleidomastoid muscle at the mandibular angle. The mass enlarges slowly over time and may become painful and tender if secondarily infected.

At US, a second branchial cleft cyst is seen as a sharply marginated, round to ovoid, centrally anechoic mass with a thin peripheral wall that displaces the surrounding soft tissues. The mass is compressible and shows distinct acoustic enhancement. Occasionally, fine, indistinct internal echoes, representing debris, may be seen. The 'classic' location of these cysts (at either CT or MR imaging) is at the anteromedial border of the sternocleidomastoid muscle, lateral to the carotid space and at the posterior margin of the submandibular gland. The cyst typically displaces the sternocleidomastoid muscle posteriorly or posterolaterally, pushes the vessels of the carotid space medially or posteromedial and displaces the submandibular gland anteriorly. It may also be seen more medially within the parapharyngeal space after extending through the stylomandibular tunnel and middle constrictor muscle.

MR imaging better depicts the deep tissue extent of a second branchial cleft cyst, which allows accurate preoperative planning. The cyst fluid varies from hypointense to slightly hyperintense relative to muscle on T1-weighted images and is usually hyperintense on T2-weighted images. Mural thickness and enhancement vary, depending of the presence and severity of any associated inflammatory process. Occasionally, a 'beak sign' may be seen on axial CT or MR images. This sign represents a curved rim of tissue or 'beak' pointing medially between the internal and external carotid arteries. It is considered a pathognomonic imaging feature of a second branchial cleft cyst.

Koeller KK, et al. Congenital cystic masses of the neck: Radiologic – Pathologic correlation. *Radiographics.* 1999;19:121–46.

48. C. Sacrococcygeal bony defect

Anterior sacral meningocele may occur as part of the Currarino triad, also known as the *ASP triad* (anorectal malformation, sacrococcygeal osseous defect and presacral mass), a rare syndrome characterised by autosomal dominant genetic inheritance in more than 50% of cases.

The presacral mass in those affected may be a teratoma, anterior sacral meningocoele, dermoid cyst, hamartoma or enteric duplication cyst, or more than one of these types of masses may be present.

Kocaoglu M, Frush DP. Pediatric presacral masses. *Radiographics.* 2006;26(3):833–57.

49. C. Anechoic mass in the midline

On all radiologic images, a thyroglossal duct cyst manifests as a cyst-like mass either in the midline of the anterior neck at the level of the hyoid bone or within the strap muscles just off the midline.

At US, the finding of an anechoic mass with a thin outer wall in this characteristic location easily establishes the diagnosis of a thyroglossal duct cyst. However, this 'classic' appearance is seen in less than half (42%) of cases. More commonly, these cysts manifest as hypoechoic masses, often with increased through-transmission. They may be either homogeneous or heterogeneous in appearance with variable degrees of fine to coarse internal echoes. There is no correlation between the sonographic appearance and pathologic evidence of infection and inflammation. Heterogeneity seen in thyroglossal duct cysts on sonograms is more likely due to the proteinaceous content of the fluid secreted from the cyst wall rather than to infection. Preoperative sonographic visualisation of normal thyroid tissue is sufficient to exclude a diagnosis of ectopic thyroid tissue and obviates routine thyroid scintigraphy.

Koeller KK, et al. Congenital cystic masses of the neck: Radiologic – Pathologic correlation. *Radiographics*. 1999;19:121–46.

50. E. RUL lung primary and SVC obstruction

Obstruction of the superior vena cava results in impaired venous drainage of the head and neck and upper extremities. Clinical manifestations include facial and neck swelling, distended neck veins, headache due to cerebral oedema, dyspnoea, stridor and altered mental status. Cancer is the most common underlying cause of superior vena cava obstruction and this includes lung cancer, mediastinal tumours, lymphoma/lymphadenopathy and mesothelioma, either directly or through malignant mediastinal lymphadenopathy. Other causes include catheter-induced iatrogenic SVC obstruction, fibrosing mediastinitis and Behcet's disease.

Sheth S, et al. Superior vena cava obstruction evaluation with MDCT. *AJR Am J Roentgenol*. 2010;194:W336–46.

51. B. Angiodysplasia

The clinical history and findings on angiogram suggest angiodysplasia. There is no history of atherosclerosis elsewhere to suggest ischaemic colitis. The major mesenteric vessels are usually patent in ischaemic colitis. The exception to this rule would be in a case of possible superior mesenteric artery obstruction. Angiodysplasia can be part of the hereditary haemorrhagic telangiectasia syndrome. The condition results from a chronic intermittent obstruction of the veins where they penetrate the circular muscle layer of bowel. Distorted dilated vascular channels replace the normal mucosal structures. Endovascular treatment is an option. The findings on angiography do not point to colon carcinoma, diverticulitis or haemorrhoids.

Hastings GS. Angiographic localization and transcatheter treatment of gastrointestinal bleeding. *Radiographics*. 2000;20:1160–8.

52. E. Trabeculated bladder with decreased capacity

Neurogenic bladder can be caused by meningomyelocele, spinal trauma, diabetes, multiple sclerosis, polio and herpes infection. It is a heterogeneous condition: for example, it can cause incontinence owing to detrusor over-activity, difficulty in passing urine owing to detrusor underactivity or retention with overflow incontinence. Most commonly, the bladder eventually becomes trabeculated with decreased capacity, but very large atonic bladders can also be seen. The detrusor muscle is innervated by the sympathetic nerves originating from S2–S4, therefore, neurogenic bladder is a common problem in spinal trauma. Indwelling urethral or suprapubic catheters may be seen and can be associated with stone disease and infection, including pyelonephritis. Treatments that may be seen on imaging include urinary diversion and continent pouch formation.

Brant WE, Helms CA. *Fundamentals of Diagnostic Radiology*, 3rd edn. Philadelphia, PA: Lippincott Williams & Wilkins, 2006:899.

Dähnert W. *Radiology Review Manual*, 7th edn. Philadelphia, PA: Lippincott Williams & Wilkins, 2011:960.

53. D. MRI of the wrist

The patient's presentation is a classic description of a hook of hamate fracture. These often occur during racquet, bat or club sports. A fracture of the hook of hamate can narrow Guyon's canal, compressing the ulnar neurovascular bundle and causing distal neuropathy of vascular compromise. Conventional radiographs even with multiple dedicated views only have a sensitivity of 72% for diagnosing this carpal fracture. CT with multiplanar reformatting would be a reasonable next investigation; however, in view of this patient's neurological signs of ulnar nerve compression, MRI is the imaging modality of choice. This gives better soft-tissue definition while still having a sensitivity and specificity approaching 100% for diagnosing fractures.

Powell A. *Hamate Fracture*. emedicine.medscape.com/article/97813-overview [accessed on 16 March 2017].

54. B. Rectal duplication cysts are high signal on T1W images.

Anterior sacral meningocoele may be accompanied by other anomalies or syndromes, too, including uterine, renal and bladder malformations; Marfan syndrome; and Type 1 neurofibromatosis.

Benign sacrococcygeal teratomas are predominantly cystic; have attenuation similar to that of fluid on CT scans; and may include bone, fat and calcification. Cystic areas typically have the appearance of fluid on T1-weighted and T2-weighted MR images. Areas of fatty tissue demonstrate high signal intensity on T1-weighted images, whereas calcification and bone are depicted as areas of signal void. The coccyx is always involved, even in benign sacrococcygeal teratoma. Malignant teratomas have a predominant solid component, and haemorrhage and necrosis are common.

Enteric cysts are rare and may arise in locations between the rectum and sacrum. They are classified according to their histologic basis as either tail-gut cysts or rectal duplication cysts. Duplication cysts on MR imaging demonstrates well-marginated, thin-walled lesions with low signal intensity on T1-weighted images and high signal intensity on T2-weighted images. Mucoid contents of tail-gut cysts cause them to have high signal intensity on T1-weighted images.

On MR images, cystic lymphatic malformations appear as areas of homogeneous high signal intensity on T2-weighted images and have the signal intensity of fluid on T1-weighted images. A fluid–fluid level can be seen in the setting of acute haemorrhage.

Kocaoglu M, Frush DP. Pediatric presacral masses. *Radiographics*. 2006;26(3):833–57.

55. D. Tuberous sclerosis

The US images suggest renal cysts, bilateral angiomyolipomas and splenic hamartoma. Polycystic kidney disease PCKD1 gene lies next to Tuberous sclerosis gene TSC2 and renal cysts are common in TS.

TS is an autosomal, dominant, inherited neurocutaneous syndrome characterised by a variety of hamartomatous lesions in various organs. Classically, TS demonstrates a triad of clinical features (Vogt triad): mental retardation, epilepsy and adenoma sebaceum. PHACE syndrome constitutes, posterior fossa malformations–hemangiomas–arterial anomalies–cardiac defects–eye abnormalities–sternal cleft and supraumbilical raphe syndrome. Typically infants have large plaque like facial haemangiomas.

Umeoka S, et al. Pictorial review of tuberous sclerosis in various organs. *Radiographics*. 2008;28(7):e32

56. D. CD4 <200

Knowledge of the CD4 count when reporting a chest X-ray in an AIDS patient is important as opportunistic infections present at different count levels. A CD4 count lower than 200 is regarded as indicating a potentially life-threatening complication of *Pneumocystis jiroveci* infection.

CD4 >500: No risk of opportunistic infection
CD4 200–500: Candidiasis, Kaposi's sarcoma
CD4 100–200: *P. jiroveci*, histoplasmosis, coccidioidomycosis, PML
CD4 50–100: Toxoplasma, cryptosporidiosis, cryptococcosis, CMV
CD4 <50: *Mycobacterium avium* complex (MAC)

Dähnert W. *Radiology Review Manual*, 7th edn. Philadelphia, PA: Lippincott Williams & Wilkins, 2011:468.

57. E. Pericolic focal hyperattenuation with a central area of fat density

Epiploic appendagitis is most common in the sigmoid colon or caecum, where the appendages are most prominent. Most cases resolve spontaneously in about 2 weeks. It is therefore an important diagnosis to make, as it does not require surgery. It can appear on ultrasound as a non-compressible pericolic hyperechoic ovoid mass immediately under the abdominal wall. The accordion sign is seen in pseudomembranous colitis on post-contrast CT. Ascites is a non-specific sign that can be seen in a variety of conditions, including liver failure, trauma and pseudomembranous colitis. Mucosal wall thickening with air-filled outpouchings is characteristic of diverticulitis.

Ng KS, et al. CT features of primary epiploic appendagitis. *Eur J Radiol.* 2006;59:284–8.

58. C. The upper pole moiety is often associated with an ectopic ureterocoele.

Ureteric duplication is seen in around 1%–2% of the population and is usually unilateral. The upper pole moiety inserts inferiorly and is often associated with an ectopic ureterocoele, which is more likely to obstruct, causing upper pole calyceal dilatation. The lower pole ureter inserts horizontally into the bladder, making it prone to vesicoureteric reflux, which can lead to scarring and deformity of the obstructed kidney's lower pole. Intravenous urography may show poor or no function in the dilated obstructed upper pole. An MR or CT Urogram may also demonstrate the 'drooping lily' sign caused by the lower pole moiety being displaced inferiorly.

Brant WE, Helms CA. *Fundamentals of Diagnostic Radiology*, 3rd edn. Philadelphia, PA: Lippincott Williams & Wilkins, 2006:889.

59. E. Nail–patella syndrome

Nail–patella syndrome is a rare autosomal dominant disorder characterised by symmetrical mesodermal and ectodermal abnormalities. Radiographic abnormalities include bilateral posterior iliac horns in 80% (diagnostic), flared iliac crests with protuberant anterior iliac spines, genu valgum owing to asymmetrical development of the femoral condyles, prominent tibial tubercles, fragmentation/hypoplasia/absence of the patella, radial head/capitellum subluxation with dislocation of the radial head dorsally, short fifth metacarpal, clinodactyly of the fifth finger, scoliosis and, occasionally, mandibular cysts. Protrusio acetabuli and bipartite patella are not disease entities as such; they are radiological descriptions of the acetabular floor bulging into the pelvis and a congenital fragmentation or synchondrosis of the patella, respectively. Diastrophic dysplasia refers to severe rhizomelic dwarfism, and Osgood–Schlatter refers to rupture of the growth plate at the tibial tuberosity secondary to an apophyseal traction injury.

Dähnert W. *Radiology Review Manual*, 7th edn. Philadelphia, PA: Lippincott Williams & Wilkins, 2011.
Raman D, Haslock I. The nail-patella syndrome – A report of two cases and a literature review.
  Br J Rheumatol. 1983;22:41–6.

60. B. Fatty atrophy of the right masticator muscles

Denervation and fatty atrophy of the pterygoid muscles occurs due to involvement of the motor portion of cranial nerve V supplying the muscle of mastication. This nerve runs through the foramen ovale.

Laine FJ, et al. CT and MRI imaging of the central skull base. Part 2. Pathologic spectrum. *Radiographics.* 1990;10:797–821.

61. B. Routine urinary tract ultrasound within 6 weeks

Recommended Imaging Schedule for Infants Younger than 6 Months

Test	Responds well to treatment within 48 hours	Atypical UTI	Recurrent UTI
Ultrasound during the acute infection	No	Yes	Yes
Ultrasound within 6 weeks	Yes	No	No
DMSA 4–6 months following the acute infection	No	Yes	Yes
MCUG	No	Yes	Yes

Recommended Imaging Schedule for Infants and Children between 6 Months and 3 Years

Test	Responds well to treatment within 48 hours	Atypical UTI	Recurrent UTI
Ultrasound during the acute infection	No	Yes	No
Ultrasound within 6 weeks	No	No	Yes
DMSA 4–6 months following the acute infection	No	Yes	Yes
MCUG	No	No	No

Recommended Imaging Schedule for Children 3 Years or Older

Test	Responds well to treatment within 48 hours	Atypical UTI	Recurrent UTI
Ultrasound during the acute infection	No	Yes	No
Ultrasound within 6 weeks	No	No	Yes
DMSA 4–6 months following the acute infection	No	No	Yes
MCUG	No	No	No

Atypical UTI includes the following:

Seriously ill, poor urine flow, abdominal or bladder mass, raised creatinine, septicaemia, failure to respond to treatment with suitable antibiotics within 48 hours, infection with non-*E. coli* organisms.

Recurrent UTI includes the following:

Two or more episodes of UTI with acute pyelonephritis/upper urinary tract infection, or one episode of UTI with acute pyelonephritis/upper urinary tract infection plus one or more episode of UTI with cystitis/lower urinary tract infection, or three or more episodes of UTI with cystitis/lower urinary tract infection.

Urinary tract infection in under 16s: diagnosis and management.
Clinical guideline [CG54] Published date: August 2007. https://www.nice.org.uk/guidance/cg54 [accessed on 22 February 2017].

62. A. T1 MR hypointense; T2 MR hyperintense; contrast enhancement on CT avid

Benign mesothelioma is otherwise known as solitary fibrous tumour of the pleura. Unlike malignant mesothelioma, it has no recognised association with asbestos exposure. It is usually solitary and more commonly arises from the visceral pleura. It is asymptomatic in 50% and is a recognised cause of finger clubbing, hypertrophic pulmonary arthropathy and episodic hypoglycaemia. It is usually sessile but may be pedunculated, in which case shape and location may vary with the patient's position. Imaging characteristics are as above, and contrast enhancement may be heterogeneous if there is myxoid degeneration and haemorrhage. About 14%–30% undergo malignant degeneration. Surgical excision is curative.

Dähnert W. *Radiology Review Manual*, 7th edn. Philadelphia, PA: Lippincott Williams & Wilkins, 2011:524.

63. D. Dilated transverse colon with mucosal islands

Toxic megacolon and perforation are major complications that account for most ulcerative colitis-related deaths. Toxic megacolon is a fulminant form of colitis where inflammation becomes transmural and ulceration leads to neuromuscular degeneration and loss of muscle tone.

The transverse colon is the least dependent part of the colon in the supine patient and therefore gas collects in this location. Dilatation occurs and perforation is likely. Radiographic findings include marked dilatation of the colon with absence of haustral markings, oedema and thickening of the colon wall, pneumatosis coli and perforation. Barium studies should not be performed because of the risk of perforation.

Brant WE, Helmes CA. *Fundamentals of Diagnostic Radiology*, 3rd edn. Philadelphia, PA: Lippincott Williams & Wilkins, 2007:856.

64. C. Inferior mesenteric artery

As the horseshoe kidney ascends, the isthmus comes in contact with the inferior mesenteric artery and halts it, causing the renal pelves to lie inferior and anterior to their normal position. Horseshoe kidney is the most common renal fusion abnormality, which is seen in 1–4 per 1,000 individuals. It occurs when the two kidneys are attached in the midline by their lower poles. There is an increased risk of calculi and infection because of urinary stasis. The risk of trauma is also increased, as in compressive injuries of the abdomen the midline isthmus of the horseshoe is compressed against the spine. In addition, as the kidney is lower-lying than normal, it is less protected by the thoracic cage. There is a three to four times greater risk of malignancies including transitional cell carcinoma, Wilms and occasionally carcinoid.

Brant WE, Helms CA. *Fundamentals of Diagnostic Radiology*, 3rd edn. Philadelphia, PA: Lippincott Williams & Wilkins, 2006:875.

Dähnert W. *Radiology Review Manual*, 7th edn. Philadelphia, PA: Lippincott Williams & Wilkins, 2011: 948–9.

65. C. Type III

The Schatzker classification grades tibial plateau fractures in order of increasing severity based on the pattern of injury.

Type I: Lateral tibial plateau split fracture, no depression

Type II: Lateral tibial plateau split with depression; most common type

Type III: Lateral tibial plateau pure depression only

Type IV: Split and/or depressed fracture of medial tibial plateau

Type V: Fracture of both medial and lateral tibial plateau with the metaphysis still in continuity with the diaphysis

Type VI: Fracture of both tibial plateau and transverse subcondylar tibial fracture with separation of the metaphysis from the diaphysis

Markhardt BK, et al. Schatzker classification of tibial plateau fractures: Use of CT and MR imaging improves assessment. *Radiographics*. 2009;29(2):585–97.

66. A. Increased size of her uterine fibroids

Tamoxifen has weak oestrogen agonist effects in the uterus despite working as an oestrogen antagonist in the breast, to treat breast cancers. Uterine fibroids are oestrogen sensitive and therefore instead of regressing postmenopausally, these women may experience an increase in symptoms because of their fibroids (as many women taking hormone replacement therapy). Tamoxifen can also cause endometrial hyperplasia and an increased risk of endometrial carcinoma.

Formation of multiple ovarian cysts occurs in ovarian hyperstimulation syndrome as a result of clomifene therapy (taken for infertility) and in polycystic ovary syndrome where multiple cysts are characteristically seen around the periphery of enlarged ovaries.

Dähnert W. *Radiology Review Manual*, 7th edn. Philadelphia, PA: Lippincott Williams & Wilkins, 2011:1031.

67. B. Agger nasi cell

Agger nasi is a Latin term literally meaning 'nasal mound'. At rhinoscopy, the agger nasi appears as an eminence located on the lateral nasal wall at the leading edge of the middle turbinate; it represents the intranasal portion of the frontal process of the maxilla. As noted earlier, the agger nasi serves as the anterior limit of the frontal recess. Pneumatisation of the agger nasi (resulting in the so-called agger nasi cell) occurs in 78%–98.5% of individuals.

When present, agger nasi cells are considered the most anterior of all ethmoid cells and can pneumatise posteriorly to narrow the frontal recess. Coronal and sagittal reformatted CT images are most helpful in identifying the agger nasi cell. On coronal images, the agger nasi appears as a laterally placed sinus below the frontal sinus and anterior to the middle turbinate. Sagittal images demonstrate the anterior location of the air cell. Haller cells are extramural ethmoidal air cells extending to the inferomedial orbital floor. Onodi cells are posterior-most ethmoidal cells which lie superolateral to the sphenoid sinus in close relation to the optic nerve and internal carotid artery.

Huang BY, et al. Failed endoscopic sinus surgery: Spectrum of CT findings in the frontal recess. *Radiographics*. 2009;29:177–95.

68. C. Curvature of the interventricular septum to the right

Constrictive pericarditis is most common in men aged 30–50 years. It most commonly occurs following cardiac surgery although it is often idiopathic, with other aetiologies including viruses such as Coxsackie B, tuberculosis and uraemia. The computed tomography scan may show a normal-sized heart with superior vena cava, inferior vena cava and azygos vein dilatation. There is flattening of the right ventricle and curvature of the interventricular septum to the left (rather than to the right) because of high right-ventricular filling pressures. Pericardial thickening and calcification is a feature, as are pleural effusions. Treatment involves surgical stripping of the pericardium. If untreated, protein-losing enteropathy may occur as a result of raised inferior vena cava and portal venous pressures.

Dähnert W. *Radiology Review Manual*, 7th edn. Philadelphia, PA: Lippincott Williams & Wilkins, 2011:641.

69. A. Ascending cholangitis

The overwhelmingly important diagnosis not to be missed in this scenario is ascending cholangitis. This is because ascending cholangitis needs immediate treatment with broad-spectrum antibiotics and biliary drainage via either cholecystectomy or acute laparoscopic cholecystectomy. Although a sonographic-positive Murphy's sign and pericholecystic free fluid suggest a diagnosis of acute cholecystitis, this should not distract the clinician from the presence of cholangitis, which is confirmed by the presence of fever and jaundice and is primarily a clinical diagnosis rather than a radiological one. Acute cholecystitis is not a clinical emergency and in this case is an associated finding that likely predates ascending cholangitis.

Dähnert W. *Radiology Review Manual*, 7th edn. Philadelphia, PA: Lippincott Williams & Wilkins, 2011:710–11.

70. C. Histiocytic response

Histiocytic response describes a macrophage reaction to any component of the arthroplasty (e.g. metal, cement, plastic spacer). The condition tends to occur within 1–5 years after surgery and the characteristic radiographic finding is smooth endosteal scalloping. There is an increased risk of fracture through the affected bone and therefore close follow-up is required. Computed tomography may show a soft-tissue component and appearances can be aggressive.

Stress shielding refers to areas of lucency often in the femur following THR secondary to alterations in bone loading. It predisposes the patient to both periprosthetic fractures and loosening and is more common in uncemented prostheses.

Keogh CF, Munk PL, Gee R, Chan LP, Marchinkow LO. Imaging of the painful hip arthroplasty. *AJR Am J Roentgenol*. 2003;180:115–20.

71. D. Odontogenic keratocyst

Odontogenic keratocysts (OKC) are most commonly located in the body or ramus of the mandible. Most OKCs possess destructive potential, with a high recurrence rate after resection. OKCs develop from the dental lamina, which is found throughout the jaw and overlying alveolar mucosa and is lined by stratified keratinising squamous epithelium. Thus, the cysts can occur throughout periapical or primordial regions. Unlike follicular cysts, OKCs can expand cortical bone and erode the cortex. Fortunately, malignant transformation of these lesions is rare. The lesion is multiloculated, often with daughter cysts that extend to the surrounding bone.

Multiple OKCs in a young patient should raise the possibility of basal cell nevus syndrome (Gorlin–Goltz syndrome). Associated findings with this autosomal dominant disorder include midface hypoplasia, frontal bossing and prognathism, mental retardation and calcification of the falx cerebri.

Dunfee BL, et al. Radiologic and pathologic characteristics of benign and malignant lesions of the mandible. *RadioGraphics*. 2006;26:1751–68.

72. C. If physiological periosteal reaction is present, it is typically asymmetric.

Periosteal bone formation may be due to either physiologic or pathologic causes.

Physiological periosteal new bone formation is seen in up to a third of infants during the first few months of life. They are benign, usually symmetric and involve the long bones (femur, tibia and humerus). Radiographs demonstrate one or more dense lines of periosteal reaction along the diaphyses.

Pathologic bone formation generally results from an adjacent inflammatory process or a hypoxic or toxic stimulus. Common causes of pathologic periosteal reaction in children include trauma to the underlying bone. However, other causes such as hypervitaminosis A, prostaglandin therapy, cortical hyperostosis (Caffey's disease), hypertrophic osteoarthropathy (primary and secondary), osteomyelitis, leukaemia, trauma and syphilis must also be considered. The last four are usually associated with some degree of bone destruction, whereas in the first four diseases the underlying bone is left radiologically intact.

New born periosteal reaction. Paediatric Radiology. School of Medicine, University of Virginia. https://www.med-ed.virginia.edu/courses/rad/peds/ms_webpages/ms6cnewperrxn.html [accessed on 27 September 2016].

Ved N, et al. Periosteal reaction with normal-appearing underlying bone: A child abuse mimicker. *Emerg Radiol*. 2002;9(5):278–82.

73. E. Adamantinoma

Adamantinoma appears as a well-circumscribed, slightly expansile lesion, usually with a narrow zone of transition, a finding consistent with its indolent nature. It is often multilocular, with sclerosis and lysis seen in a 'soap bubble' pattern. The lesion is typically oriented longitudinally along the anterior tibial diaphysis, with an average length of 10 cm.

MR imaging is the best modality for delineating the extent of adamantinoma in the medullary cavity, soft tissues and satellite lesions. These tumours typically demonstrate intermediate signal intensity relative to muscle on T1-weighted images and intensity similar to that of fat on T2-weighted images obtained without fat saturation. Static-enhanced images demonstrate intense homogeneous enhancement within the lesion.

Camp MD, et al. Best cases from the AFIP: Adamantinoma of the tibia and fibula with cytogenetic analysis. *Radiographics*. 2008;28(4):1215–20.

74. E. Ground-glass and solid components to the nodule

A variety of features of solitary pulmonary nodules suggest a benign aetiology. If computed tomography scans have been performed pre- and post-contrast administration, assessment of the degree of enhancement can be performed. Enhancement of less than 15 Hounsfield units strongly favours benignity, whereas enhancement of greater than 15 Hounsfield units could represent malignancy or an inflammatory process. A peripheral rim of enhancement implies benignity but can occur with cavitating tumours such as squamous cell carcinoma. A flattened nodule (axial: craniocaudal diameter ratio of >1.78:1) is also indicative of a benign aetiology, as is central calcification. Partly solid nodules (i.e. solid and ground-glass components) are more likely to represent malignancy, in particular bronchioloalveolar cell carcinoma.

Pretorius ES, Solomon JA. *Radiology Secrets*, 2nd edn. Philadelphia, PA: Elsevier Mosby, 2006:506–8.

75. A. Yersinia

Yersinia enterocolitica is the most common cause of non-stenotic ulcers of the small bowel. It is a Gram-negative organism that causes fever, right iliac fossa pain and diarrhoea. It most commonly affects the terminal ileum. As a human pathogen, *Y. enterocolitica* is most frequently associated with acute diarrhoea, terminal ileitis, mesenteric lymphadenitis and pseudoappendicitis. It may be complicated by abscess formation and has been associated with reactive arthritis. Tuberculosis and lymphoma are also differential diagnoses; however they are less common than yersinial infection. Occasionally, they can only be differentiated by direct visualisation and biopsy rather than by imaging characteristics.

Dähnert W. *Radiology Review Manual*, 7th edn. Philadelphia, PA: Lippincott Williams & Wilkins, 2011:796–7.

Khan ZZ, et al. *Yersinia enterocolitica*. emedicine.medscape.com/article/232343-overview [accessed on 22 February 2017].

76. C. Detachment of a large submucosal fibroid following embolisation

Uterine artery embolisation is an increasingly popular treatment that is used for the treatment of troublesome uterine fibroids; however, complications have been reported. Fibroid passage is one such complication; this is defined as detachment of the treated uterine fibroid. An increased risk of fibroid passage is seen in fibroids abutting the endometrial cavity (e.g. submucosal fibroids). Fibroid passage can precipitate severe pain, infection or recurrent bleeding. In this case, fibroid passage has caused cervical obstruction and pyometra. Cervical carcinoma and a large endometrial polyp can both cause cervical stenosis and consequent pyometra, but they are both much less likely in this circumstance.

Kitamura Y, et al. Imaging manifestations of complications associated with uterine artery embolization. *Radiographics*. 2005;25:S1129–32.

77. D. Homolateral Lisfranc fracture dislocation

Lisfranc injury is a fracture dislocation of the tarso-metatarsal joints in a dorsolateral direction. The second metatarsal is held in a mortise formed by the medial and lateral cuneiform bones. Transverse metatarsal ligaments, both on the plantar and dorsal surfaces, connect the second to fifth metatarsals proximally. There is no transverse ligament between the first and second metatarsal. The plantar ligaments are stronger; hence most dislocations occur dorsally. If there is medial dislocation of the first metatarsal and lateral dislocation of the remaining metatarsals, it is considered a divergent type of Lisfranc injury. If the alignment of the first metatarsal is normal, or if it displaces laterally along with the remaining metatarsals, it is considered the homolateral type. On AP radiography of the foot, the medial aspect of the second metatarsal and middle cuneiform bone should align and, on the oblique view, the medial aspect of the third metatarsal and the lateral cuneiform bone should align.

March fracture is another name for stress fracture, which commonly occurs at the distal shafts of the second and third metatarsals. They may appear on plain radiograph as a lucent line or their presence may be noted secondary to faint periosteal reaction or callus formation. If not visible on plain films and clinical suspicion persists, MRI or radionuclide scan may be helpful.

Lover's fracture is another term for fracture of the calcaneus. Jones fracture occurs in the proximal shaft of the fifth metatarsal. It has a high rate of non-union and is found within 1.5 cm of the fifth metatarsal tuberosity.

Dahnert W. *Radiology Review Manual*, 6th edn. Philadelphia, PA: Lippincott Williams & Wilkins, 2007.

78. C. Tornwaldt's cyst

Tornwaldt's cyst or pharyngeal bursa is an epithelial cyst that is related to the embryogenesis of the notochord. The incidence of Tornwaldt's cysts has been reported in 4% of autopsy specimens and from 0.2% to 5% on MR observation. They occur in the posterior wall of the nasopharynx.

Although Tornwaldt's cysts are present in all age groups, the peak incidences have been reported to occur in various age groups.

The three major symptoms are persistent, noticeable nasal discharge; obstinate occipital headaches; and halitosis and an unpleasant taste in the mouth. According to researchers who have used MR imaging to study Tornwaldt's cyst, this lesion has characteristic high signal intensity on T1-weighted and T2-weighted images.

Ikushima I, et al. MR imaging of Tornwaldt's cysts. *AJR Am J Roentgenol*. 1999;172:1663–5.

79. E. Mastocytosis

Multifocal histiocytosis has a triad (only 10% of patients) of calvarial lesion, exophthalmos and diabetes insipidus. About 40% of patients with Hand–Schüller–Christian disease (multifocal histiocytosis) have destructive lesions affecting the alveolar margins on the mandible. The surrounding radiolucent matrix gives the appearance of floating teeth.

Other conditions such as leukaemia, multiple myeloma and Burkitt lymphoma can also give the appearance of floating teeth. Mastocytosis can cause focal or diffuse sclerotic lesions and does not give the appearance of floating teeth.

Keusch KD, et al. The significance of 'floating teeth' in children. *Radiology*. 1966;86(2):215–19.

80. A. Raised serum calcium levels

The aetiology of alveolar microlithiasis is uncertain, and the condition is characterised by multiple tiny intra-alveolar opacities known as *calcospherites*. The peak age of those affected is 30–50 years, although onset is at a young age, with antenatal onset having been reported. On biochemical profiling, serum calcium and phosphate levels are both normal. There is diffuse involvement of both lungs by submillimetre micronodulations. Uptake on bone scintigraphy is intense. The majority of patients are asymptomatic, although shortness of breath on exertion, cyanosis and digital clubbing may be present. Lungs may appear more dense than the heart shadow on a chest radiograph, and radiographic features are disproportionate to the degree of symptoms.

Dähnert W. *Radiology Review Manual*, 7th edn. Philadelphia, PA: Lippincott Williams & Wilkins, 2011:470.

81. A. Adenocarcinoma of the small bowel

Crohn's disease is a risk factor for the development of small bowel tumours, including lymphoma and small bowel adenocarcinoma. Lymphoma, however, is usually associated with lymphadenopathy and rarely involves the duodenum, being more common in the ileum or stomach. It is also more commonly extraluminal. In contrast, adenocarcinoma is most commonly intraluminal. Hamartomatous polyps are benign polyps usually associated with Peutz–Jeghers syndrome, which is also a risk factor for small bowel adenocarcinoma. Gastrointestinal stromal tumours are usually extramural exophytic masses. Pancreatic carcinoma is not usually associated with Crohn's disease but could cause a bulky tumour mass in this region, although it should arise from the pancreas and invade the duodenum.

Dähnert W. *Radiology Review Manual*, 7th edn. Philadelphia, PA: Lippincott Williams & Wilkins, 2011:813.
Weissleder R, et al. *Primer of Diagnostic Imaging*, 4th edn. Philadelphia, PA: Mosby Elsevier, 2007:196.

82. E.   Papilloma

Papillomas are benign lesions (hyperplastic epithelium on a stalk) usually found in an ectatic subareolar major duct. They are the most common cause of blood or serous discharge. Papillomatosis refers to multiple peripheral papillomas that are located in the duct lumen just proximal to the lobule; it carries an increased risk of malignancy. Ductal ectasia is a benign entity that represents accumulation of cellular debris in enlarged subareolar ducts. Presentation is usually with non-bloody discharge and/or pain. It is the second most common cause of blood or serous discharge. Plasma cell mastitis refers to an inflammatory component associated with extensive secretory calcification.

Weissleder R, et al. *Primer of Diagnostic Imaging*, 4th edn. Philadelphia, PA: Mosby Elsevier, 2007:752.

83. C.   Sjogren's syndrome

Most high-grade mucoepidermoid carcinomas, undifferentiated carcinomas, adenocarcinomas and squamous cell carcinomas of the major salivary glands have low to intermediate signal intensity on long repetition time images. Some malignancies, however, exhibit elevated signal intensity on T2-weighted images. Most commonly, this is seen in low-grade mucoepidermoid carcinomas, in some adenoid cystic carcinoma, and rarely in adenocarcinomas. Among benign masses that are not hyperintense on long repetition time images, Warthin's tumour, the second most common benign mass in the adult parotid gland, is often of intermediate, low or mixed signal intensity on T2-weighted images.

The chronic sialadenitis, such as Sjögren disease, Mikulicz disease (also known as Sjögren Type 1 or sicca syndrome without a connective tissue disorder) and radiation sialadenitis may also appear hypointense on T2-weighted images. In most series, these exceptions account for the 25% error rate that occurs if one relies solely on signal intensity on T2-weighted images to predict histologic diagnosis.

Yousem DM, et al. Major salivary gland imaging. *Radiology*. 2000;216:19–29.

84. A.   Cartilage injury

Conventional radiographs demonstrate physeal widening, irregularity and fragmentation. MR imaging can be used to further characterise the injury by demonstrating oedema in the adjacent bone on T2-weighted or STIR MR images and focal extensions of unmineralised cartilage into the metaphysis, which appear as 'tongues' of high signal intensity on T2-weighted, STIR and gradient-recalled echo (GRE) images and as intermediate signal intensity on T1-weighted images. Continued overuse leads to further physeal widening, irregularity and occasionally bone bridging.

Jaimes C, et al. Taking the stress out of evaluating stress injuries in children. *Radiographics*. 2012; 32(2):537–55.

85. D.   Pars flaccida (attic) cholesteatomas are located at the lower one-third portion of the tympanic membrane.

Cholesteatomas can be classified as either congenital or acquired, though the origins are indistinguishable with histology and imaging. Only the location of the lesion, the clinical history of the patient, and the otologic status of the tympanic membrane (TM) give some idea how to differentiate these two types of cholesteatomas.

Congenital cholesteatomas develop from embryonic epithelial rests and can be located anywhere in the temporal bone: in the middle ear, in the mastoid, in the petrous apex in the squama of the temporal bone, within the TM or in the external auditory canal (EAC). Furthermore, the same histologic entity can arise in other areas of the skull, in the extracranial soft tissues or in an intracranial extra-axial location, where it is referred to as *epidermoid cyst*. Middle ear congenital cholesteatomas represent approximately 2% of all middle ear cholesteatomas. Primary acquired cholesteatomas (80% of all middle ear cholesteatomas) develop behind an apparently intact TM, usually in the region of the pars flaccida.

Secondary acquired cholesteatomas (18% of all middle ear cholesteatomas) grow into the middle ear through a perforated TM, usually through the pars tensa and sometimes the pars flaccida. Pars flaccida (attic) cholesteatomas are located at the upper one-third portion of the TM.

Pars tensa (sinus) cholesteatomas develop most often through a defect of the lower two-thirds portion of the TM.

Barath K, et al. Neuroradiology of cholesteatomas. *AJNR Am J Neuroradiol.* 2011;32:221–9.

86. B. Round and hypoechoic node

US criteria for benign versus malignant nodes:

	Benign	Malignant
B mode scan criteria		
Size	Small	Large >1 cm/>1.5 cm short-axis diameter (SAD); size is a poor predictor on its own
Shape	Oval	Round
Hilum	Present	Absent
Echogenicity	Iso to slightly hypo	Markedly hypo
Margins		
Focal cortical nodules	Absent	Present
Intranodal necrosis	Absent	Present
Reticulation	Absent	Present
Calcification	Absent	Present
Matting	Absent	Present
Doppler criteria		
Flow	Absent	Present
Vessel location	Central	Peripheral
Vascular pedicle	Single	Multiple
Vascular pattern	Regular	Chaotic
Impedance values	Low	High

Dudea SM, et al. Ultrasonography of superficial lymph nodes: Benign vs. malignant. *Med Ultrason.* 2012; 14(4):294–306.

87. C. Ankylosing spondylitis

Ventilation in the lungs is better in the upper zones than in the lower zones. By contrast, perfusion is better in the lower zones than in the upper zones. Accordingly, there is a tendency for occupational dust exposure to cause interstitial fibrosis with a predominantly upper zone distribution (although asbestosis is a notable exception, with a lower zone distribution). Ankylosing spondylitis also has an upper zone distribution. Lower zone fibrosis tends to arise as a result of haematogenous factors. Hence, drug-induced fibrosis (e.g. that caused by methotrexate) and collagen vascular diseases (such as systemic lupus erythematosus, rheumatoid arthritis and scleroderma) show lower zone predominance. Idiopathic pulmonary fibrosis is the most common cause of lower zone interstitial fibrosis.

Pretorius ES, Solomon JA. *Radiology Secrets*, 2nd edn. Philadelphia, PA: Elsevier Mosby, 2006:517–27.

88. D. Malignant GIST (gastrointestinal stromal tumour)

Gastrointestinal stromal tumours are the most common mesenchymal tumours of the gastrointestinal tract. They are usually found around the stomach and are often exophytic in nature. Commonly, they are found incidentally and can become very large before causing symptoms. These are difficult to distinguish from leiomyomas, leiomyosarcomas, schwannomas and neurofibromas radiologically and are characterised on immunohistochemistry by their expression of the KIT gene. It is important to appropriately identify GISTs as these can be treated successfully with tyrosine kinase inhibitors (Glivec®). Gastrointestinal stromal tumours can metastasise to the liver and peritoneum but lymphadenopathy is very uncommon. Once these tumours are over 5 cm malignancy becomes more likely.

Lymphoma would usually be associated with lymphadenopathy. A gastric adenocarcinoma of this size would also be likely to have associated lymphadenopathy. Gastric lipoma should not enhance and be of low attenuation. Ectopic pancreas is usually endoluminal with an ill-defined border and is more often found in the antrum of the stomach and duodenum.

Dähnert W. *Radiology Review Manual*, 7th edn. Philadelphia, PA: Lippincott Williams & Wilkins, 2011:853–4.
Kim HC, et al. Gastrointestinal stromal tumours of the stomach: CT findings and prediction of malignancy. *AJR Am J Roentgenol*. 2004;183:893–8.
Kim HC, et al. Ectopic pancreas: CT findings with emphasis on differentiation from small gastrointestinal stromal tumour and leiomyoma. *Radiology*. 2009;252:92–100.
Weissleder R, et al. *Primer of Diagnostic Imaging*, 4th edn. Philadelphia, PA: Mosby Elsevier, 2007:177.

89. B. The absence of the lateral epicondyle ossification centre is often a normal finding in a 12-year-old.

The ossification centres occur in order of appearance according to the commonly recited mnemonic CRITOE – capitellum, radial, internal (medial epicondyle), trochlear, olecranon and external (lateral epicondyle). Although the associated age groups are commonly stated as 1, 3, 5, 7, 9 and 11 years of age, respectively, there is actually some variability, particularly as the final ossification centres appear. As such, the lateral epicondyle ossification centre may not appear until age 13. Medial epicondyle avulsion injuries are far more common than lateral epicondyle avulsion injuries. The common extensor tendon inserts onto the lateral epicondyle and the common flexor tendons insert onto the medial epicondyle.

Dahnert W. *Radiology Review Manual*, 6th edn. Philadelphia, PA: Lippincott Williams & Wilkins, 2007.

90. D. Gymnast's wrist results in negative ulnar variance

In Little Leaguer's shoulder, excessive overhead throwing leads to widening and irregularity of the proximal humeral physis on radiographs and MR images. In gymnast's wrist, repetitive weight-bearing on the wrist can lead to physeal stress changes of the distal portion of the radius and, occasionally, the ulna. Abnormal distal radial growth produces positive ulnar variance. At a later stage, this could be associated with injury to the TFC complex. The valgus stress of the cocking and acceleration phases of pitching results in a traction injury to the medial epicondyle that is known as *Little Leaguer's elbow*. MR imaging is more sensitive than conventional radiography for detecting physeal changes.

Jaimes C, et al. Taking the stress out of evaluating stress injuries in children. *Radiographics*. 2012; 32(2):537–55.

91. B. Two-chamber view in mid-diastole

In cardiac CT imaging, standard views include the four-chamber (both atria and ventricles), three-chamber (left ventricle and atrium and aortic root), two-chamber (left atrium and ventricle) and short axis projection views. Five-chamber views (both atria and ventricles and aortic root) can also be used. These views are usually formulated using maximal intensity projection technique on source images, with two-chamber, three-chamber and four-chamber views obtained by rotating the imaging plane along the left ventricle's long axis. Combinations A through E will all demonstrate the mitral valve, but the two-chamber view taken in mid-diastole is the optimal view and timing for the assessment of the mitral valve.

Chen JJ, et al. CT angiography of the cardiac valves: Normal, diseased and postoperative appearances. *Radiographics*. 2009;29:1393–412.
Halpern EJ. *Clinical Cardiac CT: Anatomy and Function*. New York: Thieme, 2008:146–9.

92. E.   Haemochromatosis

The patient is likely to have undetected haemochromatosis; the dense liver will be caused by iron deposition and this would give a low signal on T2-weighted (especially T2*) magnetic resonance images. Deposition in the pancreas and gonads can cause diabetes, erectile dysfunction and hypogonadism, respectively. Haemochromatosis is often termed *bronze diabetes*, as there is hyperpigmentation in the skin because of the deposition of iron. It is known to cause osteoarthritic changes at many joints because of iron deposition, and the most characteristic place for this to occur is the metacarpo-phalangeal joints, especially the second and third, where there may also be hook-like osteophytes.

Amyloidosis causes a decrease in the liver density. Wilson disease can give a dense liver and is associated with arthropathy, although this is usually of the large joints and spine; it does not cause diabetes and more often causes neuropsychiatric complaints. Haemophilia would tend to present as an arthropathy first involving multiple joints and at a younger age. The dense liver may be caused by repeated blood transfusions but is less likely to be associated with diabetes in this case. Gaucher disease (the most common glycogen storage disease) tends to present earlier in life, although late cases are not unheard of. They tend to present with splenomegaly, lytic bone lesions and haematological upset.

Chapman S, Nakielny R. *Aids to Radiological Differential Diagnosis*, 4th edn. London: Saunders Elsevier, 2003;297:555–6.

Georgiades CS, et al. Amyloidosis: Review and CT manifestations. *Radiographics*. 2004;24:405–16.

Weissleder R, et al. *Primer of Diagnostic Imaging*, 4th edn. Philadelphia, PA: Mosby Elsevier, 2007:214.

93. C.   Radionuclide imaging using an analogue of guanethidine such as metaiodobenzylguanidine (MIBG)

An MIBG scan will help evaluate an extra-adrenal paraganglioma. Radionuclide imaging using an analogue of guanethidine such as MIBG is concentrated in sympatho-adrenal tissue and is thus used to image adrenal medullary disorders.

Adam A, et al. *Grainger & Allison's Diagnostic Radiology: A Textbook of Medical Imaging*, 5th edn. New York: Churchill Livingstone, 2008;1723:1729–30.

94. C.   Prostate cancer metastases

Metastases to bone are 15–100 times more common than primary skeletal neoplasms and are found at sites of dominant haematopoietic marrows because of its rich haematopoietic marrow. In adults, this includes the calvarium, spine, flat bones and proximal humeral and femoral metaphyses. Focal sclerotic lesions are hypointense on T1 and T2-weighted sequences. The most common metastases in adult men are due to prostate carcinoma. Renal metastases are usually lytic. Haemangiomas are hyperintense on both T1 and T2-weighted sequences.

Dähnert W. *Radiology Review Manual*, 7th edn. Philadelphia, PA: Lippincott Williams & Wilkins, 2011.

95. B.   Premaxillary and retro-antral fat are rarely involved.

The combination of necrotising granulomatous lesions of the upper and lower respiratory tracts, generalised necrotising vasculitis of arteries and veins and glomerulonephritisis is called Granulomatosis and polyangitis (previously called Wegener's granulomatosis). The disease may affect the eyes, skin, joints, muscles and cardiac system as well as the paranasal sinuses, lungs and kidneys.

Advanced Wegener's granulomatosis may lead to destructive lesions of the hard palate, sinonasal-oral fistulas or complete nasal septal destruction.

The premaxillary soft tissues, retro-antral fat, pterygopalatine fossa, infratemporal fossa and orbits are commonly involved. Sarcoidosis may have a similar appearance.

When a destructive mass in the nasal septum extends into the orbits, Wegener's granulomatosis should be considered in the differential diagnosis. Intracranial involvement may also result, usually in the anterior cranial fossa, owing to the spread of the disease through the cribriform plate.

As the disease becomes chronic, the walls of the residual paranasal sinuses (particularly the maxillary sinuses) become markedly thickened while the sinus volume is gradually reduced, and the nasal septum may completely disappear.

Valencia MP, Castillo M. Congenital and acquired lesions of the nasal septum: A practical guide for differential diagnosis. *Radiographics*. 2008;28:205–23.

96. D. Absence of drop metastases on MRI spine imaging

The description would fit with a medulloblastoma. Drop metastases are commonly found at presentation, and complete imaging of the neuraxis is strongly recommended at diagnosis.

Cerebrospinal fluid (CSF) seeding, with the resultant formation of spinal intradural 'drop metastases', is a well-known mode of dissemination for many intracranial neoplasms. This manner of tumour spread is most commonly observed in medulloblastoma. Ependymomas, anaplastic gliomas, germinomas, choroid plexus tumours and pineal parenchymal tumours (pineoblastomas and pineocytomas) are other intracranial tumours that frequently deposit metastases in the spinal canal.

Intradural metastases may also occur as a result of haematogenous spread from extracranial neoplasms, most commonly lung and breast adenocarcinoma and from haematological malignancies.

Ahmed A. MRI features of disseminated "drop metastases." *S Afr Med J*. 2008;98(7):522–3.

97. B. Grade 2

The most common location for injury to the premature brain is the periventricular white matter, with ischaemic parenchyma manifesting as periventricular leukomalacia (PVL). Initial sonograms show hyperechogenic globular change in the periventricular regions, and MR images depict areas of T1 hyperintensity within larger areas of T2 hyperintensity. Subsequent cavitation and periventricular cyst formation, features that are required for a definitive diagnosis of PVL, develop 2–6 weeks after injury and are easily seen on sonograms as localised anechoic or hypoechoic lesions. The progressive change ventricular dilatation occurs, described as end-stage PVL.

Subsequent reperfusion to the ischaemic tissues in the setting of weakened capillaries and increased venous pressure result in germinal matrix haemorrhage, ranging in severity from subependymal haemorrhage (Grade 1) to intraventricular haemorrhage without (Grade 2) and with (Grade 3) ventricular dilatation, to parenchymal extension and coexisting periventricular venous infarction (Grade 4).

Chao CP, et al. Neonatal hypoxic-ischemic encephalopathy: Multimodality imaging findings. *Radiographics*. 2006;26(Suppl 1):S159–72.

98. B. Presence of microcalcification

These are general recommendations for adult patients who have a thyroid nodule on US images, regardless of how the nodule was initially detected.

The recommendations may not apply to all patients, including those who have historical, physical or any other features suggesting they are at increased risk for cancer or who have a history of thyroid cancer.

Part I

The following are general recommendations for nodules 1.0 cm or greater in largest diameter:

Solitary nodule:

Strongly consider FNA for (1) a nodule 1.0 cm or more in largest diameter if microcalcifications are present and (2) a nodule 1.5 cm or more in largest diameter if any of the following apply: (a) nodule is solid or almost entirely solid or (b) there are coarse calcifications within the nodule.

Consider FNA for (1) a nodule 2.0 cm or more in largest diameter if any of the following apply: (a) the nodule is mixed solid and cystic or (b) the nodule is almost entirely cystic with a solid mural component; or (2) the nodule has shown substantial growth since prior US examination. FNA is likely unnecessary if the nodule is almost entirely cystic, in the absence of the above-listed features.

Multiple nodules:

Consider FNA of one or more nodules, with selection prioritised on the basis of the previously stated criteria in the order listed above. FNA is likely unnecessary in diffusely enlarged glands with multiple nodules of similar US appearance without intervening normal parenchyma.

Note that these recommendations are not absolute or inflexible. In certain circumstances, the physician's clinical judgment may lead him or her to determine that FNA need not be performed for nodules that meet the recommendations above. In others, FNA may be appropriate for nodules that do not meet the criteria listed above.

Part II

The recommendation for non-diagnostic aspirates from initial FNA is as follows: Consider a second FNA of nodules meeting the criteria for FNA of solitary nodules, as outlined above.

Part III

The presence of abnormal lymph nodes overrides the US features criteria and should prompt biopsy of the lymph node and/or (if necessary) of an ipsilateral thyroid nodule.

Frates MC, et al. Management of thyroid nodules detected at US: Society of radiologists ultrasound consensus conference statement. *Radiology*. 2005;237:794–800.

99. A. Transection of the proximal thoracic duct

Disruption of the thoracic duct results in a chylothorax. The thoracic duct measures 45 cm and commences at the level of T12, ascending on the right side of the aorta, crossing the midline at the level of T5 and ascending in the left hemithorax to drain into the confluence of the left subclavian and internal jugular veins. Accordingly, disruption of the proximal thoracic duct results in a right-sided pleural effusion, and disruption of the distal thoracic duct causes a left-sided pleural effusion. Dissecting aneurysm of the thoracic aorta and traumatic rupture of the aorta both result in left-sided effusions, as does spontaneous oesophageal rupture (Boerhaave syndrome) and gastric carcinoma. Pancreatitis can give rise to bilateral or unilateral pleural effusions, with more than two-thirds of pancreatitis-related effusions occurring on the left.

Dähnert W. *Radiology Review Manual*, 7th edn. Philadelphia, PA: Lippincott Williams & Wilkins, 2011:445.

100. A. In-phase and out-of-phase T1-weighted images

The hyperechoic area seen on ultrasound anteriorly within Segment 4 is most commonly caused by focal fatty infiltration and is a common finding at ultrasound and is more common in heavy drinkers, hyperlipidaemia and in obese patients. It is also commonly seen at the portal bifurcation. Although all of the above sequences will be important in accurately defining the lesion, the most useful sequence when this is likely to be focal fatty infiltration will be the in-phase and out-of-phase T1-weighted images. Focal fat should lose signal between the in-phase T1-weighted images and the out-of-phase T1-weighted images.

Middleton WD, et al. *Ultrasound: The Requisites*, 2nd edn. St Louis, MO: Mosby, 2004.
Sohn J, et al. Unusual patterns of hepatic steatosis caused by the local effect of insulin revealed on chemical shift MR imaging. *AJR Am J Roentgenol*. 2001;176:471–4.

101. C. MIBG, an analogue of guanethidine, is used to image adrenal cortical disorders.

All the statements are correct except option C. MIBG, an analogue of guanethidine, is used to image adrenal medullary disorders. [18]F FDG has been reported to be able to differentiate between benign adenomas and metastases.

Adam A, et al. *Grainger & Allison's Diagnostic Radiology: A Textbook of Medical Imaging*, 5th edn. New York: Churchill Livingstone, 2008;1723:1729–30.

102. E. The AC ligament and CC ligament are ruptured with detachment of the deltoid muscle.

The Rockwood classification is used to classify ACJ injuries. Lifting of the clavicle above the superior border of the acromion implies a severe strain injury with typical complete derangement of the internal attachments and stabilising structures (Grade III injury). Grade IV–VI injuries also imply the same degree of soft-tissue injuries, but there is accompanying complete dislocation with the clavicle displacing into various positions.

Grade I injuries have an intact CC with AC ligament strain. Grade II injuries (elevation of the clavicle but not above the superior border of the acromion) have a ruptured AC ligament and joint capsule, with strain of the CC ligament.

Rockwood CA, et al. Acromioclavicular injuries. In: Rockwood CA, et al., eds. *Fractures in Adults*, 4th edn. Vol I. Philadelphia, PA: Lippincott-Raven, 1996:1341–413.

103. D. Mounier–Kuhn disease

Tracheobronchomegaly, known as *Mounier–Kuhn disease*, is a rare condition, usually affecting men in the fourth and fifth decade of life. It is characterised by marked dilatation of the trachea and bronchi. Patients typically present with recurrent respiratory infections and bronchitis. It is caused by atrophy and dysplasia of the tracheal wall and the tracheal diameter is usually more than 3 cm.

Tracheopathia osteoplastica is a rare benign disease affecting the trachea and characterised by multiple submucosal osteocartilaginous growths within the anterior and lateral walls. This condition, as the others listed above (relapsing polychondritis, tracheal Wegener's granulomatosis, tracheal sarcoidosis), cause significant narrowing of the tracheal diameter with wall thickening and symptoms of stridor, wheeze, cough and dyspnoea.

Kwong JS, et al. Diseases of the trachea and main-stem bronchi: Correlation of CT with pathologic findings. *Radiographics*. 1992;12:645–57.
Weissleder R, et al. *Primer of Diagnostic Imaging*, 4th edn. Philadelphia, PA: Mosby Elsevier, 2007:49.

104. D. Carcinoid syndrome

Carcinoid syndrome is a collection of symptoms that are caused by a small proportion of carcinoid tumours. This nearly always occurs following metastasis to the liver, although it can happen if a carcinoid tumour occurs outside the gut and its excreted chemicals (adrenocorticotropic hormone, histamine, serotonin, etc.) bypass liver metabolism. These chemicals cause recurrent diarrhoea, bronchospasm, flushing and right-sided heart failure. A spiculated mesenteric mass with calcification and a desmoplastic effect on the adjacent bowel in a patient with these symptoms is characteristic of carcinoid syndrome. These tumours are often hyperintense on T2-weighted magnetic resonance imaging as they are very vascular. They also produce hypervascular metastases. If there is carcinoid syndrome, the carcinoid tumour is usually located in small bowel.

Malignant melanomas are often bright on T1 and do not usually give a desmoplastic mesenteric reaction or give flushing. Cholangiocarcinomas produce hypervascular liver metastases but mesenteric deposits are unusual and the biliary tree appeared normal in this case. Retractile mesenteritis would not cause liver lesions. Mesenteric abscesses from cholecystitis would be rare and only the rim should enhance with gadolinium. This condition would also not be expected to produce a desmoplastic reaction.

Bader TR, et al. MRI of carcinoid tumours: Spectrum of appearances in the gastrointestinal tract and liver. *J Magn Reson Imag*. 2001;14:261–9.

Dähnert W. *Radiology Review Manual*, 7th edn. Philadelphia, PA: Lippincott Williams & Wilkins, 2011:826–8.
Horton KM, et al. Carcinoid tumours of the small bowel: A multitechnique imaging approach. *AJR Am J Roentgenol*. 2004;182:559–67.
Weissleder R, et al. *Primer of Diagnostic Imaging*, 4th edn. Philadelphia, PA: Mosby Elsevier, 2007:191.

105. E.   Uraemic cystic disease

About 40% of patients with end-stage renal disease develop renal cysts. The incidence increases with time on dialysis so that incidence of uraemic cystic disease is 90% in patients 5 years on dialysis. Associated complications include haemorrhage within the cysts and rarely malignancy. Cysts regress after successful transplantation.

Weissleder R, et al. *Primer of Diagnostic Imaging*, 4th edn. Philadelphia, PA: Mosby Elsevier, 2007:289.

106. D.   Cervical spine CT.

In high-risk patients or patients with limited physical examination, given the relative insensitivity of plain films, CT should be performed. In a rheumatoid patient there is an increased risk of cervical injury. Repeat views would not be of benefit.

Age and mechanism of injury would indicate CT cervical spine according to NICE guidelines.

Blackmore CC, et al. Cervical spine screening with CT in trauma patients: A cost-effective analysis. *Radiology*. 1999;212:117–25.
Head injury: Assessment and early management. NICE guidelines [CG176], https://www.nice.org.uk/guidance/cg176 [accessed on 22 February 2017].

107. B.   Stress fracture of the femoral neck involves the superior surface.

The most common cause of stress fractures is a chronic and repeated workload. Children with extremity malalignment or abnormal weight-bearing also are at increased risk. Typical locations of stress fractures in children include the tibia, fibula, femur and tarsal and metatarsal bones. MR imaging is currently the best diagnostic modality for stress fractures.

Stress fractures of the femur tend to occur after skeletal maturity and resemble adult injuries, affecting the inferior surface of the neck, the shaft and the distal metaphysis. This injury is most common in endurance athletes, such as runners, triathletes or soccer players but also occurs in association with abnormal weight-bearing, such as with a coxa vara deformity.

The most common site for stress fractures in the adolescent athlete is the tibia. Tibial stress fractures occur with activities requiring sudden stops or changes in direction, such as football, soccer and tennis.

Stress also can result in shin splints, which are probably an early stress response secondary to periosteal traction. In cases of stress fractures, MR imaging shows diffuse and irregular bone marrow oedema, whereas in shin splints, the area of high signal intensity often is more linear and is limited to the medial aspect of the tibia.

Spondylolysis is a stress injury of the pars interarticularis that is due to repetitive extension and torsion of the trunk. Usually occurring in the lower segments of the lumbar spine, stress injuries of the pars interarticularis have been observed in young female gymnasts, college football players and wrestlers.

Jaimes C, et al. Taking the stress out of evaluating stress injuries in children. *Radiographics*. 2012; 32(2):537–55.

108. B.   Destruction of underlying bone is normally seen at presentation on plain radiography.

If joint inflammation is limited to a single joint, infection must first be carefully excluded. The cause of septic arthritis is usually related to haematogenous seeding owing to staphylococcal or streptococcal microorganisms.

The radiographic features of a septic joint encompass those of any inflammatory arthritis – namely, periarticular osteopenia, uniform joint space narrowing, soft-tissue swelling and bone erosions. Not all findings may be present simultaneously, and, acutely, bone erosions may not be evident. Furthermore, the joint space may be initially widened owing to the effusion. Joint space widening may also be seen with more indolent and atypical infections, such as those related to tuberculosis and fungal agents.

The Phemister triad describes these findings classically seen in tuberculous arthritis: juxta-articular osteopenia, peripheral bone erosions and gradual narrowing of the joint space.

The presence of anterior capsular distension was noted as convexity of the anterior recess and compared to contralateral normal side in equivocal cases.

Bhargava S, Bhargava SK. Infective arthritis of hip: Role of sonography. *JIMSA*. 2013;26(1):15–16.

Jacobson JA, et al. Radiographic evaluation of arthritis: Inflammatory conditions. *Radiology*. 2008;248(2):378–89.

109. A. Malignant melanoma

About 90% of all tracheal tumours are malignant and of those metastases are the most common group. Malignant melanoma, renal cell tumour, breast carcinoma and colonic adenocarcinoma are the most common sources of haematogenous metastatic spread to the tracheal mucosa. The lesions are usually multiple, polypoid, well defined and without tracheal wall thickening or extratracheal extension, as commonly seen in primary tracheal tumours. Cancers of the thyroid, oesophagus, larynx and lung may invade the tracheal wall by direct extension from the primary source, and this type of spread is the most common in secondary tracheal malignancies. The symptoms of tracheal malignancies are non-specific and include haemoptysis, dyspnoea, chest pain, cough and wheeze.

Dähnert W. *Radiology Review Manual*, 7th edn. Philadelphia, PA: Lippincott Williams & Wilkins, 2011:455.

110. A. Hashimoto thyroiditis

Hashimoto thyroiditis, also known as *chronic autoimmune lymphocytic thyroiditis*, is a disease with a typical clinical presentation of painless diffuse enlargement of the thyroid gland accompanied by hypothyroidism and thyroid autoantibodies. The sonographic appearance of Hashimoto thyroiditis is well recognised. The gland is often diffusely enlarged, and the parenchyma is coarsened, hypoechoic and often hypervascular. A micronodular pattern on ultrasound is highly diagnostic of Hashimoto thyroiditis with a positive predictive value of 95%. Discrete nodules may, however, also occur within diffusely altered parenchyma or within sonographically normal parenchyma. The nodular form of Hashimoto thyroiditis has not received nearly as much analysis as the diffuse form, and the reported findings have been variable.

Anderson L, et al. Hashimoto thyroiditis: Part 1, sonographic analysis of the nodular form of hashimoto thyroiditis. *AJR Am J Roentgenol*. 2010;195:208–15.

111. D. Atrophic gastritis

Atrophic gastritis has a high association with B12 deficiency. It occurs in the older population and is often caused by autoimmune disease. However, it can also be caused by *Helicobacter pylori*, leading to chronic inflammation of the gastric mucosa and eventually fibrosis. Atrophic gastritis particularly affects the chief and parietal cells, resulting in achlorhydria and B12 deficiency, and causes the classic featureless stomach. It is associated with an increased risk of gastric carcinoma.

Infectious gastritis, Ménétrier disease and eosinophilic gastritis are often associated with thickened folds. Linitis plastica would have a history of weight loss and iron deficiency anaemia as opposed to B12 deficiency.

Adam A, et al. *Grainger & Allison's Diagnostic Radiology: A Textbook of Medical Imaging*, 5th edn. New York: Churchill Livingstone, 2008:635–7.

112. C. Transvaginal ultrasound

This patient has a suspected ectopic pregnancy, which is a potentially fatal gynaecological emergency. Transvaginal ultrasound (TVUS) can detect intrauterine pregnancy 1 week sooner than transabdominal ultrasound (TAUS). If no intrauterine pregnancy (IUP) is seen on TAUS, you should therefore confirm that there is no IUP by TVUS where possible. The free fluid in this case is the result of a ruptured bleeding tube secondary to an ectopic pregnancy; the fluid may be echogenic because of blood content. TVUS is preferable to CT, as the patient may have a viable early pregnancy. In hospitals where TVUS is not available, emergency laparoscopy may be considered. However, MRI is not a safe environment for a potentially unstable patient.

Chapman S, Nakielny R. *Aids to Radiological Differential Diagnosis*, 4th edn. London: Saunders Elsevier, 2003:496.

Dähnert W. *Radiology Review Manual*, 7th edn. Philadelphia, PA: Lippincott Williams & Wilkins, 2011:1054–5.

113. C. Periarticular osteoporosis

Degenerative arthritis and *osteoarthritis* are interchangeable terms that can be used to describe the clinical and radiographic joint changes associated with ageing.

Early changes include damage to the articular cartilage with progressive damage to and loss of the ground substance that eventually leads to the subchondral bone being exposed.

Clinically, patients present with joint pain worsened with use and the joint may be found on examination to be enlarged, deformed, tender with crepitus and possibly display joint effusion.

The five radiographic hallmarks are asymmetrical joint space narrowing, subchondral sclerosis, subchondral cysts, osteophytes and lack of osteoporosis. Periarticular osteoporosis is much more characteristic of rheumatoid arthritis.

Weissleder R, et al. *Primer of Diagnostic Imaging*, 4th edn. Philadelphia, PA: Mosby Elsevier, 2007:450–2.

114. C. There is associated dilatation of the superior ophthalmic vein.

Graves' disease of the orbit is also known as *thyroid ophthalmopathy* or *endocrine exophthalmos*. It is produced by long-acting thyroid stimulating hormone, probably due to cross reactivity against antigens shared by thyroid and orbital tissue. Signs and symptoms usually develop within 1 year of hyperparathyroidism. It is the most common cause of unilateral/bilateral proptosis in adults. It commonly involves the inferior rectus first (mnemonic – I'M SLOW). The superior ophthalmic vein is dilated due to compromised orbital venous drainage at the orbital apex. There is increased density of the orbital fat late in the disease.

Dähnert W. *Radiology Review Manual*, 7th edn. Philadelphia, PA: Lippincott Williams & Wilkins, 2011:348–9.

115. C. Squamous cell carcinoma of the urethra

Primary urethral carcinoma is rare. About 50%–75% occur in the bulbar urethra and nearly 90% are squamous type, particularly if there has been a stricture in the past. Urethral carcinoma is often advanced at diagnosis, explaining the weight loss. Primary transitional cell carcinomas (TCC) are closer to the bladder neck, although secondary TCCs can occur anywhere in the urethra when seeded from the bladder in patients with a bladder TCC history, when they are often multiple (these are the most commonly encountered male urethral tumours). Adenocarcinomas are extremely rare and tend to occur at the prostatic utricle or glands of Littre. Haematogenous metastases to the urethra are exceedingly rare but are most likely to be from melanoma. Prostatic carcinoma would be more likely to involve the prostatic urethra. Benign strictures can appear a little irregular, but weight loss would not be expected.

Lynch D. *Carcinoma of the Urethra*. American Medical Network. http://www.health.am/cr/urethral-carcinoma/ [accessed on 24 February 2017].

Weissleder R, et al. *Primer of Diagnostic Imaging*, 4th edn. Philadelphia, PA: Mosby Elsevier, 2007:318–19.

116. C. Tracheomalacia

Weakening of the tracheal walls associated with posterior tracheal wall collapse during expiration is a recognised complication post-intubation and tracheal tube placement, when the cuff pressures exceed 25 cmH$_2$O. This condition is often underdiagnosed as it can present with non-specific symptoms such as shortness of breath, wheeze, stridor and recurrent chest infections. Dynamic CT scan during inspirational and expirational phases is the modality of choice for its diagnosis, and it is considered positive when the AP diameter of the trachea decreases more than 50% during expiration. Tracheomalacia may also be a complication of chronic obstructive pulmonary disease (COPD), relapsing polychondritis and recurrent infections.

Tracheal diverticulum and saber-sheath trachea (decreased coronal diameter of trachea) are conditions associated with COPD, and carrot-shaped trachea refers to a narrowing of the tracheal diameter in the caudal direction as a result of an aberrant left pulmonary artery.

Webb EM, et al. Using CT to diagnose nonneoplastic tracheal abnormalities: Appearance of the tracheal wall. *AJR Am J Roentgenol.* 2000;174:1315–21.
Weissleder R, et al. *Primer of Diagnostic Imaging*, 4th edn. Philadelphia, PA: Mosby Elsevier, 2007:107.

117. C. Small bowel lymphoma

Small bowel lymphoma is a soft pliable tumour and therefore can often be quite large in size without causing a bowel obstruction. Characteristically, it destroys Auerbach's plexus, leading to aneurysmal dilatation of the small bowel; however, this is a rare finding. It often fistulates, mimicking Crohn's disease, but there would be more likely to be skip lesions with Crohn's disease. Tuberculosis can have similar appearance, but these patients will often be from an endemic area or have HIV; fever and night sweats will also be more prominent, although these symptoms can also occur in lymphoma.

Adam A, et al. *Grainger & Allison's Diagnostic Radiology: A Textbook of Medical Imaging*, 5th edn. New York: Churchill Livingstone, 2008:668–9.
Annand MKN, et al. *Gastrointestinal Tuberculosis.* emedicine.medscape.com/article/376015-overview [accessed on 24 February 2017].
Dähnert W. *Radiology Review Manual*, 7th edn. Philadelphia, PA: Lippincott Williams & Wilkins, 2011:867.

118. B. Liposarcoma

Liposarcoma is a malignant tumour of mesenchymal origin; it is the second most common soft-tissue sarcoma in adults after malignant fibrous histiocytoma (now called pleomorphic undifferentiated sarcoma or PUS). It usually presents in the fifth to sixth decade. On CT, it is seen as a non-specific soft-tissue mass, as the fat content is usually not radiologically detectable. On MRI, because of the high content of myxoid cells (the most common type of liposarcoma), it is low signal on T1-weighted sequences and high signal on T2-weighted sequences.

A lipoma would not be expected to enhance post-contrast. A large lymph node would be unlikely to reach the sizes described and additionally may be hyperintense to muscle on T1-weighted sequences. A soft-tissue fibroma would have a small hypointense nodule on all sequences. Lipoblastoma usually affects children less than 3 years of age.

Dähnert W. *Radiology Review Manual*, 7th edn. Philadelphia, PA: Lippincott Williams & Wilkins, 2011.
Kransdorf MJ, et al. Imaging of fatty tumors: Distinction of lipoma and well-differentiated liposarcoma. *Radiology.* 2002;224:99–104.

119. D. The beta angle can help to determine the dysplasia subtype.

The Graf method for ultrasound classification system for developmental dysplasia of the hip (DDH) in infants combines both the alpha and beta angles. The alpha angle is formed by the acetabular roof to the vertical cortex of the ilium.

The normal value is greater than or equal to 60 degrees. Less than 60 degrees suggests acetabular dysplasia.

The beta angle is defined as the angle formed between the vertical cortex of the ilium and the triangular labral fibrocartilage (echogenic triangle). There is a great deal of variability in the beta angle and is not universally used.

The beta angle is necessary to determine the subtype of hip dysplasia.

Acetabular angle is a radiographic assessment for dysplasia. It is formed by a horizontal line connecting both triradiate cartilages (Hilgenreiner line) and a second line which extends along the acetabular roofs.

Graf R, et al. *Hip Sonography, Diagnosis and Management of Infant Hip Dysplasia.* Berlin: Springer Verlag, 2006.

120. C. Pott's puffy tumour

Pott's puffy tumour is defined as a subperiosteal abscess of the frontal bone with frontal osteomyelitis.

Frontal sinus infection can spread directly through the thin bone wall of this sinus or through the network of small veins that drain its mucosa. Today, this is a rare complication, given the widespread use of antibiotics. Trauma and frontal sinusitis are the most common causes of this condition. The bacteria causing Pott's puffy tumour usually reflect the type of bacterial species responsible for community-acquired chronic sinusitis.

The most common causal organisms are streptococci, staphylococci and anaerobic bacteria. Cultures frequently reveal polymicrobial involvement. The infection may spread as a thrombophlebitis from the frontal sinus through the diploic veins, involving the intracranial space with consequent epidural or subdural empyema, meningitis, brain abscess and venous sinus thrombosis.

Morón FE, et al. Lumps and bumps on the head in children: Use of CT and MR imaging in solving the clinical diagnostic dilemma. *Radiographic.* 2004;24:1655–74.

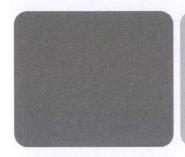

CHAPTER 13
TEST PAPER 7

Questions

Time: 3 hours

1. A middle-aged patient who sustained RTC 6 months ago presents with progressive visual loss and exophthalmos on the right. MRI demonstrated a dilated superior ophthalmic vein with flow voids in the cavernous sinus. What is the likely diagnosis?
   A. Buphthalmos
   B. Carotid-cavernous fistula
   C. Orbital pseudotumour
   D. Arteriovenous malformation
   E. Dural fistula

2. A preterm neonate on the intensive care unit develops gross abdominal distension and bleeding per rectum. A supine abdominal radiograph is performed demonstrating multiple loops of dilated bowel loops.
   Given the likely diagnosis, all of the following would be expected findings on the supine radiograph, except:
   A. Mottled gas shadows within the bowel wall
   B. Branching gas pattern overlying the liver shadow
   C. Foci of calcification projected over the renal angles
   D. Generalised lucency overlying the liver shadow
   E. Rounded area of lucency within the central abdomen

3. Which of the following is a recognised cause of a 'bone within bone' appearance?
   A. Renal osteodystrophy
   B. Paget's disease
   C. Hyperparathyroidism
   D. Melorheostosis
   E. Osteopathia striata

4. A 25-year-old woman with recurrent urinary tract infections and post-void dribbling attends the urology clinic. The urologist suspects a urethral diverticulum. What is the most appropriate first-line test?
   A. Micturating cystourethrogram
   B. Urodynamics
   C. Transvaginal ultrasound
   D. Double-balloon catheter positive pressure urethrography
   E. Pre- and post-void magnetic resonance imaging of urethra

5. A 40-year-old male and intravenous drug user, is on your barium list. The history on the card says 'c/o dysphagia. Exclude pouch!'. During the barium swallow, you notice no oesophageal pouch but there are at least three giant 3- to 4-cm flat ulcers noted within the oesophagus near

the gastro-oesophageal junction. The intervening oesophagus appears normal. Which of the following is the most likely diagnosis?

A. Cytomegalovirus oesophagitis
B. Caustic oesophagitis
C. Candida oesophagitis
D. Behçet's disease
E. Crohn's disease

6. A 16-year-old girl with a history of recurrent bronchitis undergoes chest X-ray. The lungs are clear but there is tracheal deviation to the left, with a focal indentation of the right wall of the trachea. Underlying vascular anomaly is suspected, and the patient undergoes a magnetic resonance imaging scan for further evaluation. All of the following will explain the above Chest X-ray appearance, except:

A. Double aortic arch
B. Right aortic arch with aberrant left subclavian artery and patent ductus arteriosus
C. Aberrant left pulmonary artery
D. Left aortic arch with aberrant right subclavian artery and patent ductus arteriosus
E. Common origin of innominate and left common carotid artery

7. A 50-year-old man was recently diagnosed with a thyroid cancer following an ultrasound-guided FNA of a thyroid lesion. Regarding malignant thyroid nodules, which of the following statements is true?

A. Punctate calcification is a feature of papillary carcinoma.
B. Anaplastic carcinoma is associated with MEN syndrome.
C. Echogenic foci seen in medullary carcinoma are due to calcitonin deposits.
D. Characteristic lymphadenopathy in medullary carcinoma is hypoechoic to muscle.
E. Follicular carcinoma can be differentiated from follicular adenoma on US.

8. A 6-year-old boy presents with a 1-month history of progressive left-sided proptosis. An orbital MRI reveals a large, lobulated, retro-orbital mass without any intracranial or globe invasion. The mass is isointense to muscle on T1 and hyperintense on T2 with uniform enhancement post-contrast. The patient is afebrile, and inflammatory markers are not significantly raised. What is the most likely diagnosis?

A. Dermoid cyst
B. Orbital cellulitis with abscess formation
C. Lymphangioma
D. Capillary haemangioma
E. Rhabdomyosarcoma

9. A 30-year-old woman was involved in a severe road traffic accident and sustained direct high-energy trauma to her pelvis. Among other injuries, she was found to have a fracture on her left sacroiliac joint and left ischiopubic ramus. What type of fracture has she sustained?

A. Open book
B. Straddle
C. Bucket handle
D. Duverney
E. Malgaigne

10. A patient undergoes a routine abdominal ultrasound for generalised abdominal pain. Unfortunately, the spleen cannot be detected. Which of the following is the least likely cause for this?

A. Myelofibrosis
B. Sickle cell anaemia

C. Polysplenia syndrome
D. Traumatic fragmentation of the spleen
E. Wandering spleen

11. A 6-year-old boy presents with adrenal insufficiency and developmental delay. Magnetic resonance imaging demonstrates diffuse T2 hyperintensity in the deep white matter, most predominant in the posterior parieto-occipital region and splenium of the corpus callosum. Which of the following is the most likely cause for this finding?
A. Metachromatic leukodystrophy
B. Acute disseminated encephalomyelitis
C. X-linked adrenoleukodystrophy
D. Alexander disease
E. Canavan disease

12. A 26-year-old woman who had an intrauterine contraceptive device (IUCD) coil inserted 6 years ago presents to her general practitioner complaining of right iliac fossa pain, constipation, night sweats and fevers. The practitioner refers her for a transvaginal ultrasound, which shows a right-sided convoluted cobra-shaped structure containing fluid echogenicity and some polypoidal outgrowths from the wall. Adjacent to this is a cystic left adnexal mass containing internal echoes. Which of the following is the likely diagnosis?
A. Actinomycosis
B. Appendix abscess
C. Diverticulitis with pericolic abscess
D. Migrated IUCD causing hydroureter
E. Salpingitis secondary to tuberculosis

13. A 75-year-old man had a history of dyspnoea associated with haemoptysis and weight loss. Computed tomography (CT) showed a 1.5 cm spiculated mass in the anterior segment of the right upper lobe, 5 cm deep to the pleural surface on a background of widespread emphysematous change. The case was referred for discussion at multidisciplinary team meeting to consider safety of undergoing a CT-guided lung biopsy. In this patient's case, which of the following statements concerning CT-guided lung biopsy is correct?
A. The patient carries a 10%–15% risk of developing pneumothorax.
B. As the lesion is not contiguous with the pleural surface, there is a lower risk of pneumothorax.
C. The patient carries an increased risk of developing pulmonary haemorrhage post-procedure.
D. If a pneumothorax were to develop as a complication, he is less likely to require subsequent intercostal drain insertion.
E. The procedure is relatively contraindicated because pulmonary function tests revealed a forced expiratory volume in 1 second (FEV$_1$) of 45% predicted.

14. A 58-year-old man, who underwent coronary artery bypass grafting 8 years ago, presents to the cardiology clinic with symptoms of progressive shortness of breath on exertion, associated with increase in abdominal girth and peripheral oedema. Clinical examination elicits raised jugular venous pressure, with bibasal fine inspiratory crackles, shifting dullness and bilateral ankle pitting oedema. Elective ecg-gated spin-echo cardiac MRI demonstrates limited ability of the right ventricle to distend during filling (diastole), assuming a tubular shape, with limited change in cavity size during the end-systolic phase. Pericardial thickening of 6 mm and calcification is evident, with a moderate pericardial effusion and

dilated superior vena cava and azygos vein. Which of the following is the most likely diagnosis?

A. Cardiac tamponade
B. Restrictive cardiomyopathy
C. Constrictive pericarditis
D. Dressler syndrome
E. Hypertrophic cardiomyopathy

15. An 8-month-old boy presents with a right upper quadrant mass. Blood results reveal a raised alpha-fetoprotein (AFP). Ultrasound of the abdomen demonstrates a large 7-cm, hypervascular, heterogeneous hyperechoic mass in the liver with a few cystic regions. There is no vascular invasion. No renal or suprarenal lesions are present. Which of the following differential diagnoses is most likely?

A. Hepatoblastoma
B. Infantile haemangioendothelioma
C. Hepatic haemangioma
D. Mesenchymal hamartoma of the liver
E. Fibrolamellar hepatocellular carcinoma

16. What is the purpose of the heel–toe manoeuvre in ultrasound examination of the shoulder?

A. To decrease the beam angle incidence
B. To minimise anisotropy
C. To increase the field of view
D. To minimise posterior reverberation artefact
E. To minimise beam width artefact

17. A 23-year-old woman presents with left iliac fossa pain. The uterus and both ovaries are within normal limits. There is an anechoic left adnexal cyst adjacent to the uterus that appears separate from the ovary. You note that the patient has had a previous ultrasound for left adnexal pain, and that a left adnexal cyst with similar dimensions was noted then. Which of the following is the most likely diagnosis?

A. Theca lutein cyst
B. Paraovarian cyst
C. Endometrioma
D. Adenomyosis
E. Dermoid cyst

18. A patient undergoes pancreatic transplantation. Which of the following statements is least likely?

A. The transplanted pancreatic duct is normally dilated.
B. Indistinct pancreatic margins on ultrasound may indicate graft rejection.
C. Most patients have a simultaneous renal transplant.
D. The donor pancreas is normally grafted onto the external iliac vessels.
E. Most patients achieve insulin independence.

19. A 30-year-old woman presents with bilateral foot drop 2 days post-partum. What finding on MRI would explain this?

A. Posterior disc protrusion at L3/L4
B. Bilateral common peroneal nerve entrapment
C. Bilateral sciatic nerve compression
D. Paracentral disc protrusion at L3/L4
E. Spinal canal stenosis at L3/L4

20. On an antenatal ultrasound, a foetus is found to have an intracranial anomaly. At birth, the cranial ultrasound reveals a large cystic mass in the posterior fossa communicating with the fourth ventricle with hypoplasia of the cerebellar vermis.

    What other associated abnormality would you not expect to be associated with the underlying condition?
    A. Subependymal calcification
    B. Corpus callosum agenesis
    C. Grey matter heterotopia
    D. Schizencephaly
    E. Occipital encephalocele

21. A 13-year-old boy presents with symptoms and radiographic evidence of a slipped capital femoral epiphysis (SCFE). It is noted on his radiographs that the physes are generally wide with flaring of the metaphyses. Which of the following is the most likely diagnosis?
    A. Rickets
    B. Hypophosphatasia
    C. Blount's disease
    D. Achondroplasia
    E. Renal osteodystrophy

22. A 76-year-old woman is having a pelvic magnetic resonance imaging (MRI) scan to assess for a possible hernia. She is noted to have a 6 cm very low intensity lesion within the right ovary on both T1 and T2. Some fluid is also noted within the pelvis. Which of the following is the most likely diagnosis?
    A. Ovarian mucinous cystadenoma
    B. Krukenberg tumour
    C. Ovarian fibroma
    D. Dermoid cyst
    E. Clear cell carcinoma of the ovary

23. You are reviewing the X-rays of a 44-year-old male patient who has complained of mild breathlessness and a cough but otherwise well. Several chest radiographs performed over an 18-month period demonstrate diffuse ground glass shadowing with several scattered confluent areas of air-space consolidation. The lung changes do not appear to have any zonal predilection, and no mediastinal, hilar or cardiac abnormality is evident. HRCT also showed fairly extensive smooth interlobular septal thickening. The intervening lung appears normal, and there is sharp demarcation between the abnormal and normal lung parenchyma. Which of the following is most likely given the radiological findings described?
    A. Pulmonary vasculitis
    B. Pulmonary oedema
    C. Primary tuberculosis
    D. Alveolar proteinosis
    E. Extrinsic allergic alveolitis

24. An otherwise healthy 44-year-old patient presents acutely unwell with new-onset epigastric pain and is found to have a significantly raised amylase level. Which of the following clinical scenarios is least likely?
    A. Alcoholic patient, recent 48-h binge
    B. Previous bouts of right upper quadrant abdominal pain
    C. Recent flu-like symptoms
    D. Computed tomography report describing a 6 cm pseudocyst
    E. Fulminant haemolytic–uraemic syndrome

25. A 73-year-old woman with weight loss, previous history of endometriosis and a CA-125 of 983 µg/mL, attends for an magnetic resonance imaging (MRI) scan of the pelvis after a cystic mass with nodules was noted in the left adnexa on ultrasound. There is a 6 cm predominately unilocular cystic mass in the left adnexa, which is bright on T1W & T1W fat-saturated images with enhancing solid mural nodules along its wall. It remains high signal on fat-saturated imaging. Which of the following is the most likely diagnosis?
    A. Dysgerminoma
    B. Brenner tumour of the ovary
    C. Endometrioma
    D. Ovarian dermoid
    E. Clear cell carcinoma of the ovary

26. A 32-year-old lady presents with acute sudden onset headache to the A&E department. CT shows haemorrhage within the fourth ventricle. Which vessel is most likely to be involved?
    A. Anterior cerebral communicating artery
    B. Anterior cerebral artery
    C. Posterior cerebral artery
    D. Posterior cerebral communicating artery
    E. Posterior inferior cerebellar artery

27. A 4-year-old child undergoes a CXR for suspicion of chest infection. The request mentions that the child has a congenital cardiac anomaly, which is, as yet, untreated. No further information regarding the type of anomaly is provided. The only abnormalities you can detect on the CXR include mild generalised cardiomegaly and increased pulmonary arterial flow. You note from the A&E department notes that the child is not cyanosed. What is the most likely diagnosis?
    A. Ebstein anomaly
    B. Ventricular septal defect
    C. Tetralogy of Fallot
    D. Atrial septal defect
    E. Truncus arteriosus

28. An elderly patient presents to the orthopaedic clinic with progressive hip pain. He has a history of a hip replacement performed 5 years ago. A radionuclide bone scan is ordered and demonstrates increased uptake around the proximal aspect of the prosthesis. This finding is sensitive and specific for which of the following conditions?
    A. Prosthetic fracture
    B. Mechanical loosening
    C. Periprosthetic fracture
    D. Particle disease
    E. None of the above

29. A 68-year-old male patient presents with painless jaundice. Abdominal ultrasound reveals both intrahepatic and extrahepatic biliary dilatation. The gallbladder is thin-walled and there are no gallstones. No other significant abnormality is detected, but the report mentions that '… the pancreas was not visualized due to overlying bowel gas …'. What is the most likely underlying diagnosis?
    A. Pancreas divisum
    B. Pancreatic acinar cell carcinoma
    C. Pancreatic adenocarcinoma
    D. Pancreatic islet cell tumour
    E. Pancreatic pseudocyst

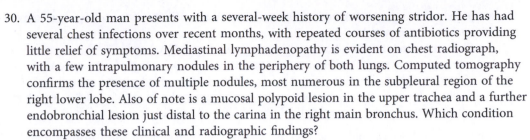

30. A 55-year-old man presents with a several-week history of worsening stridor. He has had several chest infections over recent months, with repeated courses of antibiotics providing little relief of symptoms. Mediastinal lymphadenopathy is evident on chest radiograph, with a few intrapulmonary nodules in the periphery of both lungs. Computed tomography confirms the presence of multiple nodules, most numerous in the subpleural region of the right lower lobe. Also of note is a mucosal polypoid lesion in the upper trachea and a further endobronchial lesion just distal to the carina in the right main bronchus. Which condition encompasses these clinical and radiographic findings?
    A. Amyloidosis
    B. Alveolar proteinosis
    C. Pulmonary vasculitis
    D. Histoplasmosis
    E. Hydatid disease

31. A neonate is noted to be markedly cyanosed, worsening when she cries. A CXR performed on day 1 is normal. Which of the following types of congenital cardiac anomaly is most likely?
    A. Patent ductus arteriosus
    B. Ebstein anomaly
    C. Coarctation of the aorta
    D. Tricuspid atresia
    E. Tetralogy of Fallot

32. Pick's disease affects which of the following?
    A. Fronto-parietal lobe
    B. Temporo-parietal
    C. Temporo-frontal
    D. Parieto-occipital
    E. Frontal

33. A 36-year-old woman is being investigated for possible renal stones with CT KUB. An incidental "polka-dot" appearance to the T12 vertebral body is noted on the axial CT images. MRI at the same level shows characteristic high signal in the vertebral body on T1 and T2W images. All of the following statements regarding this entity are true, except
    A. They may extend to involve the posterior element.
    B. They are commonly multiple.
    C. Compressive lesions are common in the lumbar spine.
    D. Low T1W lesions are more likely to be active.
    E. Most are asymptomatic.

34. An alcoholic patient is referred for an ultrasound from the A&E department of your hospital. The request states that the patient has deranged liver function tests and raises the possibility of underlying liver cirrhosis. Which of the following findings would not help you to confirm this diagnosis?
    A. Caudate lobe hypertrophy
    B. Increased echogenicity of the liver parenchyma
    C. Coarse echotexture to the liver
    D. Decreased resistive index in hepatic artery
    E. Hepatofugal flow within the portal vein

35. A 53-year-old man is assessed by the receiving surgeon, having presented with severe chest pain, vomiting and sepsis. Mediastinal emphysema is evident on chest radiograph and

computed tomography confirms oesophageal perforation. Which of the following statements is incorrect with regard to this condition?

A. Plain chest radiography is normal in approximately 10% of cases.
B. Iatrogenic injury is the most common single cause of oesophageal perforation.
C. Upper oesophageal perforations typically result in right-sided pleural collection.
D. In blunt chest trauma, the perforation usually occurs in the lower third of the oesophagus.
E. Water-soluble contrast agents should be used for fluoroscopic assessment.

36. A normally well 8-year-old child presents to the A&E department short of breath and pyrexial complaining of joint pain. Chest X-ray shows an enlarged heart with upper lobe venous blood diversion and small bilateral pleural effusions. No focal collapse/consolidation is evident, but there are patchy interstitial infiltrates in a perihilar distribution. Further questioning reveals that the child recently had a sore throat. What is the most likely underlying diagnosis?

A. Toxic synovitis
B. Juvenile rheumatoid arthritis
C. Reiter's disease
D. Rheumatic fever
E. Septicaemia

37. All the following cause basal ganglia calcification except?

A. Pseudohypoparathyroidism
B. Lead poisoning
C. Ageing
D. Hypothyroidism
E. Wilson's disease

38. An 82-year-old woman presents with postmenopausal bleeding. Transvaginal ultrasound shows a thickened endometrium and a left adnexal lobulated multicystic lesion, which has some solid elements. Some of the cysts contain fluid–fluid levels and have thick septa. Which of the following is the most likely diagnosis?

A. Endometriosis
B. Granulosa cell tumour
C. Endometrial hyperplasia and haemorrhagic corpus luteal cyst
D. Serous cystadenocarcinoma
E. Fibrothecoma

39. A 33-year-old woman with progressive increase in back pain and perineal pain was sent for further evaluation to the spinal surgeons. Axial and coronal reformatted CT image showed a well-defined lytic lesion of the right upper part of the sacrum with extension through the right sacroiliac joint and absence of a sclerotic rim. All the following are features of this lesion except?

A. Most commonly affected bone is sacrum.
B. Extension into intervertebral disc helps to differentiate GCT from ABC.
C. Septa show intense enhancement post-contrast injection.
D. Doughnut sign on scintigraphy usually suggests an alternate diagnosis.
E. Fluid–fluid level is not specific for this lesion.

40. A 38-year-old woman is undergoing investigations for infertility. She is otherwise asymptomatic. On hysterosalpingography, there is a large filling defect within the uterine fundus with a linear defect that extends into the filling defect. She subsequently has an MRI scan, which demonstrates a myometrial mass with indistinct margins, which abuts the junctional zone and has lower signal on T2 when compared with the adjacent myometrium. There are a few focal high T2 signal intensity areas within, some which

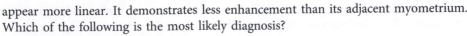

appear more linear. It demonstrates less enhancement than its adjacent myometrium. Which of the following is the most likely diagnosis?

A. Leiomyosarcoma
B. Leiomyoma
C. Endometrial carcinoma
D. Adenomyosis
E. Hydatidiform mole

41. Before being referred for a CT colonography, a patient asks to speak with a radiologist to clear up a few points regarding colon cancer; Of the following statements, which is most correct?

A. Smaller polyps are more likely to be malignant than larger ones.
B. Most colonic polyps are malignant.
C. Gardener syndrome carries an increased risk of cancer but Peutz–Jeghers syndrome does not.
D. Most colon cancers start as an adenomatous polyp.
E. Inflammatory bowel disease carries no increased risk of cancer.

42. A 75-year-old man presents with abdominal pain after eating and mesenteric angina is suspected. You decide to perform a celiac axis angiogram using a mechanical contrast pump. What is an appropriate volume and flow rate of contrast to use?

A. 32 mL @ 8 mL/s
B. 20 mL @ 20 mL/s
C. 40 mL @ 20 mL/s
D. 30 mL @ 20 mL/s
E. 20 mL @ 6 mL/s

43. A 62-year-old postmenopausal woman has a magnetic resonance imaging (MRI) scan to look for a hernia. In the right ovary is a 1 cm sharply demarcated low T1 and T2 signal solid mass with adjacent calcification. There is also a multilocular cystic lesion within the same ovary, containing multiple thin-walled septa. Which of the following is the most likely cause of the well-demarcated low-signal lesion?

A. Ovarian fibroma
B. Ovarian Brenner tumour
C. Ovarian dermoid cyst
D. Endometrioma
E. Corpus luteal cyst

44. Which of the following is specific for osteomalacia?

A. Brown tumour
B. Looser zones
C. Cloaca
D. Cyclops lesion
E. Wimberger's sign

45. AP radiograph of the leg of a 3-year-old girl shows periosteal reaction in the mid-fibula. Exuberant periosteal reaction was worrisome for malignancy, and MRI was performed. Coronal STIR images showed a low signal intensity fracture line surrounded by extensive soft-tissue and bone marrow oedema. No mass was depicted. Other sites commonly affected in toddlers fracture include all the following, except:

A. Tibia
B. Humerus
C. Talus
D. Calcaneum
E. Cuboid

46. A 63-year-old man presents with progressive vertical gaze abnormality and cognitive symptoms. MRI of the brain demonstrates volume loss of the mid brain, which was described by the reporting radiologist as Hummingbird sign. What is the diagnosis?
    A. Multisystem atrophy
    B. Progressive supranuclear palsy
    C. Parkinson's disease
    D. Shy–Drager syndrome
    E. Amyotrophic lateral sclerosis

47. A patient is diagnosed with *Helicobacter pylori* infection. Which of the following findings would you not expect?
    A. Gastric ulcer
    B. Duodenal ulcer
    C. Linitis plastica
    D. Polypoid gastritis
    E. Thickened gastric folds

48. You performed a catheter angiogram and angioplasty for right popliteal stenosis on a patient in the vascular ward and are there to review him the following day. The nurse asks you to prescribe him some analgesia because, overnight, his limb has become painful and pale with loss of power and intolerable tingling. Which of the following is your next step?
    A. Review the puncture site (you find no significant haematoma) and prescribe analgesics
    B. Arrange for the patient to be taken back to the suite for further angiography
    C. You immediately page the vascular surgeon on call
    D. Organise urgent CTPA to exclude pulmonary embolism
    E. You start the patient on low molecular weight heparin and organise US leg veins

49. A 72-year-old poorly controlled diabetic gentleman with multiple foot ulcers undergoes an MRI examination to exclude osteomyelitis. All of the following are MR features of osteomyelitis of bones of the forefoot, except
    A. Low signal intensity in infected bone marrow on T1W images
    B. Contrast enhancement of bone marrow
    C. Decreased signal intensity of bone marrow on STIR images
    D. Increased signal intensity of bone marrow on T2W images
    E. Contrast enhancement of adjacent soft tissues

50. A *malformation* is defined as a congenital morphologic anomaly of a single organ or body part due to an alteration of the primary developmental program caused by a genetic defect. All of the following are examples of posterior fossa cystic malformation, except
    A. Blake's pouch cyst
    B. Dandy–Walker malformation
    C. Arachnoid cyst
    D. Rhombencephalosynapsis
    E. Giant cisterna magna

51. Which of the following combination of MRI signal is characteristic for cerebral abscess?

	DWI	ADC
A.	Low	High
B.	High	High
C.	High	Low
D.	Low	Low
E.	Isointense	High

52. A 37-year-old woman, with a previous history of cervical carcinoma and radiotherapy, presents with abdominal pain. On magnetic resonance imaging, there is a large cystic midline structure, which has high T1 signal and some internal debris, extending anteriorly and superiorly from the cervix. Coincidentally, in the cervical region, there is high/intermediate T2 signal surrounding the endocervical canal and disruption of the low-intensity cervical stromal ring. Which of the following is the most likely diagnosis?
    A. Cervical carcinoma recurrence causing haematometra
    B. Cervical carcinoma with invasion of the uterus
    C. Radiotherapy-induced cervical stenosis causing haematometra
    D. Cervical carcinoma recurrence with metastasis to ovary
    E. Imperforate hymen

53. Which of the following statements is most accurate regarding the use of endoscopic ultrasound?
    A. It is superior to cross-sectional imaging for local staging of oesophageal cancer.
    B. It is superior to cross-sectional imaging in the assessment of liver metastases.
    C. It is less effective than cross-sectional imaging for local staging of rectal cancer.
    D. It is less effective than traditional endoscopy for assessing submucosal masses.
    E. It is not useful in the assessment of a primary pancreatic mass.

54. You are called to perform a catheter angiogram on a 26-year-old biker who was involved in a road traffic accident. You are told that he has suffered a dislocated knee. The clinician informs you that his foot is perfused but has sluggish capillary refill. He has a palpable dorsalis pedis pulse but no posterior tibial pulse. Which of the following would you expect to find on the angiogram?
    A. Severed anterior tibial artery
    B. Severed tibioperoneal trunk
    C. Traumatic popliteal artery dissection
    D. Atheromatous plaque at the peroneal origin
    E. Normal anatomy

55. A 13-year-old post-pubescent girl presents to the emergency department with acute abdominal pain sited predominantly within the right iliac fossa. An ultrasound scan is performed. This reveals an echogenic mass within the right side of pelvis measuring approximately 4 cm. The sonographer thinks it is adjacent to and inseparable from the right ovary. What is the most likely diagnosis?
    A. Acute appendicitis
    B. Ovarian dermoid
    C. Ovarian torsion
    D. Ectopic pregnancy
    E. Haemorrhagic ovarian cyst

56. A young adult presented with complex partial seizures and amnesia. His MRI scan demonstrated T2 hyperintensity within the medial right temporal lobe, loss of hippocampal head digitations and dilatation of the ipsilateral temporal horn of lateral ventricle. Which of the following is the most likely diagnosis?
    A. Herpes simplex encephalitis
    B. Choroidal fissure cyst
    C. Mesial temporal sclerosis
    D. Early-onset Alzheimer's disease
    E. Post-seizure appearance

57. A 32-year-old man presented to the A&E department after injuring his great toe. No fracture was demonstrated on plain X-ray performed, but incidental note was made of a flattened and

sclerotic metatarsal head with subchondral collapse compatible with chronic changes of avascular necrosis (AVN). Which metatarsal is the most common site of Freiberg disease?

A. First
B. Second
C. Third
D. Fourth
E. Fifth

58. A 39-year-old woman taking human menopausal gonadotrophins presents with pelvic pain, bloating and weight gain. On transvaginal ultrasound, both ovaries are enlarged and contain multiple bilateral cysts, some of which are 8 cm. There is also free fluid within the pouch of Douglas and surrounding the uterus. Which of the following is the most likely diagnosis?

A. Large corpus luteal cysts
B. Endometriomas
C. Polycystic ovarian syndrome
D. Ovarian hyperstimulation syndrome
E. Ovarian torsion

59. You are asked to perform an ultrasound scan on an asymptomatic 30-year-old pregnant woman 4 weeks after the obstetrician incidentally notes a 3 cm hyperechoic lesion in the right lobe of the liver. On today's scan, you notice a 7 cm hyperechoic lesion involving segments VI & VII of the liver and subcapsular fluid. What is the most likely diagnosis for this lesion?

A. Focal nodular hyperplasia
B. Liver haemangioma
C. Metastasis
D. Hepatic adenoma
E. Hepatic abscess

60. A 72-year-old man presents with recurrent episodes of flash pulmonary oedema. Magnetic resonance angiography shows bilateral renal artery stenosis with atherosclerotic disease at both renal artery ostia. Which of the following do you advise?

A. No endovascular option
B. Bilateral renal artery radiofrequency (RF) denervation
C. Bilateral renal artery angioplasty and stenting
D. Continue with best medical management
E. Refer to vascular surgeons for bilateral renal artery endarterectomy

61. A 7-year-old boy who is otherwise well is being investigated for chronic right-sided hip pain. Which of the following diagnoses is most likely?

A. Septic arthritis
B. Perthes disease
C. Slipped upper femoral epiphysis
D. Juvenile rheumatoid arthritis
E. Developmental dysplasia of the hip

62. Which one of the following is the incorrect association?

A.	Astrocytoma	Intramedullary
B.	Abscess	Extradural
C.	Nerve sheath tumour	Intradural extramedullary
D.	Dermoid	Extradural
E.	Meningioma	Intramedullary

63. A 10-year-old girl of Jewish descent presents with pain in her left thigh. A radiograph revealed diffuse medullary osteoporosis, a 'flask-shaped' distal femur, a serpentine area of sclerosis

within the femoral metaphysis, and a sharply circumscribed endosteal lytic lesion in the distal femur with a pathological fracture. Clinical examination reveals splenomegaly. Which of the following is the most likely diagnosis?

A. Thalassemia
B. Osteopetrosis
C. Diaphyseal aclasis
D. Gaucher disease
E. Rickets

64. A 29-year-old woman attends for a transvaginal ultrasound for dyspareunia. While passing the probe, you notice an anechoic cystic lesion in the lower vagina within the posterolateral wall. Which of the following is the most likely diagnosis?

A. Lipoma
B. Nabothian cyst
C. Gartner duct cyst
D. Bartholin's cyst
E. Squamous cell carcinoma

65. A previously healthy 36-year-old woman presents with acute hepatic failure of unknown cause. Her international normalized ratio (INR) is 2.6 and fails to normalise despite treatment. An ultrasound scan shows ascites. The liver team asks you to consider a liver biopsy. Which of the following is the most appropriate reply?

A. Unable to perform because of INR and ascites
B. Advise the patient of the increased risk of bleeding and go ahead with liver biopsy
C. Drain the ascites and the perform the biopsy
D. Perform transjugular liver biopsy
E. Perform transarterial liver biopsy

66. A 79-year-old diabetic patient presents with right short-distance calf claudication. Magnetic resonance angiography shows focal stenosis of the right popliteal segment, and a decision is made to proceed to angiography and endovascular treatment. Which of the following is the best approach for catheter angiography?

A. Right common femoral artery (CFA), retrograde
B. Left CFA, retrograde
C. Right CFA, antegrade
D. Right popliteal puncture under ultrasound scan
E. Left CFA, retrograde

67. A 2-year-old boy is referred for a painless lump in the right supraorbital region. The lesion is fluctuant on clinical examination. On ultrasound, it demonstrates low internal echoes and scalloping of underlying bone. What is the most likely diagnosis?

A. Angular dermoid
B. Haemangioma
C. Neurofibroma
D. Lymphangioma
E. Aneurysmal bone cyst

68. Which of the following is an absolute contraindication to vertebroplasty?

A. Symptomatic vertebral haemangioma
B. Metastasis
C. Multiple myeloma
D. Infection
E. Severely painful osteoporosis

69. An elderly man presents to his GP with pain in his left middle finger in the region of the nail bed. This has worsened over the past 2 months. Plain film reveals a destructive lytic lesion within the distal phalanx of his left middle finger. What is the likely diagnosis?
    A. Breast cancer metastasis
    B. Renal cancer metastasis
    C. Lung cancer metastasis
    D. Gastric cancer metastasis
    E. Pancreatic cancer metastasis

70. A 34-year-old pregnant woman with severe abdominal pain attends for an MRI scan after an ultrasound showing a uterine mass. As well as the normal gestational sac, on T1W imaging there is a low-signal mass noted within the posterior myometrial wall, which displaces the uterine cavity anteriorly. This mass has a high T1 signal intensity rim. On T2W images, this lesion is intermediate to low signal and has a low-signal rim. Which of the following is the most likely diagnosis?
    A. Non-degenerated leiomyoma
    B. Hyaline degeneration within a leiomyoma
    C. Red degeneration within a leiomyoma
    D. Myxoid degeneration within a leiomyoma
    E. Cystic degeneration within a leiomyoma

71. You are performing a tunnelled dual lumen dialysis line via a right jugular approach on a 50-year-old with chronic renal failure. As you are peeling the sheath, you hear a hushing sound and the patient suddenly becomes agitated, with an acute decrease in his partial oxygen saturation pressure. Which of the following is the most appropriate immediate management?
    A. Perform needle decompression in the right mid-clavicular line, 2nd interspace
    B. Obtain a chest X-ray
    C. Inject 10 mL of contrast down the sheath and look for extravasation
    D. Put the patient head down and give fast intravenous crystalloid
    E. Administer high-flow oxygen and put the patient in the left lateral position.

72. The surgeons want you to review the CT of a young man at an X-ray meeting. A young patient had been admitted with acute abdominal pain and intussusception was diagnosed on pre-operative CT scan. Regarding this condition, which one of the following statements is incorrect?
    A. A lead point is rarely the underlying cause in adult cases.
    B. The intussusceptum is the entering limb of bowel.
    C. Ileocolic intussusception is the most common type in children.
    D. The CT appearance is of multiple concentric rings.
    E. Intussusception is the leading cause of acquired bowel obstruction in childhood.

73. A 10-year-old girl of African origin presents with colicky right upper quadrant pain and deranged liver function tests. Ultrasound of the abdomen demonstrates acute calculus cholecystitis. What is the most likely diagnosis?
    A. Sickle cell anaemia
    B. Familial hypercholesterolaemia
    C. Inflammatory bowel disease
    D. Choledochal cyst
    E. Thalassaemia minor

74. A 60-year-old non-smoker presents with a history of increasing headaches and loss of consciousness. An unenhanced CT of the brain is performed which demonstrates high

attenuation lesions within the cerebellum. All of the following may appear hyperdense on non-contrast CT, except

A. Bronchogenic metastases
B. Melanoma metastases
C. Renal cell metastases
D. Prostate metastases
E. Thyroid carcinoma metastases

75. On an AP skull radiograph, there are fractures of the pterygoid plate, maxilla and nasal septum. What is the best classification for this type of injury?

A. Le Fort I facial fracture
B. Le Fort II
C. Le Fort III
D. Depressed skull fracture
E. Pyramidal fracture

76. A 56-year-old woman with known pancreatic cancer is brought from home by ambulance with haematemesis and melaena. After stabilisation, she undergoes endoscopy, which reveals isolated gastric fundus varices with a normal oesophagus. She also undergoes abdominal computed tomography, which shows echogenic material in one of the splanchnic veins, consistent with thrombosis. Which of the splanchnic veins is most likely to be associated with isolated gastric fundus varices rather than gastro-oesophageal varices?

A. Superior mesenteric vein
B. Inferior mesenteric vein
C. Portal vein
D. Splenic vein
E. Hepatic veins

77. A 40-year old with recurrent pulmonary emboli is due to have a hip replacement and it is decided to deploy a temporary inferior vena cava (IVC) filter. What is the preferred site of deployment of an IVC filter?

A. Suprarenal IVC
B. Infrarenal IVC
C. Proximal to the clot load, no matter the level
D. At the confluence of common iliac vessels
E. At the junction of IVC and right atrium

78. Which of the following is an appropriate puncture site for a percutaneous nephrostomy in a patient with normal sonographic anatomy? (You anticipate no need for further intervention.)

A. Posterior calyx, middle/lower pole
B. Posterior calyx, upper pole
C. Direct puncture of the renal pelvis
D. Anterior, middle pole calyx
E. Anterior calyx, upper pole

79. An 18-month-old toddler with a history of prematurity presents with an acutely distended abdomen and vomiting. He has not passed flatus for 24 hours. On examination, the referring accident and emergency registrar is concerned that the patient may have a torted testis, which he believes is causing the abdominal pain. An ultrasound demonstrates mixed echogenicity in the right scrotum. The testis could not be identified. What is the most likely diagnosis?

A. Acute testicular torsion
B. Testicular carcinoma

C. Inguinal hernia

D. Femoral hernia

E. Sacro-coccygeal teratoma

80. A 31-year-old presented with a 3-month history of progressive leg weakness, sensory disturbance, urinary hesitancy, urgency and erectile dysfunction. He had treatment for sputum positive pulmonary TB 1 year ago. MRI of the spine shows clumping of nerve roots within the thecal sac and empty thecal sac sign. Intradural cysts are also seen. What is the most likely diagnosis?

A. Discitis

B. Cauda equina

C. Arachnoiditis

D. Diastomatomyelia

E. Arachnoid cyst

81. A healthy 12-year-old boy presents with painful ankles (no history of trauma). A plain radiograph of his ankles demonstrates bilateral symmetrical periosteal reaction of his tibia and fibula. His father reports similar symptoms in adolescence but never had it investigated. No treatment is given. The boy had a further plain film performed after a football injury to his ankle at the age of 15 years. No periosteal reaction was seen at this time. Which of the following is the most likely diagnosis?

A. Thyroid acropathy

B. Pachydermoperiostosis

C. Hypertrophic pulmonary osteoarthropathy

D. Hypervitaminosis A

E. Venous insufficiency

82. A 40-year-old man presents with postprandial abdominal pain and 10 kg weight loss. A computed tomography scan with arterial phase imaging shows an indentation at the proximal coeliac axis caused by the low insertion of the median arcuate ligament. Which of the following is the most appropriate treatment option?

A. Catheter angiography and stenting

B. Open surgical management

C. Refer for laparoscopic division of the ligament

D. Catheter angiography and stenting

E. No indication for treatment

83. Which one of the following is not an indication for upper urinary tract drainage (nephrostomy or stent) in the presence of renal failure and hydronephrosis?

A. Retroperitoneal fibrosis

B. Mid-ureteric calculus

C. High-pressure chronic retention

D. Mid-ureteric stricture

E. Advanced pelvic malignancy

84. A 65-year-old female patient with known disseminated renal cell cancer presents with increasing abdominal pain and distension. A computed tomography (CT) scan is performed which reveals moderate ascites and mild hepatomegaly. Portal venous phase images show geographic liver and hyperenhancement of a normal-size caudate lobe. On delayed images, a characteristic 'flip-flop' pattern of enhancement is observed. Which of the following is the most likely underlying diagnosis?

A. Portal vein thrombosis

B. Acute Budd–Chiari syndrome

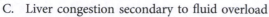

C. Liver congestion secondary to fluid overload

D. Peliosis hepatis secondary to chemotherapy

E. Chronic Budd–Chiari syndrome

85. A 47-year-old obese male patient with long-standing fatty liver infiltration and a strong family history of hepatic cirrhosis underwent liver biopsy, which confirmed the diagnosis of non-alcoholic steatohepatitis (NASH). He is to be followed up with imaging to exclude progression to cirrhosis. Which radiological feature is not typical for NASH?

A. Low attenuation of the liver on computed tomography

B. High signal of liver on T1W magnetic resonance imaging

C. Irregular liver contour

D. Hepatomegaly

E. High echogenicity of the liver parenchyma on ultrasound

86. A 70-year-old woman has a computed tomography scan for diverticulitis. An incidental 18 mm aneurysm in the mid-portion of the splenic artery is identified on the scan. Which of the following is the most appropriate treatment for this patient?

A. Catheter angiography

B. Catheter angiography and coil embolisation

C. Catheter angiography and stenting

D. Percutaneous thrombin injection

E. Conservative management and repeat scan in 6 months

87. Which of the following is not a feature of holoprosencephaly?

A. Single ventricle

B. Fused thalami

C. Absent corpus callosum

D. Tectal beaking

E. Hypoplasia of the optic nerves

88. A 69-year-old man with a chronic headache underwent an MRI brain and MR cerebral venogram, which showed a chronic thrombosis of the left transverse and sigmoid sinuses with evidence of recanalisation. As far as diagnosis of cerebral venous sinus thrombosis is concerned, which of the following statement is false?

A. Polycythemia can cause positive delta sign.

B. Unenhanced MRI is more sensitive than unenhanced CT.

C. Slow flow mimics sinus thrombosis on contrast-enhanced MRV.

D. Turbulent flow is more of a pitfall on TOF MRV.

E. Irregular sinus and intrasinus channels suggest recanalisation.

89. Which of the following statements is incorrect as regards the anatomy and imaging findings of the seminal vesicles and vasa deferens?

A. The seminal vesicles are located posterior to the bladder and distal ureters.

B. Normal seminal vesicles appear hypointense and hyperintense on T1W imaging and T2W imaging respectively.

C. The seminal vesicle joins the distal portion of the vas deferens, becoming the ejaculatory duct, and then drains into the prostatic urethra.

D. The distal portions of the seminal vesicles and vas deferens are intraperitoneal.

E. The seminal vesicles initially increase in volume with age, but then steadily reduce in size with advancing age.

90. A 65-year-old smoker presents with an achy pain around both his ankles. The GP orders ankle radiographs to look for degenerative change. The report comes back describing 'smooth,

lamellar periosteal reaction with new bone formation in the distal diametaphyses of both tibiae'. Which of the following is the most likely cause?

A. Systemic lupus erythematosus
B. Low-grade chronic osteomyelitis
C. Rheumatoid arthritis
D. Hypertrophic osteoarthropathy
E. Reiter syndrome

91. You are performing a varicocele embolisation. The patient suddenly develops left loin pain. He remains haemodynamically stable, but you notice contrast extravasation proximal to the coils. Which of the following is the most appropriate management?

A. Inject polyvinyl alcohol (PVA) at the extravasation site
B. Stent grafting to exclude the extravasation site
C. Alert the surgical team – need to proceed to laparotomy
D. Take the patient for a computed tomography scan of the abdomen/pelvis
E. Conservative management

92. Chest radiograph of a 12-year-old boy shows a cystic lesion with air–fluid level in the right upper lobe. CT scan confirms the presence of a thin-walled cystic lesion. Rest of the lungs are clear. There is no lymphadenopathy in the chest. Quantiferon test was negative, and there are no features of infection or signs of inflammation. What is the diagnosis?

A. TB
B. Intrapulmonary bronchogenic cyst
C. Hydatid cyst
D. Infected bulla
E. Congenital lobar emphysema

93. A 40-year-old man presents with acute onset of III cranial nerve palsy. The unenhanced CT shows subarachnoid blood. Where is the aneurysm likely to be?

A. Anterior communicating cerebral artery
B. Anterior cerebral artery
C. Middle cerebral artery
D. Posterior cerebral artery
E. Posterior communicating cerebral artery

94. A 7-year-old girl presents with abdominal pain, which has come on and off over the past year, and failure to thrive. An X-ray performed revealed dense metaphyseal bands in both lower limbs. The blood profile was unremarkable. What is the most likely diagnosis?

A. Leukaemia
B. Lead poisoning
C. Congenital rubella
D. Osteopetrosis
E. Osteopathia striata

95. A 63-year-old man is diagnosed with sigmoid adenocarcinoma with no metastatic spread identified on initial staging computed tomography (CT) scan. After a course of neoadjuvant chemotherapy, he is considered for tumour resection and undergoes a repeat CT scan. New hepatic lesions suspicious for metastases are identified. All of the following are criteria for resectability, except:

A. Less than three hepatic lesions
B. At least three segments spared from metastatic involvement
C. No visible nodal involvement

D.   At least one main portal vein branch must be spared

E.   At least one hepatic vein must be spare

96. A taxi driver is brought to the accident and emergency department after a high-speed road traffic accident. The fire brigade needed 2 hours to extricate him from his wrecked car. On arrival, he is hypothermic but stable, complaining of severe abdominal pain. An urgent contrast enhanced CT scan is performed and the radiologist on call issues a report describing features suggestive of mesenteric injury with segmental small bowel ischaemia. Which finding is the most specific for a mesenteric injury with associated bowel wall ischaemia?

A.   Generalised increased bowel wall enhancement

B.   Patchy and irregular Localised bowel wall enhancement

C.   Localised bowel wall thickening

D.   Decreased or absent bowel wall enhancement

E.   segmental bowel dilatation

97. A 4-week-old neonate is being investigated for neonatal jaundice. Post-feed ultrasound of the abdomen demonstrates a normal looking distended gallbladder and no focal hepatic abnormality. A cholescintigraphy scan, also known as hepatobiliary iminodiacetic acid (HIDA) or mebrofenin scan, demonstrates isotope in the urinary bladder at 24 hours. What is the most likely diagnosis?

A.   Choledochal cyst

B.   Transient neonatal hyperbilirubinaemia

C.   Biliary atresia

D.   Idiopathic hepatitis

E.   Cystic fibrosis

98. Which of the following is not an angiographic sign of active bleeding?

A.   Contrast extravasation

B.   Vessel spasm

C.   Vessel cut-off

D.   Early venous filling

E.   Vessel dilatation

99. A 5-year-old girl presents with left-sided abdominal pain. On examination, there is a palpable mass in the left flank. Computed tomography demonstrates a well-circumscribed multiseptated cystic renal mass, which is replacing the lower pole of the left kidney. The intervening septa are thick and enhance post-contrast, and the cysts appear to be herniating into the renal pelvis. Which of the following is the most likely diagnosis?

A.   Multicystic dysplastic kidney

B.   Multilocular cystic nephroma

C.   Nephroblastomatosis

D.   Polycystic kidney disease

E.   Mesoblastic nephroma

100. A 54-year-old woman is having an MRI for suspected cerebral venous sinus thrombosis. With regard to parenchymal abnormalities associated with venous thrombosis, all are true, except

A.   Parenchymal changes are better depicted on MRI.

B.   DWI helps distinguish between types of cerebral oedema.

C.   Parenchymal changes may not correlate with location of venous occlusion.

D.   Parenchymal abnormalities secondary to venous occlusion are irreversible.

E.   Brain swelling with normal parenchymal signal is well recognised.

101. A 24-year-old man sustained an injury to his wrist following a fall while skiing. There is tenderness in the anatomical snuffbox, particularly on ulnar deviation. Plain radiograph

performed in casualty revels a scaphoid fracture. Which one of the following statements regarding fractures of the scaphoid bone is true?

A. The distal fragment is at risk for avascular necrosis when the waist of the scaphoid is fractured.
B. They usually are the result of a direct blow to the wrist.
C. Fractures of the distal pole are less common than fractures of the proximal pole.
D. Fractures involving the proximal pole invariably lead to avascular necrosis of the proximal fragment.
E. Fractures through the waist of the scaphoid do not displace because of the strong supporting intercarpal ligaments.

102. A 71-year-old man with biopsy-proven Gleason grade 8 adenocarcinoma and a PSA level of 5.65 ng/mL is sent for an MRI prostate for local staging. T2W axial MR image shows that the dominant tumour is within the left peripheral zone extending from the apex to the base with features indicative of extracapsular extension. All the following suggest extracapsular extension, except

A. Broad contact (>12 mm) of tumour with capsule
B. Obliteration of rectoprostatic angle
C. Asymmetry of the neurovascular bundle
D. Nodes in the perivescical fat
E. Irregular capsular bulge

103. An 8-month-old child is investigated for a 5-month history of respiratory symptoms. Chest X-ray shows a right upper zone mass. MRI confirms the presence of a low T1, high T2 signal, well-defined mass displacing the trachea to the left. There is homogeneous internal signal; the lesion is separate from the spinal canal. There is no associated vertebral anomaly and no widening of the neural foramina. The patient is afebrile. What is the most likely diagnosis?

A. Neurofibromatosis
B. Lateral meningocele
C. Neuroenteric cyst
D. Lung abscess
E. Foregut duplication cyst

104. A 10-year-old boy has a 48-hour history of drowsiness and decreasing GCS. In the previous week, he was unwell with a chest infection. The MRI demonstrates multiple areas of hyperintensity on T2 and FLAIR within the white matter. Contrast enhancement demonstrates 'open ring sign'. What is the most likely diagnosis?

A. Multiple sclerosis
B. Acute disseminated encephalomyelitis
C. Multiple cerebral abscesses
D. Herpes encephalitis
E. CMV encephalitis

105. You notice an area of focal dissection at the site of angioplasty of a left common iliac lesion during your completion run. Which of the following is the next step?

A. Reinflate the angioplasty balloon
B. Deploy a stent
C. Measure the pressure gradient
D. Deploy a covered stent
E. Report the finding and finish the procedure

106. A 32-year-old man who fell of his bike in mid-air during a motor cross championship was brought into casualty with weakness of all four limbs and GCS of 10 out of 15. Initial CT showed

a fracture dislocation at C7/T1. An MRI was organised given that there were clinical features of acute spinal cord injury. All of the following findings are expected on the MRI, except
A. Hyperintensity on T2W images
B. Swelling of the spinal cord
C. Hypo intensity on T2W images suggesting haemorrhage
D. Occasional contrast enhancement
E. Atrophy of the spinal cord

107. A 21-year-old man, who presented with a growing mass in the left testis of 2–3 months duration with a palpable, non-tender, firm nodule on the surface of the left testicle, on physical examination showed a well-circumscribed hypoechoic mass with a concentric lamellar pattern of alternating hyper-and hypoechoic rings on US. What is the diagnosis?
A. Tunica albuginea cysts
B. Simple cyst of testis
C. Epidermoid cyst
D. Intratesticular varicocele
E. Intratesticular spermaocele

108. A 2-year-old toddler is brought to the accident and emergency department by his mother with constant vomiting. During clinical examination the toddler is restless, dehydrated and shows the signs of peritonitis. The examining doctor also notices multiple bruises of different ages, skin lacerations and scars. Visceral trauma on a background of non-accidental injury (NAI) is suspected. Which of the following is not a common bowel injury associated with non-accidental trauma?
A. Small bowel rupture
B. Shocked bowel syndrome
C. Intramural mesenteric haematoma
D. Boerhaave syndrome
E. Duodenal contusions

109. You are asked to review the chest X-ray of a postoperative patient, now in intensive treatment unit. The patient has a number of lines and tubes. Which of the following positions suggests incorrect placement?
A. Endotracheal tube with the tip 2 cm above the carina
B. Central venous catheter with the tip in the junction of the superior vena cava/right atrium
C. Nasogastric tube with the tip below the diaphragm overlying the stomach
D. Peripherally inserted tunnelled central venous catheter with the tip in the superior vena cava
E. Intra-aortic counter pulsation balloon pump in the descending aorta distal to the origin of the left subclavian artery

110. A 2-year-boy presents with a 2-week history of melena culminating in an acute episode of bright red blood per rectum. Ultrasound was unremarkable. Upper gastrointestinal endoscopy was negative. Technetium pertechnetate demonstrates increased uptake in the left upper and right lower quadrants. What is the most likely diagnosis?
A. Acute appendicitis
B. Intussusception
C. Meckel's diverticulum
D. Gastrinoma
E. Non-specific inflammatory bowel disease

111. The following are appropriate MR spectroscopy findings, except
A. Canavan disease characteristically demonstrates reduced NAA.
B. Decreased NAA and higher Cho/Cr ratio signifies high-grade malignancy.

C. Lipid peaks suggest infracted brain.

D. Absent choline can distinguish toxoplasmosis from lymphoma.

E. PML may demonstrate elevated myo-inositol.

112. A 44-year-old man with chronic back pain underwent a spinal X-ray, which showed extensive marginal osteophytes with flowing ossification along the anterior aspect of more than four vertebrae with no significant facet joint arthropathy. Intervening disc spaces were maintained with no loss of disc height. In the extremities, generally symmetric enthesophytes are seen most commonly in the

A. Metacarpals, metatarsals and terminal tufts

B. Calcaneus, patella and olecranon

C. Lesser trochanter and acetabulum

D. Medial and lateral epicondyle of humerus

E. Glenohumeral joint and greater tuberosity

113. A 69-year-old man with a history of non-muscle invasive urothelial carcinoma of bladder treated with transurethral resection and intravesical BCG therapy presented with a firm palpable nodule on PR examination. MRI showed a low T2 signal lesion with high signal on DW MR, low signal on ADC map and non-enhancement on subtracted contrast-enhanced images in the peripheral gland at 4 'o' clock. The findings were stable on an MR repeated at 9 months.

A. Prostatic carcinoma

B. Post-inflammatory scar

C. Post biopsy haemorrhage

D. Granulomatous prostatitis

E. Post-radiotherapy change

114. A 14-year-old boy who accidentally fell from a second floor window underwent an urgent computed tomography scan. It revealed diffuse small bowel wall thickening with increased enhancement of bowel wall following intravenous contrast. A flattened inferior vena cava and retroperitoneal oedema were also noted in the radiological report. What is the most likely diagnosis?

A. Small bowel wall contusion

B. Isolated mesenteric haematoma

C. Incomplete jejunal wall tear

D. Complete ileal wall tear

E. Shocked bowel syndrome

115. A 65-year-old man with recurrent bouts of acute red hot swollen 1st MTPJ of the right foot showed classic features of gout on plain radiograph. Which one of the following statements regarding the radiographic appearance of gouty tophi is false?

A. They can contain some degree of calcification.

B. They are asymmetric soft-tissue masses.

C. They may form in bursae.

D. Tophaceous deposits in tendons may result in tendon rupture.

E. They classically are intra-articular in location.

116. A 9-month-old boy with recurrent urinary tract infections and renal pelvis dilatation is referred for a micturating cystourethrogram (MCUG). The patient is currently taking a prophylactic dose of trimethoprim.

With regard to performing an MCUG in this patient, which of the following instructions would you give his mother?

A. The patient should continue on his current regime of antibiotics until his physicians advise him to stop.

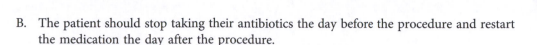

B. The patient should stop taking their antibiotics the day before the procedure and restart the medication the day after the procedure.

C. The patient should take a course of treatment dose trimethoprim, starting on the day of the procedure for 3 subsequent days.

D. The patient should take a 5-day course of treatment dose trimethoprim, starting on the day before the procedure.

E. The patient should stop their antibiotics the day before the procedure and take a 3-day course of treatment dose gentamicin.

117. Which of the following is incorrect?

	Supratentorial tumour	Features
A.	Astrocytoma	Solid with a necrotic centre or cystic with a mural nodule. Associated with NF1
B.	Craniopharyngioma	Cystic or solid tumour with a partially calcified suprasellar mass presenting with endocrine abnormalities
C.	PNET	Heterogeneous hemispheric mass. Necrosis, haemorrhage and enhancement are common
D.	Choroid plexus papilloma	Poorly circumscribed and poorly enhancing tumours
E.	Ganglioglioma	Well-circumscribed peripheral tumour that often presents with seizures

118. A chest X-ray is performed on a patient 1 week following a left pneumonectomy for bronchogenic carcinoma. Which of the following would you not normally expect to see?
    A. Loss of volume of the left hemithorax
    B. Mediastinal shift to the left
    C. Tracheal shift to the right
    D. An enlarging left-sided hydrothorax
    E. Elevation of the left hemidiaphragm

119. A 74-year-old man with painless haematuria and weightloss with irregular thickening of the bladder wall on US underwent an MRI for staging. MRI revealed focal plaque-like thickening in the bladder wall and areas of thin calcification on plain film. All of the following are recognised findings in squamous cell carcinoma of the bladder, except
    A. Single enhancing bladder mass
    B. Papillary tumour with pure intraluminal growth
    C. Sessile enhancing tumour mass
    D. Calcification related to tumour
    E. Mass in a diverticula

120. A restrained driver of a car involved in a high-speed road traffic accident is brought to the emergency department. He is hypovolaemic, tachycardic and has a very tender abdomen. After stabilisation, an urgent intravenous contrast-enhanced CT scan is performed which show features of significant mesenteric injury and the patient is immediately taken to theatre. Which CT sign is not specific for significant mesenteric injury?
    A. Mesenteric contrast extravasation
    B. Mesenteric fat infiltration
    C. Mesenteric vascular beading
    D. Termination of mesenteric vessels
    E. Bowel ischaemia

CHAPTER 14
TEST PAPER 7

Answers

1. B. Carotid-cavernous fistula

Carotid-cavernous fistula (also described as caroticocavernous fistula) is an abnormal communication between the internal carotid artery (ICA) and the veins of the cavernous sinus. It is mostly due to trauma with laceration of the ICA within the cavernous sinus usually due to a skull base fracture or penetrating trauma. Ultrasound and MRI usually show arterial flow in the cavernous sinus and superior ophthalmic vein.

Dähnert W. *Radiology Review Manual*, 7th edn. Philadelphia, PA: Lippincott Williams & Wilkins, 2011:346.

2. C. Foci of calcification projected over the renal angles

The main observations to be made on the plain abdominal radiograph relate primarily to the presence, amount and distribution of gas, which includes intraluminal gas, intramural gas, portal venous gas and free intraperitoneal gas. From observations of the intraluminal gas, it may sometimes be possible to make inferences regarding the presence of bowel wall thickening, free fluid and focal fluid collections.

Dilatation with loss of the mosaic pattern and the development of rounded or elongated loops is more suggestive that an abnormality is present. On plain abdominal radiographs, intramural gas may be diffuse or localised and appears as linear or rounded radiolucencies. Extensive intramural gas can result in a mosaic pattern or bubbly appearance. Portal venous gas appears as branching, linear, radiolucent vessels that may extend from the region of the main portal vein towards the periphery of both hepatic lobes.

On the supine view, large amounts of gas may give rise to the 'football' sign, where the gas outlines the whole of the peritoneal cavity, the undersurface of the diaphragm and the falciform ligament (the lacing of the football). In this view, even smaller amounts of free gas may be detected when both sides of the bowel wall are outlined (Rigler's sign).

Epelman M, et al. Necrotizing enterocolitis: Review of state-of-the-art imaging findings with pathologic correlation. *Radiographics*. 2007;27(2):285–305.

3. B. Paget's disease

A 'bone within bone' appearance describes the radiographic appearance whereby a bone appears to have another bone within it, which results from endosteal new bone formation. Recognised causes include Paget's disease, sickle cell disease, thalassemia, Gaucher's disease, acromegaly, hypervitaminosis D, scurvy and rickets, among many others. It can also be a normal finding in infants, particularly in the thoracolumbar spine.

Dähnert W. *Radiology Review Manual*, 6th edn. Philadelphia, PA: Lippincott Williams & Wilkins, 2007:75.

4. E. Pre- and post-void magnetic resonance imaging of urethra

Female urethral diverticula are thought to be caused by obstruction of Skene's glands. Rarely, carcinoma (usually adenocarcinoma) or calculi can form within them. The gold standard imaging investigation is double-balloon catheter positive pressure urethrography; however, this is invasive and uses ionising radiation. The best first-line test is a pre- and post-void magnetic resonance imaging (MRI) of the urethra, as this avoids ionising radiation and does not involve invasive placement of catheters, and the patient can empty her bladder in private between scans. Positive pressure urethrography is reserved for cases where MRI is equivocal. The remaining options are inappropriate: transvaginal ultrasound may show a lesion but will not clearly demonstrate its relationship to the urethra; micturating cystourethrogram would have a high likelihood of a false negative, requires catheterisation, uses ionising radiation and requires the patient to void in the presence of the radiologist; urodynamics are a functional examination.

Patel AK, Chapple CR. Female urethral diverticula. *Current Opinion in Urology* 2006;16:248–54.
Weissleder R, et al. *Primer of Diagnostic Imaging*, 4th edn. Philadelphia, PA: Mosby Elsevier, 2007:319.

5. A. Cytomegalovirus oesophagitis

Cytomegalovirus oesophagitis almost always occurs exclusively in human immunodeficiency virus (HIV)-positive patients. Barium swallow or endoscopy appearances are of giant ovoid flat ulcers >2 cm near the gastro-oesophageal junction or less commonly, smaller superficial ulcers. Giant ulcers can also be seen in HIV at the time of seroconversion. Caustic ingestion would usually have a different clinical history and tends to produce stricture of the oesophagus. Candida tends to involve the upper oesophagus, has linear plaques and is associated with abnormal motility. Behçet's disease (a rare immune-mediated systemic vasculitis) produces aphthous ulcers. Crohn's disease rarely affects the oesophagus and also would produce aphthous ulcers.

Adam A, et al. *Grainger & Allison's Diagnostic Radiology: A Textbook of Medical Imaging*, 5th edn. New York: Churchill Livingstone, 2008:623.
Dähnert W. *Radiology Review Manual*, 7th edn. Philadelphia, PA: Lippincott Williams & Wilkins, 2011:846–8.
Vossough A, Levine MS. Infectious oesophagitis imaging. Candida oesophagitis. emedicine.medscape.com/article/376127-overview [accessed on 26 February 2017].
Weissleder R, et al. *Primer of Diagnostic Imaging*, 4th edn. Philadelphia, PA: Mosby Elsevier, 2007:165.

6. C. Aberrant left pulmonary artery

Double aortic arch variants and right aortic arch with aberrant left subclavian artery and patent ductus arteriosus are the two most common types of vascular rings which encircle the mediastinal airways. Both these conditions cause leftward deviation of the trachea and indentation of the right tracheal wall visible on the chest X-ray together with a large posterior oesophageal impression visible on oesophagogram. Left aortic arch with aberrant right subclavian artery is the most common vascular anomaly of the aortic arch, but only in the extremely rare association with patent ductus arteriosus will it cause similar appearances.

A less common vascular anomaly, which may cause a similar appearance of the trachea but does not cause any oesophageal indentation, is a common origin of innominate and left common carotid artery. Aberrant left pulmonary artery causes posterior tracheal indentation and anterior oesophageal impression.

Dähnert W. *Radiology Review Manual*, 7th edn. Philadelphia, PA: Lippincott Williams & Wilkins, 2011:598–9.
Yedururi S, et al. Multimodality imaging of tracheobronchial disorders in children. *Radiographics*. 2008;28:e29.

7. A. Punctate calcification is a feature of papillary carcinoma.

Thyroid calcifications may occur in both benign and malignant diseases. Thyroid calcifications can be classified as microcalcification, coarse calcification or peripheral calcification. Microcalcifications are found in 29%–59% of all primary thyroid carcinomas, most commonly in papillary thyroid carcinoma. Their occurrence has been described in follicular and anaplastic thyroid carcinomas as well as in benign conditions such as follicular adenoma and Hashimoto's thyroiditis.

At US imaging, microcalcifications appear as punctate hyperechoic foci without acoustic shadowing. Coarse calcifications may coexist with microcalcifications in papillary cancers, and they are the most common type of calcification in medullary thyroid carcinomas. Inspissated colloid calcifications in benign thyroid lesions may mimic microcalcifications in thyroid malignancies, but the former can be distinguished from malignant calcifications by the observation of ring-down or reverberation artefact. Peripheral calcification is one of the patterns most commonly seen in a multinodular thyroid but may also be seen in malignancy.

US features that should arouse suspicion about lymph node metastases include a rounded bulging shape, increased size, replaced fatty hilum, irregular margins, heterogeneous echotexture, calcifications, cystic area and vascularity throughout the lymph node instead of normal central hilar vessels at Doppler imaging.

Hoang JK, et al. US features of thyroid malignancy: Pearls and pitfalls. *Radiographics*. 2007;27:847–65.

8. E. Rhabdomyosarcoma
Rhabdomyosarcoma is the most common mesenchymal tumour in children. Rhabdomyosarcoma is an aggressive, rapidly growing tumour and most often manifests with rapidly progressive proptosis or globe displacement. Orbital cellulitis is differential, but patients are afebrile and inflammatory markers are normal. On CT images, orbital rhabdomyosarcoma generally appears as an extraconal, irregular ovoid, well-circumscribed, homogeneous mass that is isoattenuated relative to muscle. Calcification is usually seen only in association with bone destruction. At MRI, they are isointense to muscle or brain with T1-weighted sequences and variably hyperintense to muscle and brain with T2-weighted pulse sequences. They enhance uniformly with contrast.

Dermoid cyst is the most common orbital mass in children. Imaging features that suggest a dermoid include a cystic appearance, internal fat attenuation or signal intensity (T1 hyperintensity) and internal calcification, all of which are uncommon in rhabdomyosarcoma.

On images, vascular malformations are often cystic and multiloculated with ill-defined borders. They frequently contain fluid–fluid levels because of haemorrhage into the cysts, whereas fluid–fluid levels are quite uncommon in rhabdomyosarcoma. Peripheral enhancement can be seen around cystic area, which is uncommon in rhabdomyosarcomas.

Chung EM, et al. From the archives of the AFIP: Pediatric orbit tumors and tumorlike lesions: Nonosseous lesions of the extraocular orbit. *Radiographics*. 2007;27(6):1777–99.

9. E. Malgaigne
Pelvic fractures can be divided into stable and unstable fractures. The Malgaigne, open book, straddle and bucket-handle fractures are all unstable, as the pelvic ring is interrupted in two places. The Malgaigne fracture is described in this case. The open book fracture implies fracture/diastasis of both ischiopubic rami and sacroiliac joints, the straddle fracture involves both obturator rings and the bucket-handle fracture refers to an SI joint fracture with a contralateral ischiopubic ramus fracture. Patients with unstable fractures are at significant risk of pelvic organ injury and haemorrhage. Duverney fracture is an isolated fracture of the iliac wing and is a stable fracture.

Weissleder R, et al. *Primer of Diagnostic Imaging*, 5th edn. Philadelphia, PA: Mosby Elsevier, 2011.

10. A. Myelofibrosis
Myelofibrosis causes splenomegaly and therefore make splenic detection easier. All of the other options provided are potential causes of a non-visualised spleen. Polysplenia syndrome (also known as bilateral left-sidedness) is, as the name suggests, actually associated with

multiple spleens, but these are usually in the wrong place (in addition to a vast array of other intra-abdominal anomalies). A wandering spleen relates to the condition where the spleen is attached to an abnormally long and mobile pedicle, which means that the spleen can be found in places other than in the left upper quadrant.

Dähnert W. *Radiology Review Manual*, 7th edn. Philadelphia, PA: Lippincott Williams & Wilkins, 2011:130–1.

11. C. X-linked adrenoleukodystrophy

Dysmyelinating diseases, or leukodystrophies, encompass a wide spectrum of inherited neurodegenerative disorders affecting the integrity of myelin in the brain and peripheral nerves. Most of these disorders fall into one of three categories – lysosomal storage diseases, peroxisomal disorders and diseases caused by mitochondrial dysfunction – and each leukodystrophy has distinctive clinical, biochemical, pathological and radiological features. X-linked adrenoleukodystrophy is an inherited white matter disorder caused by gene mutation (*ALD* gene) resulting in abnormal formation of myelin. The childhood cerebral form (CCALD) is the most common and affects males aged between 4 and 10 years. Hyperpigmentation can occur as a result of adrenal insufficiency. The diagnostic clue is symmetric, peritrigonal white matter abnormality involving the splenium. Alexander disease characteristically involves the frontal white matter preferentially, and Canavan disease causes diffuse white matter abnormality.

Moore KR, et al. *Diagnostic Imaging: Paediatric Neuroradiology*, 1st edn. Salt Lake City, UT: Amirsys, 2007.

12. A. Actinomycosis

Pelvic actinomycosis is a rare chronic bacterial infection but is commonly seen in the setting of a long-standing IUCD. It can also be associated with recent surgery. It often causes abdominal pain, low-grade fever and an abdominal or pelvic mass/abscess, which can mimic a malignant mass as it can get quite large if left untreated. The earlier it is diagnosed and treated, the less likely the patient will require surgery. The cobra-shaped structure is an infected dilated tube. Endometriosis can give cysts containing low-level echoes but fever would be unusual with pain. Appendix and diverticulitis can cause irritation of the adjacent tube but the clue is the long-standing IUCD.

Dähnert W. *Radiology Review Manual*, 7th edn. Philadelphia, PA: Lippincott Williams & Wilkins, 2011:48.
Lely RJ, van Es HW. Case 85: Pelvic actinomycosis in association with an intrauterine device. *Radiology*. 2005;236:492–4.
Maloney JJ, Cho SR. Pelvic actinomycosis. *Radiology*. 1983;148:388.

13. C. This patient carries an increased risk of developing pulmonary haemorrhage post-procedure.

Studies have identified lesion depth as being the most important risk factor for pulmonary haemorrhage, with an increased risk in lesions deeper than 2 cm. The incidence of pneumothorax is reported to be between 22% and 45%, of which 3.3–15% will require a chest drain. The risk of developing pneumothorax increases significantly if the lesion is not contiguous with the pleural surface. Studies have shown that the presence of chronic obstructive airway disease increases the necessity of chest drain insertion, although this does not necessarily hold for risk of pneumothorax. Although there are no definite absolute contraindications to CT-guided lung biopsy, there are, however, several relative contraindications. Patients should not undergo the procedure without adequate prebiopsy assessment or if they plan to fly within 6 weeks of the procedure. The risk is increased by abnormalities of lung function, respiratory failure (including mechanical ventilation), arterial and venous pulmonary hypertension and coagulation abnormalities. The balance of benefit against risk for the procedure should be assessed at a multidisciplinary meeting. Previous contralateral pneumonectomy precludes needle biopsy; however, if the lesion abuts the pleural surface and can be accessed with no needle traversing lung tissue, then the risk of pneumothorax is very low and may not, therefore, be considered as a contraindication. Patients should not undergo needle biopsy without further multidisciplinary team assessment if pulmonary function tests demonstrate an FEV_1 of <35%.

Anderson JM, et al. CT-guided lung biopsy: Factors influencing diagnostic yield and complication rate. *Clin Radiol.* 2003;58:791–7.
Manhire A, et al. Guidelines for radiologically guided lung biopsy. *Thorax.* 2003;58:920–36.

14. C. Constrictive pericarditis

Constrictive pericarditis is a recognised complication of cardiac surgery, with recent evidence showing an incidence of 0.2%. The most common cause, however, would be idiopathic, thought to result from an occult viral pericarditis, with tuberculosis being the most common cause worldwide. Clinical symptoms attributed to both left- and right-sided heart failure are usually present.

The hallmarks of pericardial constriction are pericardial thickening, pericardial calcification and abnormal diastolic ventricular function. Other findings associated with raised right-sided pressure such as dilatation of the superior vena cava and azygos vein help support the diagnosis. Constrictive pericarditis can be distinguished from restrictive cardiomyopathy on the basis of pericardial thickness measuring more than 4 mm in the presence of characteristic haemodynamic findings.

Dressler syndrome typically occurs 3 weeks to several months, not years, after cardiac surgery.

Adam A, et al. *Grainger & Allison's Diagnostic Radiology: A Textbook of Medical Imaging,* 5th edn. New York: Churchill Livingstone, 2008:934–6.
Dähnert W. *Radiology Review Manual,* 7th edn. Philadelphia, PA: Lippincott Williams & Wilkins, 2011:641.

15. A. Hepatoblastoma

Hepatoblastoma is the most common primary hepatic tumour in children. Hepatoblastoma has been associated with several syndromes, including Beckwith–Wiedemann syndrome, Gardner syndrome, familial adenomatous polyposis, type 1A glycogen storage disease and trisomy 18.

Heptoblastomas are most often hyperechoic relative to adjacent liver on US. A spoke-wheel appearance with areas of alternating echogenicity may be seen at antenatal imaging. CT shows a sharply circumscribed mass that is slightly hypoattenuating relative to the adjacent liver on unenhanced and contrast-enhanced images. Epithelial hepatoblastomas demonstrate a more homogeneous appearance, while mixed tumours are more heterogeneous in attenuation. Speckled or amorphous calcification is seen in more than 50% of lesions. The tumour enhances slightly, but less than adjacent liver.

At MR imaging, epithelial hepatoblastomas are homogeneously slightly hypointense on T1-weighted images and hyperintense on T2-weighted images relative to adjacent liver parenchyma. Mixed tumours demonstrate more heterogeneous signal intensity characteristics. Fibrotic septa are hypointense on both T1- and T2-weighted images and enhance after intravenous administration of gadolinium contrast material.

Infantile haemangioendothelioma (IHE) is a vascular tumour and enhances much more than adjacent liver, while hepatoblastoma typically enhances much less than adjacent liver. Occasionally, the peripheral rim enhancement on arterial phase images seen in hepatoblastoma may suggest IHE, but IHE is distinguished by intense nodular or corrugated peripheral enhancement with centripetal fill-in on delayed phase images. Mesenchymal hamartoma of the liver (MHL) is a benign tumour that manifests in the same age group as hepatoblastoma. It can usually be distinguished from hepatoblastoma by normal serum AFP levels in MHL, predominantly cystic appearance and age at diagnosis >5 years (cf. hepatoblastoma generally diagnosed <5 years).

Chung EM, et al. From the archives of the AFIP: Pediatric liver masses: Radiologic-pathologic correlation. Part 2. Malignant tumors. *Radiographics.* 2011;31(2):483–507.

16. B. To minimise anisotropy

The purpose of the heel–toe manoeuvre in ultrasound is the same in all situations regardless of the site being imaged. It is to reduce anisotropy artefacts that result when the probe is not perpendicular to the structure being imaged. Similarly, reducing beam angle incidence would increase such artefacts. Reducing probe compression reduces posterior reverberation artefact. Placing the structure of interest within the central region of the probe and placing the focal zone at the region of interest reduce beam width artefact.

Taljonovic MS, et al. Artefacts in musculoskeletal ultrasonography. *Semin Musculoskel Radiol.* 2014;18:3–11.

17. B. Paraovarian cyst

Paraovarian cysts are responsible for about 10% of adnexal masses. They do not usually change in size. They are susceptible to torsion or bleeding which can cause pain but are usually asymptomatic. They are congenital, occurring from embryonic Wolffian or mesonephric duct remnants within the broad ligament, and are separate from the ovary. Theca lutein cysts are usually bilateral.

Endometriomas usually contain low-level echoes and there is often more than one deposit; they are also less likely to remain static over time. Adenomyosis is a uterine abnormality that involves abnormal glandular tissue within the myometrium and causes thickening of the myometrium. An ovarian dermoid would usually be hyperechoic or contain mixed elements, giving it a heterogeneous appearance.

Dähnert W. *Radiology Review Manual*, 7th edn. Philadelphia, PA: Lippincott Williams & Wilkins, 2011:1075.
Thickman D, Gussman D. Magnetic resonance imaging of benign adnexal conditions. In: Colletti PM, Gussman D, Kanal E, et al. eds. *MRI Clinics of North America: The Female Pelvis*, Vol. 2: no. 2. Philadelphia, PA: WB Saunders, 1994:275–90.
Weissleder R, et al. *Primer of Diagnostic Imaging*, 4th edn. Philadelphia, PA: Mosby Elsevier, 2007:349.

18. A. The transplanted pancreatic duct is normally dilated.

Pancreatic transplant is a potentially curative treatment option predominantly for Type 1 diabetes. The pancreas is normally grafted onto the external iliac vessels. In most cases, the procedure is combined with a simultaneous renal transplant. Exocrine pancreatic secretions can be redirected either into the bladder (easier with simultaneous renal transplant) or bowel. There are advantages and disadvantages of both approaches; redirection to the bladder enables close monitoring of secretions but can lead to acidosis. Radiological input is usually required in postoperative monitoring. Ultrasound scanning can reveal peripancreatic collections/pseudocysts, vessel thrombosis and other signs of acute rejection (indistinct pancreatic margins, acoustic inhomogeneity of the pancreas and dilatation of the pancreatic duct).

Dähnert W. *Radiology Review Manual*, 7th edn. Philadelphia, PA: Lippincott Williams & Wilkins, 2011:755.
Kaufman DB. Pancreas transplantation. emedicine.medscape.com/article/429408-overview.

19. B. Bilateral common peroneal nerve entrapment

Common peroneal neuropathy (CPN) is the most common mononeuropathy in the lower extremity. In most cases, CPN neuropathy occurs in the knee region, whereas neuropathy of the superficial peroneal nerve (SPN) and deep peroneal nerve (DPN) occurs more distally in the leg, ankle or foot.

The CPN is particularly prone to entrapment because it is fixed in position at the greater sciatic foramen (peroneal division) and around the fibular head. There are two common compression sites of the CPN. The nerve may be compressed as it crosses the fibular neck, owing to its superficial location, or as it travels under the origin of the peroneus longus muscle. Injury to the nerve at these locations may be the result of extrinsic compression, stretch injury or direct trauma.

Extrinsic compression of the CPN can be the result of external compression by various agents such as short-leg cast, crush injury, surgery, tumour, osteochondroma, synovial cyst, intraneural and extraneural ganglia, varicosities, aberrant muscle, prolonged immobilisation (Saturday night palsy), prolonged squatting (strawberry pickers' palsy) and extended lithotomy position due to childbirth or obstetric surgery will typically produce bilateral CPN entrapment. Diabetic patients are at an increased risk for entrapment of the CPN within the fibrous tunnel underneath the peroneus longus muscle.

Patients with CPN often present with frequent tripping related to a foot drop. Pain may be present at the site of compression. Sensory disturbances include paraesthesia and anaesthesia along the lateral lower leg and dorsal foot. On physical examination, patients demonstrate foot drop, weak foot extension (anterior tibial muscle), weak foot eversion (peroneus longus and brevis muscles) and loss of sensation in the lower lateral two-thirds of the leg and the dorsum of the foot.

Donovan A, et al. MR imaging of entrapment neuropathies of the lower extremity. Part 2. The knee, leg, ankle, and foot. *Radiographics*. 2010;30:1001–19.

20. A. Subependymal calcification

Dandy–Walker malformation is the most common posterior fossa malformation. The key neuroimaging features are hypoplasia (or, rarely, agenesis) of the cerebellar vermis (whose inferior portion is typically affected, possibly in combination with its superior portion), which is elevated and upwardly rotated; and dilatation of the cystic-appearing fourth ventricle, which consequently may fill the entire posterior fossa.

Additional malformations, including dysgenesis or agenesis of the corpus callosum, occipital encephalocele, polymicrogyria and grey matter heterotopia, may be present in 30%–50%. Hydrocephalus is associated in about 90% of patients.

Subependymal calcification is a feature of tuberous sclerosis.

Bosemani T, et al. Congenital abnormalities of the posterior fossa. *Radiographics*. 2015;35(1):200–20.

21. A. Rickets

Rickets is the paediatric equivalent of osteomalacia. It affects the metaphysis of bones as these are the most metabolically active sites. Common sites of involvement include proximal humerus, proximal tibia and proximal and distal femur. Appearances include widened and irregularly shaped physeal lucencies and metaphyseal flaring. There may be long bone deformation with lower limb bowing. Patients with rickets are at increased risk of Salter–Harris I fractures of the epiphyses that most commonly occur at the proximal femur (SCFE).

While Blount's disease is often associated with bow legged-ness in infants and children, it is an abnormality at the knee with an increase in the tibial metaphyseal angle. There are a few cases in the literature of SCFE in association with Blount's disease.

While hypophosphatasia may give similar findings to rickets, its incidence 1:10 0000 is several orders of magnitude less than rickets (1:100–1:1000).

Manaster BJ, et al. *The Requisites: MSK Imaging*, 3rd edn. Philadelphia, PA: Mosby, 2007:380–1.

22. C. Ovarian fibroma

Ovarian fibromas typically arise in postmenopausal women and are usually asymptomatic. Rarely, they can cause pressure-type symptoms if they get large enough, or tort causing pain.

Ovarian fibromas are classically known to cause Meigs syndrome, which is the combination of ascites, pleural effusion and a benign ovarian tumour. The ascites and pleural effusion often resolve after tumour removal. They are also more common in Gorlin (basal cell naevus) syndrome, where they tend to occur at a younger age and are more likely to be bilateral. Owing to their highly fibrous component, they have a similar intensity to uterine fibroids, being low on T1 and T2-weighted sequences. On ultrasound, they are often hypoechoic with attenuation of the ultrasound beam as it passes through the lesion. About 1% can undergo malignant transformation to a fibrosarcoma.

Krukenberg tumours result from ovarian metastases, classically from the stomach; however, colon, breast, lung, gynaecological tumours, sarcomas and melanoma can also spread to the ovary.

These tumours would less likely be so low intensity on T1 and T2-weighted images and there may be a history of cancer. Ovarian mucinous cystadenomas tend to contain a jelly-like fluid, so are usually cystic on imaging, but can contain solid components. A dermoid cyst usually contains mixed elements including fat and would not usually cause ascites. Clear cell carcinoma is an aggressive ovarian lesion associated with endometriosis and a poor prognosis; these often have cystic and solid components.

Dähnert W. *Radiology Review Manual*, 7th edn. Philadelphia, PA: Lippincott Williams & Wilkins, 2011:1074.
Thickman D, Gussman D. Magnetic resonance imaging of benign adnexal conditions. In: Colletti PM, Gussman D, Kanal E, et al. eds. *MRI Clinics of North America: The Female Pelvis*, Vol. 2: no. 2. Philadelphia, PA: WB Saunders, 1994:275–90.
Weissleder R, et al. *Primer of Diagnostic Imaging*, 4th edn. Philadelphia, PA: Mosby Elsevier, 2007:355.

23. D. Alveolar proteinosis

Alveolar proteinosis is a rare disorder that is characterised by the abnormal accumulation of proteinaceous material in alveoli, secondary to altered surfactant homeostasis. It affects young to middle-aged adults and is more common in men. There is a strong association with cigarette smoking. Clinical features are variable, with symptoms usually being of gradual onset. Chest radiography typically demonstrates bilateral air-space opacity with either an ill-defined nodular or ground-glass pattern. An important discriminator from pulmonary oedema is the presence of perihilar lung changes in the absence of cardiomegaly, pulmonary venous hypertension and pleural effusions. Similarly, while sarcoidosis can mimic many lung conditions, the absence of lymphadenopathy is an important feature to note in alveolar proteinosis. The classic computed tomography finding is known as crazy paving – the description given to the combination of patchy ground-glass opacities with smooth interlobular septal thickening in a geographical distribution.

Dähnert W. *Radiology Review Manual*, 7th edn. Philadelphia, PA: Lippincott Williams & Wilkins, 2011:471.

24. D. Computed tomography report describing a 6 cm pseudocyst

The clinical scenario presented is that of new-onset acute pancreatitis. Pseudocysts are encapsulated collections of pancreatic fluid found in a peripancreatic position. Classically, these take 4 weeks to develop. The other options provided are all potential causes of acute pancreatitis. Alcoholism and cholelithiasis are the most common causes. Recent viral infection (e.g., mumps, hepatitis, glandular fever), trauma, structural anomalies (pancreas divisum), some drugs (e.g., steroids, azathioprine, diuretics) and multisystem conditions (shock, haemolytic–uraemic syndrome, systemic lupus erythematosus) are all recognised causes of pancreatitis. In a large number of patients, no definite cause is ever identified (idiopathic).

Dähnert W. *Radiology Review Manual*, 7th edn. Philadelphia, PA: Lippincott Williams & Wilkins, 2011:755–7.

25. E. Clear cell carcinoma of the ovary

Clear cell carcinoma and endometrioid carcinomas are commonly found in patients with previous endometriosis. Clear cell carcinoma is an aggressive carcinoma. It is frequently cystic with enhancing mural nodules. The cystic and solid components are high signal on both T1- and T2-weighted images. Brenner tumour of the ovary is low signal on T1- and T2-weighted imaging. Endometrioma may have a bright T1 signal but should not have enhancing mural nodules or be associated with weight loss. Dysgerminoma is a solid germ cell tumour of the ovary, typically solid with a fibrous capsule and fibrous septa. Ovarian dermoid should contain fat and would not be associated with weight loss.

Imaoka I, et al. Developing an MR imaging strategy for diagnosis of ovarian masses. *Radiographics*. 2006;26:1431–48.
Matsuoka Y, et al. MR imaging of clear cell carcinoma of the ovary. *Eur Radiol*. 2001;11:946–51.

26. E. Posterior inferior cerebellar artery

With posterior inferior cerebellar artery (PICA) aneurysms, the rate of intraventricular haemorrhage is high due to reflux of blood. If there is an isolated intraventricular haemorrhage, a peripheral PICA aneurysm, lying in or near the fourth ventricle, may be suspected.

Urbach H, et al. Posterior inferior cerebellar artery aneurysm in the fourth ventricle. *Neuroradiology.* 1995;37 (4):267–9.

27. B. Ventricular septal defect

Congenital cardiac anomalies can be categorised according to whether or not the child is cyanosed. Thereafter, assessment of both heart size and pulmonary arterial flow allows considerable shortening of the differential diagnosis:

Pulmonary arterial flow	Cyanosed		Not cyanosed
Increased	Truncus arteriosus		Left to right shunt (VSD, ASD, PDA)
	Total anomalous pulmonary venous return		
Normal/variable	Transposition of the great arteries		Obstructive lesions (coarctation, aortic/pulmonary arterial stenosis)
	Tricuspid atresia		
Decreased	Enlarged heart	Normal size heart	
	Ebstein anomaly	Tetralogy of Fallot	
	Pulmonary atresia with intact ventricular septum		

In the case provided, the only conditions not associated with cyanosis are ventricular septal defect (VSD) and atrial septal defect (ASD). VSD is the most common congenital heart anomaly.

Donnelly LF. *Pediatric Imaging: The Fundamentals.* Philadelphia, PA: Saunders Elsevier, 2009.

28. E. None of the above

A cemented component in a total hip joint replacement (THR) will demonstrate increased uptake on a radionuclide bone scan for up to 1–2 years. Following this time, increased uptake is good evidence to support mechanical loosening or infection with a 50%–100% sensitivity. It is, however, not specific and therefore correlation with the patient's clinical presentation and plain radiography is required. Aspiration under fluoroscopic guidance may be required to diagnose or exclude infection. An arthrogram can be performed at the same time, which may allow a confident diagnosis of mechanical loosening to be made; however, a negative arthrogram does not exclude this.

Cementless THR components may have persistently increased radionuclide uptake. This is secondary to bone ingrowth into the prosthesis and needs to be differentiated from pathology.

Weissman BN. Imaging of total hip joint replacements. *Radiology.* 1997;202:611–23.

29. C. Pancreatic adenocarcinoma

Painless jaundice commonly occurs secondary to tumours in the head of pancreas. The most common pancreatic tumour, by far, is adenocarcinoma. All the other tumours described are rare by comparison. Pancreas divisum is an anatomical variant relating to pancreatic duct morphology where rather than having a single pancreatic duct, the patient has two (embryologically, there is a failure of fusion); it has an association with idiopathic, recurrent pancreatitis but not with bile duct obstruction. Pancreatic pseudocyst is an encapsulated collection of pancreatic fluid found either within the pancreas or in a peripancreatic position. It most commonly occurs secondary to acute pancreatitis.

Dähnert W. *Radiology Review Manual*, 7th edn. Philadelphia, PA: Lippincott Williams & Wilkins, 2011:750–1.

30. A. Amyloidosis

Amyloidosis is a rare condition, which can affect one specific organ, or present as a systemic illness. The disease is characterised by the deposition of proteinaceous material either in a focal, tumour-like lesion or an infiltrative fashion. Within the chest, cardiac involvement is the most commonly seen, with patients presenting with variable symptoms ranging from arrhythmias to cardiac failure. Pulmonary involvement is typically in the setting of multiple previous chest infections. Computed tomography often demonstrates 'tree-in-bud' opacity, usually in a peripheral location, at sites of previous pneumonia. Within the tracheo-bronchial tree, mass-like lesions are seen arising from the internal wall, often significantly compromising the airway lumen. While the other conditions listed could result in scattered intrapulmonary nodules, the additional endobronchial abnormality makes amyloidosis more likely.

Georgiades CS, et al. Amyloidosis: Review and CT manifestations. *Radiographics*. 2004;24:405–16.

31. D. Tricuspid atresia

Congenital cardiac anomalies can be categorised according to whether or not the child is cyanosed. Thereafter, assessment of both heart size and pulmonary arterial flow allows considerable shortening of the differential diagnosis:

Pulmonary arterial flow	Cyanosed		Not cyanosed
Increased	Truncus arteriosus		Left to right shunt (VSD, ASD, PDA)
	Total anomalous pulmonary venous return		
Normal/variable	Transposition of the great arteries		Obstructive lesions (coarctation, aortic/pulmonary arterial stenosis)
	Tricuspid atresia		
Decreased	Enlarged heart	Normal size heart	
	Ebstein anomaly	Tetralogy of Fallot	
	Pulmonary atresia with intact ventricular septum		

In the case provided, the child is cyanosed; this excludes patent ductus arteriosus and coarctation as the cause. Ebstein anomaly classically produces a grossly enlarged heart. While tetralogy of Fallot is the most common congenital cardiac anomaly to cause cyanosis, it has characteristic CXR features; upturned cardiac apex and deficient main pulmonary artery creates a 'boot-shaped' heart. In addition, there is usually decreased pulmonary vascularity associated with Fallot's tetralogy.

Tricuspid atresia is the third most common congenital cardiac cause of cyanosis after tetralogy of Fallot and transposition of the great vessels.

Dähnert W. *Radiology Review Manual*, 7th edn. Philadelphia, PA: Lippincott Williams & Wilkins, 2011.
Donnelly LF. *Pediatric Imaging: The Fundamentals*. Philadelphia, PA: Saunders Elsevier, 2009.

32. C. Temporo-frontal

Pick's disease is a neurodegenerative disease, and one of the tauopathies (group of neurodegenerative diseases characterised by abnormal metabolism of tau proteins leading to intracellular accumulation and formation of neurofibrillary tangles, similar to Alzheimer's disease) characterised by the accumulation of the Pick bodies. It is sometimes used synonymously with fronto-temporal lobar degeneration (FTLD), although strictly it is incorrect since all causes of FTLD isn't pathologically Pick's disease.

The primary imaging abnormality is that of cortical atrophy of the frontal and temporal lobes. These changes can be markedly asymmetric and affect one region much more than another. Volume of the head of the caudate nucleus may also be reduced. Differentials include Alzheimer's disease and corticobasal degeneration where parietal lobe involvement is more pronounced.

Levine R. Fronto-temporal dementia-Picks disease. In: *Defying Dementia, Understanding and Preventing Alzheimer's and Related Disorders.* Levine R (ed.). Westport, CT: Praeger Publishers, 2006:67–78.

33. C. Compressive lesions are common in the lumbar spine

Vertebral haemangiomas are a hamartomatous lesion. Spinal haemangiomas are common and frequently multiple. The prevalence of haemangiomas seems to increase with age and is greatest after middle age, with a slight female predilection. Most haemangiomas are seen in the thoracic and lumbar spine. They are usually confined to the vertebral body, although they may occasionally extend into the posterior elements. Most spinal haemangiomas are asymptomatic. Occasionally, vertebral haemangiomas may increase in size and compress the spinal cord and nerve roots. Compressive vertebral haemangiomas can occur in patients of any age, with a peak prevalence in young adults and preferentially occur in the thoracic spine.

CT shows the pattern as multiple dots (polka-dot appearance). At scintigraphy, the appearance of osseous haemangiomas ranges from photopenia to a moderate increase in radiotracer uptake. The presence of high signal intensity on T1-w and T2-weighted MR images is related to the amount of adipocytes or vessels and interstitial oedema, respectively.

Fatty vertebral haemangiomas (high on T1-weighted MR) may represent inactive forms of this lesion, whereas low signal intensity at T1-weighted MR imaging may indicate a more active lesion with the potential to compress the spinal cord.

Rodallec MH, et al. Diagnostic imaging of solitary tumors of the spine: What to do and say. *Radiographics.* 2008;28(4):1019–41.

34. D. Decreased resistive index in hepatic artery

There are many features of liver cirrhosis identifiable with ultrasound. Most commonly, these include an echo bright, irregular, shrunken liver (late stage) with a coarse echotexture and hypertrophy of the caudate lobe (earlier in the disease the entire liver can hypertrophy). Isoechoic regenerative nodules may be apparent. If measured, there should be an increase in the resistive index (RI) of the hepatic artery. Reversal of portal venous flow (hepatofugal), portalisation of the hepatic veins, ascites and splenomegaly are extrahepatic signs that are commonly identified. Hepatocellular carcinoma is a major complication of cirrhosis that should always be borne in mind when examining these patients.

Dähnert W. *Radiology Review Manual*, 7th edn. Philadelphia, PA: Lippincott Williams & Wilkins, 2011:719–21.

35. D. In blunt chest trauma, the perforation usually occurs in the lower third of the oesophagus.

Oesophageal perforation is a surgical emergency that carries a high mortality. Oesophageal instrumentation, biopsy, balloon dilatation and attempted intubation (iatrogenic) are the most common causes of rupture and typically result in lower oesophageal injury. Spontaneous rupture, also known as Boerhaave syndrome, arises when intraluminal pressure is elevated during sudden and severe vomiting episodes. While oesophageal rupture in blunt chest trauma is rare, this typically results in upper oesophageal injury and resultant right-sided hydrothorax.

Chest radiography signs include mediastinal and neck emphysema, mediastinal widening and hydrothorax. Barium can be used in the assessment of patients with possible oesophageal perforation, but only after water-soluble contrast swallow has not shown an abnormality.

Dähnert W. *Radiology Review Manual*, 7th edn. Philadelphia, PA: Lippincott Williams & Wilkins, 2011:844.

36. D. Rheumatic fever

The imaging features described are those of acute congestive heart failure. In the context of joint pain following a recent sore throat and with no previous cardiac history, rheumatic fever should be considered.

Rheumatic fever commonly causes a pancarditis with valve insufficiency that can lead to acute congestive heart failure in severe cases. This follows a streptococcal pharyngitis. Chronically, rheumatic heart disease can cause valve stenosis with varying degrees of regurgitation, arrhythmias and ventricular dysfunction. Rheumatic fever as a child is the most common cause of valvular heart disease in adults in the western world. The mitral valve is the most commonly affected. Currently, the disease rarely affects children in the West, but the condition remains common in the developing world.

Chin TK, et al. *Pediatric Rheumatic Heart Disease*. emedicine.medscape.com/article/891897 [accessed on 27 February 2017].

37. E. Wilson's disease

Basal ganglia calcification:

Common causes: Hypoparathyroidism, pseudohypoparathyroidism, idiopathic, normal variant, physiologic with ageing.

Uncommon causes: AIDS encephalopathy, atherosclerosis, birth anoxia, hypoxia, carbonic anhydrase II deficiency, carbon monoxide intoxication, Fahr disease (ferrocalcinosis), familial idiopathic symmetrical basal ganglia calcification and microcephaly, Hallervorden–Spatz disease, haemorrhage, hyperparathyroidism, hypothyroidism, cretinism, Kearns–Sayre syndrome, lead encephalopathy, lipoid proteinosis, MELAS syndrome, methotrexate therapy for childhood leukaemia, oculodento-osseous dysplasia, parasitic disease (e.g., toxoplasmosis, cysticercosis), parkinsonism, phenylketonuria variants, pseudopseudohypoparathyroidism, radiation therapy, Down's syndrome, tuberous sclerosis, viral encephalitis.

Reeder MM. Gamut A-49; Basal Ganglia Calcification. Reeder and Felson's Gamuts in Radiology (2003); A. Skull & Brain. Page 40. Springer-Verlag New York, Inc.

38. B. Granulosa cell tumour

Many ovarian tumours produce oestrogen, the most common being granulosa cell tumour. This results in postmenopausal bleeding, irregular bleeding in premenopausal women and precocious puberty in prepubertal girls. Breast tenderness is another sign, particularly in postmenopausal women. The fluid levels are caused by haemorrhage into the tumour cysts. Endometriosis tends to improve in postmenopausal women as there is no longer oestrogen being produced; it should not cause a thickened endometrium. Endometrial hyperplasia and haemorrhagic corpus luteal cyst are related to ovulation, so do not occur in postmenopausal women. Serous cystadenocarcinomas may produce adnexal masses but do not produce oestrogen, so do not cause endometrial thickening. Fibrothecomas can produce oestrogen and cause endometrial thickening but tend to be solid hypoechoic lesions.

Imaoka I, et al. Developing an MR imaging strategy for diagnosis of ovarian masses. *Radiographics*. 2006;26:1431–48.

Tanaka YO, et al. Functioning ovarian tumours: Direct and indirect findings at MR imaging. *Radiographics*. 2004;24:S147–66.

Weissleder R, et al. *Primer of Diagnostic Imaging*, 4th edn. Philadelphia, PA: Mosby Elsevier, 2007:1045.

39. C. Septa show intense enhancement post-contrast injection.

Giant cell tumour of the spine occurs in the 2nd–4th decades of life, more frequently in females. Sacrum is affected in 90% of such cases. It is usually located in the upper sacrum and sacral wing. Extension to the iliac wing through the sacroiliac joint is possible. Lumbar, thoracic and cervical spine may be affected. It usually predominates in the vertebral body, with frequent involvement of the posterior arch. Extraosseous involvement of the soft tissues is common. Intervertebral disk invasion and extension into an adjacent vertebra are possible.

In radiography, they appear as lytic lesion with cortical expansion. CT demonstrates lack of a sclerotic rim. Bone scintigraphy shows increased radiotracer uptake. The tumour usually has low-to-intermediate signal intensity on T1-weighted MR images. Areas of high signal intensity suggest haemorrhage. More specifically, they have low to intermediate signal intensity on T2-weighted images, caused by haemosiderin and high collagen content. Enhancement reflects its vascular supply. Cystic areas, haemorrhage, fluid–fluid levels and a peripheral low-signal-intensity pseudocapsule may also be seen.

ABC occurs between 5 and 20 years but can manifest at any age. There may be a slight female predilection. Thoracic spine is most commonly affected. Spinal involvement is typically in the posterior elements, although extension into the vertebral body is common. Spinal ABC may extend into the adjacent vertebrae or intervertebral disk, ribs and the paravertebral soft tissue. CT and MR imaging typically show a well-defined lesion with internal septation. Fluid–fluid level is better seen on MRI. The predominant bone scintigraphic pattern is moderate to intense radiotracer accumulation at the periphery with little activity at its centre ('doughnut sign'). Post-contrast images show intense enhancement of the septa. Solid components suggest secondary ABC.

Rodallec MH, et al. Diagnostic imaging of solitary tumors of the spine: What to do and say. *Radiographics*. 2008;28(4):1019–41.

40. D. Adenomyosis

Adenomyosis can be focal or diffuse, the latter being the more common. The aetiology is unclear, but prominent endometrial glands extend into the myometrium with adjacent smooth muscle hyperplasia. Leiomyoma tends to be sharply demarcated as opposed to ill-defined and tends to have low-intensity T1 and T2 signals, although multiple signal characteristics are seen. It would be unusual for leiomyomas to have linear bands extending from the endometrium; this is more commonly seen in adenomyosis. Leiomyoma and leiomyosarcomas cannot be differentiated accurately on imaging; secondary features of lymphadenopathy or metastasis can help raise the suspicion of leiomyosarcoma. Endometrial carcinoma usually presents in an older age group and tends to present with symptoms of irregular bleeding, which is why it is often diagnosed at an early stage. There would likely be endometrial thickening also. Hydatidiform moles would usually be identified clinically, particularly in a patient being investigated for infertility, as she would have raised beta-human chorionic gonadotrophin levels.

Dähnert W. *Radiology Review Manual*, 7th edn. Philadelphia, PA: Lippincott Williams & Wilkins, 2011:1046–7.
Weissleder R, et al. *Primer of Diagnostic Imaging*, 4th edn. Philadelphia, PA: Mosby Elsevier, 2007:344.

41. D. Most colon cancers start as an adenomatous polyp.

The vast majority of colon cancers begin as an adenomatous polyp (>90%), although the vast majority of polyps are benign (>90%). With increasing size comes an increased risk of malignant change. In addition, of the three recognised pathological subtypes (tubular, tubulovillous and villous), villous adenomas carry the greatest risk of malignant transformation. There are a large number of other risk factors for developing colon cancer but among them are the hereditary polyposis syndromes (Peutz–Jeghers syndrome is less commonly related as the polyps are more likely in the small bowel) and the inflammatory bowel diseases 'Crohn's disease and ulcerative colitis'.

Dähnert W. *Radiology Review Manual*, 7th edn. Philadelphia, PA: Lippincott Williams & Wilkins, 2011:812–13.

42. A. 32 mL @ 8 mL/s

The aim is to closely replicate the natural blood flow in the vessel. A hand-injected test run is essential before a pump run to highlight the anatomy and confirm that the catheter tip is not in a subintimal position. An 8/32 injection delivers 8 mL of contrast per second to a total of 32 mL and lasts 4 s. The patients are usually asked to keep as still as possible and hold their breath to minimise artefact caused by motion.

43. B. Ovarian Brenner tumour

Brenner tumours are uncommon tumours that are almost always benign. These tumours have a large fibrous component and therefore have a similar appearance to an ovarian fibroma (low signal on T1- and T2-weighted imaging) on both ultrasound and MRI. Brenner tumours are commonly found with an adjacent epithelial tumour of the same ovary (usually mucinous cystadenoma); hence, in this case, the diagnosis of Brenner tumour is more likely than ovarian fibroma. An ovarian dermoid would usually contain fat but would also be in the differential diagnosis. However, the patient is postmenopausal and so endometrioma and corpus luteal cyst are unlikely.

Dähnert W. *Radiology Review Manual*, 6th edn. Philadelphia, PA: Lippincott Williams & Wilkins, 2007:1048.
Imaoka I, et al. Developing an MR imaging strategy for diagnosis of ovarian masses. *Radiographics*. 2006;26:1431–48.

44. B. Looser zones

Looser zones are a highly specific radiographic feature of osteomalacia. They are sometimes referred to as pseudofractures and are focal linear areas of undermineralised osteoid at sites of mechanical loading. They are often seen bilaterally as linear lucencies that run perpendicular to the bone cortex and do not involve the whole bone width. Common locations include the medial cortex of the femoral necks, the inferior scapula and the ribs.

These need to be differentiated from bisphosphonate fractures, which start at the lateral cortex of the proximal femur, are often bilateral and are termed as atypical fractures in patients on bisphosphonate therapy.

Brown tumours are lucent lesions seen in hyperparathyroidism. Cloacas are seen in established osteomyelitis. Wimberger's sign refers to localised bilateral metaphyseal destruction of the medial proximal tibias. It is a pathognomonic sign for congenital syphilis. Wimberger's ring sign (sometimes also called just Wimberger's sign to create confusion) is a radiographic sign seen in scurvy, showing thin pencil-like sclerosis along the epiphyseal margins. The cyclops lesion is an intra-articular mass of fibrotic tissue that may be seen post-anterior cruciate ligament (ACL) graft repair.

Jain TP, Thorn M. Atypical femoral fractures related to bisphosphonate therapy. *Indian J Radiol Imaging*. 2012;22(3):178–81.
Manaster BJ, et al. *The Requisites: MSK Imaging*, 3rd edn. Philadelphia, PA: Mosby, 2007:367–9.

45. B. Humerus

Stress fractures of the lower extremities associated with the onset of ambulation are called toddler's fractures. These fractures typically occur in children between 9 months and 3 years of age, manifest with a refusal to bear weight and are not preceded by a recognised acute traumatic event.

A similar injury can result from subtle torsional forces, such as those occurring in a toddler who stumbles and falls on a positioned foot.

The typical toddler's fracture is a non-displaced oblique fracture of the distal portion of the tibia. Although other locations are less common, weight-bearing can also account for toddler's fractures of the fibula, posterior aspect of the calcaneus, the base of the cuboid and the talus.

Jaimes C, et al. Taking the stress out of evaluating stress injuries in children. *Radiographics*. 2012;32(2): 537–55.

46. B. Progressive supranuclear palsy

Conventional MRI is usually not helpful in the diagnosis of early Parkinson's disease because it most often yields normal findings. In advanced disease, abnormalities of the substantia nigra, including volume loss, decreased T2 signal reflecting iron deposition and blurring of the margins, can be seen. However, the primary role of MRI is to exclude structural abnormalities that potentially mimic Parkinson's disease (e.g., NPH – normal pressure hydrocephalous, intracranial mass and bilateral subdural haematomas).

FDG PET images are most often normal and show preserved metabolism in the putamen and globus pallidus. This is a defining feature of Parkinson's disease and allows differentiation from both PSP (progressive supranuclear palsy) and MSA (multisystem atrophy, Shy–Drager syndrome), which commonly demonstrate reduced basal ganglia FDG activity.

In patients with MSA–Parkinson's type, abnormalities are confined to the putamen and include atrophy, symmetric hypointensity on T2 and T2*-weighted images and 'slitlike' marginal T2 hyperintensity. Putaminal atrophy appears to help discriminate MSA from Parkinson's disease, whereas T2 hypointensity is a non-specific sign that can be seen in PSP, Wilson's disease, neurodegeneration with brain iron accumulation and other acquired conditions.

Patients with PSP exhibit atrophy of the midbrain and tegmentum, manifesting as third ventricular dilatation, reduced midbrain AP diameter or flattening of the superior midbrain. Reduced midbrain AP diameter at the level of the superior colliculi on axial images gives rise to the Mickey Mouse sign. Midbrain atrophy with relative preservation of pons produces the hummingbird sign or penguin sign. Additional findings include superior cerebellar peduncle atrophy and increased FLAIR signal, both of which have reasonably high sensitivity and specificity in distinguishing PSP from Parkinson's disease and MSA.

Broski SM, et al. Structural and functional imaging in parkinsonian syndromes. *Radiographics*. 2014;34(5): 1273–92.

47. C. Linitis plastica

Helicobacter pylori infects the gastric mucosa. In most cases, it is asymptomatic but can be associated with epigastric pain and dyspepsia. Imaging can demonstrate the sequelae of gastritis (thickened folds, polypoidal changes and enlarged areae gastricae), but most commonly patients have either a gastric or duodenal ulcer (or both!). *Helicobacter pylori* is the most common cause of both gastric and duodenal ulcer diseases.

Linitis plastica (also known as leather bottle stomach) is a form of gastric stenosis that leads to narrowing of the stomach and which occurs secondarily to a number of conditions but is most frequently seen secondary to malignancy.

Dähnert W. *Radiology Review Manual*, 7th edn. Philadelphia, PA: Lippincott Williams & Wilkins, 2011:855.

48. C. You immediately page the vascular surgeon on call

You have just heard the dreaded symptoms and signs of compartment syndrome. The patient needs urgent surgical fasciotomy to prevent muscle necrosis. Any salvage treatment can be planned after that.

Muscle oedema will raise the intracompartmental pressure in the calf fascial compartments. If it is not released promptly, it will lead to muscle necrosis. The patient must have suffered an embolus during the angioplasty procedure. This is a medical emergency and needs urgent treatment. The team can consider revascularisation options after this is done.

Kessel D, Robertson I. *Interventional Radiology: A Survival Guide*, 3rd edn. London: Churchill Livingstone, 2010.

49. C. Decreased signal intensity of bone marrow on STIR images

Osteomyelitis is the infection of bone of which the primary modes of pathogenesis are through haematogenous spread, direct spread through trauma or iatrogenic source and extension from adjacent soft-tissue infection. MR is highly sensitive in the diagnosis of osteomyelitis of which the loss of the normal T1-weighted bone marrow fat signal is the most sensitive finding. Other additional findings include increased T2-weighted and STIR signals from the oedema and inflammation. Post-contrast studies may reveal a rim enhancing intraosseous abscess, which would warrant surgical intervention.

Dahnert. *Radiology Review Manual*, 6th edn. Philadelphia, PA: Lippincott Williams & Wilkins, 2007:137–8.

50. D. Rhombencephalosynapsis

Dandy–Walker malformation is characterised by hypoplasia or agenesis of cerebellar vermis and cystic dilatation of the 4th ventricle, which can result in enlargement of the posterior fossa.

Blake's pouch cyst is a result of absence of communication between the 4th ventricle and the subarachnoid space leading to tetraventricular hydrocephalus. The cerebellum has a normal size and shape. Typical neuroimaging findings include the presence of a cyst in a retro/infracerebellar location, which is essentially a diverticulum of the enlarged 4th ventricle.

Giant cisterna magna is an enlarged cisterna magna (≥10 mm on mid-sagittal images) with an intact vermis, normal 4th ventricle and, in some patients, an enlarged posterior fossa. Consistent presence of hydrocephalus allows the differentiation of Blake's pouch cyst from mega cisterna magna.

Arachnoid cysts are well-defined CSF density extra-axial lesions in the posterior fossa, which do not communicate with the 4th ventricle or the subarachnoid space. They may enlarge during infancy and produce mass effect on the cerebellum and vermis, which may cause a secondary obstruction of the ventricular system, hydrocephalus and/or remodelling or thinning of the overlying occipital bone.

Isolated hypoplasia of the inferior vermis with normal 4th ventricle has been described variably in literature as Dandy–Walker variant.

Rhombencephalosynapsis is characterised by the absence of the vermis and continuity of the cerebellar hemispheres, dentate nuclei and superior cerebellar peduncles, which creates a horseshoe-shaped arch across the midline, resulting in a keyhole-shaped fourth ventricle. It is a key feature of Gómez–López–Hernández syndrome (parietal alopecia, trigeminal anaesthesia and craniofacial dysmorphic signs) and may be seen with VACTERL.

Posterior coronal T2-weighted images show the horizontal folial pattern.

Bosemani T, et al. Congenital abnormalities of the posterior fossa. *Radiographics*. 2015;35(1):200–20.

51. C. High   Low

The typical appearance of a brain abscess at conventional MRI is that of a ring-enhancing lesion, with high signal intensity on T2-weighted images and low or intermediate signal intensity on T1-weighted images. A mature abscess has a low-signal-intensity capsule on T2-weighted images.

However, the presence of a ring-enhancing lesion in the brain is not diagnostic of abscess and must be distinguished from a necrotic neoplasm and other cystic lesions. Data from recent studies suggest that DWI is more sensitive than conventional MRI in distinguishing brain abscesses and cystic tumours. Pus in brain abscesses is strongly hyperintense on trace DWI and has a reduced ADC. On the contrary, most necrotic or cystic brain tumours have intermediate signal intensity on DWI and elevated ADC values.

Cartes-Zumelzu FW, et al. Diffusion-weighted imaging in the assessment of brain abscesses therapy. *AJNR Am J Neuroradiol.* 2004;25(8):1310–17.

52. A. Cervical carcinoma recurrence causing haematometra

Cervical carcinoma tends to be of higher signal on T2 than the surrounding cervical stroma and, in the above case, there is also disruption of the cervical stromal fibrous ring, increasing the likelihood of microscopic parametrial invasion. In this case, the cervical tumour is causing a malignant cervical stenosis and haematometra (high T1 signal is consistent with haemorrhage; tumour is usually intermediate signal/hypointense, similar to myometrium on T1 imaging).

After radiotherapy to the cervix, cervical stenosis with haematometra can occur; however, post radiotherapy, the cervix becomes low signal because of fibrosis. Ovaries usually lie to either side of the midline, and it would be unusual for a cervical carcinoma metastasis of the ovary to have a high T1 signal. Imperforate hymen is congenital and is normally picked up either neonatally or at the time of menarche, if the latter commonly presents with haematometrocolpos; it would be inconsistent with a cervical cancer history, as this tumour is not seen in patients who are virgo intacta.

Dähnert W. *Radiology Review Manual*, 7th edn. Philadelphia, PA: Lippincott Williams & Wilkins, 2011:1049–50.

Nicolet V, et al. MR imaging of cervical carcinoma: A practical staging approach. *Radiographics*. 2000;20:1539–49.

53. A. It is superior to cross-sectional imaging for local staging of oesophageal cancer.

Endoscopic ultrasound (EUS) involves the addition of an ultrasound probe in the endoscopy apparatus. This has a number of clinical uses, which are currently being developed. Evidence already exists that EUS is superior to cross-sectional imaging in the local staging (for assessment of both the primary tumour and local nodes) of oesophageal, pancreatic and rectal cancer. By visualising the wall layers of the gastrointestinal tract, it is the modality of choice for assessment of submucosal lesions. EUS can be combined with interventional techniques such as drainage or fine needle aspiration cytology. It is useful for differentiating inflammatory and neoplastic pancreatic masses. Cross-sectional imaging remains superior in the assessment of liver metastases.

Hawes RH. *The Evolution of Endoscopic Ultrasound: Improved Imaging, Higher Accuracy for Fine Needle Aspiration and the Reality of Endoscopic Ultrasound-guided Interventions.* www.medscape.com/viewarticle/729124 [accessed on 28 February 2017].

54. B. Severed tibioperoneal trunk

The most common anatomical configuration of the popliteal trifurcation is the anterior tibial (AT) artery branching off first and terminating as the dorsalis pedis artery. The tibioperoneal trunk arises distal to the AT origin and gives rise to the peroneal artery and posterior tibial (PT) arteries.

Ryan S, et al. *Anatomy for Diagnostic Imaging*, 2nd edn. Philadelphia, PA: Saunders, 2008.

55. E. Haemorrhagic ovarian cyst

Acute pelvic pain in adolescent girls is a common problem, but ultrasound scanning is very useful in differentiating the many possible causes. Haemorrhagic ovarian cysts are a common cause of pelvic pain in adolescent girls and appear as an echogenic mass in relation to the ovary.

Acute appendicitis is likely to occur as a blind-ending tubular structure. This may appear like a 'target lesion' in cross section and there may be fluid/collection adjacent to it. An acute appendix should be clearly distinct from the right ovary.

Ovarian dermoids are usually predominantly fat filled and therefore echogenic on ultrasound, but these tend to be a painless, incidental finding.

Ovarian torsion can certainly produce an echogenic mass within the right pelvis, but this is less common than haemorrhagic cysts and would not appear distinct from the ovary.

Ectopic pregnancy usually appears as a 'doughnut'-shaped complex mass in relation to one of the uterine tubes; a foetal heartbeat may be present.

Donnelly LF. *Pediatric Imaging: The Fundamentals.* Philadelphia, PA: Saunders Elsevier, 2009.

56. C. Mesial temporal sclerosis

Mesial temporal sclerosis typically demonstrates an atrophic, T2 hyperintense hippocampus on imaging. Other pathology affecting the temporal lobe including infection and tumour would cause enlargement of the hippocampus. Alzeheimer's dementia results in medial temporal atrophy, but T2-weighted hyperintensity is not a feature. Herpes encephalitis is caused by *Herpes simplex virus*

(HSV) type 1 in adults and HSV type II in children. It involves the limbic lobe (hypothalamus, parahippocampal gyrus, cingulate gyrus); and typically appears bilateral but asymmetric. Gyriform enhancement and haemorrhage are late features. Choroidal fissure cyst is a benign incidental finding, similar to arachnoid cysts in the brain. These occur in the region of the hippocampal fissure.

Osborn AG, et al. *Diagnostic Imaging: Brain*, 1st edn. Altona: Amirsys, 2004.

57. B. Second

Frieberg disease is essentially osteochondrosis of the metatarsal head, of which the 2nd metatarsal is most commonly affected, and less commonly in the 3rd and 4th metatarsal. Ten percent of cases are bilateral. MRI findings of subchondral fracture of the metatarsal head with severe marrow oedema-like pattern suggest early-stage changes. Metatarsal head collapse with subchondral sclerosis and mild or absent marrow oedema-like pattern suggests late-stage changes.

Torriani M, et al. MRI of metatarsal head subchondral fractures in patients with forefoot pain. *AJR Am J Roentgenol.* 2008;190(3):570–5.

58. D. Ovarian hyperstimulation syndrome

Human menopausal gonadotrophins are an infertility drug, which contains follicle-stimulating hormone and luteinising hormone, derived from the urine of postmenopausal women and given as an injection. One of its main side effects is ovarian hyperstimulation syndrome, which can also occur because of high levels of beta-human chorionic gonadotrophin seen in multiple pregnancies and hydatidiform moles. Typical symptoms are those mentioned in the question, vomiting and nausea. Corpus luteal cysts are singular and usually unilateral. Ovarian torsion is more common in infertility treatment but is usually unilateral, with a very oedematous ovary containing small, subcentimetre cysts arranged around its periphery. Polycystic ovarian syndrome causes bilaterally increased ovarian volume, but cysts are usually small and subcentimetre. Endometriomas usually contain low-level echoes.

Cornfeld D, Scoutt L. Torsion of a hyperstimulated ovary during pregnancy: A potentially difficult diagnosis. *Emergency Radiology.* 2007;14;331–5.
Dähnert W. *Radiology Review Manual*, 7th edn. Philadelphia, PA: Lippincott Williams & Wilkins, 2011:1074.
Graif M, et al. Torsion of the ovary: Sonographic features. *AJR Am J Roentgenol.* 1984;143:1331–4.

59. D. Hepatic adenoma

Hepatic adenomas are benign encapsulated liver lesions, which are usually 8–15 cm in diameter but can grow up to 30 cm. They are associated with the oral contraceptive pill and can often increase in size during pregnancy. They appear as hyperechoic lesions on ultrasound and are usually of low density on plain computed tomography and enhance in the arterial phase with rapid washout. They have a risk of haemorrhage and, if rupture occurs, can develop into a subcapsular haematoma. Focal nodular hyperplasia, haemangiomas and metastases would not be expected to grow this fast. Hepatic abscesses can grow quickly but the patient would be unwell, especially with spread into a subcapsular collection.

Brant WE, Helms CA. *Fundamentals of Diagnostic Radiology*, 3rd edn. Philadelphia, PA: Lippincott Williams & Wilkins, 2006:767–70.

60. C. Bilateral renal artery angioplasty and stenting

The results of the ASTRAL trial have shown no benefit of endovascular treatment when compared with best medical management of hypertension. However, recurrent flash pulmonary oedema is a good indication for intervention. Surgical endarterectomy is a procedure that carries huge risks and has no role in this case. Radiofrequency (RF) denervation is a relatively new method. The renal arteries are catheterised via a common femoral artery approach. Using an

RF generator, the artery is denervated, excluding the kidneys, from the sympathetic control. The long-term results are unknown.

The ASTRAL Investigators. Revascularization versus Medical Therapy for Renal-Artery Stenosis. *N Engl J Med.* 2009;361:1953–62.

61. B. Perthes disease

There are a large number of potential causes for hip pain in children. However, many of the conditions have common presenting age ranges, which makes creation of a differential diagnosis difficult.

Perthes disease is an idiopathic condition where avascular necrosis affects the femoral head leading to chronic destruction of one or both heads of femur. It tends to affect boys between the ages of 5 and 8 years.

Septic arthritis occurs at any age but would not be expected to present as a chronic finding, especially as many children have associated septicaemia.

Slipped upper femoral epiphysis affects adolescent children (12–15 years) and is usually associated with childhood obesity or in those who perform high-impact activity.

Juvenile rheumatoid arthritis is similar to the adult form of the disease in that it is idiopathic but tends to affect the large joints of which the hip is not the most common. In addition, there are often other systemic features of the disease as well as multiple joint involvement. Finally, this condition tends to present in younger children (1–3 years).

Developmental dysplasia of the hip presents in infancy but if undetected will lead to chronic hip problems.

Donnelly LF. *Pediatric Imaging: The Fundamentals.* Philadelphia, PA: Saunders Elsevier, 2009.

62. E. Meningioma Intramedullary

Lesions of the spinal canal can be divided into three categories:

Intramedullary lesions:

Ependymoma, astrocytoma, ganglioglioma, haemangioblastoma, PNET, metastasis, lymphoma, lipoma, epidermoid, abscess, vascular malformation, MS plaques, infarction, myelomalacia, sarcoidosis

Intradural extramedullary:

Nerve sheath tumour, meningioma, lipoma, dermoid, metastasis from outside CNS, ependymoma of filum terminale, arachnoid cyst, neuroenteric cyst

Extradural:

Dermoid, epidermoid, lipoma, lymphoma, metastasis, drop metastasis, meningioma, disc material, arachnoid cyst, infection

Dahnert W. *Radiology Review Manual, 5th edn.* Philadelphia, PA: Lippincott Williams & Wilkins, 2003:186–7.

63. D. Gaucher disease

Although the Ashkenazi Jews are particularly predisposed to this hereditary condition, Gaucher disease is not confined to any particular ethnic group or sex. Splenic enlargement is detected in up to 95% of cases. There is abnormal modelling of the distal femur and proximal tibia secondary to marrow infiltration, leading to an 'Erlenmayer flask' deformity. This feature is, however, not diagnostic for Gaucher disease and may be seen in all the other answer options. Diffuse medullary osteoporosis, bone infarcts and sharply circumscribed endosteal lytic lesions (owing to marrow replacement) can also be seen. The combination of Jewish ancestry, the radiographic features described and splenomegaly, makes Gaucher disease the most likely diagnosis.

Dahnert W. *Radiology Review Manual,* 7th edn. Philadelphia, PA: Lippincott Williams & Wilkins, 2011.
Sutton D. *Textbook of Radiology and Imaging,* 7th edn. Edinburgh: Churchill Livingstone, 2003.

64. D. Bartholin's cyst

Bartholin's glands secrete mucous to lubricate the vagina and are equivalent to the male Cowper glands (adjacent to urethra, producing pre-ejaculate). They lie within the posterolateral portion of the lower vagina. Bartholin's cysts occur when the small duct becomes obstructed; superadded infection can occur, leading to an abscess. Nabothian cysts are small mucous-filled cysts on the cervix and are very common. Gartner duct cysts are a Müllerian duct remnant and are uncommon; they have a typical location within the anterolateral proximal third of the vagina. Squamous cell carcinoma would usually appear as a thickened vaginal wall on ultrasound, if seen at all. Usually, the proximity of the probe to the lesion can make it difficult to assess, so this is better demonstrated with magnetic resonance imaging. A lipoma would have the appearance of other superficial lipomas and characteristically would be hyperechoic.

Dähnert W. *Radiology Review Manual*, 6th edn. Philadelphia, PA: Lippincott Williams & Wilkins, 2007:1032.

Siegelman ES, et al. High-resolution MR imaging of the vagina. *Radiographics*. 1997;17:1183–203.

65. D. Perform transjugular liver biopsy

This is a commonly occurring scenario. Liver biopsy is contraindicated in the presence of ascites and coagulopathy. The transjugular approach is a good alternative where available. The right internal jugular vein is punctured and a catheter is advanced into a hepatic vein, usually the right. Through this, a long specially designed biopsy needle is introduced and a biopsy is taken. The method is used for generalised liver disease and not for a focal lesion. An alternative method is the plugged liver biopsy; here the biopsy is done over a sheath, and coils are dropped after the core is taken to plug the hole.

Grainger RG, et al. (eds.). *Grainger & Allison's Diagnostic Radiology. A Textbook of Medical Imaging*, 4th edn. London: Churchill Livingstone, 2001:1309.

66. C. Right CFA, antegrade

The 'down the leg', antegrade, approach via a right common femoral artery puncture is the easiest and most direct approach. Retrograde puncture is usually used for angiography and intervention at the iliac systems, aorta and aortic branches. Ultrasound scan is commonly used to visualise the vessels during puncture. The puncture can also be safely performed using anatomical landmarks and feeling for the femoral pulse. The CFA can be found in the mid-point between the anterior superior iliac spine and the symphysis pubis. By using USS, the local anaesthetic can be accurately placed around the vessel, ensuring good analgesia. The profunda femoris artery can also be visualised and hence minimise the chance of accidental puncture. The popliteal artery can be punctured using ultrasound guidance at the popliteal fossa, but it would not be preferred in this case.

Kessel D, Robertson I. *Interventional Radiology: A Survival Guide*, 3rd edn. London: Churchill Livingstone, 2010.

67. A. Angular dermoid

The location of this lesion at the angle of the eye brow with ultrasound imaging features such as contiguous bone scalloping, fluctuance and presence of mobile debris within the lesion is reassuring and points to a diagnosis of an angular dermoid. T1 hyperintensity demonstrated on MRI consistent with a fat signal is diagnostic of this lesion. As the lesion may also contain debris, this may result in an inhomogeneous signal on MRI. A haemangioma would be expected to demonstrate flow voids and increased vascularity on ultrasound and MRI. The location is very unusual for a lymphangioma.

Weissleder R, et al. *Primer of Diagnostic Imaging*, 5th edn. Philadelphia, PA: Mosby Elsevier, 2011.

68. D. Infection

Percutaneous cementoplasty (vertebroplasty) with acrylic cement, PMMA (polymethylmethacrylate), is a procedure aimed at preventing vertebral body collapse and pain in patients with pathologic vertebral bodies.

Indications:
- Symptomatic vertebral angioma.
- Painful vertebral body tumours and acetabular tumours.
- Severe painful osteoporosis with loss of height and/or with compression fractures of vertebral bodies.

Contraindications:
- Haemorrhagic diathesis.
- Infection.
- Lesions with epidural extension. These require careful injection to prevent epidural overflow and spinal cord compression by the cement or displaced epidural tissue.

The absolute contraindications are haemorrhagic diathesis and infection. Patients with more than five metastases or diffuse metastases are not candidates for vertebroplasty.

Gangi A, et al. Percutaneous vertebroplasty: Indications, technique, and results. *Radiographics*. 2003;23(2):e10.

69. C. Lung cancer metastasis

The most common sites for bone metastases are bones that contain red bone marrow. Hence, bone metastases have a predilection for the axial skeleton. Peripheral metastases are rare, and 50% of these are caused by lung cancer. The other options are also known causes of lytic metastases, but would be less likely to affect the hands.

Adam A, et al. *Grainger & Allison's Diagnostic Radiology: A Textbook of Medical Imaging*, 5th edn. New York: Churchill Livingstone, 2008.

70. C. Red degeneration within a leiomyoma

Fibroids (leiomyomas) are benign tumours made of smooth muscle. Afro-Caribbean women are more prone than Caucasian women to developing fibroids. Fibroids can outgrow their blood supply and undergo degeneration causing them to look very different on MRI depending on the type of degeneration that they undergo. Typically, a non-degenerated fibroid is a well-defined low-intensity lesion on T1 and T2-weighted images, and enhances post contrast injection. Hyaline degeneration is caused by necrotic central change and increasing collagen content; this causes variable signal on T1-weighted images but low signal on T2-weighted images. With calcific degeneration, the fibroid has similar signal characteristics on T1 and T2 to typical non-degenerative fibroids. Cystic degeneration can produce areas of fluid signal within the fibroid, which does not enhance. Myxoid degeneration results in a very high T2 signal with a little enhancement. Red degeneration is a very rare type of degeneration; it typically causes severe pain and can cause a fever. It is the result of thrombosis of the vessels surrounding the fibroid leading to the high T1 and low T2 signal rim, and it usually occurs in pregnancy.

Dähnert W. *Radiology Review Manual*, 7th edn. Philadelphia, PA: Lippincott Williams & Wilkins, 2011:1087–9.
Murase E, et al. Uterine leiomyomas: Histopathologic features, MR imaging findings, differential diagnosis and treatment. *Radiographics*. 1999;19:1179–97.

71. E. Administer high-flow oxygen and put the patient in the left lateral position.

This scenario describes an iatrogenic air embolism. This is an uncommon complication that has an incidence of around 0.13%. Treatment includes high-flow oxygen and placing the patient in the left decubitus position. This would allow the air to rise in the right atrium where it can be aspirated using a transjugular approach.

Needle decompression in the right mid-clavicular line is the treatment for a tension pneumothorax. A chest X-ray might show air in the right heart but will not help in the immediate management. Injecting 10 mL of contrast down the sheath is performed when you are suspecting extravasation and placing the patient head down and giving fast intravenous crystalloid is the treatment for hypotension.

Vesely TM. Air embolism during insertion of central venous catheters. *J Vasc Interv Radiol.* 2001;12:1291–5.

72. A. A lead point is rarely the underlying cause in adult cases.

Intussusception refers to the telescope-like invagination or prolapse of an intestinal segment into the lumen of an adjacent loop. Approximately 95% of cases occur in children, usually affecting those under the age of 2 years. A lead point is an unusual finding in this age group, with mucosal oedema and lymphoid hyperplasia secondary to viral gastroenteritis often being the underlying issue. Conversely, while intussusception in adults is uncommon, a lead point is far more commonly present. Lesions such as polyps, small bowel tumours, postsurgical changes and foreign bodies are recognised precipitants. In children, reduction of intussusception using either water or air can be attempted, provided that there is no initial evidence of perforation. A rule of '3s' is well known, whereby a maximum of three attempts at reduction with 3 minutes separating each attempt and a hydrostatic pressure equivalent to an infusion bag 3 feet (91.4 cm) above the patient is observed. Surgical intervention may be required if such techniques are unsuccessful.

Dähnert W. *Radiology Review Manual,* 7th edn. Philadelphia, PA: Lippincott Williams & Wilkins, 2011:861–2.

73. A. Sickle cell anaemia

Gallstones are an uncommon occurrence in childhood irrespective of the symptomatology and therefore should always raise the possibility of a background predisposing condition leading to their formation. In the African population, sickle cell anaemia is the most likely diagnosis. One must also consider other conditions such as malabsorption, Crohn disease, thalassemia major (in patients of Mediterranean origin), total parenteral nutrition (TPN), cystic fibrosis and short gut syndrome. The radiologist is often the first to raise the possibility of a predisposing condition. Children are at risk of the same gallstone-related complications as adults, including severe acute pancreatitis, which may be life threatening.

Dähnert W. *Radiology Review Manual,* 7th edn. Philadelphia, PA: Lippincott Williams & Wilkins, 2011.

74. D. Prostate metastases

Brain metastases may be solitary or multiple. Some tumours including breast, renal cell, colon and thyroid cancers are more commonly solitary, while others such as lung cancer and melanoma tend to be multiple.

Imaging characteristics of metastases may suggest an underlying pathologic diagnosis. Metastases that classically haemorrhage include melanoma, choriocarcinoma, renal cell carcinoma and thyroid cancer. Lung metastases are also known to haemorrhage. In the absence of haemorrhage, metastases may be hypodense, isodense or hyperdense compared with the brain. Acutely haemorrhagic metastases appear hyperdense to brain. Melanoma metastases tend to be hyperdense to brain on CT even in the absence of haemorrhage.

Fink KR, Fink JR. Imaging of brain metastases. *Surg Neurol Int.* 2013;4(Suppl 4):S209–19.

75. A. Le Fort I facial fracture

All Le Fort fractures involve the pterygoid plate. In addition, Le Fort I involves maxilla and nasal septum. Le Fort II involves nasal bones, frontal process of maxilla, maxillary sinus, medial and inferior orbital wall. Le Fort III, in addition to II, involves lateral orbital wall and zygomatico-frontal suture. Le Fort II fracture is also called pyramidal fracture.

Dahnert W. *Radiology Review Manual*, 6th edn. Philadelphia, PA: Lippincott Williams & Wilkins, 2007:208.

76. D. Splenic vein

The splanchnic circulation includes the superior mesenteric vein, inferior mesenteric vein and splenic and portal veins. Hepatic veins do not form part of the splanchnic circulation as they do not drain to the portal vein but drain directly to the inferior vena cava (IVC).

Chronic thrombosis of portal or superior and inferior mesenteric veins is often associated with gastro-oesophageal varices, owing to collateral circulation to IVC from submucosal veins of the oesophagus. Isolated splenic vein thrombosis causes only gastric fundal varices, formed by short gastric vessels serving as collaterals. This is known as left-sided portal hypertension. Left-sided portal hypertension is often associated with pancreatitis or pancreatic cancer.

Adam A, et al. *Grainger & Allison's Diagnostic Radiology: A Textbook of Medical Imaging*, 5th edn. New York: Churchill Livingstone, 2008:641.

Corr C, Callaway M. *RITI 3_116: Liver: Vascular Disorders of the Liver and Splanchnic Circulation*. London: The Royal College of Radiologists, 2010 (portal.e-lfh.org.uk).

77. B. Infrarenal IVC

In the presence of normal anatomy, IVC filters should be placed inferior to the renal veins. This is to avoid potential clot propagation and renal vein thrombosis. If the patient has aberrant anatomy such as double IVC, a single suprarenal filter or twin IVC filters can be placed. Access is via a right internal jugular puncture or a right femoral vein puncture. A cavogram is performed to visualise the renal veins and to look for aberrant anatomy as described above. Indications for IVC filter include deep vein thrombosis where anticoagulation is contraindicated, where the patient is non-compliant with medical treatment or when there is free-floating thrombus in the IVC. Retrievable devices are available and should be removed within 14 days from insertion. Pulmonary embolism can still occur despite an IVC filter with an incidence of 2.7%–4%.

Brant WE, Helms CA. *Fundamentals of Diagnostic Radiology*, 3rd edn. Vol. 3. Philadelphia, PA: Lippincott Williams & Wilkins, 2006.

78. A. Posterior calyx, middle/lower pole

When further intervention such as antegrade stent placement or percutaneous nephrolithotomy is anticipated, a posterior upper pole calyx may be appropriate. Effort should be made to puncture below the 12th rib to avoid traversing the pleura. However, this is not always possible and puncture between the 11th and 12th ribs can also be used with care. Direct puncture of the renal pelvis should be avoided as the adjacent vessels here are large. Anterior calyces should also be avoided, as puncturing these from a posterior approach increases the risk of renovascular injury because of the volume of renal parenchyma traversed.

Brant WE, Helms CA. *Fundamentals of Diagnostic Radiology*, 3rd edn. Philadelphia, PA: Lippincott Williams & Wilkins, 2006:725.

79. C. Inguinal hernia

The child in this scenario has acute bowel obstruction, which can sometimes be missed on initial assessment. When assessing plain films, the hernial orifices should be remembered as an important 'review area' as inguinal hernia are common and should not be missed, both in children and adults alike. In this case, an ultrasound was performed first but the same principles apply and bowel loops in the scrotum are diagnostic. The radiologist may be the first to raise this possibility.

An incarcerated hernia associated with obstruction or strangulation is an acute surgical emergency and requires urgent surgical intervention. Femoral hernia is uncommon in children. Acute testicular torsion may have a similar presentation and should always be considered. At least some part of a testis should be identifiable in case of torsion, tumour or injury. Non-visualised testis strongly suggests hernia.

Dähnert W. *Radiology Review Manual*, 7th edn. Philadelphia, PA: Lippincott Williams & Wilkins, 2011.

80. C. Arachnoiditis
Infectious aetiologies for arachnoiditis include bacterial, viral, fungal and parasitic agents. Non-infectious aetiologies include surgery, intrathecal haemorrhage and the administration of intrathecal agents, such as myelographic contrast media, anaesthetics and steroids. Neoplastic causes include metastasis from breast and lung carcinoma, melanoma and non-Hodgkin lymphoma or direct seeding of the CSF from primary CNS tumours like glioblastoma multiforme (GBM), medulloblastoma, ependymoma and choroid plexus carcinoma.

MRI is the most sensitive modality for diagnosis of arachnoiditis. Although arachnoiditis can be present throughout the subarachnoid space, it is most easily seen in the lumbar region where the cauda equina usually floats in ample CSF. In arachnoiditis, the nerve roots are irregularly thickened and clumped together, often stuck to the dura, resulting in an empty thecal sac sign.

Morisako H, et al. Focal adhesive arachnoiditis of the spinal cord: Imaging diagnosis and surgical resolution.
    J Craniovertebr Junction Spine. 2010;1(2):100–6.
Ross JS, et al. MR imaging of lumbar arachnoiditis. *AJR Am J Roentgenol*. 1987;149(5):1025–32.

81. B. Pachydermoperiostosis
Pachydermoperiostosis is a self-limiting condition with similar radiological findings to those of hypertrophic osteoarthropathy: symmetrical bilateral periosteal reaction. It is seen in adolescents and is of autosomal dominant inheritance pattern. Males tend to be affected more often than females. Differential diagnoses of these radiological findings include thyroid acropachy, hypervitaminosis A, hypertrophic osteoarthropathy, metastases and chronic venous insufficiency. All of the above require treatment before resolution of the periosteal reaction.

Hypertrophic osteoarthropathy is caused by many pulmonary and non-pulmonary diseases such as benign and malignant thoracic tumours, chronic infection/inflammation (bronchiectasis and lung abscesses), cyanotic congenital heart disease, inflammatory bowel disease and liver cirrhosis. In HOA, resolution of the radiological findings is only really seen following treatment of the underlying condition.

Dähnert W. *Radiology Review Manual*, 7th edn. Philadelphia, PA: Lippincott Williams & Wilkins, 2007:110.

82. C. Refer for laparoscopic division of the ligament
The symptoms and radiological findings are consistent with median arcuate ligament syndrome, the compression of the coeliac axis by the median arcuate ligament of the diaphragm. The median arcuate ligament passes superior to the coeliac axis in 10%–24% of the population. It can cause haemodynamically significant compression in a small subgroup. Treatment is controversial but benefit can be seen in cases where there is weight loss, post-stenotic dilatation along with postprandial pain. Laparoscopic ligation is the preferred method.

Horton KM, et al. Median arcuate ligament syndrome: Evaluation with CT angiography. *Radiographics*.
    2005;25:1177–82.

83. C. High-pressure chronic retention
High-pressure chronic retention is a cause of bilateral hydronephrosis. It is usually caused by prostatic hypertrophy. The patient typically has a non-compliant bladder with incomplete emptying, although its overall capacity is often normal or may even be below normal. The high pressure in the bladder causes functional obstruction of the upper tracts, and hence causes upper

tract dilatation and impairment of renal function. Treatment is by catheterisation, thus decompressing the bladder and upper tracts, and interval transurethral resection of the prostate if there is any recoverable bladder function. The other answers are valid indications for upper tract de-obstruction.

Kessel D, Robertson I. *Interventional Radiology. A Survival Guide*, 3rd edn. Oxford: Churchill Livingstone, 2010.

84. B. Acute Budd–Chiari syndrome

Acute hepatic venous obstruction (Budd–Chiari syndrome) can be associated with disseminated malignancies. In addition to ascites and hepatomegaly, characteristic CT features are geographic liver (mottled liver enhancement) and a flip-flop pattern of enhancement (early-phase hyperenhancement of the central area of the liver with peripheral hypo-enhancement, which reverses on delayed imaging with central hypo-enhancement and peripheral hyperenhancement). The caudate lobe is spared as it has direct venous drainage to the inferior vena cava, bypassing hepatic veins. In the acute phase, the liver remains normal in size, but with chronic disease there is hypertrophy of the caudate lobe, which takes over the majority of liver function, thereby helping differentiation between acute and chronic Budd-Chiari syndrome.

Peliosis hepatis may also be associated with disseminated malignancy, but CT demonstrates multiple spherical lesions with centripetal or centrifugal enhancement because of the presence of blood-filled cavities.

Dähnert W. *Radiology Review Manual*, 7th edn. Philadelphia, PA: Lippincott Williams & Wilkins, 2011:706–7.

85. C. Irregular liver contour

Non-alcoholic liver steatohepatitis is the second stage of non-alcoholic fatty liver disease (NAFLD), a very common liver disease that affects about 30% of the western population. The most common cause for this disease is obesity and hypertriglyceridemia. The first stage of NAFLD – hepatosteatosis – is potentially reversible but when untreated, 60% progress to NASH, which also has features of fibrosis and inflammation. Hepatosteatosis and NASH are indistinguishable radiologically and NASH can only be diagnosed on biopsy, which is performed in high-risk patients. Progression to cirrhosis is observed in 10% of patients with NASH, where a small shrunken liver with irregular contour and secondary features of cirrhosis are observed.

Corr C, Callaway M. *RITI 3_114: Liver: Cirrhosis and NASH*. London: The Royal College of Radiologists, 2010 (portal.e-lfh.org.uk).

86. E. Conservative management and repeat scan in 6 months

Splenic aneurysms have an incidence of around 0.1% at autopsy. Indications for treatment include portal hypertension, size >25 mm, female patient of child-bearing age and pseudo-aneurysm. There is an increased risk of rupture in pregnancy. Interventional treatment is usually by coil embolisation although stent grafting and even transabdominal thrombin injection have been described.

Madoff DC, et al. Splenic arterial interventions: Anatomy, indications, technical considerations, and potential complications. *Radiographics*. 2005:25(Suppl 1),S191–211.

87. D. Tectal beaking

Holoprosencephaly results from a lack of normal cleavage of the forebrain. The septum pellucidum is always absent in this condition. Holoprosencephaly may be divided into alobar, semilobar and lobar forms depending on the degree of abnormality. Tectal beaking is a feature of Chiari II. Single ventricle, fused thalami, absent corpus callosum and hypoplasia of the optic nerves are all features of the various forms of holoprosencephaly. In its mildest form, lobar holoprosencephaly, absence of the septum pellucidum may be the only abnormality. The lobar form may be associated with septo-optic dysplasia and the two conditions overlap. The degree of facial abnormality and mental retardation mirrors the severity of the intracranial abnormality.

Donnelly LF. *Pediatric Imaging: The Fundamentals*. Philadelphia, PA: Saunders Elsevier, 2009.

88. C. Slow flow mimics sinus thrombosis on contrast-enhanced MRV.

The classic finding on unenhanced CT is a hyperattenuating thrombus in the occluded sinus (delta sign). However, this is seen in only 25% cases. Increased attenuation in the venous sinuses may also be seen in patients with dehydration, an elevated haematocrit level, or a subjacent subarachnoid or subdural haemorrhage. On contrast-enhanced CT/MRI, the empty delta sign is seen, a central intraluminal filling defect that represents a thrombus surrounded by contrast-enhanced dural collateral venous channels and cavernous spaces within the dural envelope. Unenhanced MRI is more sensitive for the detection of venous thrombi than is unenhanced CT. The absence of a flow void and the presence of altered signal in the sinus is a primary finding. Slow or turbulent flow also may cause a signal intensity alteration in the sinus.

The signal intensity of venous thrombi on T1- and T2-weighted MR images varies according to the interval between thrombus formation and the time of imaging. Time-of-flight (TOF) MR venography is the method most commonly used for diagnosis. Contrast-enhanced MRV utilises the paramagnetic effect of intravenous gadolinium to shorten T1 relaxation time and provide positive intravascular contrast enhancement. Small-vessel visualisation is improved at contrast-enhanced MRV. Depiction of the dural sinuses is also superior with contrast-enhanced MR venography because of a decrease in the effects of turbulent/slow flow on vessel contrast.

An irregular appearance of the sinus with multiple intrasinus channels and dural collateral vessels on MRV is characteristic of incomplete recanalisation. Complete recanalisation occurs more often in superior sagittal and straight sinus thrombosis than transverse and sigmoid sinuses after anticoagulation therapy.

Leach JL, et al. Imaging of cerebral venous thrombosis: Current techniques, spectrum of findings, and diagnostic pitfalls. *Radiographics*. 2006;26(Suppl 1):S19–41; discussion S42–3.

89. D. The distal portions of the seminal vesicles and vas deferens are intraperitoneal.

The seminal vesicles are paired, elongated septated structures that lie above the prostate and abut the posterior wall of the bladder. Their fluid accounts for around 50%–80% of ejaculate. The seminal vesicle joins the distal vas deferens, forming the ejaculatory duct, which drains into the prostatic urethra at the verumontanum. The proximal portion of the vas deferens lies within the spermatic cord. The seminal vesicles and vasa deferentia are extraperitoneal structures. Seminal vesicle abnormalities are invariably found as incidental findings on imaging studies, although patients may present with haematospermia or infertility. Primary tumours of the seminal vesicle are very rare indeed, with the majority of neoplasia occurring from local spread of prostate, bladder or rectal malignancies.

Kim B, et al. Imaging of the seminal vesicle and vas deferens. *Radiographics*. 2009;29:1105–21.

90. D. Hypertrophic osteoarthropathy

Hypertrophic osteoarthropathy, or HOA, is characterised by smooth periosteal new bone formation, usually in the diametaphysis of the long bones. The tibia, fibula, radius and ulna are most commonly involved in ~80% of cases with patients usually describing painful, swollen joints. When present, caution must be given to look for an underlying thoracic cause of which the most common aetiology is bronchogenic carcinoma. In such instances, it is commonly referred to as hypertrophic pulmonary osteoarthropathy, or HPOA. Extrathoracic causes of HOA include inflammatory bowel disease and liver cirrhosis.

Dahnert W. *Radiology Review Manual*, 6th edn. Philadelphia, PA: Lippincott Williams & Wilkins, 2007:106.

91. E. Conservative management

Varicocele is a commonly identified correctable cause of male factor infertility. Surgical correction has a failure rate of less than 5%. An alternative to surgery is the selective catheterisation and embolisation of the gonadal vein. The gonadal vein is catheterised via a common femoral vein puncture and embolic material is introduced. Indications include symptomatic varicocele, recurrence of varicocele post treatment and varicocele with associated infertility. Complications include pain, recurrence and reaction to iodinated contrast. Rupture of the testicular vein is a known complication, but it needs no specific treatment. Unlike surgery, embolisation is not associated with postoperative hydrocele or testicular loss from inadvertent injury to testicular artery. However there are case reports of renal loss from coil migration.

Cassidy D, et al. Varicocele surgery or embolization: Which is better?. *Can Urol Assoc J.* 2012;6(4): 266–268.

92. B. Intrapulmonary bronchogenic cyst

Bronchogenic cysts (BCs) are congenital lesions. They are usually found in the mediastinum or pulmonary parenchyma and, less commonly, cysts may be found in the neck, pericardium, pleura, diaphragm or abdominal cavity. Intrapulmonary cysts are most common in the lower lobes. Intrapulmonary BCs are usually sharply defined, solitary, non-calcified, round or oval opacities confined to a single lobe. These can present as a homogeneous water density, an air-filled cyst, or with an air–fluid level. Signal on MRI depends on the content, and fluid-containing lesions are low on T1-weighted and high on T2-weighted images; however, proteinaceous content makes them high on T1-weighted imaging.

The differential diagnosis of intraparenchymal BCs must include acquired cystic lesions, such as a lung abscess, a hydatid cyst, infection with nocardia, an infected bulla, congenital lobar emphysema, fungal diseases and tuberculosis, especially when the lesions manifest as air-filled or have an air–fluid level.

Odev K, et al. Cystic and cavitary lung lesions in children: Radiologic findings with pathologic correlation. *J Clin Imag Sci.* 2013;3:60.

93. E. Posterior communicating cerebral artery

The third nerves exit the brain stem medial to the cerebral peduncles, and course forward and laterally in the interpeduncular cistern between the posterior cerebral arteries–posterior communicating arteries (PcomA) above and superior cerebellar arteries below. The pupillary fibres are located dorsomedially and peripherally at this segment.

Common pathologies involving this segment include aneurysm at PcomA or basilar tip, dolichoectatic vessels, microvascular ischaemia, SAH, meningitis, neoplasms (leukaemia, lymphoma, neurogenic tumours and leptomeningeal carcinomatosis), inflammatory disease (neurosarcoidosis, Wegener's granulomatosis), demyelinating disease, transtentorial herniation (from supratentorial tumour, haemorrhage or brain swelling) and head trauma with nerve avulsion (usually at the posterior petroclinoid ligament where the third nerve is stretched because of downward displacement of the brain stem at the time of impact).

Lo C-P, et al. Neuroimaging of isolated and non-isolated third nerve palsies. *Br J Radiol.* 2012;85(1012): 460–7.

94. B. Lead poisoning

The differential list for dense metaphyseal bands is plenty but includes normal variant in neonates, growth acceleration lines (usually in patients with chronic illnesses like diabetes, asthma), treated rickets, chronic anaemia, scurvy and lead poisoning. Recurrent abdominal pain is associated with lead poisoning. None of the other conditions, except for leukaemia, is associated with abdominal pain, but the dense metaphyseal band sign is acknowledged only in treated leukaemia rather than active leukaemia. Although the blood profile is often normal, the patient may sometimes have a mild microcystic, microchromic anaemia.

Raber SA. The dense metaphyseal band sign. *Radiology*. 1999;211:773–4.

95. A. Less than three hepatic lesions

Liver metastases from colorectal cancer are among the most common hepatic secondary tumours. This is also the only type of metastatic deposit for which resection has shown a survival benefit. If liver metastases from colorectal cancer are to be resected, several radiological criteria must be met.

There is no strict limit to the number of lesions that can be resected, but it is unlikely that more than six lesions will be removed. Compare this with hepatocellular carcinoma where only a solitary lesion can be surgically explored. If at least three segments of the liver are spared, there are enough hepatocytes to provide liver function following surgery; preoperative selective portal vein embolisation can be used to increase the volume of the remaining liver through hypertrophy.

Corr C, Callaway M. *RITI 3_111: Management of Hepatic Malignancies*. London: The Royal College of Radiologists, 2010 (portal.e-lfh.org.uk).

96. D. Decreased or absent bowel wall enhancement

Abnormalities in bowel wall enhancement after administration of IV contrast are very common and important positive findings in the evaluation of abdominal CT in a trauma scenario and should always be assessed. Generalised increased enhancement is typical for bowel wall injury with vascular involvement but without ischaemia, and is thought to be caused by increased permeability of the hypoperfused wall.

Localised, patchy and irregular hyperenhancement is suggestive but not diagnostic of a full-thickness tear. Areas of decreased or absent enhancement in a segment of a bowel are indicative of bowel ischaemia; lack of enhancement is considered to be highly specific.

Brody JM, et al. CT of blunt trauma bowel and mesenteric injury: Typical findings and pitfalls in diagnosis. *Radiographics*. 2000;20:1525–36.
Brofman N, et al. Evaluation of bowel and mesenteric blunt trauma with multidetector CT. *Radiographics*. 2006;26:1119–31.

97. C. Biliary atresia

Failure of gallbladder emptying following a feed and failure of isotope (HIDA) excretion into the bowel is a typical finding of biliary atresia. The presence of tracer in the urinary bladder implies that there is no hepatic excretion of tracer, only urinary excretion; this only occurs with sustained systemic levels as HIDA is preferentially excreted hepatically. The gallbladder is not visualised in some cases of high biliary atresia and cystic fibrosis. Transient neonatal hyperbilirubinaemia should resolve spontaneously by 2 weeks of age. Ultrasound imaging may demonstrate a triangular cord or tubular echogenic structure in the porta hepatis owing to fibrous tissue. When identified, this is pathognomonic of biliary atresia.

Huisman AGM. *Pediatric Imaging: Case Review Series*, 2nd edn. Philadelphia, PA: Mosby Elsevier, 2010.

98. E. Vessel dilatation

The rest are angiographic signs of active bleeding; vessel dilatation is not.

Radiology – Integrated Training Initiative (R-ITI). 1c_016 – Acute Adult GI Bleeding: Imaging and Intervention. portal.e-lfh.org.co.uk/LearningContent/Launch/310763

99. B. Multilocular cystic nephroma

Multilocular cystic nephroma is a benign renal tumour that occurs in children and, less commonly, adult women. There is no known association with Wilms' tumour. It is usually a unilateral abnormality that replaces an entire renal pole and presents as a large mass, often around 8–10 cm in diameter. Radiological appearances, while not entirely specific, can help to differentiate this lesion from other renal mass lesions. A sharply well-circumscribed, multiseptated cystic mass is typical, with a thick surrounding capsule. The cysts may appear to herniate into the renal pelvis – an appearance that is relatively specific. Unsurprisingly, these lesions are excised as a definitive radiological differentiation from malignancy is often not possible. Multilocular cystic nephroma can be differentiated from multicystic dysplastic kidney by the presence of normal functioning renal parenchyma and symmetrical renal excretion. Polycystic kidney disease involves the entire kidney, unlike multilocular cystic nephroma, which tends to be localised around a renal pole.

Dähnert W. *Radiology Review Manual*, 7th edn. Philadelphia, PA: Lippincott Williams & Wilkins, 2011:957.

100. D. Parenchymal abnormalities secondary to venous occlusion are irreversible.

Parenchymal lesions are better depicted and more commonly identified at MR imaging than at CT. Focal oedema (without visible haemorrhage) is visible on CT images in approximately 8% of cases and on MR images in 25% of cases. Diffusion-weighted MR imaging techniques allow sub-classification of parenchymal abnormalities as either primarily vasogenic oedema (with increased ADC values presumably related to venous congestion) or primarily cytotoxic oedema (with decreased ADC values related to cellular energy disruption). Haemorrhage may occur with both types of oedema. In contrast with arterial ischaemic states, many parenchymal abnormalities secondary to venous occlusion are reversible. Although parenchymal changes may occur in areas of the brain that are directly drained by the occluded venous sinus, in some patients, the parenchymal changes may not closely correlate with the location of venous occlusion. Parenchymal swelling without abnormalities in attenuation or signal intensity on images may occur in as many as 42% of patients with cerebral venous thrombosis. Sulcal effacement, diminished cistern visibility and a reduction in ventricular size may occur.

Leach JL, et al. Imaging of cerebral venous thrombosis: Current techniques, spectrum of findings, and diagnostic pitfalls. *Radiographics*. 2006;26(Suppl 1):S19–41; discussion S42–3.

101. C. Fractures of the distal pole are less common than fractures of the proximal pole.

Scaphoid fractures are common injuries but can have long-standing implications if not treated in a timely manner because of the risk of avascular necrosis and early development of osteoarthritis in cases of mal- or non-union. Scaphoid fractures most commonly occur within the waist of the scaphoid (70%), with the remaining occurring in the proximal pole (20%) and distal pole (10%). Due to the nature of the scaphoid blood supply, it is the proximal fracture fragment that is at risk of avascular necrosis. A fall on the outstretched hand is the most common mechanism. Fracture displacement and scapholunate ligamentous disruption with widening of scapho-lunate distance, ('Terry Thomas' sign) are common associated findings.

Brydie A, Raby N. Early MRI in the management of clinical scaphoid fracture. *Br J Radiol*. 2003;76 (905):296–300.

102. D. Nodes in the perivescical fat

The strength of MRI in evaluation of prostate cancer is in the diagnosis of extracapsular and seminal vascular invasion. The criteria used for the detection of extracapsular extension of tumour (on T2-weighted images) include: irregular capsular bulge, obliteration of rectoprostatic angle, asymmetry of the neurovascular bundle, angulation or step-off appearance of the prostate contour, focal capsular thickening or retraction, broad (>12 mm) capsular tumour contact and breech of capsule with evidence of direct tumour extension.

Adam A, et al. *Grainger & Allison's Diagnostic Radiology: A Textbook of Medical Imaging*, 5th edn. New York: Churchill Livingstone, 2008:907.

103. E. Foregut duplication cyst

Foregut duplication cysts usually occur on the mesenteric aspect of the alimentary canal and may be associated with other gastrointestinal anomalies. The absence of any spinal involvement and the late presentation seen here rule out other differential diagnoses. Other more likely differentials would include bronchogenic cyst and pericardial cyst, and these are often very difficult to differentiate even on computed tomography (CT) and MRI. Duplication cysts occur most commonly in relation to the small bowel, in particular the ileum; the oesophagus is, however, the second most common location. When identified, the 'muscular rim sign' on ultrasound is diagnostic. This results from an alternating echogenic inner mucosal lining and a hypoechoic outer rim signal from the mucosal lining.

Dähnert W. *Radiology Review Manual*, 7th edn. Philadelphia, PA: Lippincott Williams & Wilkins, 2011.

104. B. Acute disseminated encephalomyelitis

Acute disseminated encephalomyelitis (ADEM) is a monophasic autoimmune demyelinating disease of the central nervous system that typically follows a febrile infection or vaccination. The disorder is immunologically mediated because of an autoimmune reaction to myelin. Peak incidence is in children aged 3–10 years. Typically, ADEM manifests as multifocal lesions mimicking MS. However, clinical and radiologic criteria distinguish between ADEM and MS.

ADEM typically meets at least two of the three following criteria: (a) They have clinical symptoms atypical of MS, e.g., altered consciousness, hypersomnia, seizures, cognitive impairment, hemiplegia, quadriparesis, aphasia or bilateral optic neuritis. (b) They have absence of oligoclonal bands in CSF. (c) They have grey matter involvement (basal ganglia or cortical lesions). Imaging features, such as the number of T2 hyperintense lesions and the presence of gadolinium enhancement, oedema and periventricular or brainstem lesions, cannot be used to reliably differentiate between ADEM and MS. Corpus callosal involvement is less frequent in patients with ADEM than in those with MS. Cerebrospinal fluid findings, especially the presence or absence of oligoclonal bands, remain important in the differentiation of patients with MS from those with ADEM. The best criterion is the course of the disease, with a good outcome in 57%–81% of patients with ADEM, with no new lesions and partial or complete recovery of existing lesions on follow-up MR images.

Mialin R, et al. Case 173: Acute disseminated encephalomyelitis confined to the brainstem. *Radiology*. 2011;260(3):911–14.

105. C. Measure the pressure gradient

There will be a degree of vessel dissection in all vessels after angioplasty. If there is no limitation to flow or significant pressure gradient across the lesion, then the procedure can be regarded as being successful and no further action is necessary. The pressures can be measured by connecting the end of a catheter to a transducer via a three-way tab. The catheter is placed through stenosis and the pressures are measured on either side. The difference is the pressure gradient, and it should be less than 10 mmHg.

106. E. Atrophy of the spinal cord

Spinal cord injury can have devastating impacts on patients. Acute causes generally relate to traumatic events and include cord haemorrhage, contusion and transaction. Oedema, swelling and haemorrhage (epi and intradural) are often seen in the context of an acute cord injury.

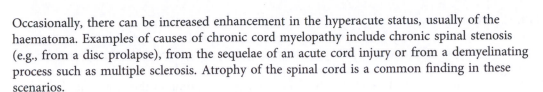

Occasionally, there can be increased enhancement in the hyperacute status, usually of the haematoma. Examples of causes of chronic cord myelopathy include chronic spinal stenosis (e.g., from a disc prolapse), from the sequelae of an acute cord injury or from a demyelinating process such as multiple sclerosis. Atrophy of the spinal cord is a common finding in these scenarios.

Chang FC, et al. Contrast enhancement patterns of acute spinal epidural hematomas: A report of two cases. *Am J Neuroradiol.* 2003;24(3):366–9.
Yu L, et al. Traumatic spinal cord injury without CT or radiographic abnormality – An under-recognized entity. *Contemp Diagn Radiol.* 2008;31(8):1–5.

107. C. Epidermoid cyst

Epidermoid cysts are also known as keratocysts. They are non-tender and usually palpable. The US appearance varies with the maturation, compactness and quantity of keratin present within the epidermoid cyst. A target appearance, a solid mass with an echogenic rim and a characteristic "onion ring" configuration with alternating layers of hyper and hypoechogenicity have been described. These cysts do not show blood flow at Doppler US examination. The constellation of an onion ring configuration, negative tumour marker status and avascularity help differentiate testicular epidermoids from other germ cell tumours.

The US findings of intratesticular varicocele are similar to those of extratesticular varicocele and include multiple anechoic, serpiginous and tubular structures of varying sizes. Colour flow and duplex Doppler US show a venous flow pattern with a characteristic venous spectral waveform, which increases with the Valsalva manoeuvre. An intratesticular spermatocele is a cystic intraparenchymal lesion that is attached to the mediastinum in the area of the rete testis.

Dogra VS, et al. Benign intratesticular cystic lesions: US features. *Radiographics.* 2001;21:S273–81.

108. D. Boerhaave syndrome

Non-accidental abdominal trauma is the second leading cause of death from child abuse after head trauma. Presentation is usually delayed with abdominal pain, vomiting, peritonism and signs of obstruction. Non-accidental visceral trauma is more common in the age group presented here than is incidental blunt abdominal injury and should always be considered as a differential diagnosis, especially if there are other associated features of NAI. Visceral perforation/laceration, intramural haematoma and shocked bowel syndrome are all within the spectrum of NAI. Boerhaave syndrome is a complete transmural oesophageal rupture caused by forceful vomiting or impacted food bolus and more commonly affects adults.

Adam A, et al. *Grainger & Allison's Diagnostic Radiology: A Textbook of Medical Imaging,* 5th edn. New York: Churchill Livingstone, 2008:1505.
Dähnert W. *Radiology Review Manual,* 7th edn. Philadelphia, PA: Lippincott Williams & Wilkins, 2011:825.

109. A. Endotracheal tube with the tip 2 cm above the carina

Close evaluation of any tubes and lines should always be performed to avoid any unnecessary complications and embarrassment. The endotracheal tube should be at least 5 cm above the carina to allow movement of the patient's body so that it never lies within the right or left main bronchus. If it does, it can cause collapse of the non-intubated lung. Central venous catheters, including peripherally inserted catheters, should have their tip within the superior vena cava or right atrium. Intra-aortic counter pulsation balloon pumps should lie within the descending thoracic aorta with the upper aspect distal to the arch vessels to avoid obstruction of blood flow.

Siela D. Chest radiograph evaluation and interpretation. *AACN Advanced Critical Care.* 2008;19:444–73.

110. C. Meckel's diverticulum

The findings on this technetium pertechnetate scan are typical of a Meckel's diverticulum containing ectopic gastric mucosa. The uptake in the left upper quadrant should not mislead the radiologist as it is the result of normal tracer uptake in the stomach mucosa. Secretions from ectopic gastric tissue in a Meckel's diverticulum can cause ulceration of the diverticulum or adjacent small bowel and can lead to bleeding, which, if profuse, can simulate an upper gastrointestinal bleed. Meckel's diverticulum may simulate acute appendicitis on clinical examination; however, a pertechnetate scan is only performed if a Meckel's diverticulum is suspected clinically.

A gastrinoma is usually located in the pancreatic islet cells, not the right iliac fossa.

Dähnert W. *Radiology Review Manual*, 7th edn. Philadelphia, PA: Lippincott Williams & Wilkins, 2011.

111. A. Canavan disease characteristically demonstrates reduced NAA.

MR spectroscopy (MRS) allows tissue to be interrogated for the presence and concentration of various metabolites.

MRS can help increase our ability to grade gliomas. As the grade increases, NAA and creatine decrease and choline, lipids and lactate increase. In recurrent tumour, choline will be elevated, whereas in radiation change, NAA, choline and creatine will all be low. With regard to ischaemic and infraction, lactate will increase as the brain switches to anaerobic metabolism. When infarction takes place, lipids are released and peaks appear. With regard to HIV, choline is low or absent in toxoplasmosis, whereas it is elevated in lymphoma, helping to distinguish the two. PML may demonstrate elevated myoinositol. Canavan disease characteristically demonstrates elevated NAA.

Al-okaili RN, et al. Advanced MR imaging techniques in the diagnosis of intraaxial brain tumors in adults. *Radiographics*. 2006;26(Suppl 1):S173–89.
Bradley WG, Bydder GM. *Advanced MR Imaging Techniques*. London: Informa HealthCare, 1997.

112. B. Calcaneus, patella and olecranon

The description is characteristic of diffuse idiopathic skeletal hyperostosis, or commonly known as DISH. The predominant finding is the calcification/ossification of the ligament and tendon entheses, most often in the spine. Within the thoracic spine, the ossification tends to occur on the right anterolateral aspect with postulated theories that the pulsations from the adjacent left-sided thoracic aorta inhibits the hypertrophic ossification. The most common diagnostic criteria employed is the involvement of at least four contiguous vertebrae (flowing ossification from calcification of the anterior longitudinal ligament) and the absence of sacroiliac inflammatory change and apophyseal joint degeneration. Recent changes have proposed reducing the contiguous vertebral segment involvement to 3 rather than 4. Extraspinal manifestations are again of calcification of the entheses and hypertrophic bone changes, with the most common sites involving the olecranon, patella and calcaneum.

Cammisa M, et al. Diffuse idiopathic skeletal hyperostosis. *Eur J Radiol*. 1998;27(Suppl 1):S7–11.
Mader R, et al. Extraspinal manifestation of diffuse skeletal idiopathic skeletal hyperostosis. *Rheumatology*. 2009;48(12):1478–81.
Resnick D, et al. Diffuse idiopathic skeletal hyperostosis (DISH): Forestier's disease with extraspinal manifestations. *Radiology*. 1975;115(3):513–24.

113. D. Granulomatous prostatitis

Granulomatous prostatitis is an inflammatory entity that often presents with a firm nodule on digital rectal examination and elevated prostate-specific antigen, thus clinically mimicking prostate cancer. Possible causes include previous intravesical BCG therapy, TB prostatitis and previous intervention such as TURP, although most cases are idiopathic. On MRI, granulomatous prostatitis may appear as a discrete mass with markedly abnormal T2 signal, DWI and ADC map. Furthermore, there may be associated infiltration of the periprostatic fat by inflammation, thus mimicking extraprostatic tumour extension. Currently, histopathologic analysis is regarded as the only means of definitively establishing the diagnosis and thereby excluding the presence of tumour; however, a suggestive history, such as prior BCG therapy, may be useful in prompting consideration of the diagnosis. In addition, the presence on MRI of large areas of non-enhancement, indicative of necrosis within the lesion corresponding with caseous abscess on pathologic evaluation, may suggest the diagnosis. A short-term follow-up MRI may be obtained after antimicrobial treatment to assess for therapeutic response.

Rosenkrantz AB, Taneja SS. Radiologist, be aware: Ten pitfalls that confound the interpretation of multiparametric prostate MRI. *AJR Am J Roentgenol.* 2014;202:109–20.

114. E. Shocked bowel syndrome
Isolated, localised small bowel wall thickening is non-specific but highly suggestive of underlying bowel wall or mesenteric injury in the trauma patient. In all of the above conditions, apart from shocked bowel syndrome, this finding may be present. Diffuse bowel wall thickening is atypical for bowel wall injury. Following trauma, in the presence of increased bowel wall enhancement, a flattened inferior vena cava, hyperenhancement of adrenal glands and pancreatic and/or retroperitoneal oedema, a shocked bowel syndrome (hypoperfusion complex) is the most likely explanation. This must not be omitted in the differential diagnosis as treatment of hypoperfusion complex is conservative and there is no need for diagnostic laparotomy.

Adam A, et al. *Grainger & Allison's Diagnostic Radiology: A Textbook of Medical Imaging*, 5th edn. New York: Churchill Livingstone, 2008:1504.

115. E. They classically are intra-articular in location.
Gout is the clinical condition of symptomatic arthritis due to the deposition of monosodium urate crystals within or around the joints due to excess serum urate levels. There is often accompanying renal disease with formation of uric acid urinary calculi. Tophaceous gout presents with an eccentric, asymmetric soft-tissue mass(es) around the joint(s) and it is this that gives rise to the typical juxta articular erosions. Intra-articular erosions can also occur, though this is less common. Large overhanging edges of bone often develop, separating the tophi from the erosions.

Llauger J, et al. Nonseptic monoarthritis: Imaging features with clinical and histopathologic correlation. *Radiographics.* 2000;20:S263–78.

116. C. The patient should take a course of treatment dose trimethoprim, starting on the day of the procedure for 3 subsequent days.
Ensure that the baby undergoing MCUG receives 4 mg/kg of trimethoprim on the day of the MCUG and for three subsequent days to prevent complication of infection. If a child is on prophylactic 2 mg/kg does of trimethoprim, full dose is required as described above to cover the MCUG.

Rennie JM, Kendall G. *A Manual of Neonatal Intensive Care*, 5th edn. Boca Raton, FL: CRC Press; 2013:326–7.

117. D. Choroid plexus papilloma   Poorly circumscribed and poorly enhancing tumours
Predominant imaging patterns of astrocytoma are mass with a enhancing or non-enhancing cyst and an intensely enhancing mural nodule, necrotic mass with a central non-enhancing zone or predominantly solid mass. They are associated with NF1.

Craniopharyngiomas are relatively benign neoplasms arising in the sellar/suprasellar region, often presenting with endocrine abnormalities. Paediatric craniopharyngiomas typically appear multicystic; the solid portions enhancing heterogeneously with characteristic calcifications in paediatric craniopharyngiomas may not be discernible without SWI. Occasionally, they are predominantly solid, typically without calcification.

PNETs arise from primitive (undifferentiated) brain cells. They are typically heterogeneous and are usually iso- to hyperdense on CT, with calcifications in 70%. On MRI, they may appear iso- to hyperintense to grey matter on FLAIR and T2-weighted images. The solid component usually has avid heterogeneous enhancement with minimal oedema. Necrosis and haemorrhage are common and are seen as restriction on DWI.

On MR images, choroid plexus papillomas appear as isointense to hypointense intraventricular masses compared with normal brain parenchyma. Flow voids, consistent with flowing blood, are common. CT show intense enhancement. Hydrocephalus is very common.

Gangliogliomas develop in the temporal lobe and are commonly associated with refractory seizures, partial complex type. Calcification is seen in 30%. Peripherally located gangliogliomas may cause scalloped pressure erosion of the calvaria. At MRI, a well-defined cystic mass with a solid mural nodule is typically seen; however, a solid mass with non-specific low-to-intermediate signal intensity on T1-weighted images and high signal on T2-weighted images is also not uncommon. Enhancement is variable, ranging from non-enhancing to ring like to intense homogeneity. There is usually little associated mass effect or oedema.

Borja MJ, et al. Conventional and advanced MRI features of paediatric intracranial tumors: Supratentorial tumors. *AJR Am J Roentgenol.* 2013;200(5):W483–503.

Koeller KK, Rushing EJ. From the archives of the AFIP: Pilocytic astrocytoma: Radiologic-pathologic correlation. *Radiographics.* 2004;24(6):1693–708.

Koeller KK, Sandberg GD. From the archives of the AFIP. Cerebral intraventricular neoplasms: Radiologic-pathologic correlation. *Radiographics.* 2002;22(6):1473–505.

Saleem SN, et al. Lesions of the hypothalamus: MR imaging diagnostic features. *Radiographics.* 2007;27(4): 1087–108.

Shin JH, et al. Neuronal tumors of the central nervous system: Radiologic findings and pathologic correlation. *Radiographics.* 2002;22(5):1177–89.

118. C. Tracheal shift to the right

Tracheal shift to the contralateral side from the pneumonectomy is an abnormal finding and along with depression of the ipsilateral hemidiaphragm may represent a bronchopleural fistula, empyema or haemorrhage. The other findings can be normally seen postoperatively following pneumonectomy. They can start to develop within 24 hours following surgery with partial and then complete filling of the thorax. The other signs such as ipsilateral mediastinal shift and elevation of the hemidiaphragm are caused by volume loss. When presented with a chest X-ray with complete white-out and ipsilateral mediastinal shift, the key to identifying pneumonectomy versus complete collapse is the presence of a posterior surgical rib defect.

Dähnert W. *Radiology Review Manual*, 7th edn. Philadelphia, PA: Lippincott Williams & Wilkins, 2011:530.

119. B. Papillary tumour with pure intraluminal growth

Squamous cell carcinoma accounts for <5% of bladder neoplasms; however, in parts of the world where schistosomiasis (bilharziasis) is endemic, it is a major health problem, accounting for over 50% of bladder cancers. Risk factors in non-bilharzial regions include chronic irritation from indwelling catheters, bladder calculi or chronic infection. All of these risk factors may be present in paraplegic patients, putting them at increased risk. Cyclophosphamide, smoking and intravesical BCG has also been implicated in the pathogenesis of squamous carcinoma of the bladder.

The imaging findings in squamous carcinoma are non-specific. Tumours may appear as a single enhancing bladder mass or as diffuse or focal wall thickening. Intradiverticular squamous tumours are soft-tissue masses, sometimes with surface calcification. In contrast to urothelial carcinoma, squamous carcinoma is sessile rather than papillary, and pure intraluminal growth is not seen. Bladder wall thickening and calcification, from chronic inflammation or infection with *Bilharzia*, may coexist and complicate the diagnosis.

Wong-You-Cheong JJ, et al. From the archives of the AFIP: Neoplasms of the urinary bladder: Radiologic-pathologic correlation. *Radiographics.* 2006;26(2):553–80.

120. B. Mesenteric fat infiltration

Significant mesenteric injury requires urgent vascular surgical treatment and, if missed, can lead to life-threatening bowel ischaemia. The most specific CT feature of significant mesenteric injury is mesenteric contrast extravasation, which is almost 100% sensitive. Other highly specific features are vascular beading (irregularity of mesenteric vessels) and termination of mesenteric vessels, which, when seen, are an indication for vascular surgery. Lack of bowel wall enhancement is highly suggestive of segmental bowel ischaemia secondary to significant vascular injury. Mesenteric fat infiltration is a common but very non-specific feature of abdominal trauma. It may be present in bowel wall laceration, contusion or incomplete bowel wall tear as well as in significant bowel and mesenteric injuries.

Brofman N, et al. Evaluation of bowel and mesenteric blunt trauma with multidetector CT. *Radiographics*. 2006;26:1119–31.

INDEX